1,000,000 Books

are available to read at

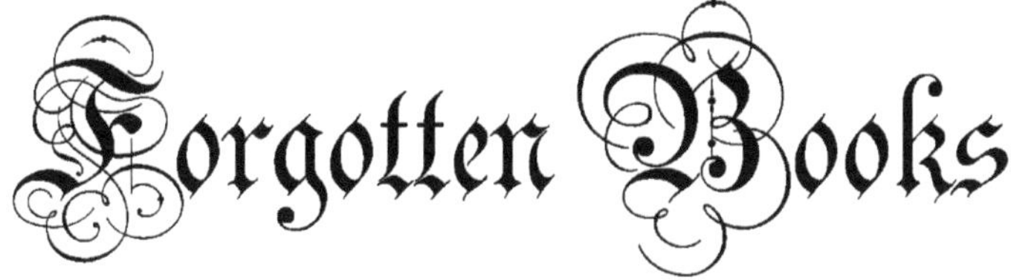

www.ForgottenBooks.com

Read online
Download PDF
Purchase in print

ISBN 978-0-259-18381-5
PIBN 10807398

This book is a reproduction of an important historical work. Forgotten Books uses state-of-the-art technology to digitally reconstruct the work, preserving the original format whilst repairing imperfections present in the aged copy. In rare cases, an imperfection in the original, such as a blemish or missing page, may be replicated in our edition. We do, however, repair the vast majority of imperfections successfully; any imperfections that remain are intentionally left to preserve the state of such historical works.

Forgotten Books is a registered trademark of FB &c Ltd.
Copyright © 2018 FB &c Ltd.
FB &c Ltd, Dalton House, 60 Windsor Avenue, London, SW19 2RR.
Company number 08720141. Registered in England and Wales.

For support please visit www.forgottenbooks.com

1 MONTH OF FREE READING

at

www.ForgottenBooks.com

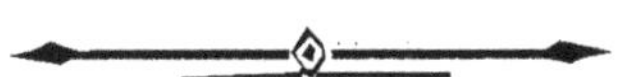

By purchasing this book you are eligible for one month membership to ForgottenBooks.com, giving you unlimited access to our entire collection of over 1,000,000 titles via our web site and mobile apps.

To claim your free month visit:

www.forgottenbooks.com/free807398

* Offer is valid for 45 days from date of purchase. Terms and conditions apply.

English
Français
Deutsche
Italiano
Español
Português

www.forgottenbooks.com

Mythology Photography **Fiction** Fishing Christianity **Art** Cooking Essays Buddhism Freemasonry Medicine **Biology** Music **Ancient Egypt** Evolution Carpentry Physics Dance Geology **Mathematics** Fitness Shakespeare **Folklore** Yoga Marketing **Confidence** Immortality Biographies Poetry **Psychology** Witchcraft Electronics Chemistry History **Law** Accounting **Philosophy** Anthropology Alchemy Drama Quantum Mechanics Atheism Sexual Health **Ancient History** **Entrepreneurship** Languages Sport Paleontology Needlework Islam **Metaphysics** Investment Archaeology Parenting Statistics Criminology **Motivational**

THE
Hahnemannia
MONTHLY.

VOLUME SECOND, NEW SERIES.

(VOLUME FIFTEENTH)

JANUARY TO DECEMBER,

1880.

E. A. FARRINGTON, M.D.,
PEMBERTON DUDLEY, M.D.,
EDITORS.

PUBLISHED BY THE
HAHNEMANN CLUB,
PHILADELPHIA.

Sherman & Co.,
Printers, Philadelphia.

INDEX

TO THE

HAHNEMANNIAN MONTHLY.

VOLUME FIFTEENTH, 1880.

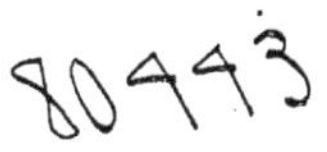

CONTRIBUTORS TO VOLUME XV.

Clarence Bartlett, M.D., Philadelphia, Pa.
James B. Bell, M.D., Boston, Mass.
B. Frank Betts, M.D , Philadelphia, Pa.
W. H. Bigler, M.D., Philadelphia, Pa.
F. F. Casseday, M.D., Stevens Point, Wis.
P. G. Clark, M.D., Unadilla, N. Y.
J. H. Clarke, M.D , Ipswich, England.
Charles H. Conover, M.D , Philadelphia, Pa.
N. F. Cooke, M.D., Chicago, Ill.
John Cooper, M.D , Alleghany, Pa
J. P. Dake, M D , Nashville, Tenn.
Pemberton Dudley, M.D , Philadelphia, Pa.
E. A. Farrington, M D , Philadelphia, Pa.
C F. Goodno, M.D., Philadelphia, Pa
W. C. Goodno, M D , Philadelphia, Pa.
H N. Guernsey, M.D , Philadelphia, Pa.
Joseph C. Guernsey, M.D , Philadelphia, Pa.
B B. Gumpert, M D , Philadelphia, Pa.
W. M. Haines, M.D , Ellsworth, Me.
E. M. Hale, M.D , Chicago, Ill.
L Hoopes, M.D., Downingtown, Pa.

George Hosfeld, M.D., Philadelphia, Pa.
John G. Houard, M.D., Philadelphia, Pa.
H. C. Houghton, M.D., New York, N. Y.
E. M Howard, M.D., Camden, N. J.
Bushrod W. James, M D., Philadelphia, Pa.
John E. James, M.D , Philadelphia, Pa.
J. B. Kniffin, M.D., Philadelphia, Pa
Aug Korndœrfer, M.D , Philadelphia, Pa.
W. F Laird, M.D., Boston, Mass.
John K Lee, M D , Philadelphia, Pa
F. Park Lewis, M D , Buffalo, N. Y.
S. Lilienthal, M.D., New York, N. Y.
H. Noah Martin, M.D , Philadelphia, Pa.
R J. McClatchey, M.D., Philadelphia, Pa
J. H McClelland, M.D , Pittsburg, Pa
J. P. McCourt, M D
W. McGeorge, M.D , Woodbury, N. J.
F R. McManus, M.D., Baltimore, Md.
C. S. Middleton, M D , Philadelphia, Pa.
Clifford Mitchell, M.D., Chicago, Ill.
J. N. Mitchell, M.D., Philadelphia, Pa.
Charles Mohr, M.D., Philadelphia, Pa
John C. Morgan, M.D , Philadelphia, Pa.
E. B. Nash, M D , Cortland, N. Y.
C. F. Nichols, M.D , Boston, Mass.
C. R Norton, M.D , Philadelphia, Pa.
G. W. Parker, M.D.. Philadelphia, Pa.
Ross V. Pitcairn, M.D., Pittsburg, Pa.
Samuel Potter, M.D , Milwaukee, Wis.
C Preston, M.D , Chester, Pa.
F. Preston, M.D., Chester, Pa.
S H. Quint, M.D , Camden, N. J.
Joseph M Reeves, M.D., Philadelphia, Pa.
A. C Rembaugh, M D , Philadelphia, Pa.
Harriet J. Sartain, M D , Philadelphia, Pa
William P. Sharkey, M D., Philadelphia, Pa
J. S. Skeels, M D., Albion, Pa
H. L Stambach, M.D , Philadelphia, Pa.
J. R Tantum, M.D., Wilmington, Del.
H. W. Taylor, M.D., Crawfordsville, Ind.
Testis Oculatus.
A. R. Thomas, M.D., Philadelphia, Pa.
C. M. Thomas, M.D., Philadelphia, Pa.
J. Sperry Thomas, M.D , Philadelphia, Pa.
W. B. Trites, M.D , Manayunk, Pa.
M. B. Tuller, M D , Vineland, N. J.
Josephine Van Deusen, M.D., Philadelphia, Pa.
M. M. Walker, M.D , Germantown, Pa
Chandler Weaver, M.D., Fox Chase, Pa.
M. S. Williamson, M D., Philadelphia, Pa.
J E. Winans, M D., Lyons Farm, N. J.
W. H Winslow, M.D., Pittsburg, Pa.
James B Wood, M.D , West Chester, Pa.

THE

HAHNEMANNIAN MONTHLY.

Vol. II., New Series. } Philadelphia, January, 1880. No. 1.

Original Department.

THE DIAGNOSTIC SIGNS AND SYMPTOMS OF PERITONITIS.

BY C S. MIDDLETON, M D,

PHILADELPHIA, PA.

(Read before the Hahnemann Club of Philadelphia.)

THE diagnostic signs of peritonitis are generally pretty clearly defined, but there are many cases, especially in young children and infants, where considerable obscurity envelops the diagnosis.

This assertion is substantiated by the fact that peritonitis is often secondary to, or follows closely, some other inflammatory condition of the abdominal organs, and consequently is overlooked ;, the results of all the abnormal or diseased state, whether of an ordinarily severe type or of the gravest character, are attributed to those other causes.

It is then apparent that peritonitis is very frequently involved with other inflammatory conditions, which will give to it a different character under different complications.

In a general way we find peritonitis characterized by pain, usually very severe, the abdomen very sensitive to touch and pressure upon it, and movements of the body are intolerable.

Peritonitis sets in with chilliness and fever, or is preceded by a severe chill followed by intense fever, hot and dry skin, high temperature, rapid and wiry pulse, distension of the abdomen, sunken and pinched countenance.

The pain usually commences in one spot, and spreads over more or less surface as the inflammation progresses, sometimes extending to all parts of the membrane. The pains are mostly sharp, lancinating, cutting and stinging, unrelenting and severe. Touch or motion, be it ever so slight, is attended with great aggravation, therefore the patient lies upon the back, as quietly as possible, usually with the limbs drawn up for the purpose of relieving tension of the abdominal muscles; indeed, the sensitiveness is so great that even the clothing is not allowed to rest upon the diseased parts.

This inflammation is soon followed by exudation of serum or lymph, or both, and in depraved constitutions sometimes blood and ichorous fluids are mixed therewith. The serum is at times readily absorbed, but not so the lymph, which often causes adhesions between different folds of the peritoneum, coils of intestine, etc. These adhesions often form little sacs, which become filled with exudation or pus. The coagulable lymph is also the means of producing the thickened and roughened condition in which the peritoneum is found in the chronic form of this disease.

Peritoneal inflammation induces paralysis of the intestines, and consequently constipation and distension by gaseous generation. Vomiting is almost always present; first, of the contents of the stomach,—if anything eaten still remain therein,—lastly, of bilions matters from the regurgitation of bile through the action of the abdominal muscles. This vomiting is always attended by aggravation of the pains for obvious reasons. Hiccough also annoys the patient if the inflammation extend to, or originate near, the diaphragm. Constipation and suppression of urine add to our list of symptoms, and as we shall find farther on the latter condition is often a complicating one.

If the peritonitis be the result of puerperal fever, phlebitis, metritis, etc., diarrhœa will usually be present, the stools being, perhaps, dysenteric in character, or, perhaps, involuntary. Frequent and painful urination will sometimes add to the torments of the sufferer.

The fever attendant upon peritonitis is graded somewhat by the extent of the inflammation. If it be severe or extensive, the higher of course will be the temperature, and the more rapid the pulse. In grave cases the fever is always intense, the pulse fails, and symptoms of collapse ensue in proportion to the degree of danger present.

In fatal cases the abdomen becomes enormously distended, cold sweats appear on the extremities, the countenance becomes pinched, the pulse flickers, the collapse is profound, and the end is accomplished.

When perforation of the intestine or stomach and extravasation has preceded peritonitis, the collapse is sudden in its onset.

Tympanitic sounds are rendered on percussion if the abdomen be distended by gas alone, but these sounds are, of course, modified by accumulation of fluid, either diffused or held in position by adhesions more or less circumscribed.

Local peritonitis is generally the result of inflammation of some abdominal organ or tissue, and is generally not so intense as primary or diffused peritonitis; but we have the same *kind* of pain and tenderness, only localized; the fever is less intense. Very frequently certain spaces limited in extent present dulness on percussion, indicating either local effusion of serum or lymph or the formation of pus. In this form of peritoneal inflammation adhesions usually result.

Chronic peritonitis may be the result of imperfect recovery from an acute attack. It is accompanied by some fever and abdominal pains, and effusions into the cavity. From this condition, occasional renewed attacks of a more acute form may arise, and, the patient becoming worn out, an exhausting diarrhœa, dropsy of the extremities, and hectic fever supervene, and the patient rapidly succumbs. Recovery may take place by the absorption of the fluid, leaving, perhaps, a thickening of the membrane.

Occasionally, however, chronic peritonitis comes on in a different manner, advancing imperceptibly, but soon manifesting a tubercular or cancerous character, accompanied by abdominal dropsy, and lasting a long time.

Puerperal peritonitis is distinguishable from acute peritonitis only by the fact of its occurrence during the puerperium. The symptoms are the same so far as the inflammatory condition of the peritoneum is concerned. But in this variety diarrhœa, which is often severe and intense, is a much more frequent accompaniment than constipation, and when such is the case the tympanitis is less.

Delirium is apt to be present under a variety of forms. Of course it must be borne in mind that disorders of the lochia often play an important part in this disease.

DIFFERENTIAL DIAGNOSIS.

Hysteria.—Among the several diseases which simulate peritonitis in some of its features, an hysterical condition referred to the abdomen may in some cases mislead us, but the history of the case alone will generally be sufficient to lead to a correct diagnosis. Furthermore, although real tenderness may be present, the pain is not increased upon deep pressure, and with the diffused and general soreness represented we should expect to find high fever and other symptoms of genuine peritonitis.

The reverse is, however, mostly true; for while we may find considerable activity of the pulse, it will not be wiry, nor will the temperature be as high as that found in peritonitis; and although there may be a tympanitic condition of the abdomen, the bowels will frequently be found regular, the urine free, pale, and watery.

Lastly, as these cases are met in women, a disturbance or absence of the menses, or some other uterine disorder, will generally account for all the hysterical manifestations, and the diagnosis will thus be established.

Metritis.—General peritonitis should be easily distinguished from metritis. In the latter the pain is located in the region of the uterus and its appendages, which can be ascertained by external examination. A still further search by examination per vaginam will reveal great tenderness upon touching the cervix uteri.

A local peritoneal inflammation is, however, almost always a concomitant of metritis; this condition being sometimes indicated by the formation of pus and its discharge per vaginam. In puerperal metritis the peritoneal inflammation is often so great as to entirely obscure the symptoms of uterine inflammation.

Cystitis.—Inflammation of the bladder may present some of the symptoms of peritonitis, but there are some well-defined distinctions by which we may differentiate.

"An acute inflammation of the bladder gives rise to frequent calls to pass urine, yet the act is performed with great difficulty, and in some cases may be impossible; the bladder distends, a sense of weight is felt in the perinæum, the region above the pubis becomes tender to the touch, and sounds dull on percussion; the sufferer is restless and distressed, and has the hot skin and excited pulse of an inflammatory fever. At times vomiting and hiccough supervene, and death is preceded by gradually deepening coma. The urine voided in peritonitis is simply high-colored, like that of any febrile state; in cystitis it contains large quantities of mucus and pus, and often blood and crystals of phosphates."

In cystitis the tenderness is localized, and the smarting in the urethra differs from that in peritonitis. These symptoms, coexisting with overdistension of the bladder, constitute an almost conclusive evidence of cystic disorder, and to these well-marked signs will be probably added the fact that the patient has not voided urine for some time, and that all distress immediately subsides upon drawing off the urine with the catheter.

Gastritis.—Vomiting is a prominent and early condition in gastritis, though pain and tenderness are easily referred to the epigastrium, and there is not so much enlargement as in peritonitis. The tongue is heavily coated, and red at tip and edges. The greater diffusion of the pain, the secondary or less prominent vomiting, rapid increase and great tenderness of the abdomen, and excessive fever will generally enable us to draw a correct conclusion.

Enteritis.—The pain of an enteritis is more paroxysmal in character, more local, usually referred to the region of the navel, generally gives rise to less distension of the abdomen and greater nausea and vomiting, and the tongue is red. It frequently happens, however, that some peritoneal inflammation is associated with enteritis, and under such circumstances it may be difficult to distinguish the indications belonging to each.

Typhlitis.—As inflammatory states of other portions of the intestines are liable to be complicated with a peritonitis more or less localized or diffused, so also do we have the same condition with typhlitis and inflammation of the cœcum. It is difficult at all times to determine the exact status of pain and tenderness in the right iliac fossa, accompanied with a fever more or less severe; but in a general way typhlitis sets in more gradually than peritonitis, especially if an impaction of fæces or the lodgment of some foreign body be the exciting cause.

In such a case constipation (or sometimes alternate constipation and diarrhœa), has preceded the attack, and a sense of weight and fulness, rather than pain and soreness accompanies it. If impaction of fæces be present there is often great enlargement in the locality, and a mass can be distinctly felt, which is dull on percussion, while around it there are the physical signs of tympanitic distension. Peritoneal inflammation, resulting from such a condition, is mostly dependent upon the length of time that the obstruction has existed, and the extent of the accumulation. The sooner it is discovered and relieved, the less will be the danger of extensive peritonitis, and *vice versa.*

Perityphlitis is so often accompanied by, or dependent upon, the above condition, that the remarks applied to typhlitis apply equally well here; but when, unassociated with typhlitis, the tissues in the iliac fossa become inflamed, there is usually less fever and pain, and no obstruction to the movement of the bowels, but more probability of abscess. If peritonitis be absent, there will be less superficial tenderness, but deep pressure increases the pain as we approach the inflamed tissues.

Colic.—The pain of colic is mostly paroxysmal, unattended with fever, and while sensitiveness to palpation is often present, greater pressure relieves the pain, while the reverse is true of peritonitis. When, however, these symptoms are attended by fever, more or less severe, and great tenderness is felt, often in some one spot, it is not improbable that the peritoneum may have become affected as a sequence to a colic from cold, the passage of a gallstone, uterine colic, etc., and these several complications should be carefully investigated.

Typhoid Fever.—Peritonitis may be secondary, but never antecedent to typhoid fever. It is usually the result of perforation of the intestine, and is recognizable by increased tenderness, great tympanitis, sunken, cadaverous expression of countenance, rapid, feeble, and sinking pulse, etc.

Inflammation and Abscess of the Abdominal Muscles.—It is not always easy to distinguish an inflammation of the abdominal walls from that of the peritoneum. Even the history of the case, which may reveal the fact that a blow or kick has been received, will often prove negative, as the violence sustained is about as likely to produce the one as the other. In fact, some of the symptoms are identical with those of peritonitis, such as fever, increased pain upon movement, coughing, etc., and great tenderness upon pressure.

The above condition is, however, most likely to be found upon one side of the abdomen, or, in case of injury, at the seat where such violence was received. Soon tumefaction and redness will be perceptible, which will either disappear by resolution, or end in suppuration and discharge of pus, followed by immediate and great relief. This inflammation is much more slow in its course than peritonitis, and much easier to differentiate as it advances to a termination. If apparent inflammation of organs lying beneath the seat of soreness be manifested, satisfactory conclusions may be obtained by the assurance that they are or are not in their ordinary functional condition. It is sometimes impossible to distinguish between a peritoneal abscess and one within the abdominal walls. Either, and especially the latter, may occasionally be mistaken for a tumor, because of its slower growth and sometimes non-inflammatory development.

Rheumatism of the abdominal walls manifests a pain not so constant or so severe, and not always affected by motion; nor is deep pressure attended by so great pain. It is often confined to one side of the abdomen; there is usually no very marked fever, seldom distension, and vomiting is wanting.

Peritonitis in Children.—While an inflammation of the peritoneum is the same in all stages of life, it is, nevertheless, met with in young children and infants under conditions differing from those in the adult.

We not only have many of the various complications met with in older subjects to differentiate, but there are, besides, in small children, and especially in infants, a tendency to meningitis, hepatitis, tubercular disease of the mesentery, etc., which must not be overlooked.

It is also a conceded fact that infants are occasionally born with peritonitis, which, it is said, may manifest itself as early as the seventh month. When we observe in the new-born infant that the abdomen is distended and painful, and we find fluctuation, it is pretty clear that inflammation of the peritoneum is present.

There are sometimes other evidences of a dropsical condition, and it is said to be "frequently combined with other abdominal affections, such as hepatitis, rupture of the liver, hæmorrhagical effusions, hypertrophy of the spleen, etc."

Notwithstanding the above quotation to the contrary, it is quite doubtful if such a grave state of affairs could take place during intra-uterine life, so far back as the seventh month, and yet the fœtus be born alive. We do not doubt that inflammation of the liver could exist and continue till birth, at which time a rupture may have occurred, thus exhibiting the above conditions *post-partum* instead of *ante-natal.*

Peritonitis of children is divided into the acute and chronic forms as in most other diseases. It is most frequently met with in children between the ages of three and thirteen years, and infants that may have been born healthy are not exempt from it.

Peritonitis at this age of life is so frequently complicated with gastro-enteric disorders that the patient may be well on the road to an acute attack before such a condition is suspected; indeed, peritonitis in children is seldom encountered without such a complication.

Acute peritonitis in children sets in with much the same symptoms as in the adult; perhaps there may be a greater tendency to restlessness, especially in very young children.

They often desire to be changed from the arms of one nurse to another, and express the pain of movement by moaning only, as severe crying produces greater pain. (Older children prefer the supine position, and avoid movements of any kind.) The abdomen is of course much distended and sensitive; often vomiting, constipation, and other gastro-enteric symptoms prevail. The tongue is red, especially along the edges and tip. The temperature is very high, the skin hot and dry; there is great thirst; the urine is dark, scanty, or almost entirely suppressed; the pulse rapid, feeble, and wiry, and the expression of the face often indicates great agony by the distortions and knitting of the brows.

The greater the effusion into the abdominal cavity the greater the distension, and, if a fatal termination is about to succeed, the countenance becomes hippocratic, the pulse grows more and more feeble and rapid, the strength fails, the skin becomes cold, and sometimes diarrhœa and vomiting set in, and death follows.

If there be no cephalic complications the patient may remain conscious to the last, but otherwise a soporific condition is most likely to precede the closing scene.

The above characterizes acute peritonitis as generally found without complications, but when, as before remarked, we take into consideration the readiness with which children are seized with enteric and cephalic inflammations, we must expect to meet these complications very frequently.

The great point, therefore, is to be on our guard, to be careful in our examinations of children that present symptoms leading us to suspect brain complications, especially where the latter are the more prominent, as under such circumstances the usual inflammatory symptoms, such as tenderness and pain on pressure, are less marked.

With inflammatory complications of the gastro-intestinal tract, there may be greater obscurity, or at least greater difficulty of determining just how much of the illness and danger is to be attributed to the one or to the other. The differential points have been set forth in the first section of this paper, and apply as well to children as to adults, but of course greater difficulty will be experienced in their application.

Chronic peritonitis may be the result of an imperfect recovery from an acute attack, or it may set in so mildly as to mislead one to the conclusion that the illness is gastric disturbance alone; but when at a later stage, distension of the abdomen, effusion therein, tenderness to touch, accompanied by slimy diarrhœa and emaciation, present themselves, we may rest assured that the diagnosis cannot longer be mistaken.

In this form we often find a complication with scrofulous inflammation and induration of the mesenteric glands. This latter condition is most likely to precede the peritoneal inflammation. Under such circumstances children are found to have been more or less restless and sleepless, to have lost flesh, which will be most readily noticed about the neck, and by the hollow eyes; to have been more voracious than usual, and to have suffered from diarrhœa, thus presenting the well-recognized symptoms of marasmus infantum.

With this condition we find post-mortem evidences of tubercular peritonitis, and the membrane and contents of the abdomen present the same characteristics of adhesions and plastic deposits, sacs of pus, etc., that have been described in the peritonitis of adults.

In *hepatic* complications, great prominence of symptoms pointing to the disordered or inflammatory condition of the liver, are mostly present. The jaundiced appearance of the skin and eyes, bilious vomiting and diarrhœa, or great heat and intense soreness in the hepatic region will aid in forming correct conclusions. Infants born with imperforate anus are often carried off by peritonitis after a surgical operation has apparently placed them in a proper condition to live.

NOTE ON THE TREATMENT OF PERITONITIS.

It will detract nothing from the value of the above paper if we presume to add a few therapeutic hints. In no disease is it more important to observe strictly every homœopathic rule of prescribing; for the vital forces are quickly and profoundly depressed, and a mistake in the choice of the remedy may precipitate a fatal termination. Local symptoms must be carefully compared with the general condition, especially with the state of the circulation, the bodily temperature, and what is of equal importance, the mental state.

Mucilaginous drinks acidulated with tamarinds or lemon-juice are often grateful and soothing to the irritated stomach. If the lemonade be made *hot* and then allowed to cool it is less likely to cause intestinal griping. Effervescing drinks may increase the tympany, and should usually be avoided. During the early stages, when the fever runs high, farinaceous foods may be given; but if the liver is so diseased as to interfere with biliary secretion, starchy and oily foods will not be readily digested, and must be mainly substituted by mutton, beef, or chicken broth. In such a contingency the broth should be allowed to cool first, that all the fat may be skimmed off. In large cities poultry is brought to market so poorly and improperly fed, that great care is needed in its purchase.

Alcoholic drinks should be interdicted except in advanced cases, in which the vitality is very low, or where blood-poisoning demands them.

ACONITE.—Burning-cutting pains, worse from the slightest motion and from lying on the right side; hard, frequent pulse; skin hot and dry. Abdomen hot and sensitive to touch. Face anxious; restlessness; fear of death. Caused by checked sweat, exposure to dry, cold winds, drinking ice-water while fatigued and hot. Puerperal cases, especially in full-blooded women, when violent emotions seem to have caused a checking of the lochia. Hahnemann's advice here is imperative, not to give Aconite simply because there is fever or because there is synochal fever, but to be guided by the infallible accompaniments of restlessness and mental agony.

Verat. viride has come into fashion as a rival of Aconite. It is selected in the beginning of inflammations by the pulse, which is said to express *great arterial excitement.* But the two remedies are really not at all similar. The Veratrum rather pictures asthenia,—fever of a low type. Congestions and inflammations are accompanied by delirium, great prostration, and, what is very characteristic, A RED STREAK DOWN THE CENTRE OF THE TONGUE. It has no action on serous membranes, like Aconite.

BELLADONNA.—Abdomen distended, hot, and exquisitely sensitive to touch or to the least jar of the bed; pains in sudden attacks, which come and go suddenly; or, less frequently, gradually increase and gradually decrease (see Allen, vol. ii, p. 102). Sometimes enteritis coexists, with clutching as from nails at the navel; bloody, slimy diarrhœa. Bodily temperature very high. On raising the bedclothes a hot steam rises. Head very hot and dry; or, hot and yet bathed in sweat. Feet cold, head hot. This is not the coldness indicative of collapse, but of upward congestion. Urine scanty and sometimes golden-yellow. Delirium, varying from simple starts in sleep to furor, with red, congested face and throbbing carotids. The face instead of being red, may appear pale, hot, and expressive of deepseated distress. Drowsiness and stupor, but easily aroused.

Belladonna especially attacks the uterus and ileo-cœcal region, and should be studied in metritis with peritonitis, and also in typhlitis. In the former case the lochia will be checked or hot, and occasionally in offensively smelling clots. There is also backache; she feels as if her back was broken.

CANTHARIS.—That portion of the peritoneum which covers the bladder is particularly affected; frequent and painful urination; the urine passes in drops and may be bloody; tenesmus vesicæ and burning cutting continue after micturition. Cutting, griping, burning, and wandering pains, worse in the lower abdomen. Face indicates extreme suffering, eyes sunken. Also indicated when effusion has taken place; and still more when collapse results from internal suppuration; surface cool; he lies unconscious with outstretched arms, which occasionally jerk; convulsions; suppressed urine.

Bryonia, Cantharis, Merc. corros., Apis, and Sulphur are useful, especially when exudation has taken place. It would be an egregious mistake to select one of these, or of any other group, merely because they have been known to produce seroplastic effusions. The individual symptoms must always determine the choice.

BRYONIA acts well, especially in rheumatic patients, and when the diaphragm is attacked, as shown by stitches with each breath or motion of the body. Tongue dry, and possibly white down the centre. There is none of the restlessness and agony of Aconite. He desires to lie perfectly still and be quiet. Still, his face is a perfect picture of anguish; he breathes in quick, short inspirations, which oppress him, and in some instances he is impelled by his distress to move, but desists, for the pains become thereby aggravated. The fever runs higher than with Cantharis, and the urine is scanty, dark red, and clear.

MERC. CORROS. has produced in toxic doses peritoneal effusion. The exudate is purulent, and is accompanied with creeping chills, sweat without relief, and cutting, stabbing, griping pains. There is less of the well-defined stitch which characterizes Bryonia. Both Merc. corros. and Cantharis have strangury with intense burning, and if enteritis complicates, both may have slimy, bloody stools. The latter, however, is relieved by perspiration.

Apis mel. is recognized by a distressing aching soreness of the abdomen, which will tolerate no pressure; burning stinging pains, or sudden knifelike thrusts through the abdomen. Urine scanty, dark, and often albuminous. Absence of thirst, or drinks little and often. Œdematous puffiness of the face.

In bad cases, with enteritis combined, he passes thin yellow stools with every motion of the body, as though the anus and rectum were paralyzed. Infants and those predisposed to tuberculosis scream out in their sleep,—a sudden shrill cry from cerebral irritation. Face looks distressed, he feels as if he would die; but he is not so full of fear as to indicate Aconite. Sleepy but cannot sleep. This differs from Belladonna; the Apis patient can't sleep because he feels so nervous and fidgety.

When typhoid symptoms develop, Rhus tox., Lachesis, Lycopodium, Arsenic, and Baptisia stand foremost.

RHUS TOX. is the most frequently indicated. Tongue red, dry; red at the tip; tympany; restless change of place; change of position relieves his pains, though it increases his weakness and compels him to desist. Muttering, not violent, delirium. His dreams are full of laborious effort; he thinks he is swimming, climbing hills, etc. If enteritis is present the stools are bloody, and each movement is accompanied with tearing down the thighs.

BAPTISIA deserves the preference when he is confused as to his personal unity,—thinks himself double, scattered in pieces, etc. Tongue is brown, especially down the centre. Stools dark, bloody, painless. Fever and temperature show decided evening exacerbation.

LACHESIS inflames the cœcum. Even if unconscious, he will resist the slightest touch to the abdomen; parts most distant from the heart are cool; pulse rapid, feeble, or intermittent; arouses from sleep smothering. This smothering may also suggest Baptisia, but the conditions are different. Tongue trembles and catches behind the lower teeth.

LYCOPODIUM.—Rumbling in the splenic flexure. Diaphragmitis, with feeling of a cord marking the costal attachments of the diaphragm; tympany. Especially useful when the brain shows signs of giving out; he becomes more and more drowsy; eyes half open, expressionless, and covered with a film; lower jaw tends to drop; one foot cold and the other warm; no urine in the bladder, or it passes involuntarily and stains the sheets with a red sand.

ARSENIC is invaluable when the patient is pale and hot, eyes half-open, with absence of winking; "gum" on the eyes; restlessness or great anguish after 12 P.M. These symptoms are not uncommon in infants.

Hyoscyamus must be remembered when there are spasmodic jerkings; delirium; she suddenly sits up, looks around and lies down again; uncovers herself; lascivious talk; or, stupor, stool and urine involuntary; the urine leaves streaks of red sand on the clothing.

Terebinthina.—Burning in the uterus; tympany; tongue dry and smooth; urine scanty, dark, smoky, with strangury.

Kali carb.—Stitching pains all over the abdomen; tympany; urine scanty, dark. Nervous; easily startled if touched, especially if the feet are touched; unconsciousness in puerperal peritonitis; or, stupid, cares for nothing; when questioned is at a loss what to reply; pulse rapid, weak, or intermittent.

In peritonitis of infants, generally tuberculous, compare with the above, SULPH., SILICA, CALC. OSTR., CALC. PHOS., *Phosph.*, *Iodine*, Ars. iod., Baryta, *Psorin.*, etc.

CALC. OSTR., general symptoms agreeing, must be remembered when, in child or adult, the abdominal pains are relieved by cold applications. This exceptional symptom of lime is recorded in Raue's *Pathology*, and may be inferred from the provings. In Allen, vol. ii, p. 365, we read: "Frequent attacks of colic after the disappearance of a severe coryza that had lasted two days, with great weariness and sickly look of the face, lasting several days, and then suddenly and completely *relieved by bathing in cold water.*"

For typhlitis, which frequently leads to peritonitis: BELLAD., Laches., Mercur., Merc. corros., RHUS TOX., *Nux vom.*, Ginseng, Hepar, Opium, Plumbum, Rhamnus Frangula, etc.

The tympany which so annoys the patient is a very dangerous symptom when occurring late in the disease. Compare: OPIUM, LYCOPOD., Kali c., Terebinth., *Rhus tox.*, *Colchic.*, CARBO VEG., *Phosph.*, CINCHONA, Verat. alb., Cocculus.

Raphanus produces distended abdomen; no emission of flatus either upwards or downwards. Dr. Bell's case confirming this symptom is suggestive, and should lead us to a careful study of the drug.

E. A. F.

SURGICAL CLINIC OF PROF. CHARLES M. THOMAS, M.D.

(Hahnemann Medical College, Philadelphia, Tuesday, December 22d, 1879.)

GENTLEMEN: This man you will recognize as the one from whom at the last clinic, four days ago, I removed an epitheliomatous carcinoma of the lower lip. You will remember that we operated by the V-shaped incision, and that the cuts through the lip were made well off from the edge of the growth, in order that if possible none of the cancerous infiltrated tissue should be left in the contiguous parts. This obliged us to take with the growth, fully one-half of the lower lip, but in spite of this, you saw how readily, owing to the elasticity of the tissues of this region, the edges of the wound were brought together.

The progress of the case has been an uninterruptedly good one. The edges, united with the pin and wire sutures, were covered with a compress of lint wet in a Calendula solution, and the same remedy given internally; he was placed upon liquid diet, of milk, meat broth, etc., and forbidden to move his lip or jaw. On the third day the two pins, which afforded the main support for the wound, were withdrawn, and I will, now before you, remove the three stitches of fine silver wire which hold the superficial edges together.

You will please notice that the cut surfaces have united accurately, and without a sign of suppuration, but that on each side, at the point of entrance and exit of the upper pin, there is a small ulcerating spot; this is due to the pressure of the pin, and can usually be avoided by its early removal. I believe it better, on this account, to take away a pin suture in many cases as early as forty-eight hours after its introduction. These were allowed to remain till the afternoon of the third day, and will probably leave a slight mark after the healing, which you can understand would not be a desirable result in the case of a woman, however slight the blemish.

RODENT ULCER.

Mrs. ——, æt. 55 years. I bring this lady before you, gentlemen, for the purpose of illustrating the difference in appearance between the epithelioma and the so-called rodent ulcer, of which this is a striking example.

About eight years ago she noticed what she supposed to be the mark of a mosquito-sting upon the side of the nose.

From scratching, this became raw, and from that time on, there has been a slow but steadily progressive destruction of the surrounding tissue, until now, as you see, all of the soft parts of the nose excepting the tip have been destroyed, and the line of ulceration is extending into the cheeks and lower eyelids. The surface of the ulcer presents a smooth, almost glazed appearance, the discharge is scant and thin, the edges are irregular in outline though but slightly raised, and with apparently no infiltration of the structures in advance of them.

As I pick up the tissues just at the margin of the ulcer, I

find them almost as pliable as farther out upon the cheek. There is no offensive odor to the discharge, and the patient complains of little or no pain. Although she has now been afflicted with this for several years, she does not find that her general health has in any way suffered from it.

Clinically considered this affection presents much that is similar to the epitheliomatous cancer, which we considered at some length last Friday, and indeed by many it has been looked upon as closely allied to the cancerous degenerations, not only in appearance but in structure. Thus we have both attacking, by preference, superficial skin surfaces, and confining their ravages to this tissue mainly, only passing to deeper and more dense structures in the later stages of the disease. They both most frequently appear first as a small tubercle or warty elevation, which, breaking down, starts the progress of ulceration. The extension of the ulceration is usually slow but constant in both, and seldom affects the general health in either until the later stages, and, finally, they are both affections of middle or old age. These resemblances might lead one to suspect a close relationship between them, but if we examine them more closely we shall find sufficiently well-marked differences to render a confounding of the two improbable. One of the most important distinctive points is the almost constant surrounding infiltrative induration in the epithelioma, and its general absence in rodent ulcer. In the progress of the latter there seems to be a simple destruction or smelting down of the invaded tissue, while in the former the ulceration is always preceded by an advancing wall of cancerous infiltration. The surface of a skin cancer is, by contrast with the smooth, flat, glossy rodent ulcer, more irregular, elevated, and covered with a more abundant and consistent discharge. Again, the rodent ulcer appears to be an entirely local affection, and does not, as in the epithelioma, involve the lymphatic glands of the neighborhood, or attack through the lymphatics the internal organs. Finally, gentlemen, it has been found, on microscopic examination, that there is, in the elevated margin of the rodent ulcer, an almost entire absence of the peculiar epithelial elements of carcinoma.

Our results of the *treatment* of the affection, as also in epithelioma, are, I am sorry to say, not brilliant. There are but few authentic cases of cure on record from the use of internal remedies alone; perhaps more from careful internal treatment combined with thorough local destruction of the disease, either with the knife or strong caustic, such as the pastes of Zinc chloride and Arsenic. The actual or thermo-cautery has also been found to be of service.

This lady has been under the care of a number of skilful physicians, but, as you see, with no good result. She has received at my hands only internal treatment, mainly Lycop., Hydras., Thuja, and Nitric acid. The latter she has been taking for some weeks, and, as there is still an uninterrupted progression of the ulceration, I shall now recommend to her the extirpation with the knife, followed immediately by a careful cauterization of the whole surface with the thermo-cautery at a high heat.

EPITHELIOMA OF THE NOSE.

Mrs. ——, æt. 45 years. As a continuation of the subject of malignant ulceration of the integuments, I am glad to be able to bring before you this lady, who has had for a long time an elevated, dirty, half-scabbed, ulcerating surface upon the side of the nose. It has lately been growing with unusual rapidity. It is now as large as my thumb-nail, and surrounded by a wall of induration. From these appearances I feel justified in pronouncing it a case of *epithelioma.*

As she comes from a distance, asking for immediate relief at our hands, and as lately it has been growing more rapidly than at any other time, we will etherize her without delay and remove the growth with the knife. In extirpating such a diseased mass, you will please notice that I run the knife well to the outside of its margins and cut, as nearly as I can judge, in healthy tissue, in order that I may not leave behind any of the cancerous elements, from which a recurrence of the growth would be almost certain to take place.

Even when the extirpation has been most radical, we should never insure the patient against a repetition of the growth, for although the results of operation in this variety of cancer are more favorable than in any other, we must not forget that a recurrence after a longer or shorter time is the rule, while total immunity is the exception.

So soon as the bleeding has somewhat subsided, this raw surface shall be covered with a compress of lint soaked in carbolized oil, held in place by turns of a roller bandage, and this or a similar dressing continued till the resulting sore has healed by granulation.

SARCOMA OF THE THIGH.

A. B., æt. 18 years, was attacked eighteen months ago, while working in the coal mines near Wilkesbarre, with what he supposed to be rheumatic pains in the left thigh. These continued with more or less severity for about six months, when he noticed the outer side of the thigh growing harder and larger. Since that time the pain has not been so severe, but the swelling has gradually increased, involving the whole circumference of the thigh, until, as you see now, it has attained an enormous growth, and reaches from the condyles of the femur to the base of the great trochanter.

It presents to the eye a uniform, smooth, tolerably well-defined, spindle-shaped enlargement, with a largest circumference of twenty-three and three-fourths inches. On palpation some portions, particularly the outer and posterior, appear quite firm, though not bony and hard, and upon its anterior and inner face the mass gives to the examining hand an elastic or obscurely fluctuating feel. Although the growth seems to have involved all the structures up to the subcutaneous tissue, the integuments are at no point adherent to it.

The patient suffers but little pain, has a moderate appetite, but is rapidly losing flesh; his face presents a yellowish-white, so-called cachectic, appearance.

Judging mainly from its rapid growth, unattended by inflammatory symptoms, and the general emaciation and cachexy, I suppose this to be a malignant and cancerous formation; and from its rather painless character, its origin in the deeper fibrous or bony structures, its encapsulated and elastic feel, and the non-involvement of the integument, I am inclined to place it in the class of *sarcomatous* cancers, rather than the carcinomatous, which, as you know, have, as a rule, no well-defined outline, are generally painful, and tend toward early softening and involvement of the integuments.

From your knowledge of the history of such new growths, you will realize that this young man's case is probably a hopeless one. Inasmuch as the tumor already occupies the thigh to a level with the hip, and probably includes all but the most superficial tissues within its grasp, the probabilities are that an exarticulation at the hip (the only available operation for removal), would be followed by an early recurrence in the stump, even should the patient survive the effects of the amputation, which of itself (necessitating as it does the removal of at least one-fifth of the body) is followed by death in considerably more than half the cases. And, again, should he pass safely through the dangers described, he will have yet to face the possibilities of a not far distant death by deposit of the cancerous material in internal organs. If after careful deliberation and consultation the amputation should be decided upon, I hope to be able to give you an opportunity of witnessing its performance.

IMPACTED FRACTURE OF THIGH.

Mr. ——, fifty odd years of age, fell last night from his doorstep to the pavement, alighting upon his left side. He suffered very severe pain at the hip, and was for some time unable to rise, but finally he not only succeeded, but walked a short distance before being brought to our hospital.

I bring him before you more particularly to illustrate the importance of repeated and careful investigation and measurement in deepseated injuries, especially in the neighborhood of joints. From such a history one would naturally suspect a fracture at or near the neck of the femur; but, as I examine him, you will notice that there is no eversion of the foot, no crepitus, no elevation of the trochanter, and little or no shortening of the arc of rotation described by the trochanter on rolling the limb, as compared with the opposite side.

All of these you know to be important and tolerably constant signs of such a fracture. If we add to this the very unusual ability to stand and bear weight upon the affected side, I am sure you will agree with me that a fracture might with some reason be thrown out of consideration. But look with me further, and you will see that the side of the hip, or region of the trochanter, appears flatter upon the affected than upon the sound side, that the slightest pressure over the base of the trochanter causes severe pain, and, finally, that there is a shortening of fully a quarter of an inch in this limb as compared with the sound one. These three symptoms, with the history, are sufficient to lead us to the conclusion that there is after all a fracture here, but accompanied by firm inpaction or denticulation of the fragments where the neck and trochanter join.

Such an impaction much increases the chances for good union here, and should not be disturbed by unnecessary manipulation.

His treatment will consist in the application of a straight external (Liston) splint and rest in the horizontal position without extension for at least five to six weeks, when he may be allowed to go about on crutches, with a support to the hip.

A CHARACTERISTIC OF GELSEMIUM IN LABOR.

BY J. C. GUERNSEY, M D.,

PHILADELPHIA, PA.

One night last summer I was summoned to attend Mrs. H. N. in labor. On my way to the house her husband expressed deep regret that his wife always suffered during labor from such terrible backache. She had been twice delivered with instruments, though in charge of a skilful homœopathic physician; and now, at her third confinement, dreaded their presumably necessary employment. Arriving at her bedside I found labor had fairly set in, and sure enough with it her excruciating "backache." On inquiring into its nature, I at once recognized my standard Gelsemium indication: *Each pain starts all right; but, instead of extending around into the abdomen and then downwards, it turns and runs up the back.* In her two previous confinements, pain after pain of this kind, each becoming more and more severe, followed, "doing no good," until after a protracted and severe labor, forceps were called into requisition. On learning the exact nature of her pains, I gave Gelsemium 30[m] in solution, one teaspoonful every fifteen minutes. After the second or third dose the character of the pains became so natural that I stopped the medicine. In four hours, to the great joy and relief of the patient and her family, a fine large boy was born, unaided by any instruments.

In Guernsey's *Obstetrics*, 3d ed., p. 386, we read: "*Gelsemium*, cutting pains in the abdomen from before backwards and upwards, rendering the labor-pains useless; these come on with every pain." And again, page 388, "The pain extends into the abdomen from before backwards and upwards; this pain is a false pain, and is so severe as to interrupt the true labor-pains." The special point I wish to make is that the pain may locate itself entirely in the back and neutralize the true pain by *running up the back.*

It is well known by every careful homœopathic prescriber, that any case of confinement, no matter what the patient's previous record of tedious and wearisome labor may be, can be rendered natural and comparatively short and easy by an exhibition of the true similimum, provided always that there be no malformation or other mechanical obstruction.

I have found the same characteristic symptom of Gelsemium in dysmenorrhœa and at the menopause, when it is sometimes accompanied by profuse hæmorrhage.

DIPHTHERIA: ITS PATHOLOGY AND TREATMENT.

BY GEORGE HOSFELD, M.D , AND G. W. PARKER, M D.,
PHILADELPHIA, PA.

(Read before the Philadelphia County Homœopathic Medical Society.)

Diphtheria is considered one of the oldest of epidemic diseases, its history having been traced back even to the time of Homer. In the second century it is said to have appeared in Egypt, and in the early part of the sixteenth century it was epidemic in Holland. During the latter part of the same century it raged in Spain, killing a great number of persons by suffocation, whence it was called garotilla; since which time it has been observed in most of the countries of Europe, exhibiting symptoms more or less violent in character.

In the United States it was first reported as an epidemic about twenty-five years ago, and now prevails in all parts of the country.

The first accurate investigation into the nature of this disease was made in 1821 by Bretonneau, who gave it its present name. He at first regarded it as a local disease, but somewhat later modified his views and conceded that blood-poisoning was an essential characteristic. Other writers, such as Virchow, Wagner, and Buhl, held different opinions regarding the nature of diphtheria, and were upheld in their theories until Professors Oertel and Henter discovered simultaneously that the diphtheritic membranes, the subjacent diseased parts, and even the blood, contained in great numbers, vegetable organisms, to which Oertel gave the name of micrococci, and this is now considered the specific cause. The relation which the local, bears to the general disease is still a mooted point.

Professor Oertel, however, claims to have proven that the specific poison first attacks the mucous membrane of the air-passages, causing a local disease, and from this point as a centre it affects the whole system and becomes a general disease. Diphtheria, then, is an acute, specific, infectious, and contagious disease. It makes its appearance under two different series of symptoms,—as a local, and as a general disease,—and in the greater number of cases followed by a third series of disturbances, called sequelæ.

The local disease makes its appearance as an inflammatory process upon the mucous membranes and denuded parts of the skin exposed to the air, and leads to the formation upon them of a grayish-white false membranous deposit. It occurs especially on the mucous membrane of the mouth and pharynx, of the nose, the larynx and air-passages lower down, and even of the stomach and bowels. More rarely it invades the vagina and rectum, or points of transition from the skin to the mucous membrane; for instance, at the corners of the mouth, on the labia, the prepuce, the anus, or the inner surface of the puerperal uterus.

The general affection has the character of an infectious disease, and holds a position midway between simple excitement of the circulatory system and the severest forms of typhoid fever and pyæmic poisoning. The sequelæ which follow the healing of the local process and disappearance of the febrile symptoms, are, for the most part, disturbances of the muscular system, which may vary from a paralysis of single muscles to a complete ataxia. On the other hand, in a few cases, extreme disease of the kidneys, with dropsy and changes in the formation of blood and lymphatic growths have been observed.

Diphtheria occurs sporadically as well as epidemically, and may, in certain localities especially favorable to it, become an endemic disease.

Regarding the conditions under which this disease manifests itself the following points are offered as compiled by the English writer, Ellis, from reports upon different epidemics:

1. The period of incubation is three or four days.

2. Diphtheria may occur in every locality and under every condition.

3. It attacks indiscriminately rich and poor, the well fed and the poorly nourished. Except that a porous soil with an understratum of clay appeared rather to favor its development, geological strata appear to have no relation to its prevalence.

4. While bad hygienic conditions of necessity promote the virulence by lowering vitality, etc., good hygienic conditions afford no exemption from its attack.

5. Temperature has little effect; the moist cold weather preceding the winter was the time of its greatest prevalence.

6. Even diathesis seems to make little difference, though some of the physicians considered struma as a predisposing cause.

7. Children from 3 to 8 years are the most frequent subjects. Children at the breast rarely suffer.

8. The duration in favorable cases is from 10 to 15 days. Terminatio in death or recovery becomes apparent in seven days. n

9. Recurrence in the same individual is not the rule, and recurrent cases are less severe than the original attack.

10. As a singular fact, the public institutions (with one exception) were remarkably free, and the Chinese race possessed absolute immunity.

The severity of an attack of diphtheria will depend upon the character of the epidemic, the influences by which it is governed, together with the susceptibility of the individual to the disease, and the existing state of the general system at the time; hence different varieties or forms of the disease will occur. The first or the mildest form is termed the catarrhal.

Here the local and general symptoms may be trifling in character; the exudation may be entirely absent or exhibit itself by small grayish-white spots on one or both tonsils, and on points in the region of the fauces; these spots may remain separate, but in more marked cases they coalesce or form streaks of false membrane.

The general symptoms present are, slight fever, sensation of dryness and slight pain in the throat, especially on swallowing. External glands not much swollen, but tender on pressure. Exceptionally a more general disturbance may take place. In twenty-four hours all general symptoms gradually subside, followed in a few days by the disappearance of the local trouble.

The next variety is the croupous form, known as true membranous diphtheria. Here we find the local inflammation so great as to cause a fibrinous exudation on the mucous membrane. At first the throat presents a dark-red livid appearance, the tissues are swollen, and become softened and infiltrated. A few hours only are necessary to develop this false membrane, which gradually assumes a grayish-white color, and becomes thickened like leather. The constitutional symptoms are great febrile heat with drowsiness and restlessness, increased temperature, rapid pulse, pains in the head, back, and limbs, and great muscular debility. In children, nocturnal delirium and even convulsions may occur.

By continuity of the mucous surface, the false membrane may extend upwards to the nasal cavity, through the Eustachian tube to the middle ear, or it may extend downwards into the larynx, trachea, and bronchi, developing the too well-known symptoms of "diphtheritic croup." The external glands about the throat, the submaxillary and cervical, are always swollen; the degree of swelling is commensurate with the extent of the local affection on one or both sides of the throat. They are also enlarged, hard, sensitive to pressure, and at times the contiguous connective tissue more or less involved. As the disease progresses the inflammation, swelling, and exudation increase, and in proportion deglutition becomes more difficult. The salivary glands may be affected, causing salivation; the tongue is heavily coated, and the breath has a peculiar, offensive odor. There is great thirst and total loss of appetite. Vomiting of the ingesta and diarrhœa may occur, though in many cases they are not present.

The examination of the urine is important, even in the first days of the disease. As long as fever continues, the disease is on the increase, the secretion of urine is diminished, deep in color and rich in salts. The presence of albumen is not constant, in some cases only at a later period, while in bad cases it may exist from first to last. When this form is inclined to terminate favorably the healing process begins from the seventh to the tenth day. This occurs with a simultaneous improvement in the local and general symptoms. Exudation ceases, swelling diminishes, and deglutition becomes less difficult. Exfoliation of the membranes gradually takes place, and they are thrown off by the patient's efforts at coughing or clearing the throat. The subsidence of the general and subjective symptoms follows as a rule quickly. The fever yields; the temperature becomes normal; the pulse diminishes steadily or may continue quickened until complete restoration. Pain in the throat lessens, tongue clears, appetite improves, the skin grows moist, the urine becomes more plentiful and its color lighter. Sleep becomes quiet and unbroken, while the muscular weakness and the signs of exhaustion more or less marked are comparatively slow to yield. The healthy process may become complete and lasting, or a relapse take place followed again by improvement, and after apparent recovery, sooner or later signs of secondary affections and diphtheritic paralysis may set in.

We now come to the next variety, the septic form, known as malignant diphtheria.

Shortly after the appearance of the exudation, or in some cases not until the false membrane has appeared for some time, the odor of the breath becomes more and more foul-smelling, the membranes assume a dirty gray-brownish appearance, become soft and brittle, and break down at many points into a grayish-brown semi-solid greasy layer. This condition denotes disintegration and decomposition of the false membranes. The fluids of the mouth, combined with the ichorous products of the decomposing membranes, become a stinking and corroding ichor, causing reddening and excoriations on the parts over which it flows, and ultimately ulceration.

The nasal discharge, which at first consisted of a thin yellowish-white mucus, also becomes fetid, acrid, and excoriating, brownish in color, and sometimes mixed with blood. The cervical and submaxillary glands now are enormously swollen, and the surrounding connective tissue œdematous to such an extent as to quite obliterate the boundary of neck and face. The face is bloated, pale, waxlike; the pulse small, weak, irregular, and remarkably slow; the temperature slightly raised, or fallen below the normal. Prostration is extreme, but consciousness remains unclouded even to the last hours, and death ensues from œdema of the lungs or some affection of the heart.

The last form of this disease is the gangrenous. When the unmistakable signs of gangrenous disorganization appear on the mucous membrane the inflammatory and febrile symptoms commonly give place to those of general depression and collapse. The features of the face lose their character, the pulse grows frequent and small, the skin cold. Often there are marked chills, metastatic inflammation of internal organs through septicæmia or embolus, erysipelas of the skin, nervous symptoms, meteorism, and involuntary stools; death finally closing the scene.

SEQUELÆ, OR SECONDARY AFFECTIONS OF DIPHTHERIA.

Among the secondary effects of this disease we may find remaining, ulcers of the throat, abscesses in different parts of the body, most frequently in the glands about the neck, ozæna, otorrhœa, cough, etc. The most important affection, however, is the post-diphtheritic paralysis. It may be motory, sensory, or both. In whatever form this condition may present itself, partial or complete muscular paralysis may occur. It develops gradually and slowly, and the course ordinarily taken by this process is characteristic. Paralysis of the soft palate and pharynx is first noticed ; this is followed either immediately or after a short interval by disturbances of vision, while paralysis of the upper and lower extremities occur later. More rarely paralysis has been observed in the muscles of the larynx, trunk, rectum, bladder, diaphragm, and finally the face. The ordinary termination of diphtheritic paralysis is in recovery.

DIFFERENTIAL DIAGNOSIS.

We find diphtheria to bear a family resemblance to croup and scarlatina. Between croup and diphtheria the following distinctions are recognizable : In the former the inflammation is sthenic, while in the latter it is asthenic. The site of the inflammation in croup is at first confined to the larynx, extending thence to the trachea and bronchi; whereas, in diphtheria it is in the tonsils, pharynx, and soft palate, extending thence to the larynx and nares. In diphtheria there is fetid breath, sanious discharge from the nostrils, and the neighboring lymphatic glands are swollen; which symptoms are absent in croup. Moreover, croup, as a rule, is sporadic, while diphtheria is generally epidemic.

The following are the chief diagnostic points between diphtheria and scarlatina:

1. An attack from either disease confers no immunity from an attack of the other.
2. The peculiar rash of scarlatina is absent in diphtheria, though there may be in the latter an erythematous blush, evanescent and occurring in patches, but this is by no means a constant symptom.
3. Albuminuria occurs in the *course* of diphtheria, but towards the *close* of scarlatina.
4. The strawberry tongue of scarlatina and the subsequent desquamation are also points wanting in diphtheria.
5. The sequelæ are totally different in the two diseases.

Diphtheria may be complicated with scarlatina, measles, small-pox, and a low form of pneumonia.

A definite prognosis of this disease is by no means possible; much will depend upon the character of the epidemic, the age and the constitution of the patient, the form of attack, etc. While all forms of this disease may end in recovery, death generally ensues from exhaustion and blood-poisoning. Unfavorable signs are the acrid discharge from the nostrils, the invasion of the larynx or the development of diphtheritic croup, hæmorrhages from the nose and mouth, purpura, petechiæ, coldness of the external surface of the body, albuminuria, diarrhœa and vomiting, convulsions.

In preparing this paper we have drawn largely from Professor Oertel's article on Diphtheria in Ziemssen's *Cyclopædia of Medicine*, Ellis on *Diseases of Children*, and Raue's *Pathology*, while the following brief therapeutic hints embody our own personal experience in this disease.

THERAPEUTICS.

The following remedies are those which we have used with the best success:

Apis.—Great debility from the commencement; the membrane assumes at once a dirty grayish color; no thirst, etc.

Belladonna.—If the disease begins with a high fever, and severe inflammation of the tonsils, it seems to cut short the disease; but if ulceration has taken place it has to be supplemented by another medicine, generally Merc. biniod. or cyanuret.

Calc. chlor. we have used in a number of cases with very good success. The only symptom noted has been that if the throat looked very raw, and the membrane appeared transparent, it has in twenty-four hours removed all the danger; have also used it empirically with success.

Kali Muriat.—This remedy we used in two cases of the disease where the membrane invaded the larynx; both cases recovered; no other remedy was used.

Lac Caninum.—Have used this in a few light cases with apparent success.

Lachesis.—When the disease commences on the left side, and the subjective symptoms are more severe than the objective, a great deal of pain on swallowing, particularly the spittle, and worse after sleeping.

Lachnanthes has cured all cases that have come under our observation, where the neck was drawn to one side, with inability to move it without moving the whole body.

Merc. Biniod.—In the catarrhal form, where the exudation has the appearance of ulceration, this remedy appears to act like a charm, particularly after the fever has been reduced by Bellad.

Merc. Cyan.—For the malignant form of the disease this is the remedy, and if it does not help, the chances are small indeed.

Nitric Acid.—Where the disease attacks principally the nose, and produces excoriating and profuse discharges, this remedy has acted nicely.

Sulphur.—We have found this remedy capable of breaking the membrane when it assumes the croupous form, and it was ejected in pieces. It was given every two hours, a powder of the first decimal trituration. We have also cured cases which had assumed the form of true croup.

In case of blood-poisoning we use Arsenic and Brandy, as recommended by Grauvogl, and think we have seen it do good.

ADJUVANTS.

As regards local applications we have used nothing but alcohol and water, as recommended by Grauvogl, and we think it has been uniformly beneficial.

DIET.

We use milk during the fever, and light food generally. After the fever is over we use milk-punch, beef tea, etc., to sustain the strength.

PARASITIC DISEASES OF THE SKIN.

BY M. S WILLIAMSON, M D.,

PHILADELPHIA, PA.

(Read before the Philadelphia County Homœopathic Medical Society.)

THE skin from its exposed situation is subject to many diseases peculiar only to this tissue, and your attention is called especially to some of a parasitic character. A suitable soil is necessary for them to flourish in, and all are modified by temperament, inherited tendencies, exposure to heat and cold, and sometimes by the occupation of the patient.

The necessity for a correct diagnosis must be insisted upon, the treatment for the removal of the malady depending upon our knowledge of its nature and course. Many of them can be readily cured in the beginning of their course; hence the importance of an early recognition of their character. Moreover, all experience has shown that the obstinacy of these disorders is increased almost in proportion to the period of their duration. Especially is this true of those which affect the parts that are covered with hair. Still another reason for the exercise of great care in this particular is to be found in the contagious character of these complaints, as evidenced not only by their transmission from one individual to another, but also in their transfer from one part to another of the same individual. The danger to be apprehended from suppressing eruptive diseases, a matter of so much concern to physicians generally, does not present itself in the class of diseases we are considering. The microscope having revealed their true character, the destruction of the parasite by proper local measures is not regarded as being attended with danger to the patient.

The parasites are of two kinds, animal and vegetable. Dr. McCall Anderson found that in 11,000 consecutive cases, there were 656 cases of vegetable and 2905 cases of the animal form.

The principal animal parasites found in this country are the *Acarus scabiei*, or itch mite; the *Pediculus*, or louse; the *Cimex lectularius*, or bedbug; and the *Pulex irritans*, or flea.

The indication of the presence of the itch is the furrow caused by the burrowing of the female, the male remaining upon the surface hiding under dirt, scabs, etc. The eggs are deposited and the young *acari* appear, when exfoliation of the epidermis takes place; and so increasing in numbers they tend to spread the trouble upon the skin. The favorite place for them is in the folds of the skin, between the fingers and upon the anterior surface of the forearm.

The *acari* cause itching and burning; vesicles are formed, and in many places papules and ecthymatous spots are caused by the scratching. In old cases linear marks and cicatrices show where the furrows have been.

Sulphur internally and applied locally in the form of ointment, containing ʒss. to ℥j of lard, twice a day for three days, is usually sufficient to kill the *acarus*. Styrax ointment is also recommended.

Pityriasis, the name given to the condition caused by the presence of pediculi, is of three varieties, affecting the head, body, and pubes respectively, each produced by a distinct species of insect. The eggs of those affecting the head and pubes are found attached to the hairs, and are commonly called "nits." The *pediculus corporis* is larger than the others, and lives in the clothing; people who are uncleanly in their habits, both young and old, are liable to have their persons invaded by these pests. These lice, by means of the proboscis, cause red spots to appear on the skin, and in sensitive persons the irritation may bring on eczema, urticaria, papulæ, or pustules. The neck and shoulders are usually the first places attacked.

Of the many things that have been used to destroy them, one of the most effective is washing thoroughly with a five per cent. solution of Carbolic acid, followed by a hot bath, and subjecting the clothing to a high temperature.

The bite of the *Cimex lectularius* causes a hyperæmic papule with a small red spot in the centre. That of the flea produces a hæmorrhagic spot surrounded by redness, which burns, itches, and smarts for a short time.

The application of a lotion of Glycerin and water, of each

℥ij, and tincture of Calendula ʒj will be found very useful in allaying the irritation in these cases.

Children of lymphatic temperament who are not kept clean, are poorly nourished, or insufficiently clothed, and live in rooms badly ventilated, are particularly liable to vegetable parasitic diseases; and unless measures are adopted to remove the exciting causes and predisposing conditions, treatment is unsatisfactory and relapses are frequent. Isolation should be resorted to whenever such a measure is practicable.

The varieties are tinea favosa, or favus; tinea tonsurans, or ringworm of the scalp; tinea circinata, or the common form of ringworm; tinea sycosis, tinea versicolor, and onychia parasitica.

Favus is a rare disease, appearing as yellow crusts having a cup-shaped depression, in the centre of which is a hair. This eruption has a peculiar mousy smell. The hairs become loosened, dry, and brittle, from the invasion of the follicles.

In tinea tonsurans the hairy parts are affected, and in tinea circinata the other parts are attacked; the former is usually met with only in children, and both diseases are often found in one individual. The tinea tonsurans exhibits patches one or two inches in diameter, covered with fine white scales; the hairs having become brittle, are broken off, occasioning a temporary baldness of the parts.

Tinea circinata was formerly known as herpes circinata, from its ring of vesicles, but its contagious character and the presence of fungi have demonstrated its true quality, and assigned it its proper place.

There are two forms of sycosis or "barbers' itch," one parasitic and the other not. This is a pustular disease resulting from inflammation of the hair-follicles of the face. The parasitic variety may be detected by the hairs becoming brittle and loose. It is more rarely met with, and covers less surface than the non-parasitic variety. The existence of tinea decalvans as a parasitic disease has been denied by some writers, but parasites have been found by Dr. Tilbury Fox to be the cause of at least some cases of alopecia.

Tinea versicolor, which formerly was called "pityriasis versicolor," is found in parts covered by the clothing; the chest being the part most frequently attacked. The patches are slightly raised, of a yellow or fawn color, and rough to the touch. When the person becomes warm, the spots itch considerably. These are the so-called "liver spots," and have been often treated on the supposition that they were produced by some derangement of that organ.

The nails may be the only part attacked, and the disease is then known as onychia parasitica. These organs become thickened, brittle, opaque, and occasionally of a yellowish color. The nails may become contaminated in individuals already affected with tinea favosa, tonsurans, etc., or the disease may be transferred from other persons by contact of the hands with diseased parts.

In treating all these diseases the first thing to be accomplished is the destruction of the parasites. Then the general state of the system should be brought up to a more healthy standard by attention more particularly to the nutritive functions, care in the selection of diet, inculcating out-door exercise, etc. Other diseases which may have been caused by the parasitic irritation must also be included in the general system of treatment.

In applying local treatment to the hairy parts it is sometimes considered necessary that the hairs be extracted, a matter usually easy of accomplishment. Olive or almond oil should be applied to hard crusts or scabs at night, when it will be found that they are so much softened as to be easily removable the next morning. This must of course be done before the treatment for the destruction of parasites is commenced.

Of the many local remedies recommended, the use of hyposulphite of soda in the proportion of ʒij to ℥j of water is often attended with excellent effect; the bichloride of mercury gr. j to gr. ij to ℥j of water has also been used in many cases and with marked beneficial results. The baldness resulting from tinea decalvans is sometimes treated by means of lotions designed to stimulate the growth of the hair. In these lotions cantharides tincture is sometimes included as an important ingredient.

THE GERM THEORY OF DISEASE.

BY C. R. NORTON, M D.,

PHILADELPHIA, PA.

(Read before the Philadelphia County Homœopathic Medical Society.)

THIS Society had the pleasure, some months ago, of listening to a paper on the "Theories of Disease," presented by Dr. Neidhard; but he did not enter upon the question as to how disease germs act in producing the symptoms referable to their introduction into the system.

There has been a theory promulgated by Dr. Maclagan, in which he starts out with the supposition that germs do cause morbid symptoms, and deals with the subject entirely from a pathological point of view, endeavoring to show that they are competent to produce the symptoms incident to certain diseased conditions. As to the nature of the contagium he says: "All we know is, 1st. That it consists of minute solid particles. 2d. That these particles are probably organized. 3d. That in chemical composition they so closely resemble the fluids in which they occur that the chemist fails even to detect their presence; and 4th. That they are so very minute that the highest powers of the microscope fail to give us definite information regarding their nature, or even their existence.

"Beyond this point the combined efforts of the chemist, microscopist, and biologist have failed to carry us."

The eruptive fevers are taken for investigation, for they possess many points in common.

"Each has a tolerably definite period of incubation.

"Each has for its most prominent symptoms the existence of that aggregate of phenomena to which we apply the term fever.

"Each possesses a characteristic local lesion.

"Each has a pretty definite period of duration.

"Each occurs, as a rule, but once in a lifetime."

This common array of characteristics renders it highly probable that each has a similar cause.

These fevers all have a period of incubation and a febrile stage. We will first consider the *period of incubation.*

The poison or contagium (which may be called the first factor), which produces an eruptive fever, probably consists of minute organisms, which require for their growth, in common with other organisms, nitrogen and water; but these organisms, existing in a living body as they do, and dependent for nutrition and growth on live tissues, are parasitic, and consequently require a special nidus for their development. This nidus, or condition of growth, is called the "second factor," and without its presence no germ can propagate in the system.

When germs have entered the system and have found this "second factor" they begin to multiply by division, and each new organism having reached maturity gives rise to others, until at last there accumulates in the body a sufficient number to cause morbid symptoms.

The greater extent to which the "second factor" exists, the faster will be the growth and propagation of the contagia, and of course the shorter the period of incubation. The number of germs originally entering the system will also modify the term of incubation. When the number of germs has reached a certain point the symptoms, which usually precede the full development of the disease, make their appearance, though sometimes, when the number of germs introduced into the system has been very large, and the "second factor" exists abundantly, the outbreak of the fever will be sudden, owing to the very rapid increase of the contagia, which may, by a propagation which appears almost explosive, develop in vast quantities.

The febrile stage now sets in, and in its study we will only consider idiopathic fever as it occurs most typically in the eruptive fevers of the organisms which we suppose to produce the fever. It may be said that:

"They are mainly composed of albumen.

"They largely consume nitrogen.

"They largely consume water.

"They multiply by division."

The essential phenomena of the febrile stage are:

"Increased waste of nitrogenous tissues.

"Increased consumption of water.

"Increased rapidity of circulation.

"Preternatural heat."

"This juxtaposition of the chief characteristics of the contagion and of the phenomena accompanying its propagation, alone suggests a probable causal relation between the two. The propagation in the system of millions of organisms, which largely consume elements requisite for the nutrition and repair of all the tissues of the body, must be accompanied by serious disturbances. If nitrogen and water be the chief requisites for the growth of the contagium particles, the symptoms and changes referable to increased but abnormal consumption of these elements will be among the chief characteristics of the disturbance to which the propagation of the contagium gives rise."

These myriads of organisms circulating in the blood, and pervading the whole system, appropriate in their growth and multiplication most of the nitrogen which was destined for the tissues, and the retrograde metamorphosis of the nitrogenous tissues goes on much more rapidly than in health, consequently the amount of urea, which normally always corresponds exactly to the amount of nitrogenous food ingested, becomes increased (with the exceptions noted below), since there are present two sources for its production, namely, the retrograde change occurring from the consumption of the albuminous compounds by the contagia, and by that taking place in the nitrogenous tissues.

The nervous system suffers from this deprivation of the blood, and, as at the same time the water which is necessary for the performance of the digestive function is consumed by the contagia, digestion is impaired, the appetite destroyed, and the assimilation of food taken is defective. Since water is required for the nutrition of the tissues, and enters largely into the formation of their bulk, this source of wasting is also present. There is a class of cases in which the elimination of urea is diminished, and this condition can be explained by the fact that in such fevers the disease is always very severe, and the morbid processes in the system go on with greater rapidity; the fluids are more largely consumed by the contagia, and the kidneys receive too scanty a supply of water to enable them to perform their functions properly. The excess of urea in the kidneys produces in them changes similar to those found in acute nephritis; and bloody albuminous urine, sometimes containing tube-casts, is excreted.

The increased consumption of water has already been alluded to. Certainly the large quantities taken cannot be retained in the system; neither are they eliminated, for the scanty urine, dry skin, and constipation preclude the idea of elimination. What can become of the water unless it is consumed by the organisms or germs in their growth and multiplication?

The increased demand for blood in the tissues, consequent on their increased wants, and those also of the contagia, lead to an increased rapidity of the blood-current through the tissues. Such acceleration of movement in the capillaries tends to hasten the flow through the veins and to more rapid action of the heart. Thus this organ, suffering in common with the rest of the body from the lack of nutritious blood, has, in addition to its rapid action, a feeble one.

It is now generally accepted that the preternatural heat in fever is due to increased consumption of tissues, but the cause of this increased consumption is not told. We have already seen that an increased quantity of blood is sent to the tissues, and that there results from this "a corresponding increase in their retrograde metamorphosis." Thus the "propagation of the contagia becomes the cause of the increased consumption of tissue, which, in its turn, gives rise to the preternatural heat."

Thus does this theory explain the mode of production of

the most important and essential phenomena of the eruptive fevers. But there are other phenomena which occur with more or less regularity in idiopathic fever, whose cause will next be considered. These are:

"The nervous symptoms.

"The typhoid symptoms.

"The mode of death.

"The changes noted after death.

"The treatment."

Under the head of nervous symptoms we have to explain rigors, headache, delirium, convulsions and coma. The vaso-motor system, controlling as it does the muscular elements of the minute arteries, cannot fail to be affected by the increased rapidity of the blood-current and by its depraved condition. Hence, when the multiplication of the contagia has reached a certain point, there is produced a contraction of the capillaries in the efforts of the system to control the circulation, and a sensation of cold results, the effect being the same, though produced within the body, as would occur were a cold substance to be placed in contact with the skin, and the contraction of the capillaries to be brought about in that manner. We find, for the same reason, that headache due to cerebral anæmia, caused by the contraction of the minute arteries of the brain, also results. So, also, "anæmia of the spinal cord causes aching in the back and limbs. Contraction of the minute vessels of the heart and lungs gives rise to feeble pulse and oppressed breathing. . . . And the general result of this general defective supply of blood is that undefined feeling of misery and general malaise, which is one of the earliest indications of commencing illness." Owing to the increasing demand by the tissues for blood the contraction of the bloodvessels gradually gives way, and the opposite condition prevails, and there occurs a sensation of heat in the body, and, in place of the headache, wandering or delirium. The brain symptoms are now due to the mal-nutrition necessitated by the unnutrient blood; and the convulsions and coma, which may supervene, should the attack prove sufficiently grave, are thus due to an exaggeration of the same cause. These conditions may be heightened yet more by the retention in the blood of the excretory products which the kidneys fail to eliminate, these products not being of themselves intrinsically poisonous, but by their interference with tissue respiration, in the same manner that the presence of carbonic acid interferes with lung respiration. The typhoid symptoms appear to be due to a failure of all the vital energies, such as might be consequent on the propagation in the system of such organisms as we have been considering.

The mode of death is either that due to a failure of the cardiac walls, causing asthenia, or to coma, or to both of these causes combined.

The appearances after death are, in the brain, chiefly diminished bulk, such as would naturally arise from impaired nutrition, and, in the heart, softening of the walls, due to degeneration of the muscular fibres. "The fact that the most successful way of treating idiopathic fever consists in supplying the system with nitrogen and water, is an additional argument in favor of this theory, which regards the cause of the fever as something which takes these elements from the tissues; such an agency can only be a living organism."

There now arises a very serious difficulty in regard to this theory. Why do not the germs invariably go on increasing until death occurs? Why does there come at a certain definite period a cessation of the symptoms, followed by recovery? These questions can only be answered by considering the contagia as parasites. Owing to the shortness of the time which can be given for this consideration, only the conclusions drawn from the evidence in hand can be given. As regards local lesions occurring in the eruptive fevers, we have the following summary: "The poisons of the eruptive fevers are specifically distinct. They are almost certainly minute organisms. They are largely reproduced in the system. Such reproduction causes the phenomena of the eruptive fevers. The characteristic local lesions of these fevers form an essential part of the illness. The seat of the local lesion is the locality in which the fever poison is most abundant. These lesions are essentially associated with the development of organisms in the affected tissue.

"Such development bears a direct relation to the activity of the inflammatory process. The organisms are more abundant in the early than in the advanced stages of the inflammation."

As regards the "different degrees of severity of the same form of fever, . . . the view which regards the amount of the second factor as the agency which determines the severity or mildness of a particular seizure is the one which best explains the facts with which we have to deal."

The cessation of the febrile symptoms is not due to the elimination or destruction of the poison which induced them, but results from the exhaustion of that second factor which is requisite to the propagation of the contagium. So "the duration of the febrile symptoms represents the time which the contagium requires to exhaust its second factor. For this purpose the poison of typhus fever requires on an average from twelve to fourteen days; that of typhoid fever an average of from twenty to twenty-two days."

With regard to the crisis, "increased consumption of water is one of the chief phenomena of the febrile state; and its increased elimination is the chief feature of the crisis. In the eruptive fevers the former results from the growth of the contagium; the latter from the sudden cessation of that growth." The exhaustion of susceptibility in those who have suffered from eruptive fevers can be explained by the fact of exhaustion of the second factor, as has been said above.

The different degrees of contagiousness of the eruptive fevers depends on the readiness with which the second factor is reached by the first factor through the circulation.

Relapsing fever is considered last, and in its discussion it is said: "*The occurrence of the characteristic second seizure of relapsing fever is due to the circumstance that the second factor is reproduced in the blood before the first is thoroughly eliminated from it;* its early reproduction leading to the renewed development of such germs as remain, and a consequent second pyrexial attack."

The abrupt ending of this paper has been necessary, owing to the limited time allowed for its reading. I have endeavored to give an idea of Dr. Maclagan's theory, but the limits of this article preclude any extended review of the work. In its preparation I have quoted freely from the author, and it will be understood that all the views I have here presented are those of Dr. Maclagan.

VIOLA TRICOLOR OR JACEA IN THE TREATMENT OF ECZEMA INFANTILE.

BY W. H. BIGLER, M.D.,
PHILADELPHIA, PA.

(Read before the Philadelphia County Homœopathic Medical Society)

THE object of the following short paper is to draw attention to a remedy in the treatment of that sometimes troublesome disease, *crusta lactea*, which, to judge from our literature, has not been so frequently employed, nor indeed so generally known as its antiquity and its real virtues deserve,—the *Viola tricolor* or *Herba jaceæ*.

According to Porta it was known to the Greeks and Romans under the name of *Phlox*. Eminent physicians employed it in the treatment of various diseases with occasional success, and cures of asthma, epilepsy, and uterine complaints have been reported from its use; but it was regarded as specially and specifically applicable to chronic and obstinate cutaneous diseases (Matthiolus's *Comment. on Diosc.*, p. 822; Fuchsius's *Hist. Stirp.*, p. 804).

In the *New London Dispensatory* (Salmon, 1684) the following notice of *Jacea* occurs: "Silver knapweed; it is called Flaming violet also. Schroder saith it is bitterish and sharp; cleanses, pierces, and discusses; it (is a) vulnerary and sudorific; takes away clammy humors, and opens obstructions of the womb; outwardly it is cosmetic, and cures scabs, itch, etc."

But as has happened with so many other, and perhaps better remedies, its use was gradually abandoned, until towards the close of the last century *Strack*, of Mentz, sought to restore it in his *Dissertation on Crusta lactea and its Remedy* (1779). He prescribes as specific one handful of the fresh, or one-half drachm of dried leaves, to be bruised in half a pint of milk, and the whole to be taken night and morning. He says that in the first week the eruption seems to increase, and to appear in other parts of the body, but that at the same time the urine acquires a smell as of cat's urine, and at the end of a fortnight the crusts begin to fall off, and sound, healthy skin appears beneath. When the urine does not acquire this odor, but remains unchanged, he says the disease will generally be of long continuance (*London Medical Journal*, vol. ii, p. 487). Some years later his observations were confirmed by Hasse (*Diss. de Viola Tricolor*, Erlangen, 1782) and by others (Melzer, Veckrskrift, and Murray). (*Apparatus Medic.*, vol. vi, p. 33.)

Although there were some who denied the specific virtues of the herb (Mursinna, Achermann, Hemmig, *et al.*), or even (Selle) maintained that it was injurious, the majority of physicians believed that it acted on the intestinal functions as a cathartic, that it sometimes produced emesis, and that, besides increasing the flow of urine, it imparted to it a disagreeable odor like that of cat's urine, that therefore it was by no means inert, but a valuable medicine.

We find it successfully employed by *Hasse* and others in *crusta lactea with violent cough and dyspnœa*, in *impetigo of hairy scalp and face*, in *acne rosacea*, in *favus*, in *serpiginous crusts in children and adults*, in swelling and indurations of cervical glands, in *large boils* all over the body in scrofulous children, in *pustulous and ichorous exanthems* of the feet, in *squamous spots* in the skin, in *rheumatism and gout*, in *articular rheumatism* with itchlike eruptions around the joints, in an *impetiginous exanthem* on the forehead consequent on suppression of gonorrhœa, and in an induration of the testicles from the same cause, in *ichorous ulcers* with violent itching, in *blennorrhœas* of the various mucous membranes, and in *epilepsy.*

In Russia a decoction of the pansy was a popular remedy for scrofula; and it was used in 1803 by Schlegel, of Moscow, with good effect in syphilitic affections, especially venereal ulcers (Sammlg., 3, pp. 141–156; *Frank's Mag., f. A. & T.*, vol. iii, p. 655).

In 1813 Fauvergne claimed to have cured with Viola, nervous paroxysms in a young girl, which he thought had been caused by suppression of crusta lactea.

Finally, we find reference to the Herba jaceæ and its several preparations, decoctions, infusions, syrups, and unguents in the various pharmacopœias of Europe, and in the *United States Dispensatory* (Wood and Bache).

During the annual meeting of the American Dermatological Association, held in New York on August 26th, 27th, and 28th, 1879, a paper on Viola tricolor was read by Dr. H. G. Piffard, in which he quoted largely from Cazin, who has experimented considerably with the drug, and used it with success, and from a brief article written by himself in the American edition of Phillips's *Materia Medica and Therapeutics.* He says it has long been a favorite in France in the treatment of *eczema capitis and faciei*, and that he has employed it for many years with great satisfaction in chronic cases of this affection. The watery preparations have appeared to answer better than the alcoholic. He believes it to be of the greatest service in eczema about the upper part of the body, and especially the head; while when the affection was situated on the lower part of the body he has found it to be frequently aggravated by the drug. (*The Medical Record,* vol. xvi, No. 11.)

It was not to be expected that a drug so well known and promising so much would be neglected by Hahnemann, and we find in Stapf's *Archiv* (vol. vii, 2, p. 173) a proving undertaken by him in connection with Franz, Wislicenus, and Gutmann. They used a tincture made of equal parts of the expressed juice of the fresh herb and alcohol. We find here as in the case of so many other of our remedies, that it is not the symptoms obtained by the provers that have given the indications for the use of the remedy, but those obtained *ab usu in morbis*, the clinical symptoms, the much-calumniated empirical usage. After this has directed our attention to certain applications of a remedy, it is not a matter of very great difficulty to read between the lines of the provings justifications for our practice. All the characteristic skin symptoms except an indefinite itching here and there over the whole body, are taken from an allopathic source (Hufeland's *Journal*, xi, iv, p. 128, et seq.), and the keynote, "urine smelling like cats' urine," was not observed by any of the provers, but is altogether clinical (Alshop, in Murray's *Appar. Med.*, i, p. 703 (?) 33 (?), Hufeland, Strack).

In his *Lesser Writings* (p. 328), Hahnemann says of the Viola, "The pansy violet at first increases cutaneous eruptions, and thus shows its power to produce skin diseases, and consequently to cure the same effectually and permanently."

In the succeeding works on Materia Medica the original proving is repeated without additions, and with or without the clinical symptoms according to the principles of the several editors, and even Allen can find no new authorities for his *Encyclopædia*. Teste and Hughes both notice it favorably in their works on Materia Medica. Guernsey, in his *Lectures*, says its principal use is in nocturnal emissions accompanied by very vivid dreams.

In many of the works on therapeutics it is not mentioned at all among the remedies used in crusta lactea, and in others it occupies a very subordinate position. Those who speak most favorably of it are Hartman (*Therapeutics*, vol. ii, p. 39) and Hughes. The latter says that he very seldom has occasion to use any other remedy. He generally uses the 1st or 2d dilution, but has seen the 6th act well, with which attenuation Dudgeon also reports a case of cure in the *British Journal of Homœopathy*, xi, 355.

Lilienthal, in his *Therapeutics*, says under Eczema: "*Viola tric.—Milk-crust, burning and itching, especially in the night, with discharge of tough yellow pus; heat and perspiration of the face after eating.*" And in his *Skin Diseases*, "*Jacea.— Violent itching eruption, worse every night, and urine smelling like cats' urine.*" Why he has used the unhomœopathic name Jacea in this latter place I cannot understand.

I have been in the habit of using the Viola for the last 12 years, and have recommended it to many of my colleagues in the treatment of the eczema of children, and in the majority of cases its use has been attended with gratifying success. I candidly confess, however, that I am unable to give any so-called *characteristic* symptoms or keynotes, the presence of which would invariably and unmistakably point to the applicability of this herb, but the following general indications may prove as useful to others as they do to myself. We may expect the best results from the employment of Viola where the eruption is acute, and is confined principally to the face, although its extension to the scalp is no counter-indication. In eczema of the whole body I have not found it produce any good results, but others may have been more fortunate. The tendency of the disease is always rapidly to the pustular form. The crusts are of a brownish-yellow color, and the eruption is very itchy in all its stages, but the itching seems to be temporarily relieved by rubbing. The general condition of the child seems to be one of perfect health, with the exception, perhaps, of a rather thin white discharge from the nose, and may be a loose catarrhal cough. The remedy very soon produces a profuse flow of urine, but never have I had a case where either before, during, or after the administration of the medicine I could detect the characteristic smell of cats' urine. I usually have about ℥j of the dried herb (the imported, for the market is full of inferior qualities) boiled in half a pint of water, and of this tea prescribe f℥j two, three, or four times a day in milk slightly sweetened. If the patient is a child at the breast, I order the mother to drink rather larger quantities of the tea morning and evening, while the child takes nothing, and I have found this to work as well as where I, in addition, prescribed Viola^{30} for the child. Frequently, in alternation with the tea, I have given the first or second decimal dilutions twice a day, or the thirtieth, but have not been able to discover any marked difference in the course of the disease produced thereby. I have also used the various dilutions without the tea, but the effects have not been so marked, nor any more permanent. Sometimes, in aggravated cases, I have derived benefit from the external use of the tea, together with internal medication. In short, I have allowed myself considerable latitude in the mode of administration of this drug, and have every reason to be satisfied with its action. Medicinal aggravations I have observed in some few cases, but they are speedily followed by improvement and cure. Usually by the end of the first week, sometimes by the third day, a decided improvement is visible, and at the end of two or three weeks the cure is complete. If others will try this drug, not waiting for the urine smelling like cats' urine, I have no doubt they will be convinced as I am of the almost specific action of Viola tricolor in the treatment of crusta lactea.

TYPHO-MALARIAL FEVER.

BY W. C. GOODNO, M D,
PHILADELPHIA, PA.

(Read before the Philadelphia County Homœopathic Medical Society)

ALL still remember that the pleasures of the Centennial year were seriously marred by a prevailing fever of a continued type, confined chiefly to the Twenty-fourth Ward, West Philadelphia, in which was located the Centennial buildings. Much consternation was created among visitors, and many persons were deterred from visiting our magnificent exhibition by reason of it. Conflicting opinions have been expressed concerning its character and causation. Nosology has been seriously drawn upon, it having been believed to be one or the other of most of the low forms of fever. I shall endeavor to show in this paper, which is drawn from an analysis of forty-eight cases, treated during the year 1876, that the disease was essentially that known in some regions as typho-malarial fever. I hesitate somewhat in my use of this term, remembering that so distinguished an authority as Professor Stillé taught, in 1876 and 1877, that it was a misnomer—that the disease so called was not the effect of the union of the respective poisons of typhoid and malarial fevers, but was a *distinct and separate affection.* The facts that the epidemic in question was developed under conditions *peculiarly* favorable to the development of both typhoid and malarial fevers—that cases in their early stage presented all the conclusive symptoms of typhoid fever, in their later development manifested just as positively all the characteristics of malarial fever, and *vice versa*—that many cases presented many of the leading symptoms of each *simultaneously*—are the principal reasons for assuming, as I do, that there is a disease embodying the elements and manifesting the symptoms of typhoid and malarial fever, which is best expressed as typho-malarial or malario-typhoid, according as either element predominates.

Early in the spring of 1876 an unusual number of cases of typhoid and intermittent occurred. (We usually see but few cases each season.) These were marked by more or less irregularity in type. The temperature-sheet indicated unusual elevations and depressions, and the typhoid cases did not present that regularity in rise and fall which is so characteristic. With each month the number of cases increased, also their irregularity and violence, until the height of the epidemic was reached in the latter part of August and the earlier part of September. Owing to causes I shall mention later, the malignancy manifested in certain districts far exceeded that in others. In one neighborhood the characteristics of typhoid fever were more especially manifest, in another of malaria, and in still others a more thorough combination existed; and I may say that all cases that I have seen since, as late as the fall of 1877, exhibited this same irregularity of type. Not one case of typhoid in which the temperature characteristics, so accurately described by Wunderlich, have been present in their perfectness.

I have, at time of writing, a case, a woman of nineteen years, who, after a period of malaise and wretchedness, was attacked with headache, slight chills several days in succession, followed by fever and sweat. When called, I found her (on first day) with an evening temperature of 105°; no delirium; general abdominal tenderness, most marked in right iliac region, with gurgling and diarrhœa, and commencing eruption. In order to curtail the length of this paper I shall confine my attention to certain points of interest which I think merit notice.

The Temperature.—There was noted (1) a sudden elevation, the first thermometric observation, on the first or second day, indicating 102° to 104°, and in one instance 105°; (2) the absence of the characteristic change occurring from morning to evening, many cases lacking it entirely, others preserving it for a day or two, then departing, to again return. These digressions were marked by complicating symptoms, viz.: neuralgic pains located in the hand, leg, head, etc. In cases presenting more or less completely the symptoms of typhoid fever, the amount of "abnormal variation" of temperature, using this term as Rilliet and Barthez do as applied to disease, was apparently in proportion to the intensity of symptoms appearing at the time, of a malarial character.

Heart and Pulse.—In several cases the heart symptoms were notable; twice I found mitral regurgitation; in both cases a loud blowing murmur, systolic and apical; one died; the other (referred to later) only began to walk after lying in bed one year, most of the time in torturing agony, the evidence of insufficiency existing for about three months. These cases are unusual. Flint states that a "mitral systolic murmur is rarely, *if ever*, due to an abnormal condition of the blood, without any anatomical change in the valves or endocardial membrane."

Cases of regurgitation of this character, however, have been reported by Dr. Sansom, of London, and M. Hayem, of Paris.

In three cases the whole force of the disease was apparently spent upon the heart. The following case will illustrate:

Mrs. R., æt. forty-six, was taken sick upon the 15th of June. Complained only of weakness. I did not at the time examine her heart or pulse; thought there was very little the matter. Was called again five days later; found her still upon her feet, but complaining of increased debility. There was loss of appetite; tongue tremulous, dry, and furred; headache; constipation; temperature 101°, A.M.; 102.5°, P.M.; and following quite closely the typhoid type, as I learned during the next few days; pulse, 160, small and weak; heart's impulse scarcely felt. Gradual improvement occurred in the general symptoms, the patient remaining recumbent for three weeks; but four months elapsed before the pulse was reduced below 100 per minute, the patient remaining debilitated and suffering from irritable heart. There were no indications of valvular disease, and the heart occupied its normal position. The rapid, feeble heart-action accompanying such mild general symptoms is quite notable, and due probably to the action of the poison upon the upper portion of the spinal cord, and thus affecting the heart through the spinal accelerators.

Digestive Apparatus.—The digestive apparatus presented, in addition to the usual array of symptoms noted in cases of continued fever, violent pain upon the accession of the disease, or, later, in connection with bowel symptoms. One case gave all evidence of neuralgia of the solar plexus; another, upon the first day of the disease, was attacked with agonizing pain extending all over the abdomen, rather paroxysmal, and having the characteristics of neuralgia; there were no bowel symptoms of any character, and constipation prevailed throughout; they were relieved promptly by *Nux vom.*, these cases running a comparatively mild course. I will say that one of these cases was a man employed in the Photographic Building (Centennial), where sanitary care was entirely ignored. He had been unwell for days, but still attended to his business; I consequently had him under observation. Upon the first day of the disease his temperature was $105\frac{1}{5}$°, pulse 120. This case illustrates the characteristic rise in temperature which was observed in most cases presenting marked *malarial* symptoms. The bowel symptoms were essentially those of typhoid fever. One case only of severe intestinal hæmorrhage occurred. Miss P., æt. 20 years, was taken sick June 10th. It was a thoroughly mixed case, her temperature being rather high at the end of the first week (104°), reaching it by the characteristic typhoid rise. The prostration was not extreme, and I had difficulty in keeping her in bed. In the second week (twelfth day) she was seized with severe aching pain in the left shoulder; nothing was to be seen upon inspection. It was very obstinate, many remedies failing to help. The pain, however, gradually moved downward until it reached the hand and wrist. The pain was very great, causing constant suffering and wakefulness. During this period the temperature rose to 105°, and lost the typhoid character. There was very annoying soreness of the mouth, ulcers of considerable size appearing in the mouth and throat; tongue dry, brown and cracked; slight delirium and pain in the abdomen, which was somewhat swollen and tender. On the seventeenth day, after looseness of a week's duration, following imprudent getting up and eating, bloody stools appeared. The amount of blood passed the first few days was not large; it increased, however, and on the fourth day there was a profuse stool consisting almost entirely of blood, black, partly coagulated, and offensive. Six profuse hæmorrhages occurred upon this day and night. The temperature dropped; respiration hurried; surface circulation poor; skin cool; pulse weak and 140; look of anxiety in face; patient presenting all the symptoms due to profuse hæmorrhage. Dr. Raue, in consultation, prescribed Hamamelis^{200}, principally on the appearance of the blood and a *bruised, sore* feeling felt in the abdomen and hips, which appeared with the bloody passages. The symptoms were promptly relieved, no severe hæmorrhage occurring after the first dose.

Several cases of a more decidedly malarial type had frequent stools, containing small quantities of blood in spots and small clots, somewhat as in inflammatory diarrhœa of children, only darker; these lacked the iliac symptoms of typhoid fever. The blood was frequently in small black clots of considerable density, the balance of the stool being made up of fecal matter, a little bright blood, and watery fluid thoroughly stained by dark or black blood.

Cerebro-spinal System.—In some the whole "brunt of the battle" seemed to be borne by the spinal cord, particularly the *posterior columns*. F. G., æt. 17, taken in June, was not able to walk a year later. Nothing of note occurred until the beginning of the third week, when he complained of pain in the thighs, the slightest movements being attended by excruciating pains. These pains continued, but gradually decreased in severity, so that a year later he could bear his weight upon his feet with crutches. Marked tenderness of the lower dorsal and lumbar vertebræ existed during the violence of the pains, and it seems probable that there was an affection of the sensitive columns of the cord, producing excentric pains, just as we find in cases of spinal anæmia in women. I am inclined to hold the same opinion in regard to the neuralgiæ which appeared in many cases; also with the heart symptoms and attacks of pain in the abdomen; these pains continued in some instances after the patient commenced to gain flesh and look quite healthy, with a normal temperature and pulse.

It is always interesting to trace out the causes of epidemics, and it has been particularly so to me in the epidemic in question, for we have exemplified in an unusual manner the part which both the patient and the essential exciting causes play. We see the patient prepared by fatigue, mental and physical, by habits of life detrimental to physical vigor, made susceptible to the operation of certain disease-producing germs originating without the body, the result, mostly, of man's filth and neglect of proper sanitary precautions. For we must not forget that it requires fertile soil as well as good seed,—this is a matter of common observation with us all in watching the march of any epidemic in our midst. The most perfect disease germs, unless supplied with proper pabulum, cannot live and multiply in the organism, or give rise to their specific forms of disease. Our inhabitants who suffered were *largely* hard-working people, who had spent considerable time, energy, and money preparing for boarders and friends, and in their entertainment their vital energies were severely taxed, and they were mostly in a state of physical and nervous exhaustion, susceptible therefore to the effects of any exciting cause of disease. The visitors were people who had worked diligently and late, earning money and getting business affairs into proper condition for absence. Many came from malarious districts, and most were fatigued by long travel; they were careless in diet, and too many hours were spent at the grounds before sufficient rest had been obtained. There was a feverish nervous excitement manifested by all: by the hosts in the hope of gain; by the guests, as a result of the physical prostration and unnatural excitement attending the visiting of such an exhibition as the Centennial entailed. Another element of importance was overcrowding. In many four and five room houses, as many as six or eight persons were lodged in addition to the family.

The erection of the Centennial buildings necessitated the digging up of immense areas of soil, as well as the opening and grading of many streets, leading to the grounds. The turning up to the sun's intense rays of such an amount of soil laden with the products of decaying vegetation alone, was sufficient to transform this usually healthy location. Added to this, the streets of the Twenty-fourth Ward in this immediate neighborhood were loaded with filth, the gutters of Merion Avenue, Paschal and Pear streets, etc., were filled with green filth. Many slaughter-houses are in this neighborhood, their refuse being largely removed by surface drainage. The grading being often imperfect the gutters were kept filled with blood and filth of a most disgusting character. This being a newer portion of the city, the conveniences of water-closets and hydrant-water were not fully enjoyed, many (in fact, nearly all) still using outdoor privies dug out of the soil, and imperfectly bricked and cemented or not at all. In one square where thirteen cases occurred almost simultaneously there was an old privy, full to the brim, the more liquid portion of the contents flowing across the owner's lot and upon adjoining property. Many wells were in the immediate neighborhood, furnishing water for all purposes to the inhabitants (the cases in this locality were more markedly typhoid in character).

The subject of the causation of fevers of this character has attracted much attention from scientific physicians and scientists generally during the last thirty years—ever since Sir William Jenner, in 1849, published his masterly discrimination of enteric fever. The impetus given to the subject by him has gained power by the successive studies of such men as Drs. Budd and Murchison, and they have all tended with unusual uniformity to connect it in its origin with excremental filth.

INTERMITTENT FEVER, ILLUSTRATED BY CLINICAL CASES.*

BY W. K. INGERSOLL, M.D., AND C. F. GOODNO, M.D.,

PHILADELPHIA.

(Read by title before the Philadelphia County Homœopathic Medical Society.)

CASE 1.—*May 22d*, 1878. Mrs. M. S., aged 44. Chills and fever ever since last fall. They come at different times in

---

* Cases 1 to 16 treated by Dr. Ingersoll; Cases 17 to 23 treated by Dr. Goodno.

the day. "Feeling bad all over." No appetite. No sleep at night; sleepy all day. Cough worse at night; expectoration of bloody transparent phlegm. Hands and feet cold all the time. *Arsen.*^{200}. No more chills.

CASE 2.—*July 5th*, 1878. G. C., æt. 13. Has a chill every other day in afternoon, followed by heat, with headache, aggravated by moving; coughs during chill; appetite poor. *Angustura*^{200}.

July 14th. Much better in every way. *Sac. lac.*

July 18th, Sunday. Had chill at 4.30 P.M. Sweats a great deal. *Lycop.*^{200}.

July 26th. No chill. Sac. lac.

August 2d. No chill. Sac. lac.

CASE 3.—*September 2d*, 1878. W. S., æt. 6 years. Chill at half-past 11 in morning (every other day), not well-marked. Has heat lasting three or four hours. Diarrhœa; stools very dark-colored. Drinks a great deal of water, but little at a time. *Arsen.*^{200}.

September 9th. Had no chill until yesterday at 10 A.M. *Natrum mur.*^{200}.

Chills ceased.

CASE 4.—*September 2d*, 1878. M. S. (sister to the above), æt. 2 years. About the same symptoms as the boy. Chill at 10 A.M. *Nat. mur.*^{200}.

September 9th. No further chills.

CASE 5.—*September 2d*, 1878. Ellen S., æt. 2, sister to the two preceding. Dumb ague, heat well marked. Other symptoms same as in the other two children. *Arsen.*^{200}.

September 9th. Chill yesterday at 11 A.M. *Natrum mur.*^{200}. No more chills.

CASE 6.—*September 2d*, 1878. P. A. D., æt. 1 month. Mother had intermittent fever before, and after birth of the child. "Baby has a chill every other day," commences at 7 A.M., and lasts one to two hours. Heat until noon. Diarrhœa; dark-green, slimy, stringy stools, most frequent in the afternoon, and smelling like decayed meat. Starts in sleep. *Podophyl.*^{200}.

September 6th. Not any better. *Elaterium*^{200}, 3 doses.

May 14th, 1879. Had no more chills and became perfectly well.

CASE 7.—*September 9th*, 1878. Mrs. S., æt. 36. Chills came on a few days ago. 10 o'clock, chill, thirst, and headache. During chill, fever and sweat. *Natrum mur.*^{200} cured.

Case 8.—*September* 17*th*, 1878. Katie, O. F., æt. 10. Intermittent fever. Symptoms poorly defined. *Arsen.*

September 19*th*. Chill about 5 A.M. Great thirst; offensive sweat. *Conium*^{200}.

September 30*th*. Chill every day for past four days. They come at different hours in the day. Chill to-day, 4 P.M. Before chill feels a soreness around the heart; thirst. Chill begins in the neck; legs feel stiff during chill. Much thirst during heat. *Lycop.*^{200}, 3 doses.

October 2*d*. Yesterday no chill, but slight symptoms of the attack. Chill to-day about 2.30 P.M. Seems now to feel better during the apyrexia. Lycop.^{200}.

October 4*th*. Chill to-day at 1 P.M. Pain in head, body, and legs during chill, although it is light. During heat, thirst, headache, short breathing. Is flighty during sleep. Sweat not prominent. *Cactus*^{200}, dose every night.

October 7*th*. No chill since last medicine. *Cactus*^{200}, dose every night.

Case 9.—*September* 17*th*, 1878. William McN., æt. 20. "Chills for the past week." Chill in the afternoon. Commences with pain at the back of neck, which runs over to forehead. The morning after chill is sick at the stomach, and has diarrhœa; stools small, bad-smelling, and slimy; straining at stool. Tongue coated in centre. *Merc. viv.* 3^{x}, after every stool.

September 19*th*. Diarrhœa cured. Chill at 5.30 P.M. Pains in limbs before chill; fever more severe, lasting three hours. Lycop.^{200}.

September 25*th*. Well.

Case 10.—*June* 16*th*, 1879. Mrs. A. L., æt. 40. Chill every third day at 12 to 1 P.M. Preceding chill, pain in and over the spleen, with thirst; very hard chill, lasting from half to one hour, during which there is thirst and vomiting of ingesta mixed with dark blood. Fever is light (and lasts but two hours), with severe pain in temples, forehead, and top of head, which only passes off by the next day; thirst; sweat light, lasting an hour or so. *Cactus*^{200}, one dose.

June 7*th*. No chill.

June 17*th*. No chill. Pain in left side. Lach.^{200}.

July 3*d*. Has not been so well for a year or more, she says.

July 11*th*. Chill last night at 11 o'clock. Vomiting during chill. *Cactus*^{200}.

No more chills.

Case 11.—*July* 15*th*, 1879. F. M., æt. 6. Chill at 11 A.M. Chill lasts fifteen or twenty minutes; nausea during chill, and continuing all the afternoon. Headache and thirst during chill; heat and sweat. *Natr. mur.* 12ˣ.

July 17*th*. Chill at 11 o'clock again; dry cough preceding chill; great thirst, and very severe headache, going off at night, with sweat; no appetite; marked jaundice. *Hydrastis* 0.

September 1*st*. Not another chill.

CASE 12.—This case we omit.—EDS.

CASE 13.—*September* 8*th*, 1879. Al. McC., aged 3. Chills poorly defined; very fretful. Face yellow. Chill always in morning. *Hydrastis* 0.

September 11*th*. Cured.

CASE 14.—*September* 12*th*, 1879. Mary M., white, aged 5. Has had chills every other day for a month. Headache and pain in the back before chills; chill usually in the morning; pains in limbs during chills. Face cyanotic during chills. Great thirst. *Natrum mur.* 12ˣ.

September 15*th*. No chill. *Natr. mur.* 12ˣ.

September 22*d*. No chill.

CASE 15.—*September* 30*th*, 1879. Samuel ——, white, aged 10. Has had chills and fever, treated by an old-school physician. The boy has had a bad headache, and some days slight chill at 2 o'clock P.M. *Eupatorium perf.* 200.

October 7*th*. No more chills.

CASE 16.—*October* 20*th*, 1879. J. S., white, aged 9. Chills every other day for two months. Chill at 11 to 12 o'clock A.M., and lasts one hour. Commences with dizziness, headache, and pain in limbs, then chill is felt in and between the shoulders, spreading from there into the limbs; is very thirsty during and before chill. Heat lasts all the afternoon. Sweat in evening not very great. *Eupatorium perf.* 0.

No more chill.

CASE 17.—Charles B., aged 34 years. During the year 1878, while living in Brazil, S. A., he contracted intermittent fever, from which he suffered for the space of several months. According to custom he took large doses of Quinine, which would sometimes prevent an attack and sometimes would not. At last, nearly worn out by the disease, he came back to Philadelphia in the fall, and presented the following symptoms:

Tertian type of fever occurring at 12 M.

Chill: Violent; thirst; gaping; pain in head and bones.

Heat: Thirst; vomiting of bile; wants to be covered; pain in back, head, and limbs.

Sweat: Thirst; vomiting; pain in head and bones.

Apyrexia: Stiffness in joints. *Eupat. perf.* 2c.

Had no chill until the next March, when he had a light one. *Eupator perf.*^{2c}. One dose *cured.*

CASE 18.—Maggie M., aged 15 years. Chills—tertian—from 11 A.M. to 2 P.M.

During chill: Thirst for acids; pain in stomach, back, and head; smothering sensation in throat as if from smoke; nausea; eyes weak; fingers and toes get very cold. Coldness in abdomen.

During heat: Pains in head, arms, legs, body, and stomach; nausea; vomiting, especially after drinking; eyes weak; flighty; dyspnœa; restlessness.

Sweat: Cold sweat; pains all over when sweating; nausea; sleepy, but cannot sleep; eyes feel heavy.

Apyrexia: Nausea; very weak; eyes weak; very irritable; when drinking sensation as if nothing would touch the left side of throat; menses have ceased; nasal catarrh; blisters on lips; feels better from sitting up. *Arsen.*^{200} *cured.*

CASE 19.—Mrs. Kate M., white, aged 27 years. Chills—quotidian—11½ A.M., sometimes irregular as to time.

Chill: Nausea; vomiting of bile; pain in stomach, left lung, knees, elbows, and head.

Heat: Pain in head and all through the body; nausea; vomiting of bile; vertigo; dyspnœa.

No sweat.

During whole attack is very restless; thirst, drinking but little at a time; vomiting after drinking even small quantities; very weak. *Arsen.*^{200} *cured.*

CASE 20.—Mrs. Mary D., aged 41 years. Chill 12 M. every third or fourth day.

During chill: Thirst; headache; vomiting; cramps in calves.

During heat: Thirst; headache; pains in limbs; nausea and vomiting.

During sweat, which is profuse, the headache becomes less severe. *Eupat. perf. cured.*

CASE 21.—J. A. D., aged 45 years. Tertian type, occurring from 12 to 3 P.M.

Chill: Pain in legs and head.

Heat: Severe; pain in head and legs; sometimes vomits.

Sweat: Thirst; pain in head and legs. *Eupator. perf. cured.*

CASE 22.—*September* 30*th*, 1878. John H., aged 25 years. Quotidian type, occurring from 4.45 to 6.30 P.M.

Chill: Half an hour before chill the calves of legs get cold; chill lasts 1½ hours; headache; nausea.

Heat: Not severe; light sensation about heart; stomach feels sore; slight dyspnœa.

Sweat: Not prominent; thirsty.

Much belching throughout; when he takes a long breath he has a pain in the left hypochondrium; urine very red. *Lycop.*^{200} *cured.*

CASE 23.—Dr. W., dentist, aged 42 years. Quotidian type, occurring from 1 to 3 P.M.

Before the attack: Tearing cough; oppression on the chest; numbness in fingers and toes; trembling of limbs.

During chill: Nausea; sometimes vomiting; passes much red urine.

During heat: Thirst; delirium, and at times stupor; pain in head.

During sweat: Some thirst; pain in head; delirium.

Apyrexia: Depression; bitter taste; craves fruit. *Natr. mur.*^{200} *cured.*

THE PHILADELPHIA COUNTY HOMŒOPATHIC MEDICAL SOCIETY.

REPORTED BY CHARLES MOHR, M D., SECRETARY.

THIS society has recently adopted the "bureau method" of organizing its members for active work, with a prospect of adding greatly to the interest and profit of its meetings. At the monthly meeting, held December 11th, 1879, the President, Dr. E. A. Farrington, occupied the chair, and there was a large attendance of members. Several interesting papers, all of which will be found in the present number of the MONTHLY, were offered, and their reading was followed by discussion.

Dr. Charles Mohr had been himself troubled with rough, fawn-colored "liver-spots," the scales coming off under friction and leaving a denuded surface. He had at first attributed them to the excessive use of coffee. Baths, Turkish and Russian included, failed to benefit him. Recently he had a violent attack of cholera morbus, with 25 or 30 passages in 24 hours. Dr. Farrington prescribed Colchicum^{30} for it, and there has been no appearance of the liver-spots since, notwithstanding a continuance of the use of coffee.

He (Dr. M.) thought that Dr. Bigler in his paper on Viola tricolor, had made the mistake of saying that that drug is not mentioned as "*Jacea*" in our literature. It is so mentioned in Hering's *Condensed Materia Medica*, in Guernsey's *Obstetrics*, and in Bœnninghausen's *Repertory*. As to the causes of malarial disorders he wished to call attention to a view of Mr. Mahan, the distinguished botanist, that during a long drought the earth's surface becomes cracked and fissured, and these probably are filled with noxious gases from decomposition of vegetable matter, the gases being expelled when the fissures are filled with water by the first rains.

Dr. J. C. Guernsey corroborated the statement of Dr. Bigler's paper on the use of Viola in nocturnal emissions accompanied by vivid dreams; the symptoms following being that the patient feels "played-out," mad, and disgusted with himself. For the liver-spots, Sepia is indicated very often, and in such cases always acts nicely. In regard to the violent pains mentioned in Dr. Goodno's paper, he had recently learned from Dr. Lippe that when the violent pains of typhoid or typho-malarial fevers occurred, particularly in the thighs, *Taraxacum* is almost a specific. He was sorry to hear local applications recommended, such as Carbolic acid, Sulphur, Corrosive sublimate, etc., and could not see how we can consider as local the diseases mentioned in the papers. There must be a predisposition in order to allow a person to contract even an infectious malady, and that can come only from internal derangement of the vital forces.

Dr. H. Noah Martin defended the ground taken by Dr. Williamson's paper, and held that external applications should be resorted to for the purpose of destroying parasites.

The President, Dr. Farrington, asked for an expression relative to the statement in Dr. Williamson's paper that a parasitic disease cannot be suppressed.

Dr. Korndœrfer alluded to a case of vegetable parasitic disease of the scalp, which had been treated locally with Cantharides, and was thought to be cured. Three months afterwards the patient was brought to him for treatment, for a violent functional disorder of the heart. A careful examination revealing no organic disease, he attributed the disorder to the suppression of the cutaneous affection. His remedy relieved the heart symptoms, and the skin disease returned. As to the *cimex* and the *pediculus*, he thought they should scarcely be regarded, pathologically speaking, as true parasites. The *acarus scabiei* will not propagate itself in certain persons. The experiment has been tried over and over again. When that Corsican discovered the itch mite, he thought homœopathy was destroyed. He forgot that "*second* factor" that Dr. Norton's paper describes. It is against this second factor that our remedies must be directed.

Dr. M. S. Williamson did not wish to be understood as saying that no form of skin disease can be suppressed. There can be no doubt that serious illness frequently results from their suppression. Very frequently, through an error of diagnosis, local measures are resorted to in non-parasitic diseases, and serious harm may follow. The case referred to by Dr. Korndœrfer was, most probably, an eczema. As to the liver-spots, we often hear of persons affected with them being treated for disease of the liver. The discoloration caused by liver disorder is jaundice and not liver-spots. He would say as regards these latter that Sepia, even when apparently indicated, had not been to him a very satisfactory remedy.

Dr. C. E. Toothaker reported a case of crusta lactea of 3 years' standing, in a child 4 years old. The hair was off, the scab dry, of a light-cream color, and without discharge. Had been under allopathic hands for about six months. Viola tricolor[12] cured it in three weeks. Since that (his first case of crusta lactea,) he has had to prescribe the same remedy for 5 or 6 similar cases. When the eruption begins in small spots which spread and involve the whole surface, with a watery discharge from under the scabs, he did not think he had ever failed with Cantharides. But in that form which Dr. Bigler's paper describes, Viola cures promptly. Another form requires Dulcamara; still another Hepar, and some cases may present indications for Rhus tox., etc.

Dr. J. C. Morgan said that with liver derangements we certainly can have discolorations of the skin; he also reminded the Society of the formation of pigmentary matter by the spleen, and the probability of derangements of its function causing cutaneous discolorations. Mosler says intermittent fever is infectious, while H. C. Wood says there is no germ to account for it. McCall Anderson says there must be a constitutional peculiarity producing a soil for the development of parasites; (the simple fact that even mosquitoes will not trouble certain persons is well known). As a rule parasites will not remain and propagate in an unsuitable soil. He cautioned members against the danger of confounding phtheiriasis with eczema, especially when located back of the head. He believes Cocculus indicus to be the best application for the destruction of lice, fleas, and noxious insects generally. Again, Tinea decalvans must not be confounded with alopecia areata, which is non-parasitic. The distinction between parasitic and non-parasitic diseases can be safely determined by the practitioner in many cases, only by the use of the microscope.

Dr. E. B. Nash, of Cortland, N. Y., President-elect of the

Central Society of New York State, was present, and by invitation participated in the discussion. He said that in our *Therapeutics* he always felt that we must accept the causes of disease with much caution. The allopathist (in treating diphtheria for instance), thrusts the patient out of mind, and endeavors to treat the cause. His own experience in that disease had been, that the indicated internal remedy is alone useful. He recalled an epidemic of malignant diphtheria in Geneva, N. Y., where he was called to see a case in consultation with an old practitioner, who had been using the fashionable remedy, Salicylic acid, to destroy the bacteria. That physician had, hitherto, lost every case. This patient exhibited an aggravated type of symptoms, pointing conclusively to Apis mel. This was given with prompt effect, followed by a recovery. Apis was found also to suit the *genus epidemicus*, and cured every case to which it was properly applied. "Let the bacteria alone, and treat the patient."

INTEMPERANCE IN STUDY.—In an interesting article recently read before the Psychological section of the British Medical Association on the general subject of mental overwork and its effects, the author, D. Hack Tuke, F.R C.P., thus expresses himself in reference to *the present system of medical education:*

"How can it be otherwise than injurious, when we consider that during recent years the amount of knowledge which it is necessary to master has prodigiously increased, while the length of time in which to acquire it remains the same?

"In regard to some examinations, a tremendous burden is laid upon the memory. There is a long period of strain, the climax of which is reached when the period of examination arrives, during which the student's mind has to hold in solution the details of knowledge on many subjects. It is often a solution saturated with minute facts and figures, many of which are of no permanent use, and, indeed cannot be remembered any longer. The mind is cramped and narrowed by this mischievous cramming, as must necessarily happen when the issue of an examination is largely to hang upon a retentive memory.

"While no one proposes to go back to the old system of medical education, it may well be doubted whether the character of these examinations is calculated to develop the best practitioners or physicians, loading the memory as they too often do, at the expense of breadth, depth, and originality. Too rapid an acquisition of knowledge—the attempt to master too many subjects—is a part of that Jehu speed at which we are now driving, whether in business or science. Knowledge so gained 'proves but of bad nourishment in the concoction, as it was heedless in the devouring.'"—*Journal of Mental Science.*

THE

HAHNEMANNIAN MONTHLY.

A HOMŒOPATHIC JOURNAL OF

MEDICINE AND SURGERY.

Editors,

E. A. Farrington, M.D. Pemberton Dudley, M.D.

Business Manager,

Bushrod W. James, M.D.

Vol. II. Philadelphia, Pa., January, 1880. No. 1.

☞ The Editors consider themselves responsible for the maintenance of the dignity and courtesy of the journal, but *not* for the opinions expressed by its contributors.

Editorial Department.

SALUTATORY.

The Hahnemannian Monthly has become the property of an organization of homœopathic physicians, known as "The Hahnemann Club of Philadelphia." This organization has included in its membership twelve physicians, one of whom, however, Dr. John G. Houard, is now deceased. The present members are: Drs. R. J. McClatchey, President; W. H. H. Neville, Secretary; A. H. Ashton, Bushrod W. James, C. S. Middleton, M. M. Walker, Aug. Korndœrfer, B. F. Betts, J. E. James, E. A. Farrington, and Pemberton Dudley. Most of these are well known to the general profession, and all of them are engaged in active practice. They represent every variety and shade of homœopathic belief and practice, and yet during the six years of the Club's history the most perfect harmony has been maintained, notwithstanding the most free and fearless expression of opposing opinions at all times.

Besides working for the especial objects of its organization, "the improvement of its members and the advancement of medical science," the Club some three years ago established the "Children's Homœopathic Hospital of Philadelphia." This institution, with accommodations for about twenty patients, is already an assured, permanent success, and under the auspices of its founders has accomplished a vast amount of good, and added largely to the reputation of homœopathy in Philadelphia. Attached to the hospital, and under its management, there is also maintained a flourishing dispensary, in which during the year 1878, according to the last published *Annual Report,* nearly 12,000 cases were treated. Among these were 325 surgical cases, 467 ear and throat cases, and 729 eye, heart, and lung cases, *clinics* for these specialties being held almost daily under the immediate supervision of members of the Club.

This organization has now assumed the proprietorship, and undertaken the publication of the HAHNEMANNIAN MONTHLY, a journal in whose reputation and influence, from its first number to its present issue, the physicians of this city and state have always taken a just pride. Indeed, the long list of distinguished medical men, representing every portion of our country, who have contributed to its pages and helped to build up its reputation, is evidence of a very warm feeling of interest in its success. It is the purpose of its present owners to make it in all respects just what the profession would wish it to be,—a still better exponent of all that is new and useful in the science, art, and literature of medicine, and a still more earnest and powerful advocate and defender of the principles and the interests of homœopathy. To accomplish this will require the aid of the very best scholars, practitioners, and investigators that our profession can produce, and will necessitate on the part of the publishers an unceasing watchfulness and energy to secure the best possible contributions to, and the best mechanical execution of, the work before them. We therefore solicit the members of the homœopathic profession to give us the benefit of their best thought, and the results of their ripest and most carefully recorded experience. This, together with fearless criticism, impartiality, and courtesy, will fill our monthly issues brimful of interesting and instructive matters, rendering the journal indispensable to all its old-time friends; attracting to it an ever-increasing list of new subscribers and contributors; extending and strengthening its influence for homœopathy, and thus securing its highest success.

False Imprisonment in Hospitals for the Insane.—On another page mention is made of the binding over of two reputable allopathic physicians to answer for having falsely certified to the insanity of a gentleman, who, in consequence, was incarcerated in a hospital for three months. We have no opinion to express relative to the merits of the case pending the action of the court. It is well known that physicians are peculiarly liable to baseless accusations, but it is equally patent that the confinement of healthy persons in hospitals for the insane is, in this country, a not very uncommon crime. And the worst feature of the infamous business is, that the guilty parties, by urging almost any sort of shallow pretext for their misdeeds, have usually managed to escape punishment.

The laws of Pennsylvania require that the admission of an insane person to a hospital shall not be granted except upon the sworn certificate of two reputable physicians upon a personal examination of the patient, had within twenty-four hours of the date of the certificate. It must frequently happen that one of these physicians has no personal knowledge of the patient's history, and yet, notwithstanding his liability to err in his diagnosis, it is perfectly right that he should be held to a rigid accountability. But it is not so clear (to any but the judicial mind) why a physician in ordinary practice should be expected to diagnose a case of alleged insanity more accurately upon one or two examinations than a professional expert,—superintendent of a hospital,—after a residence of two or three months in the same house with the supposed patient. Yet, while a physician may be, and ought to be punished for falsely certifying to the insanity of a citizen, it seems that no responsibility whatever attaches to the hospital superintendent for illegally detaining the victim in confinement. Such, at any rate, would seem to be the fact, judging from all the surrounding circumstances of the case to which we have alluded; no criminal prosecution having as yet been instituted against the hospital authorities.

It does not well comport with our American ideas of the inalienable right of all men to personal liberty, that any person, sane or insane, should be consigned to durance vile, against his will, except after a rigid scrutiny of his case, *not* by a couple of physicians, however honest and competent, but by the constituted legal authorities. The whole system of laws and regulations under which patients are sent to and detained in hospitals, needs a careful remodeling.

Our January number has been unavoidably delayed in its issue, because the transfer of the journal was not effected until near the close of December; so late, indeed, that on the morning of the 30th of the month, the newly appointed editors were not in possesion of a single line of manuscript to be used in its publication.

Our February number we expect to issue promptly on time. Through the courtesy of our predecessor, Dr. Winslow, we have received a large amount of excellent matter, besides which, other papers of interest and value are already in hand, and still others are known to be in course of preparation; so that there will be no delay for want of an abundance of choice material.

Among the papers for February we hope to present "A Proving of Nux Moschata," by Dr. E. M. Howard; "Hydronephrosis," by Dr. McCourt; "Natrum Phos. in Goitre," by Dr. Skeels; "Clinical Cases," by Dr. James B. Bell; "The Early Recognition and Early Treatment of Hip-Joint Disease," by Professor J. E. James; some valuable papers from the Chester and Delaware County Society, "Report of a Medical Clinic of Hahnemann College of Philadelphia," by Professor A. Korndœrfer, and other matters of like interest to our readers.

To our Subscribers.—We call the attention of subscribers to the conditions of publication, viz.: that subscriptions are due and payable annually *in advance.* It is the intention of the publishers to spare no exertions that may tend to place the journal on a sound financial basis, such as will enable them to increase its value to its readers, and extend its usefulness as much as possible. For this purpose the Business Manager proposes to advance its business interests in all legitimate ways, by obtaining new subscribers and securing advertisements of a proper character. Our old friends and patrons may greatly assist him in this work by forwarding their own subscriptions promptly and securing additional subscriptions from their professional neighbors. We hope to make the journal worthy of recommendation.

Our Book Department.—It is intended to make this department of the journal a prominent and valuable feature, laying before its readers the excellencies and the defects of recent publications, with a general idea of their scope, and their value to the physician. Some interesting matters of this character will appear in our next number.

Gleanings.

A GLASS of hot milk taken at bedtime will sometimes check nightsweats in phthisis pulmonalis.

ELLIS, in his work on the *Diseases of Children*, says "the *Chinese* race seemed to possess absolute immunity" from diphtheria. What is the experience of our Pacific Coast physicians on this point?

HISTOLOGICAL.—The medical student who proposes to be satisfied with getting through college "by the skin of his teeth"—*cuticula dentis*,—has, according to Frey, a margin of about $\frac{1}{25000}$th part of an inch to play on.

FRAGARIA VESCA.—"The breasts diminished in size, and the secretion of milk ceased."—*Allen*, vol. x, p. 529. Confirmed clinically by C. Mohr, M.D.—(*Trans. Hom. Med. Soc., Penna.*, 1879.)

SPIGELIA IN CHRONIC NASAL CATARRH.—In the *Transactions of the Hom. Med. Soc. of Penna.*, 1879, Dr. Korndœrfer calls attention to the nasal and throat symptoms of Spigelia in Hahnemann's *Materia Medica*, and reports striking cures of nasal catarrh with that remedy.

INFLAMMATORY EFFECTS OF COLOCYNTH.—This drug has been recently shown to possess other than merely neurotic symptoms. Schroff produced a gastro-enteritis with it, and Hughes quotes a case of poisoning, in which there was violent enteric inflammation. The autopsy revealed peritonitis and a gluing together of the intestines. The ovaries may also be inflamed under its continued action.

DIABETES.—M. Lancereaux describes two forms of diabetes, the fat and the lean. The first is insidious, showing itself as obesity between the ages of twenty and thirty. Gradually there appear polydipsia, polyphagia, and polyuria, with slight or intermittent glycosuria. Death occurs either from carbuncle, phlegmon, or gastrorrhagia, rarely from pulmonary consumption. This form is noticed in patients with gouty or calculous heredity. The other form is characterized by rapidly appearing polydipsia, polyuria, and sugar in the urine, progressive loss of flesh, decline of sexual power, continuous course, and comparatively brief duration. Its fatal termination is frequently by phthisis pulmonalis. The etiology is obscure, but in ten cases he found destruction of the pancreas.—*Exc.*

ELATERIUM AND ITS RELATION TO THE HEPATIC SECRETION.—The experiments of Rutherford and Vignal on animals elicited the fact that *Elaterium* is a hydragogue purgative, but it always failed to act, unless there was bile in the intestinal tract. Will this explain its characteristic olive-green diarrhœa? *Croton tiglium*, which is quite similar, does not in the least influence the secretion of bile. *Gamboge* excites purging, but does not stimulate the liver; it is a purely hydragogue cathartic.

Per contra, *Aloes*, *Rheum*, *Jalapa*, PODOPHYLLUM, SENNA, LEPTANDRA, IRIS VERSICOLOR, and Euonymus increase the flow of bile.

QUILLAIA SAPONARIA AND SENEGA contain an identical alkaloid, Saponin. The *Quillaia* has long been in use out West in the incipiency of catarrhs. *Senega* must be similar. The Saponin, which belongs to both, irritates the mucous membrane of the nose, causing sneezing, stuffing up of the nostrils, dull frontal headache. If we carefully examine the provings, as recorded in *Allen*, vol. viii, we shall see that it relaxes the muscular system, causing weariness, soreness in the limbs, tingling, and numbness. This fact may explain why Senega is so useful for fat, relaxed persons. Quillaia ought to be used, like Gelsemium, for catarrhs during the relaxing weather of spring.

Oxalate of Cerium in Whooping-cough.—Dr. Morjé, Physician to the German Hospital in New York, has found in the Oxalate of cerium a remedy, which acts with wonderful rapidity and effect in whooping-cough. It lessens the frequency and intensity of the paroxysms of coughing, allowing the patient to rest better at night, preventing complications, at the same time that its application is simple and easy. He gives but a single dose daily, before breakfast. The dose he regulates according to the age of the child, giving at one year 0 03 (a little less than half a grain), and increasing with every year, until a seven year old child would receive about 0.18 (about 2¾ grains). The remedy should be continued regularly for at least one week, in order to prevent relapse.—*New York Medical Record*, No. 16. (Another specific; how long will it remain in fashion?—Eds.)

Atrophy of the Optic Nerve following Erysipelas Faciei.—In the *Archiv genère de Medic*, Parinand collects six cases of atrophy of the optic nerve following facial erysipelas, and records two new cases, and Pagenstecher a third. In some both eyes were affected, while in others only the one. In none were there any marked brain symptoms. The impairment of vision did not occur until after the disappearance of the erysipelas, but then developed very rapidly, and soon became stationary. In two cases there was a central scotoma, and in a third the field of vision was concentrically narrowed. Parinand thinks that the monocular blindness depended upon an affection of the optic nerve alone, not extending beyond the chiasm, but that the double atrophy was central in its origin.

Toxic Effects of Tea.—From experiments on himself, and from the symptoms gathered from tea-tasters, Dr. W. J. Morton, of New York, gives the following résumé of the effects of tea :

The immediate effects of moderate doses were an elevation of pulse, increase of respiration, agreeable exhilaration of mind and body, a feeling of contentment and placidity, an increase of intellectual and physical vigor, with no noticeable reaction.

The immediate effects of an excessive dose were : rapid elevation of pulse, marked increase of respiration to the extent of about one-third, increase of temperature, no period of exhilaration, but immediate and severe headache ; dimness of vision, ringing in the ears, dulness and confusion of ideas. Following that was a severe reaction : exhaustion of mind and body, tremulousness and "nervousness," and dread of impending harm, that could not be relieved by taking more tea.

The effects of continued doses were a continuance of the tremulousness, extreme susceptibility to outside impressions, diminution of urine, and marked influence (retardation), on the metamorphosis of tissue as shown by the diminution in the amount of urine.

Benzoate of Soda in the Treatment of Tuberculosis.—Although Klebs's view of the specific and infectious character of tuberculosis, based on trials with rabbits, seemed for a time to have been disproved by the experiments of Tappeiner, Lippe, Schweninger, and Schottelius, the much more carefully conducted tests of Max Schüller, of Greifswalde, have proved conclusively that, provided the animals are kept in proper healthy localities, tuberculosis cannot be produced in them by any organic or inorganic substance, unless mingled with or containing some of the tuberculous virus. This virus Klebs finds in certain bacteria (Monas tuberculosum) discovered by himself, and always present when tuberculosis was developed. Schüller found that by causing rabbits, infected with the tuberculous virus, to inhale benzoate of soda, 0.5–1.0 grm. for every kilogram of weight, the development of tuberculosis was prevented. By a human being, therefore, of 60 kilograms weight, provided the circumstances were the same, 30–60 grm. (about ℥j–℥ij) would have to be inhaled daily, but he thought that smaller doses would be found sufficient. He recommended that this required quantity should be inhaled in 2 to 4 portions during the day, for about half an hour at a time. The treatment must be kept up for weeks or for months before abandoning the hope of a cure, which his experiments render probable. Professor Procopius von Rokitansky, following these indications, tried the remedy in his hospital, and from the excellent results obtained, thinks we have found in the benzoate of soda a sovereign antidote to tuberculosis. He records a number of cases of patients who came to the hospital already much reduced, and who, after a short course of the above treatment, were discharged cured. Time and further extended experiments can alone show in how far a useful discovery has been made. Schüller himself warns against raising our expectations too high, and says that by this remedy he has fulfilled only the causal indication in the treatment of the dread disease. In the meanwhile the demand for the drug in Germany can hardly be met, so eager is the medical world to test its virtues.—*Med. Ngk.*, Nos. 45, 46; *Hom. Rosh.*, No. 11.

The Grindelia robusta is recommended as a drug which slows the cardiac and respiratory movements. Its most important uses are said to be in the treatment of respiratory neuroses. Now, this general statement assumes very serious meaning when we read further: Death ensues from paralysis of the muscles of respiration. (Bartholow's *Materia Medica*, pp. 453–4.) A few years ago Dr. Farrington proved this drug. One of the provers complained of difficult breathing; when dropping off to sleep, he would be suddenly aroused, as if his breath was stopping.

Who, in the light of such facts, could hesitate to employ Grindelia in cases of debility with dyspnœa, etc. Clinical confirmations, indeed, are not wanting. Two cures have been reported, one by Dr. Hale and the other by Dr. Egbert Guernsey.

Hahnemann stated that China increased the anxiety caused by Digitalis. Bartholow remarks on page 296 of his *Materia Medica*: "The Cinchona preparations are chemically incompatible with Digitalis."

Apropos of this latter drug, the same author recommends it in renal dropsy because, according to Brunton, Digitalis acts upon the Malpighian tufts of the kidneys. Transferring this fact to our own method of research, we recognize a valuable aid in post-scarlatinal dropsy, with scanty, dark urine, and slow or quick and weak pulse, increased by the least motion.

The Grape Cure.—Hering, in the introduction to his monograph on Typhoid Fever, advises the grapery as serviceable in modifying its progress and severity. Allopathic writers recommend grape-eating in abdominal plethora, engorged liver, chronic catarrhs, skin diseases, and debility during convalescence.

Dr. Bezencenet reports a case of ascites depending upon an enlarged liver, which, after a few weeks' use of the grape cure, fully recovered.

Perhaps it is not too much to assert that grapes have a homœopathic relation to some of the diseases which they have cured.

Take, for example, catarrhs. Now grapes eaten to excess will produce diarrhœa, excoriation of the tongue, emaciation, and an aphthous condition of the whole alimentary canal. Their vegetable acids act somewhat as do the mineral acids, though far less violently.

"Acids," says Dr. Ringer, "act on the salivary glands, gastric glands, etc." Hence he advises acidulated drinks for the dry mouth of fevers—a hint we may consistently adopt. Acid drinks used by dyspeptics, who suffer from sour stomach, should be taken *before* meals, because they lessen the gastric secretion.

News and Comments.

BUREAU OF CLINICAL MEDICINE, AMERICAN INSTITUTE OF HOMŒOPATHY.

THE Bureau of Clinical Medicine has selected as the topic for papers and discussion, at the next annual meeting,—

SCARLATINA.

1. Its History, Etiology, and Varieties, by N. F. Cooke, M.D., Chicago.
2. The Diagnosis and Course of its Varieties, Progress, and Pathology, by Samuel Lilienthal, M.D., New York.
3. Contagious Nature of, Liability to, and Exemption from, as to Age and Previous Attack, by T. F. Pomeroy, M.D., Detroit.
4. Dissimilarity to Diphtheria and to other Cutaneous Diseases, by J. P. Mills, M.D., Chicago.
5. Belladonna and other Prophylactics, and for what Varieties; Influence of Seasons, Climate, etc., by O. P. Baer, M D, Richmond, Ind.
6. Treatment of its Varieties and Symptoms, by A. Lippe, M.D., Philadelphia.

Any member or other physician having anything to communicate under either of these heads will please correspond with the member of the Bureau having it in charge, or with the chairman,

C. PEARSON, M.D.,
608 Twelfth Street, Washington, D C.

CRIMINAL CHARGE AGAINST PHYSICIANS.—Two physicians of Philadelphia have been held to answer the charge of having falsely certified to the insanity of a man, who was in consequence confined in the Pennsylvania Hospital for the Insane (Dr. Kirkbride's) for a period of three months. At the hearing the counsel for the complainant said he had intended to produce a number of reputable physicians to testify as to the sanity of his client at the time of his detention in the hospital, but that he believed the verdict of the commission appointed to inquire into the case was evidence enough of this fact.

The law of Pennsylvania in reference to this offence is as follows;

"If any physician shall falsely certify to the insanity of any person, and it shall appear in evidence that such false certificate was the result of negligence or deficient professional skill on the part of said physician, or that the said physician signed such certificate for a pecuniary reward, or for the promise of a pecuniary reward, or for any other consideration or value whatsoever other than the professional fee usually paid for such services, or in which such false certificate shall tend in any manner, directly or indirectly, to advantage said physician other than relates to said professional fee, then the said physician shall be guilty of a misdemeanor, and, on conviction, be fined not exceeding five hundred dollars, or undergo an imprisonment not exceeding one year, or both, or either (*sic*), at the discretion of the court."

HAHNEMANN MEDICAL COLLEGE OF PHILADELPHIA.—The present term presents the largest class ever assembled during the thirty years of its history. With over two hundred matriculates and seventy-five candidates for graduation, with a thoroughly organized and harmonious body of instructors, with a graded course of study, and practical instruction in most of the branches, the future of the College never looked so bright. The Alumni and other friends of the school may with reason be proud of its present prosperity, and its prospects of still more extended usefulness.

THE NATIONAL BOARD OF HEALTH in its *Bulletin* recommends the formation of volunteer sanitary associations in every town of the country for the purpose of promoting the interest in general sanitary science, and to secure an improved sanitary condition of the locality, and to provide its membership with skilled inspection of their own and neighboring premises, and securing the best sanitary conditions of the same. These citizens sanitary societies are of course entirely independent of the boards of health, either national or local.

W. H. WATSON, M.D., the distinguished homœopathic physician of Utica, New York, has been appointed Surgeon-General of the State. Such an appointment reflects as much honor upon Governor Cornell, who conferred it, as upon its recipient.

THE AMERICAN PUBLIC HEALTH ASSOCIATION, at its annual session, held at Nashville, Tenn., in November, admitted to membership Professors J. P. Dake, M.D., of Nashville, and T. P. Wilson, M.D., of Cincinnati. The latter is President of, and the former, Chairman of the Bureau of Materia Medica in the American Institute of Homœopathy. And this is the same association which, a few years ago, rejected Dr. T. S. Verdi's application for membership, on the ground that he was a homœopathist. Galileo *was* right after all.

DR. CONSTANTINE HERING.—On the evening of January 1st, 1880, Dr. Hering was made the recipient of a visit from a number of his friends, who came to extend their congratulations upon his having that day reached the eightieth anniversary of his birth. They presented him with a congratulatory poem and other tokens of their esteem and friendship, and a most delightful evening was enjoyed by the venerable doctor and his family, as well as by all who participated. The hope that Dr. Hering may yet be permitted to enjoy, in health and strength, very many happy returns of his birthday anniversary will be echoed from thousands of hearts, both lay and professional, wherever the blessings of his beloved homœopathy are known.

DR. L. A. FALLIGANT, of Savannah, Ga., has associated with himself in the practice of medicine and surgery, Dr. E. R. Corson, of New York. We congratulate both.

OBITUARY.

HARRISON V. MILLER, M.D.

DR. HARRISON VAN RENSSELAER MILLER, of Syracuse, N. Y., died at his residence in that city on November 26th, 1879, in the fifty-second year of his age. He retired to rest on Saturday evening, November 22d, in as good health apparently as usual, but during the night he had an apoplectic seizure, with resulting hemiplegia, and, without entirely recovering consciousness, quietly passed to his eternal rest in the early morning of the 26th. About four years ago the doctor had a similar seizure, from which he apparently entirely recovered, and of late appeared to have better health and to be in better spirits than he had ever enjoyed before.

Dr. Miller was born in Apulia, N. Y., on the 17th of September, 1828; received his early education in excellent neighboring academies, and graduated with honor from Hamilton College in 1851. After several years spent in teaching in the West and in California, and a few years spent on a farm in Illinois, he turned his attention to the study of medicine, became the student of Dr. A. R. Morgan, then of Syracuse, and graduated from the New York Homœopathic Medical College in 1862. He practiced for several years in other localities, but finally settled down in Syracuse in 1865, where he remained until his death. He was for three years a partner of Dr. Seward, of Syracuse. Dr. Miller succeeded in building up a large and lucrative practice, was greatly beloved by his *clientele*, and deservedly held in high esteem by his colleagues, compelling even the respect and good opinion of the old-school practitioners of his vicinity. He was an unflinching and uncompromising champion of homœopathy of the Hahnemannic school, and was ever ready, with tongue or pen, to demonstrate or defend it. He was a valued contributor to the HAHNEMANNIAN MONTHLY for several years, and his reports as Secretary, of the papers and discussions of the Central New York Homœopathic Medical Society, as published in this journal from time to time, attracted a great deal of attention, and formed one of the prominent features of the periodical.

Dr. Miller was a member of the American Institute of Homœopathy, of the New York State Homœopathic Medical Society, of the Central New York Homœopathic Medical Society, and of other organizations. He was a genial, kindly, hearty man in all his relations. When the American Institute of Homœopathy met in Philadelphia in 1871 he was the guest of the writer during the session, and his kindly and pleasant ways have been held in agreeable memory ever since. In an obituary notice in the Syracuse *Herald*, the editor writes: "Dr. Miller was the ideal physician. His nature was exceedingly sympathetic and kind, and in every case of illness and suffering his entire nature became as absorbed as though he had a personal share in the griefs of the friends who surrounded the invalid's couch. . . . . His death is a public loss. He was the model physician, the sincere friend, the practical philanthropist, and the model citizen. It will be long before we look upon his like again." Dr. E. B. Nash, of Cortland, N. Y., in a note to the writer, says: "Dr. Miller was, and had been for years my personal friend and counsellor. No terms are adequate to express my estimate of him or my grief at his loss." Doubtless this expression shows the feeling of that coterie of excellent physicians which composed the "Central" Society, and who were his immediate neighbors and intimate friends; and all who knew him will say, we are sure, that he was held in high esteem, both as a physician and as a man. R. J. McC.

AT the quarterly meeting of the Central New York Homœopathic Medical Society, held December 18th, 1879, the following resolutions, offered by Drs. Hawley, Wallace, and Gwynn, Committee on Necrology, were unanimously adopted:

"Since death has taken away our friend, and long-time faithful Secretary, HARRISON V. MILLER, M.D., it is proper that this Society, while it realizes and respects his often-expressed aversion to the usual formalities of commemorating the dead, should put on record its appreciation of his character and services, Therefore,

"*Resolved*, That HARRISON V. MILLER, as our Secretary for the last ten years, has been the life of this Society, and has done more to extend its influence and promote its usefulness than any other member.

"*Resolved*, That as a man, he commanded our respect for his integrity and unflinching obedience to his own convictions; as a student, for his diligence, fidelity, and exactitude; as a physician, for his sympathetic kindness, faithful and cheering attentions, and close prescriptions; and as a member of this Society, for his uniform urbanity, and his enthusiastic disposition to work for all that could extend its influence, or advance the Science of Medicine.

"*Resolved*, That to commemorate our respect for him, this tribute to his character shall be put on our Minutes, and published in the journals of the day.

"*Resolved*, That we tenderly sympathize with his family in their loss, and give expression to such sympathy by sending them a copy of this memento.

"Attest: C. P. JENNINGS,
Secretary."

THE

HAHNEMANNIAN MONTHLY.

Vol. II., New Series. } Philadelphia, February, 1880. No. 2.

Original Department.

NOTES ON MATERIA MEDICA.

BY CLARENCE BARTLETT, M D, PHILADELPHIA, PA.

(Read before the Philadelphia County Homœopathic Medical Society)

To give in the few following notes all that has been done in the past year for the advancement of our Materia Medica is an impossibility. I shall, therefore, mention first a few cured cases confirming symptoms known to have been produced by the curative remedy. Having completed these, I shall then call your attention to the more important provings reported in our journals during 1879.

Dr. Benjamin Simmons reports three cases cured with Hepar selected by the symptom: "Pain in the eyeballs, which feel as if they would be drawn back into the head."—*Organon*, vol. ii, No. 1. Dr. Farrington records the cure of almost the same symptom with Paris quadrifolia; the symptom in the Materia Medica under Paris reading: "Sensation as if a string were tightly drawn through the eyeball and backwards into the middle of the brain."—*Hahnemannian Monthly*, vol. i, No. 1.

Professor Farrington also reports the following cases:

Manganum Aceticum.—Deep cough without expectoration, ceasing on lying down.—*Counselor*, April, 1879.

Lithium Carb. 10[m].—Rheumatic patient, with soreness about the heart; worse when stooping, with pains in limbs; the finger-joints are tender and painful.—*Counselor*, 1879.

Aconite.—Severe cutting pain coming with each breath, running around the renal region to the hip. This same symptom reads in Allen's *Encyclopedia*: "Cutting pain extending from spine over the left hip, around to the abdomen in a circle."—*Counselor*, August, 1879.

Theridion 1^{m}.—Nausea, vertigo, and headache, all worse from motion; any noise made the dizziness and nausea much worse.—*Counselor*, October, 1879.

Abies Nigra^{6}.—Lady spits blood every morning. Feeling mid-sternum as if she had swallowed a hard substance, which was sticking there.—*Counselor*, October, 1879.

Dr. E. R. Tuller reports a case with the same sensation as that found in the above case of Professor Farrington, but differing in the locality in which it was experienced. The patient described her symptom as a "sensation of an undigested, hard-boiled egg in the stomach." The patient was promptly cured with *Abies Nigra*^{30}.—*Counselor*, May, 1879.

Dr. J. R. Arndt gives as his indications for *Mercurius cyanatus* in throat affections the following: "Fetor oris and tenderness of the salivary glands without much swelling." It fails to give relief, according to his experience when there is much enlargement of the glands.—*Counselor*, October, 1879.

Aurum^{30}.—Puerperal mania; melancholy, with disposition to commit suicide.—H. V. MILLER, *Counselor*, April, 1879.

Cocculus Indicus^{30}.—Sea-sickness when riding in a railway car.—G. B. DURRIE, *Homœopathic Times*, January, 1879.

Senega 2^{c}.—Very dry sore throat; short hacking cough, which tears and scrapes the throat, entire loss of voice; even whispering is very painful to the throat, and provokes cough, which is worse from outdoor air.—C. M. CONANT, *Counselor*, September, 1879.

Equisetum 1^{x}.—Enuresis; dreams of seeing crowds of people.—S. R. KIPPAX, *Counselor*, September, 1879.

Dr. H. N. Guernsey sends to the *Organon* the following characteristics taken from an interleaved copy of Bœnninghausen, containing the author's latest office annotations, and additions by Dr. Carroll Dunham.

Apis.—Stools involuntary, oozing or pouring from a half-open anus on any movement of the trunk; yellowish water (with drowsiness, prostration, and thirstlessness).

Colchicum.—Stools varying in color on each occasion, now green, next yellow, next reddish, then variegated; slime and fæces mixed; stools acrid, having a slightly sour odor (often associated with convulsions reflex from abdominal irritation).

Bryonia.—Stools smelling like old cheese.

Ferrum Phos.—Frequent desire to urinate, originating with pain in the neck of the bladder and end of the penis. He must urinate immediately, which relieves the pain. Urine normal (?). The above only or chiefly during the day, not at night; worse the more he stands.

Croton Tiglium.—Eczema of the scrotum, itching excessively, worse at night.

Lithium Carb.—Swelling, tenderness, and sometimes redness of the last joints of the fingers, with general puffiness of the body and limbs. Increase in bulk and weight. Clumsiness in walking at night, and weariness on standing. Sometimes intense itching of the sides of the feet and hands from no apparent cause.

Fluoric Acid.—Sensation of cool air blowing into the eyes under the lids; has to keep the eyes covered warmly.

Arnica.—Cold preceded by thirst.

Ceanothus Americanus has been very highly lauded by Drs. Hale and Burnett as a drug valuable in affections of the spleen. Dr. Dunham cured two cases of enlarged spleen with it. Dr. Burnett has used it with success in acute and chronic splenitis and in chronic hypertrophy of the spleen. In one patient to whom Dr. Burnett gave Ceanothus, it produced great nervous excitement, with chilliness and loss of appetite. The patient (a young lady) felt as if her nerves were shaken so that one day, when at dinner, she could scarcely hold her knife and fork. The chilliness was confined chiefly to the back. The medicine was discontinued, when all the symptoms disappeared only to reappear on resuming the drug. Still later her menses appeared ten days before they were due, and were then very profuse. This never occurred with her before.—*Monthly Homœopathic Review*, vol. xxiii, No. 3. Dr. Hale recommends, besides Ceanothus, for hypertrophied spleen, Polymnia uredalia.—*Investigator*, vol. x.

Dr. John Wilde mentions the case of a young lady suffering from an enormous hypertrophy of one breast, to whom had been prescribed Hydrastis ϕ, 5 drops four times per day. After taking the drug for three weeks there appeared on the hands, arms, and shoulders an eruption consisting of small boils. Some of these were yet papules, while others were ready to discharge pus. On discontinuing the Hydrastis the boils disappeared. Dr. Wilde had a servant who was suffering from large crops of blind boils. Desiring to confirm the symptom, which he supposed to have been produced by Hydrastis, he prescribed for her boils Hydrastis ϕ, 2 drops every three hours. The boils were better by the next day, but the patient was covered from head to foot with a rash resembling that of scarlatina in color, and in that it disappeared for some time on pressure. On the following day the face became affected with itching, burning, and stinging, and through scratching was much swollen. Later a stye appeared on the left eyelid. The girl had never had a stye before.—*Monthly Homœopathic Review*, vol. xxiii, No. 5.

In the years 1872 and 1874, when the money paid by France to Germany as indemnity was returned to France through mercantile transactions, the clerks who had spent several weeks in handling the silver coin were seized with a peculiar train of symptoms. Dr. J. Murray Moore quotes the symptoms of this peculiar disease from Dr. Manouvrieg's article in the *Bulletin Medical du Nord*, interpolating the numbers of those particular symptoms as given in Allen's *Encyclopedia*, under Argentum metallicum. They are as follows: "Frequent sneezing and coryza ([74 73 72]); and angina ([222 224 225 243]), and expectoration of a black color. There is also a metallic taste in the mouth, which spoils the flavor of food (Arg. nit. [293]); loss of appetite ([135 136]); colic ([156 158 159]); nausea ([128 129 131 140]) and violent thirst (Arg. nit. [244]); bowels constipated ([184 185])."—*Monthly Homœopathic Review*, vol. xxiii, No. 5. I looked for the above symptoms under Argentum and found them as Dr. Moore says. But I went farther and looked into the pathogenesis of Cuprum. There I found all of the above symptoms excepting the black expectoration, which is not found under Argentum at all. The above symptoms are stated in such a very general manner that it is probable that I should have found most of them in the pathogeneses of many of the drugs recorded in Allen's *Encyclopedia*.

Four cases of poisoning from arsenical wall-paper are reported by Mr. Jabez Hogg in the *British Medical Journal*, and reprinted in the July number of the *London Monthly Homœopathic Review*. Among the symptoms experienced by the patients were the following: Chilliness; had to use blankets, which did not relieve him. In trying to rise, he found both lower limbs paralyzed, the effort to rise producing pain in the bowels as if some one was twisting them. In the morning on rising, was covered with a peculiar dusky skin eruption; and in the arm-joints the eruptive patches ulcerated. The eyelids were affected. There were also intermittent convulsions in one of the cases. The last case which he mentions is that of Miss S., who in March last moved into a furnished house. She was soon taken with a cold and cough, but as she was subject to bronchitis she stayed in her room most of the time. She became worse, and suffered from pain in the stomach and irritation of the throat, with difficulty in breathing, and daily fainting spells. Suspecting from the bright color of her wall-paper that arsenic might have been the cause of her trouble, she changed her apartments, when all the symptoms disappeared. Some of the above symptoms may have been produced by arsenuretted hydrogen.

The history of ten cases of poisoning with arsenuretted hydrogen or arsenicum hydrogenisatum have been collected by Dr. T. M. Strong and published by him in the *North American Journal of Homœopathy*. I have arranged the symptoms produced in these cases according to the plan followed by Hering in his *Condensed Materia Medica:*

[1] *Mind.*—Extreme anxiety. Fears he will die.

[2] *Sensorium.*—Coma. Vertigo.

[3] *Inner Head.*—Sensation of pressure in head. Violent pain in head forcing him to open the windows. Intense frontal headache.

[5] *Eyes.*—Eyes sunken and surrounded by bluish rings. Conjunctivæ injected.

[7] *Nose.*—Nose felt as if dead. Nose cold. Tingling in nose, producing violent sneezing.

[8] *Face.*—Face expressive of pain; besotted appearance; earthy; of a reddish color. Œdema of face.

[9] *Lower Jaw.*—Lips discolored. Tongue and lips covered with a sootlike covering.

[11] *Tongue.*—Tongue swollen, with deep irregular ulcer on its right side. Tubercle of blackish appearance on tongue. Tongue dry. Great thirst.

[13] *Throat.*—Burning and constriction in throat. Sharp pain from pharynx to the lowest end of the alimentary canal. Painful burning along the whole alimentary canal.

[16] *Nausea and Vomiting.*—Hiccough. Nausea. Vomiting, with chilliness, of yellowish green mucus, with bitter taste; of black coffee-looking substance. Vomiting from least drink. Spasmodic eructations, with emissions of inodorous gas, not relieving the abdominal pains.

Stomach.—Feeling of fulness in epigastrium. Pains in epigastrium followed by vomiting. Tenderness of epigastrium to touch.

[18] *Hypochondria.*—Pain in right hypochondrium; pres-

sure; motion. Liver painful to touch. Liver and spleen at first diminished in size, later enlarged.

19 *Abdomen.*—Colic, with vomiting. Burning pain in lower part of abdomen, with coldness of the extremities. Very painful vague feeling as if he had a stone in his abdomen.

20 *Stool.*—Emission of flatus, followed by stool. After a dose of Castor oil and Laudanum, large clay-colored stool, containing portions of mucous membranes of the rectum, with fibrinous exudation. Obstinate constipation. Stools frequent, large and fetid. Transient pricking at the anus. Hæmorrhoidal flux of thirty years' standing was cured in one of the cases of poisoning with this gas.

21 *Urine.*—Suppression of urine. Urine of a dark-red color; composed of pure blood, forming clots in the vessel; black as ink; alkaline; containing epithelium and albumen. Painless discharge of sixty grains of pure blood from urethra. Dysuria. Ardor urinæ, with continuous severe pain in small of back. The urine did not contain blood-globules, but under the action of heat and Nitric acid deposited abundant reddish-brown coagula.

22 *Sexual Organs.*—Entire prepuce and glans were covered with pustules, which were replaced by small, circular, flat ulcers.

26 *Breathing.*—Breath has an ammoniacal odor. Progressive dyspnœa with excessive anguish. Respiration accelerated and obstructed.

28 *Lungs.*—Posterior pulmonary congestion. Feeling of constriction across base of chest.

29 *Heart, Pulse.*—Pulse imperceptible; 100 to 130.

31 *Neck, Back.*—Malaise or oppression in region of kidneys, spreading along the back to between the shoulders without giving rise to any acute pain. Continuous severe pain in region of kidneys, with ardor urinæ. Dorsal pain in evening.

32 *Upper Limbs.*—When undressing at 10 P. M., acute pains in arms and elbows. Upper extremities to middle of arms feel dead. Painful tingling of hands.

33 *Lower Limbs.*—Pains in knee-joints. Legs up to knees feel dead. Painful tingling in feet.

34 *All the Limbs.*—Limbs cold. Numbness with tingling.

36 *Nerves.*—Loss of sensation.

37 *Sleep.*—Sleepless. Great tendency to sleep, but sleep is interrupted by least noise.

40 *Fever, etc.*—General chilliness. Chill at 10 P.M. when undressing. Evening temperature increased.

[43] *Sensations.*—Numbness and tingling. Parts feel dead.

[44] *Tissues.*—Anasarca. Blister placed over stomach brought dark-red blood. Fainting fits.

[46] *Skin.*—All the hair on the dead parts became as white as snow, but resumed its normal color with convalescence. Skin of body colored brown; bronze, with discoloration of the skin; excessive itching. Urticaria.

An article on Salicylic acid by Dr. W. H. Burt, in the *Investigator* of September 1st, 1879, calls attention to many facts of interest. Through the cerebro-spinal system, Salicylic acid has three special centres of action. 1. The brain and spinal cord. It affects chiefly the cerebellum and the auditory and pneumogastric nerves. When given in large doses it produces effects similar to those derived from Cinchona. Thus there is a dull, heavy expression to the face which flushes on the least excitement. The eyes are suffused. There are also deafness and noises in the ears, frontal headache, trembling of the hands, and muscular irritability. Under toxic doses the headache becomes more intense, great muscular weakness sets in, with tingling of the extremities, huskiness of the voice, and hurried, deepened, sometimes sighing respiration. There may even be ptosis, strabismus, mydriasis, delirum, olive-green urine, and involuntary stool. The action of the drug on the auditory nerve has given rise to a series of symptoms similar to those of Menier's disease, in which disease Salicylic acid 3^x has proved curative. 2. The heart. Salicylic acid increases the arterial pressure, partly on account of increasing the energy of the heart, but chiefly as the result of excitation of the vasomotor centres. Later the arterial pressure diminishes, the heart-stroke becoming weaker and weaker. 3. Spine. It acts upon both the sensory and motor nerves, as shown by the tingling in different parts of the body with cutaneous anæsthesia, and the great muscular weakness and trembling and twitching of the legs. 4. Kidneys. Salicylic acid escapes from the body chiefly through the kidneys. The urine has an olive-green color. Dr. Weber has seen the acid produce nephritis with bloody albuminous urine, containing casts. It also produces suppression of urine and involuntary urination from paralysis of the sphincter vesicæ.

Dr. Maclagan, formerly of Dundee, now of Aberdeen, introduced the treatment of rheumatism with Salicylic acid. Dr. Gillespie, of Sterling, Illinois, in the *Chicago Medical Journal and Examiner*, of August, 1878, gives a résumé of two hundred cases of rheumatism treated with Salicylic acid. The average time sick was 13.5 days; the average time of relief of pain, 2.8 days; the average time of reduction of temperature, 30 hours.

A few days since, while reading a recent number of the *Lancet* (November, 1879), I came across an article by Dr. Maclagan on the relative virtues of Salicylic acid and Salicylin in rheumatism. He considers Salicylic acid to be unsafe in the large doses in which he has been in the habit of prescribing it (30 grs. every hour), by reason of the depressing action of the drug. He therefore prescribes for rheumatism Salicylin in large doses, persisting in the use of the drug until the patient has taken about two ounces.

To resume Dr. Burt's paper, Drs. Ebstein and Müller report the cure of two cases of diabetes mellitus with Salicylic acid.

Salicylic acid ought also to become a useful drug in the treatment of morbus Brightii, more especially in patients of a rheumatic diathesis.

Dr. E. M. Hale reports the cure of a case of vesical catarrh with this acid dissolved in glycerin and warm water, and injected into the bladder once in 6 hours. The urine was very offensive, and on examination under the microscope was found to contain pus, blood, and an abundance of mucous epithelium.

Salicylic acid will be found to be useful in dyspepsia with great accumulation of flatus and acidity of the stomach, with anæmia, great irritability, and despondency.

Dr. George W. Winterburn has instituted provings of Berberis aquifolium. He publishes his results in the *Homœopathic Times* of October, 1879. There were five provers. The preparation used was Parke, Davis & Co's. fluid extract. Berberis aq. acts prominently on the mucous membranes of the air-passages and alimentary tract. It produces in the nose a stuffed-up feeling with a greenish-yellow discharge. Going further down the respiratory tract we find a weak feeling especially in the upper part of the chest, with dry nervous cough, tenacious yellow or blood-streaked expectoration, and muffled sound to the voice. These symptoms, in conjunction with increased temperature, accelerated pulse, hollow eyes, pinched expression to the face, give a strong picture of phthisis, in which disease Dr. Winterburn has used the drug with benefit. Proceeding to its action on the alimentary canal, we find a bilious taste in the mouth after eating, the tongue is covered with a yellowish-brown or thick white pasty coating. The patient is hungry soon after eating, and yet he has a complete aversion to food. Berberis must have a strong action on the liver, as shown by the above symptoms, and by the fact that in one of the provers it caused the skin to assume a waxy hue, similar to that of commencing jaundice. It caused, also, an intense burning pain in the spleen, with a sensation as if that organ had been pounded. In the provings Berberis aq. did not give any great evidence of its utility in skin diseases. Blotches and pimples annoyed the provers, and all noticed that after the proving the skin was softer and whiter than before.

Dr. Winterburn found the drug useful in rheumatism when the affected part felt as if bruised or pounded, and when the pains were entirely absent during rest.

Other provings appeared in our journals during the past year, but of them I have not the time to speak beyond merely mentioning them. Dr. W. E. Leonard, of Minneapolis, Minn., publishes a proving of Caesium made by himself with five others. It appeared in the November number of the *North American Journal of Homœopathy.* Dr. E. Chapin, in the August number of the same journal, gives the proving of Apooynum cannabinum.

ERYTHROXYLON COCA.

(THE SACRED LIFE PLANT.)

BY B. B. GUMPERT, M.D., AND H. NOAH MARTIN, M.D., PHILADELPHIA, PA.

THIS plant is a native of Brazil, and abounds in almost every tropical portion of South America. It has been used by the natives for a long time as a masticatory, mixed with ashes or quicklime. Early travellers brought home wonderful reports of its marvellous virtues, and told of its wonderful stimulating qualities; that with a mouthful of coca and lime the Indian could endure great toil and fatigue without other food, or even sleep! Others, more truthful, tell us that the excessive use of Coca will produce effects as bad as those from the use of opium or fermented liquors.

Like tobacco, the Coca habit is as hard to change, and it is computed that upwards of thirty million (30,000,000) pounds of Coca are consumed yearly by 10,000,000 of the human race.

It is only within a few years that the attention of the medical world has been called to this drug. And, like many so-called new remedies, has received on the one hand the most laudatory encomiums of its wonderful virtues as a stimulant, tonic, and brain-food! Others give very small thanks for any active properties it may possess.

The leaves of Coca, as found in the shops, are of a light-green color, about an inch broad, two inches long, oval, oblong, pointed, with short, slender foot-stalk; when chewed, they impart a slightly astringent aromatic taste, with smarting and numbing sensation to the tongue. Their ordinary virtues are extracted by hot water and dilute alcohol.

One apothecary (D. F. Shull) gave the leaves in powder to several persons, and reports (*Druggist's Circular*), in 30 to 60 grain doses, that it acted as a gentle excitant, followed by an indisposition to sleep, not unlike the reaction from tea or coffee. He thinks it has a more decided action on the heart, increasing its action; it also has (in his opinion) a peculiar stimulating power over the digestive organs, giving relief to that depression after eating caused by indigestion. Taken in doses of 100 to 200 grains it excites the whole system, flushing the face, and imparting increased vigor to the muscles as well as the brain.

B. B. GUMPERT, M.D.

Dr. Stokes made a short proving of it in 1859, and Dr. Hering published what was known about it up to 1868 in the *American Journal of Homœopathic Materia Medica*. Dr. Allen, in his *Encyclopedia of Materia Medica*, has given us all that is more recently known up to the date of its publication.

The *Monthly Homœopathic Review*, December, 1879, contains an article by Adrian Stokes, M.D., on "Coca in Chronic Constipation," never relieved during many years except by the aid of enemata. It was accompanied by "spasmodic dyspnœa and violent palpitation of the heart from incarcerated flatus, which would sometimes pass from her with such force that it seemed as if the œsophagus would be rent by it." Many medicines had been used without benefit. He gave the lady a few leaves of Coca, with instructions to make an infusion and take a small coffee-cupful at a time twice a day after food. She very shortly began to improve, and regained her health, all her symptoms leaving her.

My student, Mr. Conover, makes the following report of a case of typhoid fever with extremely feeble heart-action. The effect upon the patient was very similar to that of whiskey, producing a sensation of warmth, increasing the circulation and causing at times slight vertigo, which, however, was very transient.

After using Coca for several days the pulse, from being soft and almost imperceptible, became more tense but not increased in frequency.

The dose used was about ʒj of tincture three times a day.

It ought to be mentioned that the tincture used was made at my request by Messrs. Cramer & Small, of Philadelphia, from the dry leaves, and contained 60 per cent. of Alcohol.

The case was a very serious one, but made a good recovery.

As to the general physical action of Coca, I make the following extracts from the remarks of several eminent men.

"Professor Colpaert says 'Coca is a very strengthening substance,' facilitates assimilation, and retards tissue waste, . . . possesses a peculiarly stimulating influence on the stomach, and reliable observers claim that it facilitates digestion and gives more real tone to the stomach than anything they have ever used previously."—DR. GOULLON.

"Possesses wonderful power in preserving strength during fatiguing exercises, exhausting diseases, and food privation."—DR. DE LA VEGA.

Dr. William S. Searle says: "The effects of the Coca upon the human system borders upon the marvellous, and if not clearly authenticated by scientists of undoubted veracity would be altogether beyond belief."

Lieutenant Herndon (United States Exploring Expedition of the Amazon) says: "Coca possesses properties so marvellous that it enables the South American Indians, without any other nourishment the while, to perform forced marches of five and six days. It is so bracing a stimulant and tonic that by merely chewing it they will perform journeys of three hundred miles without appearing in the least fatigued."

"I am clearly of the opinion that Coca is conducive to health; and from long and attentive observation I am convinced that its use in moderation is very beneficial," says Dr. Van Tschudi (*Travels in Peru*, 1847).

"Coca has really wonderful power in supporting the strength under prolonged fatigue without other food. My Indian followers have accompanied me on foot through the forests of Peru for fifty miles in one day without food or anything else except Coca leaves, which they chewed at intervals."—DR. POPPIG, German Naturalist and Explorer, *Travels in Chili, Peru, and on the River Amazon*, 1835.

"Dr. Pigeaux, of Paris, who has investigated, under the direction of the French Academy, the properties of the Coca, among other remarks, says: 'It might be made the beverage of infants, children, and brainworkers, and it ought also to be used in the army and navy, and by all hard toilers. It has long excited attention in France as possessing a peculiar stimulating power, and favoring digestion more than any known beverage. It is admitted that it enables those who use it to make greater muscular exertion, and to resist the effects of an unhealthy, malarial climate.'

"Humboldt says he has never known a case of consumption or asthma among the natives who are accustomed to its use, and that they live to a great age, retaining their mental and physical faculties to the last."—*Cosmos.*

Mr. Cramer, of Cramer & Small, druggists, tells me that large quantities of the leaves are sent to officers in our army now located in the Indian territories, and used by them while on the march and deprived of sleep.

Mr. Cramer, in addition to the tincture, which is made as all other tinctures of the dried plant are made, has prepared for me an Elixir of coca, which is made by distillation, and contains 25 per cent. of Alcohol.

I have prescribed this elixir to several patients, not to get provings, because patients will not gratify us in that way, but to test its effects as a tonic.

Mrs. F. has been treated by an allopathic physician for malaria without any result.

She is anæmic, has constant desire to lie down, tired and drowsy; pulse *very* weak, can hardly feel it, not accelerated; if she walks a square she has vertigo and weakness in her legs, and staggers like a drunken person. After taking a dessertspoonful of the elixir she felt strengthened, and was able to walk much better. On the third day after commencing it she was obliged to go to New York, where she went out shopping, and she says she walked about twenty squares without fatigue. She continues the use of it, and is constantly improving.

Mrs. A. has Bright's disease, chronic form. Is sometimes exceedingly weak. I prescribed the elixir in the same way. She describes the effects as follows.

"In a few minutes I feel a warmth in my stomach, which then spreads all over me. Then my brain feels active, and I feel able to do any work or walk any distance. It seems as though it was going to cure me."

Miss B., an old maid suffering debility, found that it produced violent vertigo, and she would not continue it.

Miss T., an old maid, and long past the climacteric period, complained of violent neuralgia in the head, and vertigo, but she persisted in its use, and describes its effects very much as Mrs. A. does. She is a long time invalid. Several other patients have taken it, and they nearly uniformly state that it has great tonic properties.

Mr. A. J., 24 years old, a hearty, robust young man, chewed the leaves. They stimulated him very much, but he complained that he "could not sleep a wink all night." This seemed to be a constant result with him. He passed great quantities of water habitually; he thought he passed less of it while chewing them.

The following very interesting case I report in full:

A gentleman about 50 years of age was attacked with vertigo and an indescribable, queer, balancing sensation in the head, preceded for many months by vertiginous feelings and occipital pains on awaking in the morning. Symptoms also similar to those described in Silicia, viz.: vertigo rising from the nape of the neck through to the vertex, and also sensation of rushing, as if water-pipes were bursting in the head.

The last serious attack was accompanied by cold clammy sweat over the whole body, cold feet and hands, vomiting of water slightly tinged with bile, and sensation as if receiving a charge of electro-galvanism, *i. e.*, a tense trembling sensation in the nerves and muscles of the arms. Perfect consciousness and loquacity. Present attack was called a bilious attack; general physical condition, cerebral anæmia.

The attack was followed by great debility, inability to walk straight. Movement was similar to that of a very old person partially paralyzed. Inability to control the legs entirely. Staggering when walking as though intoxicated, and as if the head was too heavy to balance on the shoulders. When turning the head to the right all objects pass to the left at a great velocity. Could not look up, or turn around without falling to the ground, or at least without great danger of doing so. Could not lie on the back or right side without an attack of vertigo, with a sore rushing sensation in the head. When walking, the sound of the foot touching the ground was conveyed into the brain as if the brain was solid. Upon closing the eyes, could walk straight and turn around without difficulty. Could turn to the left much better than to the right, when the eyes were open.

During sleep, when lying on the left side, numbness of the left arm and especially of the little finger of the left hand.

Head most comfortable when bending forward or stooping with the head as low as the knees. No vertigo when going up stairs or down.

Urine was examined, and found to be normal. No tenderness of spinous processes. Sometimes slight numbness in the toes, when stepping out of bed in the morning. Vertiginous feeling most likely to come when sitting still, and dissipated upon sudden changing of position. Light did not disturb vision, nor did noise or confusion disturb.

Some flatulence, and an intensely nauseous odor from the mouth, probably the stomach. Bowels tolerably regular. Voice broken and hoarse, something like the husky voice of cholera patients, especially in the evening. No difficulty of breathing, except sometimes in the night the breath would seem to stop as soon as he fell asleep, and he would gasp for breath; or, in other words, the whole function of life seemed to stop.

Pulse very weak, but about natural in frequency.

Gradual improvement in general strength continued for about two weeks, when the patient was able to be taken to Cape May by boat.

Three weeks in Cape May, four weeks at Schooley's Mountain, and four weeks in Boston did but little to improve his condition. The patient hardly able to walk three squares. While on his way home visited Dr. W. S. Searle, in Brooklyn. He suggested the chewing of Coca leaves, and provided him enough to reach Philadelphia that day. After the ride, via Pennsylvania Railroad, and the general fatigue of travelling, our patient found himself feeling able to accomplish almost any labor.

The effects were almost marvellous. The following day he visited more than twenty persons in different parts of the city, and without fatigue, and he has continued at his post, doing the duties of his profession ever since. The symptoms are gradually disappearing.

Constant and close observation in this case justifies the conclusion that Coca is a powerful tonic and brain stimulant; that its effects last at least three days without any depressing reaction; that taken in large doses it will destroy the appetite temporarily; that it increases the powers of digestion, and is an anti-malaria medicine.

In some cases it causes wakefulness and in others drowsiness; it also acts as a diuretic. As to what its homœopathic action is I am not prepared to say, because on account of the shortness of time allowed my colleague and myself, we have not been able to make any proving of it.

H. Noah Martin, M.D.

CLINICAL CASES, WITH COMMENTS.

BY JAMES B. BELL, M D.

(Read before the Maine Homœopathic Medical Society of Augusta, May 21st, 1878.)

CASE 1.—*Nausea of Pregnancy.* Mrs. R., blue eyes, brown hair, well built, very intellectual; age 28; married seven years and had three children. Has always suffered severely from nausea until quickening, and has been only partially relieved by the most skilful homœopathic prescriptions.

January 16*th*, 1878.—Is about six weeks pregnant, and began to feel ill eight days ago. Complains of an indescribable dulness, and gnawing in the sternum, about midway and deep in. I found her lying on the bed, tossing from side to side, and with one hand constantly pressing and rubbing the chest and sternum. She said it gave her a little relief, and that she *could not* keep still. She had also a faint aching about the navel as though she must eat, but at the same time loathing and disgust at the *thought, sight,* or *smell of food.* All attempts to eat cause violent nausea and vomiting. The *smell of meats and eggs* is especially repugnant. Can take oatmeal gruel best, and that helps for a little while.

Indifferent to surroundings; somewhat fretful; face flushed; glad of the pregnancy, but dreads the next three months.

Now none of the "ordinary remedies" will help this case in the least. Physicians who think, in their phrase, "that the physician's first duty is to relieve his patient," and so when the "ordinary remedies" fail, to resort to morphine and other drugs, cannot help this case.

I prescribe, however, with great confidence, *Colchicum*$^{m:00}$ in water every three hours. This remedy alone has the great sensitiveness to the smell of food, meat, eggs, and broth. This symptom is so characteristic that its presence overcomes the counter-indication, "nausea worse from motion," and also the absence from the proving of the gnawing distress in the sternum. (Allen has "feeling of orgasm in the chest, and peculiar feeling as if something alive was working in it.")

From a letter which I received from the patient a few days after, in which she desired to add to my title, "A.M., for Angel of Mercy," I judge the relief to have been very striking. This it also was. She only required afterwards one dose of Sulphur 6^{m} for a faintness, which caused her to eat every two or three hours, and a little later a repetition of the Colchicum for a slight return of the sensitiveness to smell of food; and then she remained well.

Case 2.—*Condylomata.*—Mr. A. B.; age 25; sanguine temperament; good constitution; has had gonorrhœa three times.

December 22d, 1877.—Now has had for three weeks a large number of condylomata surrounding the glans penis; they are red, pedunculated, and are growing rapidly.

These warts do not get well of themselves. I do not think they have ever been known to yield to anything in the old-school treatment but the scissors or cautery. The only symptoms were weakness of the back and frequent urination.

Because these warts were quite exuberant and dry, and followed gonorrhœa, I gave *Thuja*^{200}, a dose night and morning for two days, then placebo. Seven days after the last dose, the warts were larger, but he felt better every way. Again placebo for two weeks. The warts shrinked and dropped off. He is now in excellent health.

Case 3.—*Porrigo Decalvans.*—Boy, aged 10 years. Looks healthy; had measles and chicken-pox four years ago.

March 30th, 1877.—One year ago a little spot became bald on the back of the head. It gradually spread until it covered, or rather uncovered, the whole of his head as high as the crown and well above each ear. Some bald spots are now appearing on other parts of the scalp. The skin is almost as bare as the palm of one's hand and apparently healthy. It does not look as though hair would ever grow there again. Now, as we all know that this is a parasitic affection, and that the scalp is infected with minute spores, which are destroying the hair, bulbs, and all, so of course, we have only to avail ourselves of some of the chemical antiseptics, and thus show ourselves to be progressive physicians. Let us look a little further, however, before we desert our colors.

We find a sore place in the bend of the left knee, looking like a burn produced by a chafe, but which refuses to heal. His mother says also that other small wounds suppurate. If he gets cold he is inclined to have a discharge from his head for a long time. *Graph.* 6^{m}, night and morning, for two days. Thirty days afterward reported "hair falls off less." *Graph.* 6^{m}, a dose night and morning for a month. This was an error, both in the remedy and the repetition, and the result was no better; cracks in the nose, although his skin is healed. *Lycop.* 6^{m}, a dose night and morning, for two days. One month more and examination showed the hair coming in in the small spots and in the edge of the large one. The cure thus begun was not disturbed. Month by month the hair grew faster and thicker and of a richer color than the old, until the whole head was covered again and the boy was also well. *Cured* and not *pickled* or *poisoned.*

CASE 4.—*Cancer of the Stomach.*—*November 19th*, 1877. J. C., 75 years of age, a small, feeble old man. Had a severe attack of shingles in the spring, under allopathic treatment, and in the summer his stomach began to trouble him. Some pain there, and occasional vomiting. Since September he has had active old-school treatment, with a frequent change of internal drugs, but has steadily grown worse. He has a full, burning feeling in the stomach, with considerable pain; has vomited much all the time, and for the past two weeks has kept nothing down. He vomits much more in bulk than he takes. Has no movement from the bowels. Examinations by palpation and percussion revealed the thickened and tender pyloric end of the stomach. The diagnosis was sufficiently clear, though quite a surprise to the friends. Prognosis, death within a few months, possibly weeks, but probably relief from remedies. Gave *Nux vom.* 2^m, in water, one day, followed by a dose of *Sulph.* 6^m, and a teaspoonful of Liebig's extract of beef every hour; injections of milk per rectum every eight hours. Two days after, there was some improvement, but still burning at the stomach. Gave *Arsenicum* 8^m, a dry powder, night and morning. Two days later, much better, no vomiting, no burning. Very comfortable in every way. Continued the Arsenicum as before for three days longer, when, as he was still improving, the medicine was omitted. Five days later, and eleven days after the first visit, his only suffering was from hunger, which of course he was forbidden to satisfy. His improved strength shows the amount of nourishment he is receiving from the injection and the beef extract. He may now take a part of a raw oyster several times a day and chew some beefsteak. Tongue clean; no medicine. Twenty days from first visit felt food pass out from stomach. Had an injection of molasses and water, and brought away quite an amount of digested milk, etc. Has pricking pains about the navel, where he had the zonæ. *Graph.* 6^m, one dose. Three weeks later, six weeks after the first visit, has been very comfortable all the time. Takes four or five raw oysters a day, but not allowed anything sweet or farinaceous. Some return of the burning recently, and vomiting to-day for the first time. *Ars.* 8^m, a dose night and morning. During the last few weeks the tumor has perceptibly increased in size. He now gradually failed, vomiting some, but not as before the treatment, and much relieved at different times by *Nat. m.* 4^m, *Lycop.* 6^m,

Ars. 40^{m}, *Carb. veg.* 4^{m}. He died nine weeks after my first visit. He would hardly have lived two weeks if he had not been relieved as above. I have reported this case as a fair example of a good many like incurable cases, quite a number of which were cancer of the stomach, and in which the marvellous action of the well-selected remedy in a suitable dose has accomplished and secured far more palliation than possible by any other means whatever. You will have discovered by this time that the object of my paper is not merely to present a few clinical observations, but to illustrate and enforce the truth that in Hahnemannian homœopathy and not in eclecticism of any sort, is to be found the true application of the maxim, "The physician's highest duty is to cure his patient." Some have paraded this phrase in such wise as to make it imply that the pure and proper practice of homœopathy was a sort of dilettanteism, which gentlemen who had a taste that way might indulge in when dealing with mild and harmless cases, but which must be thrown aside at once for something tangible, ponderable, and in great variety, when the painful and troublesome cases come. The exact reverse is true. Organopathy and other loose treatment may not do a great deal of harm in the lighter cases of acute disease without much psoric complication, but when we come to deal with those ills which go deep down into the unsearchable springs of the vital forces we must have subtle and penetrating forces exactly adapted to their work. The simile as exact as possible gives us the adaptations. The potentization gives us the subtlety and the penetration.

"Men and brethren, let me speak unto you freely." Although not very old, for more than half my lifetime I have been an enthusiastic student and observer of these things, and am qualified to speak with some certainty, for the same reason that the old man was, who on his death-bed advised his son that honesty was the best policy, "for," said he, "I have tried both." During the first year of my practice, influenced somewhat by teachings in the General Hospital at Vienna, and by the low state of homœopathy as represented in our journals, I satisfied myself fully as to all the boasted results of specifics, local applications, crude doses, alternations and rotations of medicines, and various other errors which are easier, at least for a beginner, to fall into than to keep out of, but which only serve to lure us into dangerous places. Now, therefore, that for many years I have known and pursued as faithfully as I could, the better way, I suppose I may be pardoned for wishing that others may benefit by my experience.

All the arguments against homœopathy as opposed to allopathy come only from those who have tried but one. All the arguments in favor of eclecticism in homœopathy come from those who have never faithfully pursued the pure methods of Hahnemann.

Laying principle aside, if you will for the present, we may be all credited with a desire to succeed, and make good cures. Appealing then to this desire alone I am certain of my case. You will not indeed succeed in every case. In the first place patients and their friends need a great deal of instruction as to what constitutes a cure as distinguished from an antipathic palliation or suppression. Many, however, have had sufficient experience with these things to desire something better. Many other patients will advance organopathic ideas, and if they can only get you to prescribe for a certain organ will be satisfied. Such need instruction upon the nature of disease and its method of cure. It is much better, too, to tell patients with complicated chronic affections, as Hahnemann did, that a cure will take at least two years. Yet in spite of all this you will occasionally hear of a case upon which you have made faithful attempts, for a longer or shorter time, without much result, but which is said to have found great help from something else. This may or may not be true, but call it true, and the balance in the long run will be greatly in your favor, and you will become daily more convinced of the power of the true similar in the minimum dose to do all that medicine can do for suffering humanity. He who goes back after this to crude and careless prescribing must do so from pure laziness or want of backbone. He had better take a *tonic*. If these cases, which I have reported to you as illustrations, were anything but fair examples of what I daily see, I could not say to you as I do, that my daily experience long ago brought me to trust not only my professional standing but the dearest interests I have on earth to the *characteristic remedy* in the *high* and *highest potencies*.

SULPHUR IN CONSTIPATION.

BY J. H. WAY, M.D., WEST CHESTER, PA.

(Read before the Homœopathic Medical Society of Chester, Delaware, and Montgomery Counties, Pa , October, 1879.)

Mrs. M., aged 28; dark hair; blue eyes; married; no children; called to have me prescribe for constipation, which had existed from childhood. She was unable to give the character of the stools, further than to say the bowels had not moved for years without the use of a purgative dose of pills, rhubarb, or magnesia, which she took weekly.

I learned upon inquiry that she suffered with a dull feeling in the brain, a heaviness on top of the head, a weak, hungry sensation in stomach before dinner, and burning of the soles of the feet at night.

I gave Sulph.^{m} three powders, one each night, with directions to use no other medicine, and make no change in her diet. She returned in one week to say the bowels now moved naturally, and that the head, stomach, and foot symptoms had disappeared, and that she was feeling in every way much better.

In three months she called again to say that the constipation had returned during the last few days. The same remedy and potency, one dose, gave entire relief at once, since which time, eight months ago, the lady has continued well, and a thorough convert to homœopathy.

The character of the stool in Sulph. constipation gives no certain indication for the choice of the remedy. The books tell us, hard, knotty, insufficient stool. But few patients observe this carefully, and if they do, the similarity to other remedies is too great to decide the choice. A few concomitant symptoms, if they exist, furnish us a sure guide. It may be the dull and full feeling in the head, or flashes of heat, or burning of the soles at night, or the faint feeling in the stomach before dinner, and should these symptoms all exist, relief will be sure, whatever may be the nature of the malady or the pathological condition. For some years I have used the 30th and 200th, and lately the 1^{m} and ^{cm}, 1 to 3 doses, 12 to 24 hours apart, and do not repeat so long as improvement continnes.

Of the comparative value of these potencies in constipation I shall report after scores of comparisons. My experience with Sulph. quite low, is valueless, since it was used empirically, and in connection with some other remedy.

T. F. Allen, in speaking of Sulphur to his class, has said: "If I wish to make a change in the tissues, as in skin disease, I give but one dose, but in constipation I repeat daily for two weeks, but never give lower than the 30th for anything."

PSORIASIS—TINEA CAPITIS SICCA.

BY F. PRESTON, M.D , CHESTER, PA.

(Read before the Homœopathic Medical Society of Chester, Delaware, and Montgomery Counties.)

Psoriasis, Dunglison defines as "a cutaneous affection consisting of rough amorphous scales, continuous or of indeterminate outline, skin often chappy." The treatment "must be antiphlogistic, with the internal use of the fixed alkalies, Sulphur, etc.; they do better without any local application."

L. A. Duhring, Professor of Dermatology in the University of Pennsylvania, advises Arsenic, Cod-liver oil, alkalies, diuretics. "External remedies should be employed in all cases. Baths of various kinds, simple or medicated, the preparations of Tar, Mercurial ointments, Sulphur, Sapo viridis, and solutions of Caustic potassa."

These verbatim quotations are introduced particularly to show how in therapeutics, "scientific medicine" works expansively as it were, around the question at issue, covering the whole ground harmoniously and completely, from positive denial to absolute affirmation. "Freedom of medical opinion" exemplified.

Psoriasis has been known under various classifications as "Impetigo," "Scaly Tetter," "Dry Scall," "Dartre Squamense," "Psoriasis Diffusa," "Herpes Squamosus" (Alibert), "Baker's Itch," "Grocer's Itch," etc.

In the spring of 1877 a German baker, aged 23 years, who had then been under treatment fourteen months, with constantly increasing aggravation, applied to me for relief. The characteristic scaly patches were well developed on dorsa and palms of hands, and on the extensor surface of the forearm as far as the elbow. He had been unable to work at his trade since the disease first appeared. The itching was almost continuous. He said that his doctors had told him they had given him "as much arsenic as he could stand," and considered his case incurable. Fine branlike particles were detached in clouds on scratching, and the raw surface looked red and angry, but did not bleed. After a few hours the scales were apparently all renewed; they at least presented the usual appearance, and the itching began again.

I gave him Arsenicum alb. 40^{m}, 3 doses in 36 hours. Twenty-one days later no trace of the eruption remained, and he resumed work.

Mrs. W., colored. Eruption covering arms, left especially,

extensor surface of arms and dorsa of hands; palms free. Had existed six months. Presented all the peculiar appearances seen in the plate (from Duhring's Atlas). Treatment had been of various kinds, mainly of the "home" variety. Although this eruption itched violently, there was not the cloud of branlike scales detached on scratching, as in the former case. She received, however, a high dilution of Ars., but with no benefit. Rhus tox.^{cm}, a single dose, which was repeated two weeks later. In six weeks no trace of the eruption remained on the hands or arms.

Professor Duhring says: "Psoriasis is usually an obstinate disease; although never involving life, it often causes much distress to the patient. Relapses, varying greatly as to severity, are the rule, which are apt to occur from time to time during life."

In the first case detailed there has been no return of the complaint for the two years that have elapsed.

The plate which I show you, from Duhring's Atlas, is a most exact and lifelike representation of the eruption as it appeared in the cases described. The division of the diseased surface into partially defined squares, resembles most the pecnliar markings on the shell of the common tortoise. The disease is seated in the upper layers of the corium. There is inflammation, and proliferation of epithelial cells. The only possible question concerning the correctness of our diagnosis is, that the elements of "obstinacy" and "relapse" were not found.

TINEA CAPITIS SICCA.

November 1*st*, 1878.—Mrs. T., aged 25 years; eruption eight years, without amelioration; has grown steadily worse. The whole hairy scalp is covered with a dark-colored scaly eruption, thickest at the occiput; gradually thinning out until it reaches the line of the hair on the forehead. Itching is violent, but worst at the occiput. Scratching causes bleeding, and a discharge of clear non-glutinous fluid, which dries with remarkable rapidity. The hair is rapidly disappearing. The accumulated scales at the thickest part, about on a line with the mastoid processes, measure one-quarter inch in thickness. The head is generally washed with soap and water daily, detaching all the scales and leaving the scalp red and moist. After the washing there is a feeling of tension over the whole scalp, very disagreeable, and particularly so around the occiput, where it is actually painful. This daily washing was continued during treatment, as I found it impossible to prevent the patient from doing it.

The patient, who, by the way, is nursing an apparently healthy and well-nourished infant of four months, is below the medium height and slightly built, with gray eyes and dark hair. General health good. On further examination there was found to be original hypermetropia of the right eye, of a high degree; vision very much impaired. She has marginal blepharitis, and commencing ectropion of the left eye, which is already unsightly, and is becoming worse. In fact, it was for this "sagging" that she applied for treatment.

After a careful consideration of her symptoms Staph[30]. was given dry, one dose every evening for a week, one dose alternate evenings for another week, two doses during third week, and one dose during fourth week.

January 1*st*, 1879.—The scalp was perfectly clean and healthy in appearance. It remained so in May, 1879. The "sagging" of the left lower lid is now not noticeable to the casual observer. The blepharitis is so much improved that she pronounces it cured, and this although she persists in misusing her eyes, not having procured glasses as ordered. The improvement was noticeable during the first week of the administration of Staph., and continued steadily on until the eruption had entirely disappeared. The peculiar combination of eye and scalp symptoms led to its use, especially the feeling of tension in the occiput. (See sympt. 97, 98, Staph., Allen's *Mat. Med.*, vol. ix, p. 150; also, Staph., Allen & Norton's *Oph. Therapeutics*, p. 129.)

THE POTENCY QUESTION IN ITS TRUE LIGHT.

BY AUG. KORNDŒRFER, M D., PHILADELPHIA, PA.

(Read before the Hahnemann Club of Philadelphia.)

DURING the past year there has been much discussion in relation to the matter of potencies, first, as regards their power of action, and, secondly, as to the point at which the process of potentization must cease, *i. e.*, the point where matter becomes so attenuated as not to be susceptible of further subdivision. This is a subject of the most intense interest, and one which deserves the greatest possible care in its investigation,—an investigation which demands of the searcher especial preparation, as well as the setting aside of all chance or mere guesswork. Earnest inquiry should be made in the interest of real truth, not the bestowing of such frivolous efforts as would remind us of that schoolboy trick of the marble in the closed hand, shifted at will only to deceive, nor yet of the guesser who, though near the truth, may be foiled by the trick of the holder. Those who have received instruction only from the older teachers of physics must, on entering anew the field of scientific research, unlearn much of what they have been taught to regard as established. Many such supposed facts were obtained from observations made upon matter in crude mass, observations which frequently tend only to error. Others must learn that objects which, through outward relationship, appear familiar, may readily be either falsely related or improperly apprehended, either through want of training or want of ability to understand.

Many of the crude errors of the day also becloud our appreciation of truths otherwise readily understood. The true investigator must learn to loosen his grip upon the commonly accepted notions of the schools, in order that he may be able to view them from new and different standpoints. He must with effort and resolution strengthen himself to the unprejudiced reception of any truth based upon and sustained by careful observation, even though such truth be opposed to all his preconceived notions; yea, even though in opposition to theories of almost universal adoption. Such mental training, in fact, forms the first step in the development of the true scientist,—a step without which the intellectual discipline necessary to the proper investigation of nature can never be attained. It is the first approach toward that state of mental purity which alone can fit us for a full and continuous perception of the truths of science. Such a student was Hahnemann. Learned in the lore of the ancients, versed in the teachings of his day, and with a mind taught from his youth "how to think," he entered the physician's walks in eager anticipation of success. Feeling, however, the great want of a foundation *in law* for everything which he had been taught to do for the sick, he was led to search in nature's great repository for that much-needed guide.

While pursuing such investigation, with a mind prepared to accept that alone which bore the imprint of truth, he arrived at the great law of cure. With it came the need of casting away much of the then, and even now, generally accepted opinions of the action of medicines for the cure of the sick. This he faithfully performed. Then, not content to alone receive, he began to bestow. His first step was toward the establishment of the Materia Medica on a firm, true, and pure foundation. This he accomplished after long and arduous study. Then came a new difficulty: the old and long-accepted minimum dose was too violent in its action, given as it must needs be in conditions at such variance with those to which popular error had assigned each drug.

We then find him diluting his tinctures and triturating his solids for the minute subdivision of the dose, his object being but to decrease the quantity, when, behold, the development of a hitherto unknown force is made manifest. The smaller dose acted in proportionally greater intensity than the larger; thus dilution developed dynamization. Power, latent before, was now placed under a condition to manifest itself. Again his master mind triumphed. Contrary as it was to accepted physics, he saw the fact, unexplainable though it was, and felt, yea, knew it to be true.

But in this most important fact he found the greatest stumbling-block, even to the friends of the law. The fact was in opposition to long-accepted views, and these early adherents, wedded to their idols, would not give them up entirely; therefore this portion of the truth must be rejected. With energy did they refuse to receive, and yet with what folly!

As proper would it be for us to deny the fact of the intensity of the heat of the sun, simply because in our pigmy knowledge we are unable to solve the question of how it is generated. Though beyond conception is the mystery of this enormous conflagration, yet it does exist, and chemistry still leaves us completely at a loss with respect to it; yea, every discovery seems rather to render the comprehension more difficult, removing further and further the prospect of a speedy solution of this wonderful problem in nature. So may we say in relation to the question of the potentization or dynamization of matter. Chemistry affords as yet no clue, though it unfolds to our view equally wonderful truths, which are equally unexplainable, yet too palpable for denial. Who, for instance, will deny the catalytic force exerted by certain substances, theoretically explain it as they may? Here, without any appreciable change in the added substance, wonderful effects are wrought. In such instances we often find exceedingly small proportions of the catalytic body producing great changes. Thus, according to Dalton, "one part of diastase is capable of effecting the transformation of two thousand parts of starch," and this too without any discoverable change in the diastase itself. It acts as it were simply by its presence. Instances of this kind exist, and are known to every educated physician, yet we do not undertake to deny simply because we cannot explain them.

How will we explain the mystery involved in the so-called isomeric bodies, exhibiting as they do "analogous decompositions and transformations when heated or subjected to the action of the same reagents, and differing only in physical properties?" Yet such substances do exist.

So, too, with our potencies. Shall we deny because we do not understand, or shall we not rather continue our search with more vigor, inquiring of nature her ways? Not with dictatorial hand attempting to strike down the unbeliever, but saying to each, "Search." Let each take his own way; one through chemistry, another through physics, a third through logic, while still others, with no less earnestness and effort, gain much vantage by clinical observation.

Each may in some point err; then let each act as a check, the one upon the other; all in one work, though not all alike gifted; each must according to his talents strive. Let each have the credit of honest purpose, and let him earn such by giving honest investigation and trusty intelligent information, giving his best efforts to the upbuilding of the temple of true knowledge, not to its destruction.

Hahnemann through such earnest and impartial investigation was led to the recommendation of the higher potencies. Hahnemann was not always right, but Hahnemann was always honest. That many equally honest followers have been led through personal experience to adopt the high potencies, even higher than Hahnemann dared think of, may only prove that Hahnemann erred on the side of the low potencies, owing to an inability on his part to conceive of the possibility of the infinite divisibility of drug matter with its medicinal power retained. When he said, "It must stop somewhere, let us stop at the thirtieth," he fell into the error of forming a conclusion not based upon experiment, but simply upon expedience.

We speak not in censure; this wonder of knowledge, though past his fourscore years, was still working with the ardor of youth, yet with the ability of a giant intellect.

Experience has since proved that higher potencies are at times needed. Let us, therefore, bury the hatchet of discord, each going to the work of investigation in the way most suited to his abilities and tastes; then the hidden may be laid bare, the unknown become known, the undiscerned made manifest. Above all let us lay aside all guess and chance, knowing that chance has *no law*, therefore is unreliable and unworthy the scientist.

"How can a high potency act?" is constantly asked. To this we answer in Yankee fashion: How does a *low* potency act? The law is the same. We have much to learn; let it be done both by re-provings and by clinical work. Those who find these methods unsuited to their tastes may make experimental efforts in any or every conceivable line until they are fully satisfied, but with it all let them bear in mind the fact that what may prove novel or pleasant, or even profitable to them, may not possess similar qualities or offer corresponding advantages to another. Let them, therefore, not censure or speak harshly, nor yet slightingly of others. Above all, let them not impute dishonest motives, for as surely as like begets like, such charges must be born of kindred minds; the law must act.

That small doses of medicine may act is conceivable. Even the allopath prescribes the $\frac{1}{240}$th part of a grain, or even less, and finds good results to follow. Why then may not smaller, and if the smaller, why not the higher potencies?

The susceptibility of the albuminous matter to the so-called catalytic force is certainly well known, and some similar action may here be brought into play; that as out of the body, in mere dead matter, such wonderful effects are produced by exceedingly small quantities, within the living organism much more active change from infinitely smaller quantities may be wrought.

A word to the opponents of the high potencies. Carefully apply the remedy according to the law, and in the much-abused potencies in cases where the well-indicated remedy in a lower potency does not act, bearing in mind the injunction as to the first step toward the development of the true scientist, and we feel assured that success will attend your ministrations on the sick, and that as knowledge increases you will become converts to the use of such potencies. In addition we may, in our day and generation, arrive at a solution of that much-vexed problem, when to give high, and when low potencies, or even the crude drug, for the dose must be individualized as well as the remedy. In addition to all which, unity and strength will be developed within our ranks.

In conclusion, it may not be amiss to remark that from personal experience, I must advocate the use of the high potencies, these having been the instruments in the cure of a long-standing, chronic affection from which I personally suffered; a condition which baffled allopathy and the low potencies of homœopathy for many years, which under the high potencies was speedily relieved and ultimately entirely removed. Nevertheless it has been my experience in practice, that the low potencies, and even the crude drugs, are at times required. In fact, we must strive not for the discarding of this or that grade of potencies, but rather for the determination of the conditions under which one or another of the various preparations of any given drug may be indicated.

ALCOHOL IN BLOOD-POISONING.

BY TH. BRUCKNER, M.D., BASLE, SWITZERLAND.

MY friend and colleague, Dr. Grubenmann, who has a very extensive homœopathic practice at St. Gallen, related to me on my visit to him in September, 1879, that he had been very dangerously ill from having wounded himself when making a post-mortem examination. He did not take much notice of the little cut at the time of the accident, but he soon felt all the effects of a poisoned wound. His hand and arm became swollen and very painful, and a high fever set in. When he felt that he was very near losing consciousness he took fifty grams of pure undiluted alcohol. He felt no more inconvenience, however, from this large dose, than from an ordinary glass of wine. He remained in a feverish, semi-conscious state for about twenty-four hours, but the next day he felt that the fever was subsiding, and that he would recover speedily. On the third day he got up to attend to some pressing business, and a few days later was able to go out and visit his patients.

This rather wonderful and speedy cure reminded me of an account of the plague at Marseillès in the beginning of the last century, which I had read shortly before, where the following anecdote was related: An old bachelor lived alone with only one servant in a large house, which he kept entirely shut up, so as not to come in contact with any one. Nevertheless, the master and the servant fell sick at the same time, and they felt sure that they were going to die of the raging disease. Under these hopeless prospects the master ordered his servant to go down into the cellar and fetch as many bottles of the best wine as he could carry, that they might both drown their sorrows, and try to forget their hopeless condition by drinking. The servant did as he was ordered, and they both kept on drinking till they fell into a heavy sleep. When they awoke next day they felt well again. Several other cases, where a beginning pernicious fever had been cut short by large quantities of alcoholic drinks, came to my recollection, and so I asked myself: What kind of diseases have been successfully treated by alcoholic liquors?

1. *Snake Poison.*—It is well known that the most dangerous cases of snake poisoning have been successfully treated with large doses of alcoholic liquors.

2. *Cholera Asiatica.*—Dr. Rubini's treatment with large doses of saturated spirits of camphor is well known to the older homœopathic practitioners.

3. *Typhus Petechialis* (Spotted Fever).—In 1864 Dr. James, of Philadelphia, published an account of sixty cases of spotted fever treated with alcohol, of which only one died (*North American Journal of Homœopathy*, 1864, p. 236).

Dr. James says, that when given at the beginning the alcohol treatment acted like a charm.

4. Rademacher states that in 1802 there was an epidemic of very dangerous *pleurisies*, for the usual venesections proved fatal in almost every case. Rademacher cured all his patients speedily and surely with Alcohol and Ether. From these facts, which might be augmented by a good many others, it would appear that alcohol is, indeed, a very powerful and very efficient remedy in some of the most dangerous miasmatic or contagious diseases, as also in cases of poisoned wounds.

I think that in all such cases a low alcoholic dilution of the specific homœopathic remedy in large and frequently repeated doses might be given with the best effect.

Before closing this short paper, I cannot help mentioning the use of the hot bath in fevers, and particularly in typhus. I have not yet seen a single notice of it in any of the homœopathic journals, although I have sent my observations to two of them. My friend and colleague, Dr. Siegrist, of Basle, first used it in typhus fever, and from its effects as observed by him, as well as from its results in the few cases in which I have myself tried it, I am confident that it is a great and most beneficial discovery in the treatment of fevers. We have both used the cool bath, cold affusions, frictions, etc., in many cases, and there can be no doubt that this treatment often succeeds very well; but it is very disagreeable to most of the patients, and if the cases be complicated with inflammatory affections of the respiratory organs, the cold bath, cold affusions, etc., will rarely be of service. On the contrary, the warm bath of 90–100° Fahr. is highly grateful to the patient, and the higher the fever the warmer he likes the bath. I am confident that those who have tried the warm bath in typhus fever, will not return to the use of the cold bath if it can be well avoided. After the bath, the patients should be wrapped up in a dry sheet, without being first rubbed dry, placed in bed and covered up until they become dry. As a rule they soon fall asleep, and the skin remains remarkably cool for many hours; whereas, the colder the bath the sooner reaction sets in, and the temperature rises again, rendering necessary a repetition of the bath every two hours for weeks together. The warm bath needs to be repeated not oftener than twice or thrice daily, and the disease is thereby shortened, and the recuperative powers of the organism saved. I am quite confident that if this method of treatment, which is strictly homœopathic, were adopted in cases of yellow fever, that disease would be shorn of many of its terrors, and homœopathy would rapidly gain the confidence of many who might never be convinced of its efficacy by the small dose of the drug selected in conformity with the law, *similia similibus.*

INCOMPATIBLES.

BY CHARLES MOHR, M.D., PHILADELPHIA.

TWELVE months ago I wrote an article entitled "The Incompatible Remedies of the Homœopathic Materia Medica," and read it to Drs. C. Hering and H. N. Guernsey, and finally to the Philadelphia County Homœopathic Medical Society, in the hope that it might suggest to our observing practitioners the desirability of making corrections and additions. At the society meeting the paper was not discussed, showing that very little attention had been paid to this subject. Later, in August, 1879, the paper was published in the HAHNEMANNIAN MONTHLY, and reprinted (with some additions) in pamphlet form, but up to the present time has not been instrumental in bringing out any new observations. Dr. T. P. Wilson, of Cincinnati, has written me a note commendatory, and in the *Organon* for January, 1880, a reviewer says: "It is a curious *fact*, the *rationale* of which we cannot yet explain, that certain medicines do not follow each other well, the second stopping the good effects of the first. This has been denied by the unobservant and careless, but Dr. Mohr gives here some striking instances of the truth of it, followed by a table of fifty-seven remedies, with their incompatibles. This is a field of observation which we should all do well to cultivate; there is yet much to be learned on this subject, and to all *thinkers* and *workers* this pamphlet will prove invaluable." Dr. T. C. Duncan, of Chicago, has written me: "The profession have occasion to thank you for your timely article on a subject that I have wondered Hering, Lippe, or some of the other *savants* have not more fully enlightened the profession upon."

We thus see that the subject is thought worthy of consideration, but nothing new has yet been published. Dr. C. G. Raue, however, has informed me that *Rhus tox.* and *Phosphorus* are *not* incompatible, but really compatible. Both he and Dr. Hering have frequently found them useful in typhoid fever, pneumonia, etc., prescribed after each other, of course when the symptoms indicated. On the authority of Dr. C. Hering (*vide* vol. ii, *Guiding Symptoms*), *Asterias rubens* should be added to my list, the incompatibles being *Coffee* and *Nux vomica;* also *Benzoic acid*, wine being incompatible. In a case of anæmia, recently under my care, in which *Ferrum phos.* was acting nicely, I found that *Paris quad.*, given for some adventitious eye symptoms, completely upset all the good the former medicine had accomplished. Are they incompatible? How can we tell unless observations are published, so that deductions can be made from an accumulation of facts?

I commend the study of this interesting subject especially to our younger physicians, who have time to make exact observations, and trust that whenever a medicine is found to stop the good effects of another, unless some other cause is found, it will be reported in our journals; and if, as was found to be the case with *Rhus tox.* and *Phosp.*, medicines have been erroneously considered incompatible with each other, let the fact be known, so that practitioners may be enabled to apply remedies with more precision and effect.

I notice that my use of the word incompatible in this connection, has been adversely criticised; but a study of Webster, Worcester, and more especialy of Smith's synonyms, as well as Roget's *Thesaurus*, gives me sufficient reason to justify the continuance of its use. Dr. C. Hering, himself, has adopted the word instead of "inimical," as will be seen by a reference to volume ii, *Guiding Symptoms*. I regret to find that this critic believes I stooped to do a mean thing when I spoke of the *United States Homœopathic Pharmacopœia* in words of dispraise (see HAHNEMANNIAN MONTHLY, November, 1879, page 678). I had no such animus as he imputes to me. My estimate of the book in question was made as early as October, 1878, when I referred to it as the "worst book," etc., to a class of students who desired to know what pharmacopœia to purchase, pharmacy being a new field of study to them. I was really wishing I could recommend the book, as a good work on pharmaceutics was sorely needed, but an examination revealed many faults. I found medicines peculiar to homœopathic pharmacy omitted altogether, or worse, the rules given for the preparation of some were not in accordance with those approved of by *authorities* in pharmaceutics in our distinctive school. It should be remembered that it is an essential feature of homœopathy that *medicines employed to cure the sick should be prepared as were the substances used in the provings.*

If the "worst"ness is pointed out, the promise is made that "it" will be expunged in a second edition of the *Pharmacopœia.* In my own copy there are so many annotations of errors of omission and commission that I fear if they are all corrected in a second edition, the *United States Homœopathic Pharmacopœia* will be a *new* book. It seems to me that a work on pharmaceutics, to be thoroughly reliable, should be published only by the authority of some such body as the American Institute of Homœopathy, the men working on it being versed in the natural sciences, and, practical pharmacists.

A RADICAL CURE WITH KALI BICHROMICUM.

BY DR. PROELL, OF NIZZA.

(Translated by S. LILIENTHAL, M.D.)

A NORTHERN lady, twenty-six years old, was sent by her physician to Nizza on account of her throat and chest affections. At a preceding consultation a high authority on physical diagnosis had said: "Whether she goes south or not consumption will soon finish her." The patient heard of it, and was therefore the more determined to try Nizza. From her father she inherited excessive nervosity, anxiety at the least ailment, irritability, and tendency to spasm, and was of a tearful disposition. As soon as she caught cold, and this happened frequently, *coryza and cough troubled her for a long time.* Several years ago she suffered from a severe *acute gastric and intestinal catarrh with ulcerations*, for which she took very large doses of Nitrate of silver. This ulcerative intestinal catarrh left her with a *great sensitiveness in the rectum and obstinate transient rheumatic pains, also a dangerous affection of throat and chest.*

The patient is a blonde, small figure, steel-gray eyes, oxygenoid constitution; of gracile, but not phthisicky habit; face slightly flushed; nasal mucous membrane irritable, either dry or secretes copiously a yellow mucus; eyes now healthy, often catarrh in the corners; teeth all destroyed (mercurial sequela), so that she wears artificial teeth; tongue clear at the tip, which is covered with red points, the root of it covered with a thick yellow coating; mostly great dryness of the mouth, alternating with salivation; gums livid; mucous membrane of posterior fauces and pharynx covered with red granulations, interlaced with white streaks and reaching down to the œsophagus. These white lines alternate with red ones (strongly injected bloodvessels). A troublesome sensation of constant irritation, as from a foreign body in throat, sometimes severe burning and scratching; tonsils and soft palate somewhat reddened; taste sour, often metallic; appetite good; great thirst, drinks black tea thrice a day; stomach bloated, with sensitiveness, fulness, and pressure; vomits sometimes; liver and spleen normal, the region of the rectum sensitive to pressure; urine very acid; stool mostly very hard and defecation difficult, (water injections cause pains and spasms, probably unabsorbed exudations from the time of ulcerations); dysmenorrhœa; pulse and skin normal. But the second principal seat of disease, or rather its localization, appeared to be the right upper (anterior and posterior) part of the chest, where percussion gave a dull sound, especially below the right clavicle. In the apex of the right lung weak rattling murmurs; the same symptoms on the left side, only weaker; cough mostly dry, but troublesome, especially in the morning after dressing and late in the evening; sometimes thick, tough, white expectoration; sensation of heat and titillation in the larynx before coughing, making her restless and impatient.

Three months in Nizza did not improve her much, though she took the full diet and was very careful not to expose herself unnecessarily. As the climate alone had failed to be of much benefit it was necessary to try other means, and as I considered the chief focus of her disease to be the abdominal mucous membranes; her diet was more restricted; all alcoholic beverages were forbidden, she was advised to take nourishment more frequently but less at once, and to live especially on eggs and milk, some bread and butter, and once a day rare meat. To quiet her nervous irritability and tendency to spasms she took Ignatia, fifth centesimal dilution, three times a day three drops, with good effect. Our radical remedy was *Kali bichromicum*, fifth cent., three times daily (five drops in 100 grams distilled water, every three hours half a teaspoonful). After two weeks slow and steady amelioration the tongue cleared up, the granulations in the throat diminished as well as the rheuma; features brighter, only the cough would not cease, though she took the tenth and thirtieth potency for three weeks. A more thorough examination revealed an old habit of hers, to sponge her chest with cold water every morning, and then to rub hard in order to bring on a reaction. I forbade this reactionary process on account of *ubi irritat, ibi adfluxus.* She kept on taking twice a day the thirtieth potency of Kali bichromicum, and the cough left her and she returned hale and hearty to her Northern climate.—*A. H. L., No.* 23, 1879.

January 6th, 1880.—A strong, hearty Irishman, of about thirty, came to the clinic and reported that during the day he is able to work and enjoys his breakfast and lunch, but for the last three years he has a complaint for which he took a great many remedies without any benefit whatever. He takes his dinner at 6 P.M., and about three hours afterwards he is seized with waterbrash, raises phlegm continually, vomits whatever food remains in the stomach, and rarely sleeps before midnight, as the phlegm chokes him; has cough, bowels rather constipated, stools hard and passed with some exertion. I had just read the case of Dr. Proell, and studied afresh this remedy. He received twelve powders Kali bichromicum, thirtieth, with directions to take a powder morning and evening and report.

January 12th.—He reports alleviation the first night, and constant and steady improvement since. He can sleep immediately on lying down, and begs for some more powders in case the trouble should return. Twelve powders Kali bichromicum, thirtieth, were given with orders to take a powder every second or third night, according to necessity.—S. L.

A CASE OF HYDRONEPHROSIS.

BY P. J. M'COURT, M.D.

November 22d, 1878.—Mrs. W., æt. 32, medium height, sanguine temperament, a lady of fine nervous organization, and highly cultured, called on me, by request of her physician. The closest inquiry as to the history of her illness elicited only the following: During the past four years, since her second and last parturition, she has suffered from dysmenorrhœa and menorrhagia, also from progressive corpulency and excessive prostration. At no time has there been renal pain or hæmaturia. She now weighs 180 pounds, 40 pounds above her normal standard.

At present her symptoms are: Great debility; dry, harsh skin; vertigo and almost constant headache, the pains shooting, in frontal and temporal regions; almost complete blepharoptosis (due, not to œdema of the lids, but to partial paralysis of the levator palpebræ superioris); spasmodic cough, with involuntary micturition; a fierce bulimia, which cannot be appeased by any amount of food; she complains that her load of flesh is crushing her, and that she "feels like a mass of blubber." Examination reveals a state of general œdema, but no pitting; heart normal; liver slightly congested; uterus somewhat prolapsed and crowded to the left; ovaries apparently healthy. On the right side, involving the hypochondriac, iliac, and, in a less degree, the umbilical regions, I find a large, bulging tumor; it is soft, almost painless, vibratory and lobulated; percussion yields a dull sound and distinct fluctuation. The left hypochondriac and iliac regions are likewise slightly tumefied, the sound somewhat dull, but fluctuation is not perceptible. Urine scanty, albuminous; specific gravity 1020 (owing, doubtless, to the very small quantity voided); a few tube-casts only are present; no blood or pus corpuscles visible; *no calculi*, nor evidence of their presence at any time.

I think the diagnosis of that extremely rare disease, hydronephrosis (Gr., from *hydor*, water; and *nephros*, the kidney) will not be questioned, and it has been caused, presumably, by pressure upon the ureters during pregnancy. The prognosis must, of course, be unfavorable, and the lady is informed that, while hoping to afford substantial relief, I cannot encourage her to anticipate a cure.

Causticum 6x, being the only drug which covers the totality of these symptoms is given, a dose every two hours, with orders to extend the intervals to three hours when urination becomes free.

November 26th.—The bulimia, cough, involuntary micturition, and blepharoptosis have completely vanished. The flow of urine is enormous; the entire body is bathed in a viscid perspiration of strong urinous odor, and the enlargement has diminished considerably. Headache and vertigo remain. In place of the bulimia, there is now anorexia, yet she feels much stronger. Soon after this the catamenia returns, and the function is free from pain and hæmorrhage for the first time in three years. Without change of medicine the lady makes steady progress until the 7th of February, 1879, when she is discharged without apparent vestige of the disease.

March 10*th*.—On the 2d instant, while walking over ice concealed by a light fall of snow, her feet suddenly slipped, and she fell, in a sitting posture, with great violence. Immediately the skin became dry, the urine scanty, general œdema reappeared, and the intumescence on the right side is nearly as large as when I first saw her. But the concomitant symptoms then noted are not present, nor any other which may serve to indicate a particular drug. Hence, in order to furnish the *experimentum crucis* as to its curative action over the pathological condition, *Causticum* is given as before. After a few doses had been taken, the skin became moist, and a free uriniferous perspiration followed, which continued to soak her clothing for several days. During the same night an abundant flow of urine ensued, and the swelling rapidly subsided. A week later, when the tumor was scarcely perceptible, a large abscess presented on the upper third of the *right* thigh, between the pectineus and adductor longus. Notwithstanding its immoderate size, the abscess matured and discharged with but slight general disturbance, and its healing appeared to be the signal of a perfect cure.

October 20*th*.—Mrs. W. informs me to-day that her health is perfect, far better than at any previous period of her life.

INCIPIENT HIP-JOINT DISEASE.

BY PROFESSOR J. E. JAMES, M.D., PHILADELPHIA, PA.

HIP-JOINT disease is a malady of such frequent occurrence, and is in its earlier stages so amenable to treatment, that an early recognition of its presence and a prompt adoption of the measures necessary to its cure cannot be too deeply impressed upon the mind of the practitioner.

The origin of the disease, whether in the synovial membrane, in the articular surface of the bones, or in other structures in and around the joint, we do not propose to discuss, as it is foreign to the intent of this paper. The causes of this affection have formed a subject of controversy among surgeons for many years. In former times it was considered a strumous or tuberculous disease entirely, and hence the treatment used was inadequate to bring about resolution before serious destructive changes had been wrought; while in later years, through the teachings of Professors Sayre, Bryant and others, the other extreme of considering the affection a purely local one has been so generally received that the treatment used, though attended with much better results, still fails to accomplish all that ought to be desired and expected.

In accordance with my own observations and belief the disease occurs much more frequently in scrofulous children than in those not of this diathesis. By scrofulous I mean those of a sickly, weak constitution, easily and quickly reduced in strength and health, of such low vitality that the recuperative powers are exceedingly feeble, with a tendency to glandular and bone affections generally. A blow or injury to the joint is very often the direct exciting cause, sometimes the only cause. It often, however, occurs when no traumatic origin can be made out; so that the two causes, constitutional predisposing and direct exciting, are present in many if not most of the cases. While this fact is denied in the text of many modern authorities, still in the treatment recommended it is tacitly admitted or at least provided for to a certain extent.

The disease is divided into three stages: 1st. Stage of irritation and inflammation. 2d. Stage of effusion and apparent lengthening. 3d. Stage of rupture and shortening.

The recognition of the disease early is of the utmost importance, for it is then that success in bringing about complete cures by resolution is most easily attained, and the means to be used are the most simple and easily applied. But because of the great apparent similarity between rheumatism, "growing pain," and the first stage of this disease, many without a careful and systematic examination are content to call it one or the other, and only recognize it after effusion and possibly suppuration has set in, and great impairment, if not destruction of the joint has taken place. A careful study of the early symptoms will enable the physician to avoid this mistake. It is to assist in attaining this desirable result that I write this paper.

The symptoms in the first stage are often very obscure, particularly in the chronic form of morbus coxarius, or that dependent mainly upon the scrofulous diathesis. The first symptom noticed will probably be a slight lameness and stiffness of the affected limb, observed mostly after rest, with slight flexion of the knee, the patient almost unconsciously standing in that position of rest to the affected side and putting the weight mainly upon the other limb. If any pain is felt at this stage it is most frequently referred to the knee or the thigh, instead of the hip-joint. This symptom should be carefully remembered, as it is one of the most constant, and its distance from the real seat of disease is calculated to mislead the physician. Any or all of these symptoms presenting in a case should lead to a careful examination. The patient should be stripped from the waist down, and the parts carefully inspected in a standing position first, when it will be easy to observe the peculiar position of rest to the affected side, the leg slightly flexed at the knee, and the foot slightly everted or parallel, causing a drooping of the pelvis and flattening of the buttock upon that side; the gluteal femoral crease will also be found to show evidences of obliteration in that it will be shorter, lower, and less deep than upon the sound side. (Upon this latter symptom Professor Gross lays great stress.) It is not completely obliterated until effusion has set in, and probably the second stage fully inaugurated. Another symptom may also be now noticed, that is, emaciation or atrophy of the thigh or entire limb on the affected side. This is not always well marked at first, but to a degree is almost, if not always, present, and is too frequently forgotten or too little significance is given to it; careful measurements of each limb will show this symptom when the eye will not. After thus examining, place the patient upon the back upon the floor or table, when, upon straightening the legs in a direct line of centre of body, and pressing them against the table, a marked curve upward of the spine will be noticed, causing a space to appear between the table and the back in the lumbar region, into which probably the thickness of a hand may be inserted. Now, upon raising the affected leg to a slight angle, or may be to a right angle in an aggravated or advanced case, the spine will straighten out and the processes will be found to be in contact with the table in its entire length. The moving of the sound leg will not affect the position of the spine in the least, as it moves freely in the joint. Complete flexion of the thigh as well as abduction, adduction, and rotation, will each show some impairment as compared with the opposite side, that is, if any of the movements natural to the joint are attempted to completion, the pelvis will be moved from the table or out of its direct line with the body. All of these symptoms depend upon a certain amount of rigidity which is always imparted to the muscles in consequence of the inflammation in the joint, and are early present and probably constitute the truest diagnostic signs, though no one symptom is sufficient for a certain diagnosis. Again, pain or tenderness upon pressing the head of the bone against the acetabulum is generally elicited. This is accomplished by pressing the femur upwards from different positions, pressure on the trochanter, or by gently tapping the heel when the leg is extended, or knee when it is flexed. Pain at the hip other than that caused by pressure or direct injury is not common in the first stage.

With this review of the symptoms I pass to the treatment of this most important stage of the disease.

Upon a diagnosis of hip-joint disease being made out, *the first and necessary thing is rest, general as well as local.* Many cases taken early and simply kept off their feet entirely for a few weeks, with, and sometimes without, the appropriate remedy, have been cured. Yet, as a rule, general rest, that is, keeping the patient lying upon a mattress bed, is not sufficient. It is safer always to add the local rest to the joint by means of extension and counter-extension. This is usually accomplished by means of the weight and pulley, fastened to the leg by adhesive plaster, and then elevating the foot of the bed sufficiently to cause the body to gravitate towards the head of the bed, a method which accomplishes both objects very effectually.

In the after stages, when general exercise and local rest are required, the apparatus of Sayre and others now in use are well adapted.

The object of the gradual extension is, first, to keep the parts of the joint separated from each other and thus remove a constant irritating cause, and, secondly, to overcome the rigidity and contraction of the muscles, thus preventing the deformity which is liable to result, and which may continue after the inflammation has subsided. With the exception of the above mechanical treatment, which is deemed essential, no local measures are of any real value.

To our remedies we owe much of the success attending this class of cases. I shall only give those that I have found curative in several cases each, and in the order of their more frequent use in my own cases.

Belladonna.—Lameness with pain at or near knee-joint; tenderness and pain in hip-joint upon concussion; heat and swelling over joint; sensation of weakness at hip-joint; worse in afternoon and evening with fever; drowsiness with restlessness; in two cases involuntary evacuations from bowels were promptly checked; in another, involuntary micturition as well as fæcal evacuation was promptly cured.

Stramonium.—When left side is affected (I have seen it curative in two cases on right side, no other remedy used except rest without extension, but its best and most prompt action is on the left side), especially when rigidity of the muscles is marked, starting during sleep as from pain; atrophy of thigh or leg; also indicated in later stage when suppuration has taken place accompanied with intense pain.

Rhus Tox.—Mostly when right side is affected; pain at knee worse after too much exercise; pain at hip on pressure over trochanter; involuntary and unconscious limping; affected by every change in weather, and worse at night.

Colocynthis.—Sharp, cramplike pain in sacrum or hip; cutting or crampy pain from hip to knees, causing him to limp; the least motion or touch aggravates; worse after sundown; better from rest and heat.

Arnica.—Especially useful after local injury; the pain is of a bruised, sore, or tearing character; bed is too hard, requiring frequent change of position; swelling is hard, hot, and shining.

The diet in hip-joint disease is of considerable importance. The patient should have good, nourishing, but unstimulating food, and as much of it as his system requires. Let him take milk, egg, beef tea, broths of chicken or lamb, with rice, barley and potatoes. To this kind of diet should be added, when the patient is much emaciated and reduced in strength, Cod-liver oil, extract of malt and beef, etc.

In the treatment of the peculiar constitutional condition which so often constitutes a predisposing cause of hip-joint disease, as well as in the more advanced stages of the complaint, a different line of remedies will, of course, be indicated. Their consideration, however, is not within the scope of the present paper.

NATRUM PHOS. IN GOITRE.

BY J. S. SKEELS, M.D., ALBION, ERIE COUNTY, PA.

WITHIN the last three years I have treated thirteen cases of goitre in young ladies, under twenty-four years of age, with *Natrum phos.* 3^x trituration, 3 grs. dissolved in a teacupful of water; dose, a tablespoonful three times a day. I continue the medicine until the pressure of the goitre is relieved, and then give it less often.

The feeling of pressure, made by the goitre, will be relieved in from three to five days; but I have usually continued the medicine from four to six weeks, and have then discontinued it until the pressure returns, repeating with each exacerbation until it returns no more.

In some instances the tumor will be removed within two years. In all my cases the patients gained in flesh, strength, and spirits shortly after commencing to take the medicine.*

ACCIDENTAL PROVING OF NUX MOSCHATA.

BY E. M. HOWARD, M.D., CAMDEN, N. J.

A YOUNG married lady was advised by some old woman to take nutmeg and whiskey for delayed menses, with the assurance that it would bring them on, whatever might be the cause of the delay. She placed one ounce of finely ground nutmeg in half a pint of whiskey, and after letting it stand about 12 hours drank off the liquid just before retiring for the night. She went to sleep, but was awakened some time in the night with præcordial anxiety and an intense burning sensation in the pit of the stomach. She rapidly grew worse, thought she was dying, and sank into a semi-unconscious condition, in which I found her at 8 A.M. Her pulse was 130, respiration oppressed, face ashy-pale, and eyes sunken. She seemed to understand what was said to her, and would commence to answer a question, but forgot what she was saying in the middle of a sentence. Coffee, black and strong, was ordered, but it was with the greatest difficulty we could get her to take it. She said she dare not move for fear she would become unconscious. Under its use, however, she began to improve, and subsequently I obtained the following subjective symptoms which she experienced: Her memory was entirely gone, (this impairment lasted several days); she could not connect any train of thought. It seemed too much trouble to think. Voices of persons in the room sounded far in the distance, and words spoken to her seemed as if spoken a long time before. Objects in the room appeared multiplied in different sizes; for instance, she saw several bureaus, one above the other, each larger than the one below. Her head felt as if it were many times its natural size, and there was a drawing sensation in the back of the neck, drawing the head backwards. She did not dare move her head for fear she would become unconscious.

---

* In reply to our inquiry Dr. Skeels informs us that the use of the above remedy was suggested to him while treating for scrofulous ophthalmia a lady who had a large goitre. She was taking Natrum phos., and one day remarked to him: "When I take this medicine my neck feels better." "How better?" "It does not feel so pressed." Here, then, we have a clinical symptom which experience tends to confirm.—EDS.

She did not dare yield to a strong impulse to sleep from a fear that she would die. There was a sensation as though her brain was constantly whirling around, and a throbbing or pulsating feeling in every part of the body. A week afterwards this was still felt in both ovaries. She lost all feeling in every part of her body, excepting the head, only when she moved, even the eyelids, something like an electric shock would run all over her, seeming to start from the small of the back. This numb or dead feeling of the body was also relieved if any one touched her. Although she felt that she could not move, if by great effort she did so, she would be surprised at the power she had.

On the following day she complained of small, sharp, cutting pains in both ovarian regions, and of a dull pain in the small of the back. Her stomach felt empty, as though she must have something to eat, but when food was brought she could not eat it. Her bowels moved very freely and copiously. Her urine had been very profuse, and smelled strongly of nutmeg, and she had a profuse, greenish, acrid leucorrhœa. For several days subsequently her bowels were costive, and evacuations were preceded by cramps in the abdomen. The stool was small and narrow, and she seemed to have a lack of expulsive power. She also complained of deficient power in deglutition, and food would stop in the œsophagus, or go down very slowly. She had a sensation as though some one was scraping her back between her shoulders. Always when sleeping, either day or night, she was troubled with dreams of sexual excitement, and awoke weak and exhausted, with a swollen sensation in the ovaries. The throbbing continued in the ovaries, although not felt in other parts of the body, and the whirling sensation in the brain continued to a limited degree. She has also been troubled with stammering, which she had not been addicted to before. All these symptoms have gradually yielded to treatment, but the catamenial function has not yet been re-established.

HOMŒOPATHIC MEDICAL SOCIETY OF THE COUNTY OF PHILADELPHIA.

REPORTED BY C. MOHR, M D., SECRETARY.

THE regular monthly meeting of the Society was held at Hahnemann Medical College, on Thursday evening, January 8th, 1880, the President, Dr. E. A. Farrington, in the chair.

By vote the HAHNEMANNIAN MONTHLY was made the organ of the Society.

The Bureau of Materia Medica, Pharmacy, and Provings, H. Noah Martin, M.D., Chairman, made a report, embracing Notes on Materia Medica, by Clarence Bartlett, M.D., and Erythroxylon *Coca*, by B. B. Gumpert, M.D. and H. Noah Martin, M.D. (See present number.) The papers were accepted and the following discussion ensued:

Dr. Martin said the patient whose case was described in his paper was perfectly free from any lung or heart disease. He had used *Coca*^{30} in the case, but it had no apparent effect. He asked Dr. Morgan to state the results of *his* observations of the case.

Dr. Morgan stated that he had seen the patient mentioned by Dr. Martin, and found him suffering from bilious, watery vomiting, and vertigo. *Bryonia* did very well for his acute symptoms, but the patient went to work as soon as he improved. After certain movements of the head and certain uses of the eyes, there was aggravation. The patient was astigmatic, and was fitted with glasses by Dr. C. M. Thomas. He was inclined to believe that the whole trouble was due to a myopic astigmatism. *Silicia*, *Conium*, and other remedies were given to the patient with varying success. Just before the patient went North he received *Magnesia phos.*, which has been found very useful for vertiginous and other troubles connected with optical defects. He (Dr. Morgan) thought that the use of *Coca* was very promising in the treatment of progressive pernicious anæmia.

Dr. Dudley had used *Coca* in two cases of inebriation. It stopped the craving for liquor, kept the patient from going on a spree simply by its stimulating effect, acting as a temporary substitute for alcohol. He administered it in the form of fluid extract, about twenty or thirty drops at a dose.

Dr. Martin had cured a young lady of the symptom, "sensation as of a string pulling the eyeball back into the head," with *Croton tiglium* 2^c. He had also relieved the sensation as of cold air blowing under the eyelids with *Fluoric acid.*

Dr. Mohr related a case of chronic debility in a lady. Marriage and pregnancy improved her condition, and after her confinement she was making a good recovery, but during the nursing period she became again debilitated and had to wean her child. Under any excitement or exertion her face flushed and she complained of a burning spot on the right side of the spinal column in the region of the kidneys; urine normal; no heart or lung trouble. Under *Ferrum phos.*^{12} she improved, and was about well. After some weeks she again reported, suffering from a sensation as though the eyeball was drawn back into the brain. *Paris quadrifolia* was given, when all her old anæmic symptoms returned. Dr. Mohr thought that he had spoiled the case by prescribing *Paris quadrifolia.* It is a mistake to prescribe for *one* symptom of a group. *Sulphur,* which has a similar eye symptom, might have followed the first prescription well. As this sensation in the eyes is frequently complained of, it may be well to bear in mind that besides *Hepar, Paris q., Crot. tig.,* and *Sulph., Asterias, Bovista, Chamom., Plumb., Rhodo., Silica,* and *Strychnia* have each a similar symptom. Dr. Mohr also reported the case of a child suffering from symptoms which led him to give *Ipecac* with relief. They returned so frequently, however, that he made investigations, and discovered that the wallpaper of her room contained arsenic.

The President called for the experience of the members in spleen affections, a subject suggested by a remark in Dr. Bartlett's paper.

Dr. Morgan, in response, stated that a number of physicians had reported to him in favor of *Bryonia.* Dr. Mitchell, of Chicago, praises the *Arsenite of quinia. Polymnia* has also been praised. As regards *Hydrastis,* he had found developed by the drug the symptom, "small wounds bleed much."

Dr. Sartain gives *Hydrastis* in debilitated conditions, but she never gives it near the menstrual period because it is apt to bring on premature and profuse flow.

Dr. Williamson thought that it was important to know the cause of enlargement of the spleen; if from congestion, it ought to be cured; if it depends upon an attack of intermittent fever, the case is not more hopeful than the cure of amyloid degeneration due to venereal taint.

Dr. Martin finds *Hydrastis* to be a good remedy in constipation and indigestion. Often in giving *Hydrastis* for catarrhal troubles, he had found it to cure a constipation or indigestion before touching the catarrh.

Dr. Mohr mentioned a case of enlarged spleen after intermittent fever in which the patient was always worse in damp weather. *Aranea diadema,* prescribed by Dr. E. A. Farrington, reduced the size of the spleen. He thought that *Hydrastis* would eventually become one of our polychrests. He described a case of typhoid fever marked by the characteristic rise and fall of temperature, and for days before the attack a feeling of entire goneness in the pit of the stomach, with no desire for food whatever. After taking to his bed he had abdominal tenderness, gurgling in ileo-cœcal region, with bloated abdomen, delirium at night, and a feeling that he could not recover (compare *Ranunculaceæ*). *Hydrastis*[30] was given, and in less than forty-eight hours, there was a most marked improvement, and the man made a good recovery.

Dr. Morgan had been using *Hydrastis* in fissure of the anus. In one case he had used the hard-rubber pile pipe, for the purpose of keeping the anus stretched, at the same time filling the pipe with oil or Glycerin containing *Hydrastis* tincture in the proportion of four drops to the drachm, and giving the first dilution internally. He had also used *Hydrastis* in cancer of the breast. The tumor with the exception of the nucleus disappeared. The disease went on to a fatal termination from inanition.

On motion of Dr. J. C. Guernsey the discussion of the report of the Bureau of Materia Medica was closed, and the Society took up the consideration of some prevailing diseases.

Dr. Guernsey said that he would like to know what remedies were useful in the prevailing throat troubles. He had found *Lachesis*, *Mercurius sol.*, and *Lycopodium* to do very well in the majority of cases; but had just had a very stubborn case, that of a lady, subject to quinsy. She had a throbbing sensation in her throat. He gave her *Hepar sulphur*, afterwards *Lach.*, and finally *Kali bi.* Various symptoms were thereby ameliorated, but she did not get well. The voice became more and more indistinct. The pain in the throat increased. This morning she talked unintelligibly. She discovered that pieces of skin came away from her throat. Her tongue looked as if covered with mucilaginous cream, with white edges. The posterior part of the throat had a pale whitish cast. He thought of giving her *Apis*, but she lacked the *Apis* pain. He also noticed a peculiar *rattle in the mouth.* He prescribed for her *Lac caninum* 100^{m}. This evening she was much better, and showed it by a most happy expression of the face. Dr. Guernsey wanted to know if other members of the Society had observed this rattle.

Dr. Sartain asked Dr. Guernsey if the patient had regained her voice?

Dr. Guernsey said that she could talk very clearly in the evening, whereas in the morning only a word here and there could be made out.

Dr. William B. Trites gave the history of a case to which he was called on the 1st of January. The patient was a lady. She was unable to speak above a whisper. Her symptoms indicated laryngitis. On the following day, when examining the expectoration he noticed that it contained a portion of diphtheritic membrane. While visiting the patient she was seized with a suffocating attack. The face became almost black, the cough was violent, and in a little while brought up a complete cast of the trachea, at least five inches in length. After this she felt more comfortable. The next morning she brought up another cast. On Sunday she died amidst intense suffering. He would like to know the experience of the gentlemen present in regard to the value of tracheotomy in diphtheritic croup. In answer to a question by Dr. Morgan, Dr. Trites stated that there was no membrane on the fauces or pharynx.

Dr. Charles M. Thomas said that he had a number of times been called upon to tracheotomize patients affected by what was supposed to be membranous croup. He did not think the results very brilliant. Out of ten cases, two had been saved. In all cases, where death resulted, it set in as in an ordinary case of diphtheria, apparently with symptoms of blood-poisoning. There was no difficulty in breathing. After the operation, in all cases, relief was marked.

Dr. Martin, in answer to Dr. Guernsey's question, said that nearly all the cases which he had seen were those of simple sore throat. Every case which he had seen complained of great dryness of the throat, especially in the morning. The remedies for this symptom are *Apis*, *Bell.*, and *Phosphorus*. For a number of years past, when a patient sent for medicine for sore throat with no particular symptoms, he has been in the habit of prescribing *Apis*, and with uniform success.

Dr. Sartain said that she had found *Apis*, *Causticum*, and *Sanguinaria* useful in throat troubles. She also stated that she had found *Baptisia*² or ³ to abort an attack of quinsy and to render a recurrence of the disorder less probable. "It cures quinsy and the disposition to quinsy."

Dr. Morgan said *Ferrum phos.* was a good remedy in inflammation of the lungs if no other remedy was indicated; there should, however, be a little fever and a good constitution. In regard to *Lac. caninum* the characteristic of the symptoms is their erratic disposition. In regard to the milk remedies he reminded his fellow-members that, aside from their organic constituents, they contained solutions of various salts which we recognize as among our most potent remedies.

The President reappointed Dr. H. Noah Martin, chairman of Bureau of Materia Medica, etc., for another year. Adjourned.

A CASE OF HYDROPHOBIA AND ITS TREATMENT.

THE Philadelphia daily *Times* of Sunday, January 18th, 1880, contains a graphic account of a case of hydrophobia which recently occurred at Delaware City, Delaware, and which, in view of the character of the phenomena occurring in connection with it, and the nature and results of the treatment adopted, is deemed worthy of record in the pages of a medical journal. The account was, of course, prepared for general public reading, a fact which will explain the familiar nature of the phraseology in which the symptoms are presented and which we transcribe.

About the beginning of December, 1879, Mr. R. G. A., a highly respected business man, was bitten upon the cheek by a dog which proved to be rabid. At the same time another dog was bitten by the same animal, and this dog subsequently died of hydrophobia, a fact which was carefully concealed from Mr. A. It seems, however, that the victim neglected no remedies. Dr. Mitchell cauterized the wounds and would have excised portions if the patient had permitted, but the real rabies of the biting dog had not then been established, and, indeed, was not until the bitten dog was seized. He took the powerful blood alteratives prescribed, and with praiseworthy faith took two of Dr. Townsend's pills, one of which has wrought a perfect cure (?) whenever taken heretofore. Guyer's Elecampane root and milk were consumed in the prescribed doses at the proper time. His throat became a thoroughfare for every remedy that promised exemption from the disease. From the day that he was bitten it seemed as if he had made up his mind to meet any fate with resignation, and if he cherished any apprehensions nobody could detect it in his manner, which was cheerful and chatty as before.

He had undoubtedly been apprehensive about the ninth day after the biting, which popular superstition assigns as the critical period. That day past, he seemed to throw fears aside, and never entertained them again until he was already far advanced in the disease. The premonitory symptoms actually appeared on Tuesday, January 13th; he had a slight chill that day, which was followed by pains in his back. These were attributed to torpid liver and remedies were taken accordingly. Wednesday brought shortness of breath, palpitation of the heart, and a heaviness of spirits. Wednesday night he was very restless, sleeping little, but resolutely repressing his nervousness, so that his wife's rest might not be disturbed. Thursday his habitually cheerful face was clouded by a look of distress and apprehension. The morning bath was passed by. "I can't touch it!" he cried, falling back with spasmodic energy, of which he was not himself aware. The morning cup of coffee was declined with nervous loathing, and the wife's fears were excited.

When Dr. Mitchell arrived he found his patient sitting up, with an evident look of anxiety on his face, and the cheek upon which the wound was received, together with the eye on the same side, and the nose, were swollen. He felt his pulse and started to touch the cicatrix of the wound made by the dog's teeth, but Mr. A. started back with an aversion that he could not restrain. "Don't touch that side," he said hurriedly, pointing to the wounded cheek. He permitted Dr. Mitchell to touch and handle the other cheek without manifesting any distaste, but the moment his fingers moved across the nose a spasmodic jerk placed the cheek out of reach. Large doses of Morphia, Bromide, and Chloral were prescribed, but the aversion to liquids seemed to render him unable to swallow them except by a supreme effort, and three or four attempts were made before he succeeded in swallowing half the dose. When the patient had begun to feel easier from the effects of the anodyne, he went to his factory to attend to business. A customer was there to whom he sold a carriage. This transaction consumed an hour, and left him feeling much worse. He returned to the house and was persuaded to try another dose of the anodyne. The spasmodic aversion was less easily conquered, but his nerve went to the extent of swallowing half the dose. Again relief was experienced, but the patient did not feel disposed to return to business again. He complained of intense thirst, but could not conquer his aversion to water. Ice was suggested, but he had as great difficulty in carrying that to his mouth as though it had been liquid. By closing his eyes he got a lump between his teeth, which closed upon it with a snap that split it like an ice pick. He swallowed the fragments with great effort. The anxious expression had been intensified into one of agony. Starting from quiescence his eyes would roll up with terrified stare, as though he saw some frightful vision which he sought to shut out with his extended upturned hands.

From this time the anodynes were administered subcutaneously at short intervals, but without much apparent effect. The danger of violent spasms was becoming more imminent with every hour, and the Morphia was injected with greater frequency. "I am burning up inside, can't you do something for me?" he implored with vehemence. At 4 A. M. on Friday, 18th, violent convulsions suddenly set in, when Chloroform was administered and temporary quiescence secured.

When the effects of the Chloroform had passed off, he again complained of the violent burning in the stomach, and begged his attendants to kill him to relieve him of his intolerable torture. The spasms recurring, straps and bandages were resorted to to prevent him from injuring himself, and Chloroform, with hypodermic injections of Morphia, were freely used. At 11 A.M., when the sufferer was recovering from the effects of Chloroform, one-third of a grain of Woorara was injected subcutaneously. Muscular relaxation followed within ten minutes, and the best auguries were indulged in by the physicians. At the end of an hour, signs of recurring spasms led to a repetition of the Woorara, but instead of producing a cumulative relaxing effect, it at once excited him. Chloroform was again administered with some effect, and then in three-quarters of an hour after the second dose of Woorara, a third was given, containing one-half a grain. Again it proved a violent excitant, and was supplemented by Chloroform. It was exhibited five times with only cumulative exciting effect, and was then abandoned finally.

The most distressing symptoms now manifested themselves. Whenever the patient passed into his frequently-recurring spasms his jaws snapped and salivary froth spurted from his mouth. That was even while under the influence of Chloroform. On awaking from his unconsciousness his piteous prayer was still for death or some relief from the terrible internal burning sensation which tortured him. The final spasm seized him between 7 and 8 P.M. Nervous force was then nearly exhausted. The ropy, viscid, mucus-like saliva, which always characterizes the disease at some stage, began to exude and cover the lips. The patient now was fast becoming past the power of Chloroform. He yielded readily to it, but the recurrent spasms followed more closely on its administration. As the mucus collected in the throat his efforts to breathe had a sharp, yelping sound, that to the nervous might easily have been mistaken for an attempt to yelp like a dog. The physicians said that the sound had no other origin than that named. His recovery from the unconsciousness produced by the Chloroform made his breathing more labored, and the effort, clogged by the obstructions in the throat, made the sound. During his last three hours the drug was given him every ten minutes. At ten o'clock it became evident that vitality was nearly exhausted. Circulation became very slow in the extremities, the pulse was hardly perceptible, and the throbbing of the heart could hardly be detected. At 11 P.M., after all pulsation had been suspended for a minute or more, he breathed twice and his tongue protruded. The eyes, which had been strained upward and backward until little more than the whites were visible, closed naturally. The face was still distorted as it had been, but life had ceased. It was a case of death from nervous exhaustion.

The physicians have found some things to confirm and some things to contradict the dicta of the books. One thing seems clear, namely, that an inoculated human being cannot germinate the poison within thirty days, which is the short limit laid down. In Mr. A.'s case, with the favoring condition of a place well supplied with blood, it required forty-two days.

It has been thought that the nervous irritation of the wounded spot is an unvarying symptom. The exterior lesion was in the cheek, at least an inch and a half away from the nose, but all the nervous irritation was in the nose itself, although that may be accounted for to some degree by sympathetic irritation from the swelling of the cheek extending to a very sensitive surface.

At times the pulse showed surprising alternations, from 80 to 150 and back within two minutes. His case showed that Woorara, so far from being a counteracting principle, has an aggravating action in hydrophobia. More than all, it shows the hopelessness of a well-defined seizure, whether the remedies be officinal or quack.

All the physicians agree that this could not possibly have been one of the cases of hysteria and subsequent nervous collapse because of dread of inoculation. It was genuine hydrophobia, if there ever was a case.

LETTER FROM DR. CLARKE.

To the Editor of the HAHNEMANNIAN MONTHLY.

SIR: Will you allow me to apologize to your readers, as I have already done to Dr. Dudgeon, for the errors in my letter which appeared in the October issue?

For the mis-spelling of Dr. Dudgeon's name, my bad writing must share the blame with your printer's bad reading. For the rest, the blame rests with me. It was merely a *lapsus pennæ*. I wrote "*soft*," meaning, all the time, *hard*, as might have been inferred by the subsequent remarks about "secondary symptoms."

I can only account for the error by the fact that we do sometimes unwittingly say the opposite of what we mean, and put down "left," when we intend to say "right."

Apologizing for my blunder,

Yours, respectfully,

JOHN H. CLARKE.

IPSWICH, January, 1880.

LETTER FROM DR. WINSLOW.

PITTSBURGH, January, 1880.

EDITORS OF HAHNEMANNIAN MONTHLY: The ink is dry upon my editorial quill, but I have a rusty steel pen yet by me for trenchant work. It is probable the "*nullius addictus jurare*" crowd never heard of the Phœnix that arose from the ashes, or they would not have been so anxious to cremate me and scatter my dust for telling the truth about them. Fortunately for the cause of truth, I still have breath sufficient to blow off their tinsel and expose their shallow pretensions.

Though I have lent my voice to the party of progress, which shall yet purify our Materia Medica, and make homœopathy to accord with the principles of the sciences, I have also pointed out the folly of a reliance upon clinical experience alone, and the perils of palliation to the exclusion of homœopathic treatment, as recommended by some teachers. The admirable exposition of Dr. P. P. Wells in his letter to Dr. Hughes, published in the *North American Journal of Homœopathy*, had my public and hearty indorsement, and mild as was Dr. Hughes's eclecticism, I considered it my duty to oppose it. Surely I could do no less than to assail the organization known as the "Modern School," with its whitewashed allopaths and its all-kinds-of-pathic principles.

The prime movers of that delectable corporation, who think to smother criticism and annihilate opponents, have yet to learn that the homœopathic school is composed, rank and file, of as great a proportion of educated and able men as the old-school profession, and they do not intend to have homœopathy dragged in the mud by novices, nor the Buffalo school held up as a model institution of their beloved system. The Erie County Society was right in excluding persons from its membership who, according to their public avowals, were *not* homœopaths, any more than the school they manage is homœopathic in aught but the name, and this official protest against wrong ought to have the moral support of the whole profession.

What a beautiful homœopathy is set forth in "S. N. B.'s" article in the new school journal! How consistent the bold avowals of mongrelism in the introductory address are, with the name "Homœopathic!" How modest the comparisons of the initiatory struggles of the "Modern School" with those of Cornell! There is too much *consciousness* of greatness for the genuine article,—too great an *assumption* of omniscience for the presence of omnipotence. Students thirsting for the knowledge of our beautiful system may go east or west, and find bubbling springs and sparkling fountains of truth; but let them not be deluded by promises of universal medical knowledge in two terms of *four months* each; for in proportion as they acquire palliative and antipathic principles will their homœopathy deteriorate, and they be blinded to a proper appreciation of the simplicity and reliability of Hahnemannian homœopathy.

Yours, in the faith,
W. H. Winslow, M.D.

OVARIAN TUMORS.

The following letter is commended to the consideration of our readers:

Philadelphia, January 1st, 1880.

Dear Doctor: From the frequency with which small cysts are found in the ovaries of young children and infants after death, and from the difficulty experienced in tracing the origin of these tumors to any definite cause after birth, it is reasonable to suppose that they often arise from defects in the *development* of the ovaries. If this is the case it seems probable that these defects are as often corrected by homœopathic treatment as are those found in other parts of the body; and, therefore, we may infer that ovarian tumors occur less frequently amongst those who have habitually used this system of medicine from childhood than amongst those who have used the other practice. As the history of a large number of patients who have suffered from ovarian tumors is the only evidence from which correct conclusions can be drawn, you are most earnestly requested to furnish such answers to the questions annexed as will give the information necessary, and oblige,

Fraternally, B. F. Betts, M.D.,
17th and Girard Ave., Philadelphia, Pa.

1st. Name and address of patient?
2d. Character of tumor—whether cystic or solid?
3d. Treatment of—by operation or otherwise?
4th. Results of treatment?
5th. Age at which tumor was first recognized?
6th. Did the patient have homœopathic treatment during childhood, or when did she first use it habitually?
7th. Remarks.

THE

HAHNEMANNIAN MONTHLY.

A HOMŒOPATHIC JOURNAL OF

MEDICINE AND SURGERY.

Editors,

E. A. FARRINGTON, M.D. PEMBERTON DUDLEY, M.D.

Business Manager,

BUSHROD W. JAMES, M.D.

Vol. II. Philadelphia, Pa., February, 1880. No. 2.

☞ The Editors consider themselves responsible for the maintenance of the dignity and courtesy of the journal, but *not* for the opinions expressed by its contributors.

Editorial Department.

BOOK-MAKING.—Rapid progress in medicine and other sciences necessitates the frequent issue of books. And when they set forth the views of trustworthy and competent investigators, they become an indispensable addition to every physician's library. But to merit favor, books must be for the most part original, clearly written, free from pedantry, and eminently practical, rather than theoretical. Ambitious men, influenced by base pride, and a still meaner class who worship the almighty dollar, court the enviable reputation of successful publications and flood the market with trashy imitations. By means of copious quotations from standard works, together with numerous plagiarisms, they give their lucubrations the appearance of excellence and worth. Thus they succeed in deceiving many. Good advice is contained in the answer which a certain party made to the importunities of an agent for the sale of a new organ: "Well, I'll wait awhile. If your instrument is what it pretends to be, competent judges will pronounce favorably on its merits." "But," interrupted the disappointed agent, "if every one were to follow your plan, we should not sell a single instrument." "Do not fear; there are plenty foolish enough to listen to your praises, and I desire to wait and profit by their haste."

In homœopathy especially, do we fear an unwholesome spread of the mania for bookmaking. Our science is so pre-eminently practical that it cannot be expected to grow rapidly. Provings may, indeed, be multiplied almost without end, and if observers are but conscientious in their reports we shall never be at a loss for material with which to institute experiments. But the growth of confirmations and characteristics must ever be slow, and the nicest discrimination is requisite in their selection. He who has accustomed himself to weigh in the balance, drug provings and clinical cases, must have often noticed the discrepancies between them. Perhaps the remedy has cured, but not on account of the indications by which it was selected. Perhaps the clinical symptoms which have been incorporated with a drug-proving are genuine, but frequently they are not. Elated with success, the physician reviews his case to determine what wrought the happy results. He hits on certain unique or peculiar symptoms, which promptly disappeared after administering the medicine, and immediately records them as characteristics. Their publication in some journal leads to their early appropriation by the bookmaker, and thus they become a part of our literature. We are not of the number who exclude cured symptoms, but we do, nevertheless, deprecate the reprehensible practice of adopting them unqualified. They should be retained in the private collection of the physician, there to await the oft-repeated test of clinical confirmation before they can deserve public confidence.

The remedy for book plethora is to be found in the careful application of the sound principles of homœopathy, together with a consistent restraint upon self-pride and love of money. He who knows how to make characteristics is the one least likely to abuse them, for he applies them according to fixed rules. His characteristics do no violence to provings, but merely emphasize and expand what is partially expressed in them. If he adopts cured symptoms, he does so because they accord with the genius of the drug employed, and have, moreover, received additional confirmations.

A Misstatement Corrected.—Dr. E. M. Hale desires us to correct the statement made in the December Hahnemannian, page 766. He writes us that he has never recommended *Gallium* in diphtheria as there recorded.

If your "Journal" does not come regularly or properly

directed send a postal card notice of the fact to the business manager. All who have paid their subscriptions will get their receipts with the March number.

CORRIGENDA.—In January number, page 28, twenty-fourth line from top, for "pityriasis" read "phthiriasis."

On page 30, fourth line from bottom, the title of Dr. Neidhard's paper should be "*Germ* Theories of Disease."

Page 52, second line from top, for "Mahan" read "Meehan."

Book Department.

THE CLINIQUE. A monthly abstract of the Clinics and of the Clinical Society of the Hahnemann Hospital of Chicago. Published by authority of the Hospital Board. Volume I, No. 1.

There can be no doubt that one of the best methods of studying the therapeutic action of drugs, and the modes of applying surgical means to the cure of disease, is by witnessing their application at the bedside; and next to this method comes free access to the records of such applications and of their results. Our medical colleges and journals are fully alive to the importance and significance of this truth. And the managers of the Hahnemann Hospital, appreciating its force, have commenced the publication of *The Clinique*, whose title sufficiently indicates the purpose of its issue. The first number, now before us, is filled with records of cases treated in the hospital and elsewhere, and is of course pre-eminently practical. The journal presents a neat and attractive appearance, and its 32 pages monthly can be obtained at the reasonable price of $1.00 a year. Correspondents can address Dr. C. H. Vilas, Treasurer, No. 56 E. Washington Street, Chicago. We wish the new journal success.

THE NEW YORK OPHTHALMIC HOSPITAL REPORT for 1879 is before us. It shows an excellent clinical record, embracing over six thousand cases treated.

Under Appendix C we notice the announcement of the twenty-eighth course of lectures, under an able corps of professors. The school has the legal right to confer the degree *Oculi et Auris Chirurgus*. Candidates must have been in practice at least one year after graduation from some medical college.

THE MEDICAL RECORD VISITING LIST, OR PHYSICIANS' DIARY for 1880. New York, William Wood & Co.

This visiting list, besides the usual blank forms for daily practice, and alternate pages for special memoranda, vaccination, obstetric and other engagements, contains also a list of doses of drugs used in subcutaneous injections, of doses of common and rare drugs, of drugs suited for atomization, inhalation, etc. of disinfectants, etc. It also gives compact directions for the examination of urine; for antidoting poisons; for emergencies and the treatment of asphyxia; and the preparation of Lister's antiseptic solutions. An exceedingly compact and convenient book. The Philadelphia office is at 929 Chestnut Street.

TRANSACTIONS OF THE HOMŒOPATHIC MEDICAL SOCIETY OF THE STATE OF NEW YORK. 1879. Volume XV, No. 5, N. S. Price, $1.00.

This book is a compact volume of about 300 pages, plainly printed, and bound in stiff paper covers.

It contains sixty-eight articles, arranged according to subjects, in four parts. The second part contains reports of bureaus, embracing all departments of medicine, and in addition a section on necrology.

Among its many interesting papers may be mentioned an exhaustive article on "The Secondary or Immediate Causes of Death," by Dr. W. Y. Cowl; "Medical Notes on the Treatment of Mental and Nervous Diseases," by Dr. S. H. Talcott; "Fourteen Remedies in the Treatment of Insanity," by Dr. W. M. Butler; "Treatment of Iritis," by Dr. W. P. Fowler; "Duboisia," by Dr. C. Th. Liebold; "Infantile Constipation," by Dr. C. M. Conant; "Diseases of the Umbilicus," by Doctress J. G. Brinkman, etc.

Dr. H. M. Paine's article, entitled "An Examination of the Doctrine of the Minimum Dose, and the Theory of Dynamization promulgated by Dr. S. Hahnemann," occupies thirteen closely printed pages, which might have been more acceptably filled. In his violent opposition to the doctrine of dynamization, he has denounced Hahnemann as a fanciful theorist, who, mayhaps, was "endeavoring to play a huge practical joke upon his professional associates, in order to test their credulity, by reciting, Gulliver-like, an account of his fanciful musings." No more telling criticism can be made on such a paper than that which appears on page 36 of the *Transactions*. Dr. H. Amelia Wright sarcastically remarks: "It seems to me that the author has made a mistake in presenting his paper *here*. I should think that it properly belonged in the society that met here about a week ago. The doctor evidently must have been behind time."

Dr. Mitchell, in his article on Phytolacca, gives excellent indications for the employment of this drug in diphtheria, mastitis, boils, etc.

Dr. Conant differentiates carefully between Carbolic acid, Creasote, and Petroleum.

We are pleased to see so goodly a portion of the book devoted to the important subject of the management of the insane. There are five articles in this section, which will repay careful perusal. Especially suggestive are the papers on the treatment of mental aberrations. Nervous diseases are alarmingly on the increase, but with our Materia Medica well stocked with confirmed symptoms, we can promise all the benefit that can possibly accrue from medical treatment.

Specialties are the order of the day, and we observe the names of several, who have gained considerable reputation in their respective departments.

But we could have wished for more than one paper from the able Bureau of Otology. And we rather lament the status of homœopathy, as exemplified in the proffered treatment of laryngeal diseases. Some of the indications are very good, as, for instance, those calling for Arsenic, Kali bich., Carbo veg., etc.; but it is the so-called adjuvant treatment, which exposes either the inefficiency of our art or its imperfect application. We think, the latter. F.

The Physicians' and Surgeons' Investigator. A Monthly Journal, devoted to the Best Interests of the Profession. Edited by the Faculty of the College of Physicians and Surgeons of Buffalo, N. Y. S. W. Wetmore, M.D., Editor in Chief. S. N. Brayton, M.D., Managing Editor. January, 1880. Vol. I, No. 1.

The above is the title by which this new candidate for journalistic honors will be known by its publishers. By everybody else it will be called the Buffalo *Investigator*, to distinguish it from its older namesake of Chicago, a circumstance which, we think, should have been sufficient to determine the choice of some other title.

In attempting to review an uncompleted work, like the one before us, it is very desirable to learn, first of all, the circumstances and motives which have led to its publication, and, secondly, the platform or policy which is to govern its editorial management.

On page 2 of the cover we find a prospectus announcing that

"The *Physicians' and Surgeons' Investigator* is published as the exponent of Rational Homœopathy. It is the Champion of the True Science of Medicine, and will ever sustain the principles of Right, irrespective of party, pathy, creed, or dogma."

If the question "What *is* rational homœopathy?" were already solved to the entire satisfaction of the profession, or even of a majority thereof; if there were no differences of opinion amongst honest, educated physicians as to what constitutes "the true science of medicine;" if all were agreed upon the exact and unvarying principles of "right" that should govern the medical man in all his beliefs, his relations, and his actions, there could scarcely be a more firm and enduring basis upon which to build up the prosperity of a medical journal than the one thus laid down.

In the Salutatory, pages 1 and 2, we are told that

"The members of the profession who are familiar with our principles, as evinced in former monographs, will readily anticipate our object. To those unacquainted with our platform, suffice it to say that we have taken a bold step in advance of the professional vanguards, and promulgated the principles of *liberality*."

Of the "former monographs" alluded to, we happen to know of but two (unless the *First Announcement of the Homœopathic College of Physicians and Surgeons of Buffalo, N. Y.*, is to be considered an additional one). Of these, one is entitled "A Therapeutical Inquiry into Rational Medicine," by S. W. Wetmore, M.D., formerly Professor of Descriptive and Surgical Anatomy in the Medical Department (allopathic) of Wooster University, Cleveland, Ohio, and for many years Demonstrator of Anatomy in the Medical Department (allopathic) of the University of Buffalo, Member of the Erie County Medical Society, the Buffalo Medical Association, etc.

In the preface to this monograph we see that it is addressed "to the student of medicine who is searching for truth, and the reasonable, liberal, rational portion of the medical profession." Further, it interests us somewhat to observe that "it is . . . . the result of some twenty-five years of earnest pupilage and *less than two* of careful and close observation of *the law of correspondence.* It was written at the earnest solicitation of many of our old-school friends, who are desirous to disseminate the principles of modern therapeutics and the present outlook of *rational* medicine. The principal object has been to simplify as much as possible the law of *similars,* and by a few practical examples to illustrate the application of a *rational* therapeutics."

This monograph, then, appears to have been intended for old-school physicians and students, for the purpose of bringing homœopathy before them as constituting a part of a rational system of therapeutics, and the text of the monograph confirms this idea. On page 3 of this pamphlet, the writer alludes to his other paper, entitled, "What is Modern Homœopathy?" This paper was also intended for allopathists, for it was read before the Buffalo Medical Association, though it afterwards (February and March, 1878) appeared in the *American Observer.*

These two papers, then, together with the announcement of the Homœopathic College of Buffalo, an institution in which the editor of the *Investigator* holds the positions of Dean and Professor of Surgery, ought to give us a pretty good idea of the opinions which are likely to control the new journal in medical matters. Going back, therefore, to the "Therapeutical Inquiry into Rational Medicine," we find in its preface the following significant language. The italics are ours.

"We trust, however, that the few 'mile posts' we have set may serve to guide and stimulate the energetic and earnest student to his whole duty in the investigation of *all* methods of treating disease in the most thorough manner possible; in which event *he will not be apt to acknowledge that he is an exclusive,* or that he is an allopath, an eclectic, a hydropath, uropath, thermopath, electropath, *or a homœopath,* but a doctor of the rational school of medicine—a physician in the full and most noble sense of the term"

We also find in the paper entitled "What is Modern Homœopathy?" the following declaration of principles. (See *American Observer,* vol. xv, p. 137.)

"I have no penchant for homœopathy. Nevertheless, if I find by actual experience that Hahnemann's remedies, administered in accordance with his law, *or any other,* more remedial, I shall have no hesitation to bring them into requisition, whereupon some Rip Van Winkle, some inimical, captious, critical 'cuss' will probably feed me with the bread I have so often cast upon the water. *With the same propriety I might be called a hydropath, or uropath, or thermopath, as a homœopath;* the while I am still an *all*-opath, and doubtless always will be, though free to select from all sources, at the risk of being considered heretical."

We do not feel called upon to add any comments to the above quotations. Our readers are perfectly competent to judge of their force and significance for themselves. It is worth while, however, to ask how a physician whose "investigation into all methods of treating disease" have not made him willing "to acknowledge that he is an exclusive or a homœopath," should yet be willing to hold the position of Dean in a college which insists upon calling itself *homœopathic.* If the physician, who selects what seems to him best from all systems, cannot consistently take the name of homœopathist, how can his college, in which he teaches the doctrines on which his practice is based, take the name which he declines to accept? Or, remembering the statement in the Salutatory of the *Investigator*, that the "object" of the journal may be inferred from the "monographs" from which we have quoted, how can a physician who refuses to be hampered by the shackles of a homœopathic title, consent to edit a journal in the interests of "rational homœopathy" and as the champion of the "true science of medicine?"

Quoting again from the Salutatory we read as follows:

"We believe that any society, school, or sect that is fettered by any distinctive dogma, creed, pathy, or ism, so much as to ignore that which experience has taught to be good (and not unfrequently indispensable), is subject to the most severe criticism, for they certainly do not promote the best interests of humanity, the art of medicine, or the school which they represent. Believing, as we most sincerely do, that the law of similars is the true and most scientific method of treating morbid conditions, we must, as honest and honorable servants of the people, admit its limitation, for it is still in its infancy and necessarily imperfect. It will be our aim to promote the best interests of homœopathy by encouraging a more thorough education in the collateral sciences, and a more perfect understanding of the *therapeutics* of the 'old school.'"

If we understand the above syllogism it means that if we believe homœopathy to be the "true and most scientific method of treating disease," we shall "promote its best interests" by teaching our students "the therapeutics of the old school."

There are in the journal under consideration, and in the "former monographs" a number of allusions, besides those quoted, to the proud independence of all creeds and pathies which has been attained by the publishers of the *Investigator*,—the Faculty of the *Homœopathic* College of Physicians and Surgeons of Buffalo. These men "have taken a bold step in advance of the professional vanguards." It usually happens that the men who are "taking steps in advance of the vanguard" of a victorious host belong to a routed, retreating enemy.

One of the most offensive features of the new journalistic and collegiate enterprise is its pretension to what it is pleased to call "liberality." We "have promulgated the principles of liberality." "It will be seen that our platform is broad, generously liberal," etc. (see Salutatory). These men are apparently making the very common mistake of confounding a broad, perhaps an indefinite, creed with liberality. If their creed (and they must and will have one, either ready-made or home-made)—if their creed happen to be a many-colored patchwork affair, composed of fragments torn from a number of other creeds, it does not follow that those who accept it are any more liberal than the followers of the narrowest and most exclusive dogma that ever was devised. Liberality depends not on breadth of view, but upon a due deference to the opinions of men who hold different views. This true liberality is scarcely manifest in such passages as the following: "Our platform is based upon true principle;" "All candid, honest, thoroughly educated, self-thinking men can stand with us consistently;" "Our only apology for introducing ourselves to the medical profession in the garb of the schoolmen of Alexandria, when there is already a multiplicity of medical journals, is *to exhibit the 'actual truth'* which exists in the practice of the 'modern school of medicine'—*rational homœopathy*," (see Salutatory); or this from the College Announcement: "For many years the 'Queen City' has felt the necessity of a *liberal* medical school which would instruct *unbiasedly* in the system having for its guide the law of correspondence or similars;" or this from the preface to the Therapeutical Inquiry: "It is not expected that our convictions and conclusions can be transferred to the minds of others, *for they may be too timid to accept*, or *too indolent to investigate* for themselves." What do our readers think of the above as manifestations of a liberality to be bragged about?

The journal contains a readable article by Dr. A. A. Hubbell, on "Diseases of the Ear in General Practice;" also an article by S. N. B., in which the writer advocates the use of alternated remedies, and recommends the administration of Baptisia throughout the duration of typhoid fever, as a specific for the poison of the disease, while the *indications* are "met with a second or even a third medicine." We are not told whether this is a sample of "rational homœopathy" or not. In conclusion we are afraid that the physician, hungry for the nourishment that shall strengthen him for his daily work, will not be able to find in the pages of the Buffalo *Investigator*, Vol. I, No. 1, the material for a good square meal.

D.

Gleanings.

TAYUYA is recommended for scrofula and syphilis. Fifteen cases of the latter disease and one of ulceration of the lip, of uncertain origin, are reported cured.—*Exc.*

LAPARO-ELYTROTOMY.—This comparatively new operation was eminently successful under the charge of Dr. W. R. Gillette. Complications were, the subsequent need of forceps, version, and finally of craniotomy, and yet the mother recovered.—See *New York Medical Journal*, January, 1880.

RUDIMENTARY KIDNEY.—Dr. Stimson has presented to the New York Pathological Society a kidney in a rudimentary condition. There was no renal artery on the corresponding side, but there was a renal vein. The ureter measured from the bladder, six inches, and then terminated in a slender cord to the kidney.—*Exc.*

MICROSCOPIC LESIONS IN THE KIDNEYS.—Dr. Seiler is of the opinion that it is very difficult to decide in post-mortems whether organs are absolutely healthy or not. He examined a large number of human kidneys microscopically, and failed to find any perfectly healthy except those obtained from infants when they are first flushed with urine. In the adult domestic cat the kidneys are always fatty.—*Exc.*

Acute Yellow Atrophy of the Liver.—In yellow fever the liver is increased in size; in acute yellow atrophy it is diminished. The most characteristic signs of the latter malady, in addition to the size of the liver, are cerebral disturbance, scanty, albuminous or suppressed urine, epithelial and granular casts in the urine, deep jaundice, high temperature. The disease is most frequently found among women, especially during pregnancy. Dr. Loomis thinks it an albuminoid hepatitis.—*Exc.*

Delivery Impeded by Cicatricial Tissue.—The patient had convulsions. After a long time the cervix was sufficiently dilated to warrant the use of forceps. But even moderate traction brought down the uterus. Cicatricial tissue was then found extending across the upper and anterior half of the cervix, like a piece of whip-cord and undilatable. The important lesson is, caution against the rapid and violent use of the forceps.—*Exc.*

Handy Antiseptic Surgery.—A writer in the *Medical Tribune*, January, 1880, recommends the free use of dilute alcohol as a convenient antiseptic dressing for wounds, and after surgical operations. He thinks the practice of antiseptic surgery is considerably older than Lister, and cites as an example the Good Samaritan's treatment—oil and wine—of the man who "went down from Jerusalem to Jericho and fell among thieves."

Damiana in Prostatitis.—A patient was put on ℨss. doses of the fluid extract of Damiana, twice daily for impotency. At the end of three months he reported himself relieved, but "with a discharge from the genitals not unlike gonorrhœa." There was tenderness and inflammation along the whole course of the urethra, attributed by the attendant to the muco-purulent discharge from the prostate. Gelsemium, fl. ext., relieved the trouble in a few days.—See *Medical Tribune*, January, 1880.

More Allopathic Homœopathy.—Dr. Murrell, of the Westminster Hospital, reports in the *Western Lancet* having used Dover's powder in fifty-five cases of nightsweating in phthisis, with relief in all the cases but five. This report excites the *Medical Tribune* to the profound remark that "the use of a sudorific to check sweating may seem paradoxical." If the *Tribune* and the *Lancet* could only recognize the existence of a principle in nature under which all disordered actions can be similarly relieved, their patients would have cause to sing a paradoxology.

The Climate for Consumptives.—The air must be both dry and pure, and a cold bracing climate is far preferable to a warm one. Variations in temperature are altogether of secondary importance. A moderate amount of elevation above the level of the sea is also a requisite. Among the numerous locations advised is Aiken, S. C., 585 feet above the sea. The mean winter temperature is 48.59° Fahr., the soil and air are as dry as at any station east of the Rocky Mountains. The average relative humidity is 59 per cent., while that of St. Paul is 68 per cent.—*Exc.*

Tea-testing.—Dr. S. Lilienthal writes us that a patient whom he was attending in consultation, and who was a tea-tester, finally became so deranged that he was sent to the insane asylum. On the days he tested a line of Japan teas he would lie awake most of the night with excessive nervousness and irritability followed by great depression. He was also an inveterate smoker. But, as Dr. Lilienthal remarks, tobacco affects far more the cardiac nerves than the cerebrum itself. In spite of careful homœopathic treatment at the Middletown Asylum the patient has not yet improved.

Preventing Conception.—The alarming prevalence of this crime among the married, as well as among the victims of illicit intercourse, has led many of our ablest men to denounce the crime. Quite recently Dr. William Goodell has reported a case of elongated cervix uteri, traceable to this cause.

"If you ask me," he says, "what I think of this interference with the due course of nature, I tell you very candidly that I always hold it to be a very great sin. . . . . I hold that the woman who thus attempts to thwart the proper consequences of coition becomes a man's mistress, and is no longer his true wife."—*N. Y. Med. Journ.*, Jan., 1880. This noble sentiment is found also in Dr. Goodell's recent work on Gynæcology.

TYPHOID FEVER demands a diet of liquids, farinaceous food and bread in some form. Milk must not be used in unlimited quantities, as it sometimes lies in curds in the stomach and bowels, provoking vomiting, restlessness, flatulency, etc. Give freely of pure water. The frontal headache, common in the earlier stages, is sometimes relieved by cold applications, while in other cases warm are needed. When even a trace of blood is noticed in the stools, keep the patient in the recumbent position and restrain defecation as long as possible. In profuse sweating, dry the skin frequently and place dry cloths between the wet linen and the skin. Death has occurred from asthenia when the nurse has carefully covered up the sweating patient and so eveloped him in a vapor-bath. (From an address by Sir William Jenner.)

SCARLET FEVER: ITS STATISTIC FEATURES.—In an article on scarlet fever in the current number of the *Medical and Surgical Reporter* of this city, Dr. Sozinskey says:

"Scarlet fever does not come and go like Asiatic cholera, yellow fever, and several other destructive diseases; it is a lingering pestilence. For over fifty years the city of Philadelphia has never been free from it."

And the writer also says: "A remarkable feature of scarlet fever is the secular variation in its degree of prevalence from year to year, which is noticeable. In an article on epidemical cycles, in the *British Medical Journal*, September 1st, 1877, Dr. Ransome shows that this disease prevails to an unusual degree every fifth year. This law is very observable in the records of it in Philadelphia. The number of deaths from it each year, for sixteen years, is as follows:

Year	Deaths	Year	Deaths
1864	349	1872	174
1865	624	1873	319
1866	491	1874	461
1867	367	1875	1032
1868	224	1876	328
1869	799	1877	359
1870	956	1878	554
1871	262	1879	336

"The probability is very strong, then, that it will be very prevalent in 1880."

MORTALITY OF PHILADELPHIA, 1878 AND 1879.—The following statement, compiled from the weekly returns of the Board of Health, shows the number of deaths in Philadelphia during 1879 as compared with the number in 1878.

Months.	1879.	1878.	Months.	1879.	1878.
January,	1,748	1,536	July,	1,885	1,945
February,	1,363	1,225	August,	1,345	1,244
March,	1,468	1,202	September,	1,099	1,127
April,	1,250	1,222	October,	1,159	1,086
May,	1,052	1,366	November,	1,016	1,153
June,	1,006	1,200	December,	1,082	1,192
				15,473	15,498

Decrease in 1879,—25.

News and Comments.

AMERICAN INSTITUTE OF HOMŒOPATHY, BUREAU OF PÆDOLOGY.—The Bureau of Pædology of the American Institute of Homœopathy has selected "The Diseases of the Digestive Apparatus" for papers and discussions at the meeting of the Institute, to be held in Milwaukee next June. The papers of the Bureau will be presented in the following order, viz.,—

W. H. Jenney, M.D., of Kansas City, Mo., Chairman.—"Acute Gastritis," Anatomical Characteristics, Causes, and Diagnosis.

W. Edmonds, M.D.—Prevention and Treatment of the same.

J. C. Sanders, M.D.—"Stomatitis," Anatomical Characteristics, Causes, and Diagnosis.

A. M. Cushing, M.D.—Prevention and Treatment of same.

R. J. McClatchey, M D.—"Gastromalacia," Anatomical Characteristics, Causes, and Diagnosis.

W. Danforth, M.D.—Prevention and Treatment of same.

T. C. Duncan, M.D.—"Thrush," Anatomical Characteristics, Causes, Diagnosis, and Treatment.

S. P. Hedges, M.D.—"Gangrene of the Mouth," Anatomical Characteristics, Causes, Diagnosis, Prevention, and Treatment.

Mary A. B. Woods, M.D.—"Dietetic Rules to be Observed in the Treatment of Diseases of the Digestive Organs."

BUREAU OF GENERAL SANITARY SCIENCE, CLIMATOLOGY, AND HYGIENE.—The special subject for discussion at the meeting in June, 1880, at Milwaukee, will be "Quarantine."

The divisions of the subject have been assigned to members of the Bureau, and papers promised as follows:

A. R. Wright, M.D., Buffalo, N. Y., Chairman (no paper).*

1. "International Quarantine," Bushrod W. James, M.D.
2. "National Quarantine, including Seacoast Quarantine," George M. Oakford, M.D., Burlington, Vt.
3. "State and Local Quarantine," W. H. Leonard, M.D., Minneapolis, Minn.
4. "Quarantine for Refugees, Exposed to an Epidemic of any kind, by River, Railroad, or Wagon-way," D. H. Beckwith, M.D., Cleveland, Ohio.
5. "Disinfection of People, Cargo and Baggage in Quarantine," M. S. Brury, M.D., ——, Me.
6. "Summary of Quarantine Laws, Rules, and Regulations of Different Commercial Nations," E. U. Jones, M.D., Taunton, Mass.
7. "The Cordon Sanitairé," George A. Hall, M.D., Chicago, Ill.
8. "Sanitation and Location of Quarantine Stations," L. A. Falligant, M.D., Savannah, Ga.
9. "Kinds of Quarantine Required for the Different Contagions," G. W. Barnes, M D , San Diego, Cal.
10. "Quarantine of Mailable and Circulating and Easily-Transportable Material," Lucius D. Morse, M.D., Memphis, Tenn.

From these reports, synopses will be made and submitted as a basis for discussion by members of the Institute.

All the information that can be gleaned that is useful and novel upon this topic is desired by the Bureau.

BUSHROD W. JAMES, M.D.,
Chairman *pro tem.*

N. E. Cor. 18th and Green Streets, Philadelphia, Pa.
January, 1880.

---

* A. R. Wright, M.D., having resigned on account of ill-health, has no paper. Dr. B. W. James was appointed to act in his stead.

PROFESSOR LUDLAM is preparing a thorough revision of his work on the diseases of women.

HAHNEMANN MEDICAL COLLEGE OF CHICAGO.—The twentieth annual commencement exercises of the Hahnemann Medical College and Hospital of Chicago will be held on the evening of February 27th. Professor Hawkes will deliver the valedictory.

UNIVERSITY OF MICHIGAN.—Professor Charles Gatchell has resigned the chair of Theory and Practice in the above-named institution, in order to enter upon general practice in Milwaukee.

Professor T. P. Wilson, of Cincinnati, has been elected to fill the vacancy created by Professor Gatchell's resignation, and has removed to Ann Arbor with his family. He will have charge of the Eye and Ear Department of the new hospital, and engage, as formerly, in the practice of his specialty. He will also continue to edit the *Medical Advance*.

ALLEGHENY COUNTY HOMŒOPATHIC MEDICAL SOCIETY.—At the annual meeting of this Society, held December 12th, 1879, the following officers were elected to serve for the ensuing year: President, C. P. Seip, M.D.; Vice-President, R. E. Caruthers, M.D.; Treasurer, C. F. Bingaman, M.D.; Secretary. T. M. Strong, M.D.; Censors, L. M. Rousseau, M.D., W. R. Childs, M.D., and W. J. Martin, M.D.

THE HOMŒOPATHIC MEDICAL SOCIETY OF CHESTER, DELAWARE, AND MONTGOMERY COUNTIES, at their annual meeting elected officers as follows: President, Trimble Pratt, M.D.; Vice-President, W. A. D. Pierce, M.D.; Secretary, L. Hoopes, M.D.; Corresponding Secretary, R. P. Mercer, M.D.; Treasurer, C. Preston, M.D. The address of the Corresponding Secretary is Chester, Delaware County, Penna.

THE CHILDREN'S HOMŒOPATHIC HOSPITAL OF PHILADELPHIA will, by direction of the Board of Lady Managers, observe February 27th as "Donation Day." It will be just the right time for the physicians of the city and neighborhood, and their friends, to pay "that visit" to the institution, N. E. corner of Eighth and Poplar streets, in order to inspect its workings, get acquainted with its managers, make a donation suited to the needs of the hospital or the enjoyment of its little sick folks, and become a part of its organization.

NATIONAL BOARD OF HEALTH—ANNUAL REPORT.—The Board has expended to December 31st, 1879, $154,002.42. Besides this, 10,000 copies of the Report of the yellow fever experts, 1878, including maps of about one hundred cities and towns, will cost $8459.33, and the Reports of Drs. Bennis and Cochran and Colonel Hardee will cost $15,810.20, or a total of $24,269.53.

We wonder if the Report of the Homœopathic Yellow Fever Commission is to be included in this Report.

The estimates for 1880 are, to June 30th, . . .	$234,330.00
From June 30th to December 31st, ...	202,060.00
Total, ...	$436,390.00

About $290,000 of this is for quarantine maintenance and improvements.

MARRIED.—NORTON—PARTZ.—On January 7th, at the residence of Prof. Oswald Seidensticker, by the Rev. J. Richards Boyle, CLAUDE R. NORTON, M.D., of Philadelphia, to CONSTANZA L., daughter of Dr. A. F. W. Partz, of Paris, France.

MCKINSTRY—BOILEAU.—At the residence of the bride's parents, January 29th, 1880, by Rev. W. H. Conard, Dr. FRANK P. MCKINSTRY, of Bound Brook, N. J., and JENNIE K., youngest daughter of E. B. Boileau, Esq., of Southamptonville, Bucks County, Pennsylvania.

THE

HAHNEMANNIAN MONTHLY.

Vol. II., New Series } Philadelphia, March, 1880. No. 3.

Original Department.

THE MEDICAL PROFESSION IN ITS RELATION TO CRIMINAL ABORTION.

BY ROBERT J. M'CLATCHEY, M.D., PHILADELPHIA.

It is my purpose to present for your consideration this evening, the subject of the attitude assumed by, or which should be assumed by the medical profession in regard to criminal abortion, especially from two standpoints, viz., 1st, the attitude which the profession should assume towards the crime of procured abortion *per se* and in general; and, 2d, the duties of physicians in individual cases of criminal abortion. I have prepared the paper by request, and with the hope that it may enable some to more thoroughly establish themselves in the right way of thinking on this subject.

The term *Abortion* in medicine means the expulsion of the contents of the uterus before the sixth month of pregnancy; and if expulsion takes place after that period and before the ninth month is completed, the woman is said to have had a *premature labor;* but in *law* the term abortion is applied to the expulsion of the fœtus at any time prior to the full term of pregnancy, and hence is synonymous with the popular term, *miscarriage.*

The cause of abortion may be either *natural* or *violent.* The criminal abortion results only from the latter of these causes.

A very great deal has been written on the subject of Criminal Abortion, and its prevalence has been adverted to as one of the crying evils of the times. Whether it be more common now than it was a number of years ago, is a question which might be considered as disputable, but I shall not discuss it here. The generally received opinion is that it is practiced to a greater extent than ever in this country, and that in the matter of cheating the state of its population by means of procured abortion and its confederate wickedness—sexual fraud —the United States equals ancient Rome in its worst days. This much may be said on this point, however, that the medical literature of fifty years or more ago, while treating of abortion and its causes, rarely refers to criminal abortion, and it is not until many years later that we find the matter discussed. While this may be significant of the infrequency of the occurrence of criminal abortion among our ancestors, on the one hand, it may on the other simply show a want of knowledge on the part of our professional predecessors.

Let this be as it may, physicians practicing in cities or in towns or country places can all bear abundant testimony as to its very frequent procurement by physicians, midwives and others, notwithstanding that it is generally regarded as a sin, and known to be a crime in the eyes of the law. It *is* a crime against the state, inasmuch as it lessens population in a greater or less degree, and it is a crime against morals, religion and the laws of the land.

Criminal law in its relation to criminal abortion speaks very plainly: "Whoever shall unlawfully supply or procure *any poison or other noxious thing*, or *any* instrument or *thing* whatsoever, knowing that the same is intended to be unlawfully used or employed with intent to procure the miscarriage of any woman, whether she be or be not with child, shall be guilty of a misdemeanor; and being convicted thereof, shall be liable, at the discretion of the court, to be kept in penal servitude for the term of three years, or to be imprisoned for any term not exceeding two years."* "Every woman, *being with child*, who, with intent to procure her own miscarriage, shall unlawfully administer to herself any poison or other noxious thing, or shall unlawfully use any instrument or other means whatsoever with like intent, and whosoever, with intent to procure the miscarriage of any woman, whether she be or be not with child, shall unlawfully administer, etc., shall be guilty of felony."

The law was laid down thus in 1858, in England, by Baron

* Taylor's Principles of Medical Jurisprudence, vol. ii, p. 198, loc. cit.

Bramwell: "If a man, for an unlawful purpose, used a dangerons instrument, or medicine, or other means, and thereby death ensued, that was murder, although he might not have intended to cause death, although the person dead might have consented to the act which terminated in death, and although possibly he might very much regret the termination that had taken place contrary to his hopes and expectations. This was wilful murder. The learned counsel for the defence had thrown on the judge the task of saying whether the case could be reduced to manslaughter. There was such a possibility, but to adopt it would, he thought, be to run counter to the evidence given. If the jury should be of the opinion that the prisoner used the instrument not with any intention to destroy life, and that the instrument was not a dangerous one, though he used it for a lawful purpose, that would reduce the crime to manslaughter. He really did not think that they could come to any other conclusion than that the instrument was a dangerous one if at all used. Then, if it were so used by the prisoner, the case was one of murder; and there was nothing for the case but a verdict either of murder or acquittal."*

Judge King, of this city, ruled as follows: "Every act of procuring abortion, contrary to the usual interpretation of the law, is murder, whether the person perpetrating such an act intended to kill the woman, or merely feloniously to destroy the fruit of her womb."

Authorities without number might be quoted to show in what estimation criminal abortion is held by the law, but the above suffice to show that it is looked upon as a heinous crime: "a foul and unnatural crime, not only against society, but against a helpless, innocent and defenceless life—one of the most cowardly acts a man can perpetrate—since 5½ or 6 feet and ten or twelve stone are pitted against a few inches and less than half a stone in weight."† It will be seen, too, that the *intent* to procure abortion, whether it be successful or not, and whether the woman be pregnant or not, and no matter who the guilty party may be, including the woman herself, are taken into account by the law, and not with a view of lessening or condoning the offence. It is to be borne in mind, too, that it is a legal axiom that ignorance of the law is not to be pleaded as an excuse for its violation.

In view of all these circumstances, it seems strange that

---

* Woodman & Tidey's Forensic Medicine and Toxicology, p. 662.

† Loc. cit.

criminal abortion is so common, and especially strange, when we consider that this great crime is committed with the *consent*, at least, of members of that gentler sex to which crime is generally an abhorrence, and even of those who stand high in the community, and to whom the thought of crime in any other guise would never come. There are reasons for this, and they are doubtless to be found in an improper view regarding the time at which the product of conception becomes a living human being; a view which is fostered by the conversation and conduct of some members of the profession, who allow themselves, against their better judgment, to give a half or a whole consent to erroneous opinions, and who fail to do their duty in the matter of duly impressing upon the minds of their *clientèle* the true state of the case.

The opinion entertained by many women, that the embryo begins its life at the time of the so-called "quickening," is doubtless traceable to the old rulings of the English laws, which referred to the time when a woman was "quick," and when she was "not quick." This has been handed down from person to person year by year, and is at this day a popular falsehood used for base purposes; a falsehood fruitful in sin and crime, and not respectable on account of age nor because it is still recognized in some criminal codes. There are many women who give themselves up to the commission of abortion before the fruit of their womb has reached the period of "quickening," laying the flattering unction to their souls that unless that period of pregnancy has arrived the destruction of the fœtus is no great matter, who would not, under any consideration, have it performed *after* that time, as they would then regard it as murder. And those who consent to the procurement of abortion after quickening are those who are willing to be *particeps criminis* in a murder rather than carry the fœtus to term.

No opinion can be more fallacious than that which looks upon the "quickening" as the beginning of life in the fœtus. It must be either *alive* or *dead*. If there is life at the time of quickening, there must have been life from the commencement; for if, on the other hand, the embryo is not alive, but is dead, at the time of or shortly after conception, it remains dead, and there is no power on the part of the mother to impart life to it.

The learned Professor A. E. Small, of Chicago, formerly Professor of Physiology in the Hahnemann Medical College of Philadelphia, referring to the life of the fœtus, writes as follows: "In order to arrive at the conclusion that embryotic life exists from the commencement to the end of pregnancy, it is not necessary to set up the claim of sentience and will, as some writers have done. For while perfection of endowment does not exist with the embryo, its independent life can be conceded, with prophetic endowments for future development, in the womb and after birth, of all the attributes of human perfection. We must concede this, if anything, for how can the embryo merge into the fœtus without a perfectly independent excito-motory system, distinct from that of the mother? If we admit this, we are brought directly to the conclusion, that the existence of a distinct and independent nervous centre must be as self-acting and living as that of the mother.

"If we have succeeded in proving the existence of fœtal life, before quickening has taken or can take place, even though but the beginning of undeveloped faculties, the inalienable rights of a human being are implied, and this should compel us to believe that unnecessary abortion is a crime."

On this point, also, Dr. Horatio R. Storer, of Boston, writes: "Common-sense would lead us to the conclusion that the fœtus is, from the very outset, a living and distinct being. It is alike absurd to suppose identity of bodies and independence of life, or independence of bodies and identity of life; the mother and the child within her in abstract existence, must be entirely identical from conception to birth, or entirely distinct. Allowing, then, as must be done, that the ovum does not originate in the uterus; that for a time, however slight, during its passage through the Fallopian tube, its connection with the mother is wholly broken; that its subsequent history is one merely of development, its attachment merely for nutrition and shelter—it is not rational to suppose that its total independence thus once established, becomes again merged into total identity, however temporary; or that life depending on nine months' growth, or in birth, because confessedly existing long before the latter period—since quickening, at least, a time varying widely as to limits, dates from any other period than conception.

"Another argument is furnished us, but differing. The fœtus, previous to quickening, must exist in one of two states, either death or life. The former cannot take place, nor can it ever exist except as a finality. If its signs do not at once manifest themselves, as is generally the case, and the fœtus is retained in utero, it must either become magnified or disintegrated,—it can *never become vivified.* If, therefore, death has not taken place, we can conceive of no other state of the fœtus save one, and that, namely, life, must exist from the beginning.

"These reasons are strengthened by the reasoning from analogy. The utter loss of direct influence by the female bird upon its offspring, from the time the egg has left her, and the marked effect originally of the male. The independence in body, in movement and in life, of young marsupial mammals, almost from the very moment of their conception, identical analogically with the intrauterine state of other embryos—nourishment by teats merely replacing that by placenta at an earlier period; the same in birds, shown by movement in their egg, on cold immersion before the end of incubation. The permanence of low vitality or of impaired or distorted nervous force, arising from early arrest or error of development, and necessarily contemporaneous with it, are all instances in point."

Very pertinent to this matter also, are the words of the celebrated homœopathic physician and author, Dr. William H. Holcombe, of New Orleans, who says:

"The true *scientific* position is this: From the moment of conception, when the spermatozoa coalesces with the cell-wall of the ovule, the ovum is a distinct human being, with a human soul, simply attached to the mother for the attainment of nutritive material, but growing, living, organizing, by forces and powers entirely its own, and derived through nature from God.

"The true *moral* position is this: The destruction of this ovum is always homicide, justifiable, perhaps, under a few extraordinary and painful conditions, after the failure of all reasonable medical and surgical means, and then imposing such solemn and fearful moral responsibilities that it should only be accomplished after the mature deliberation and concurrent advice of several respectable members of the profession."

The above beautiful and forcible expressions of Holcombe exhibit the views that *must* be held by all physiologists, and that *should* be held by all persons. From the moment of conception, when the ovule of the mother has had brought into contact with it that necessary element to its fructifying found in the semen of the male, and fecundation has taken place, that ovule becomes a new, independent being, and through nutrition and growth is converted into the embryo, the fœtus, the babe, the child, the man, and is from the outstart the receptacle of a living soul, which grows with its growth and strengthens with its strength. To destroy its life is to murder a living human being, and there is no sophistry capable of glozing over the ruggedness of this truth, or of lessening the degree of this crime.

This is the doctrine of the Roman Catholic Church, as promulgated first, I think, by St. Augustine. It looks upon conception as the commencement of life of a new being, and the wanton destruction of that life as murder; and the members of that denomination of Christians are remarkably free from the crime of abortion, according to the testimony of a very large number of physicians.

It is the duty of physicians to instruct their patients in these matters at every fitting opportunity, and no doubt this is done by a very large majority of the members of the medical profession. But there are physicians, in good standing, who act as though it was their duty to keep the truth concealed, and even to give "aid and comfort" to such of their patients as have procured or are desirous of procuring a miscarriage. I do not now refer to that large class of miserable wretches who are known as abortionists, but to that smaller class who, while they would scorn to produce an abortion by instruments or other appliances, and who would feel that they had had a deadly insult offered them if they should be termed abortionists, would, nevertheless, under certain circumstances, do something "to bring on the courses" of a patient in whom the menstrual flux had failed to appear for two or three consecutive months.

Such a practitioner reasons with himself about as follows: Here is a patient whose menses have failed to appear for two or three months. This may be due to pregnancy, or to some other and widely different cause. Now it is a well-known fact that it is almost impossible to absolutely determine the existence of pregnancy during the first three months, and I might as well give her the *benefit of the doubt*, as she don't wish to have another child, and, in fact, should not have one, on account of her general health, or for some other reason. Therefore I will give her some medicine, and recommend hot foot-baths, or something of that sort, and then if it be simply suppression of the menses, her courses will return. In fact, if her courses *do* return, it will be clear that she was not pregnant, and if she be pregnant, then the medicine will do no harm. This is a specious argument, but it cannot be altogether satisfying to the maker of it. It has nevertheless led to many a miscarriage procured by respectable and reputable physicians. It is true that it is not possible to positively determine the existence of pregnancy during the first three months, but upon this subject a writer in the *Gynæcological Journal*, vol. iii, p. 375, makes the following pithy statement: "A married woman, with no known incapacity for fecundation, and in good health, whose menses have hitherto been regular and normal in every respect, presents herself to her physician, telling him that her terms have suddenly ceased, but that she feels no inconvenience from it, except, perhaps, a little nausea in the morning. The physician tells her at once that she is pregnant. What are the chances of his being in error? So small, in my opinion, that he might pursue such a course for a lifetime, and not injure his reputation. His mistakes would, I am sure, be few and far between."

The physician desires, he says, to give his patient the benefit of the doubt in regard to the question of pregnancy. She already has the benefit of the doubt, and it will do no harm to await the period of quickening, if the existence or non-existence of pregnancy cannot be determined sooner. By giving the medicine and the foot-bath the *doubt* is converted into a *certainty* for the benefit of a woman who does not wish to have any more children.

Professor Small, before alluded to, says: "When a woman, a wife, either with or without the consent of her husband, applies for the purpose of ridding herself of the product of conception, she will always make a show of reason for the act, by attempting to show necessity for it. She may set up the claim of being unable to have the responsibility of children; that she cannot educate them or keep them fed and clothed, or above degradation; that her own health will not permit it; that the period of gestation subjects her to confinement and keeps her from society, and she might as well be dead as alive. We have known some physicians to listen to an appeal like this, and yield to the dictates of a blind sympathy, especially when a generous fee was forthcoming to more effectually close their minds against all sense of moral obligation, and plant themselves upon the flimsy reasoning of such women, and while prostrate before mammon would write a prescription for some powerful deobstruent. But they lend countenance to crime by such acts, and become *particeps criminis* in a murderous transaction."

All honorable physicians should set their faces resolutely against this crime. They should denounce it, and show it up in its proper light, in public and in private. Above all, they should tear to pieces that flimsy pretext that there is no life until the fourth or fifth month is reached, and that to destroy the fœtus while it is yet *very small* is not a crime. This excuse is as absurd as that of the young woman called to act as wet-nurse, and who had the misfortune to have a baby without having had a husband. In reply to the upbraidings of her mistress, she offered as an excuse, "If you please, ma'am, it was such a little one."

A great deal more might be written on this subject, but my paper is already of greater length than I intended it should be, so I shall pass to the second point for your consideration, viz.:

What are the duties of physicians in individual cases of Criminal Abortion?

When a physician is called to attend a case of criminal abortion, what should he do? We are often called to attend in cases where an abortion has been committed, either by the woman herself, or by some male or female abortionist. The patient gets frightened at the pain or flow of blood or something else, and the counsel and assistance of the physician (perhaps the regular family physician) is sought. Or, again, we may be called to a case where an abortion has been procured, and the patient endeavors to conceal that fact, declaring either that she is suffering from prolonged menstruation, or that she has had a miscarriage in a natural way, while our knowledge tells us the truth. Now, under these and similar circumstances, what course of conduct should be taken.

In the first place it is clearly the duty of the physician as an act of humanity to go as soon as possible to such a case, simply because he professes to be a healer of the sick and an aider of the suffering. But it has been insisted upon by some, that, under such circumstances, and especially when the case is a doubtful one and the life of the mother seems threatened, a medical friend should be taken along, for the purpose of bearing witness to whatever may occur or be said; and this is doubtless sound advice, although it is not always necessary, and is at all times disagreeable, especially to the patient. It is, however, a measure of self-protection which is perfectly justifiable under certain circumstances, and may prevent suits against the physician for black-mailing or other base purposes. It is a well-known fact that honorable physicians, who would as soon think of murdering their own child as of destroying the life of the fœtus in útero, have been called to attend where an abortion has been committed, and have afterwards, for revenge, or from cupidity, been themselves charged with the commission of the act, and have been put to vast trouble and expense to save—and only then to half save—a before unspotted reputation. Therefore, in all doubtful cases, and in the case of persons entirely unknown to the physician called, while it is his duty as a humanitarian to attend to the cry for help, it will be well for him to secure himself against possible peril by taking a medical friend with him.

When a physician is called to a case of Criminal Abortion, what is his duty as regards the law?

In the first place it is assumed that he has the knowledge that a crime of a heinous nature has been committed, and in view of this it is his duty as a good citizen to see to it that the law is not violated with impunity if he can prevent it. Therefore, in all such cases, he should endeavor to get from the patient the name of the perpetrator, and notify the police authorities that an abortion has been committed, giving at the same time the name of the alleged perpetrator. It is important that this should be done promptly too, and more particularly if the woman's life be in danger. The police authorities have then been informed of the facts in the case, and they have a good chance to bring the criminal to justice by being able to obtain, perhaps, an ante-mortem statement from the patient, should her death be imminent, and to secure the perpetrator, together with corroborative testimony as to his guilt in the shape of instruments or drugs for the procurement of abortion, letters, notes, memoranda, visiting list, etc., all of which might be lost were there to be much delay.

A physician has no right to conceal a crime, however much it may go against the grain for him to act as an informer. There are cases in which it is very hard to do right, as, for instance, in that of an unmarried woman, or when there is a desire on the part of every one to keep the matter concealed, and a shrinking from anything like publicity. But all the conscientious physician has to do in such cases is, to inquire of himself as to what is his duty as a citizen, and what is his duty as a physician desirous of doing his share in the work of suppressing this meanest and most demoralizing of all crimes. What he *should do* is very plain; what he will do, will determine his character as to honesty and worth.

There is another and a very strong reason, however, why the police authorities should be informed of the commission of a criminal abortion, although it is not of so high an order as the former, and that is, for the sake of self-protection. If an abortion has been committed and it is discovered, either through the death of the woman, or by other means, and the physician who has been called to attend the woman takes no step to make the matter known to the proper authorities, he places himself in the position, or very nearly so, of being *accessory after the fact.* An accessory is " he who is not the chief actor in the perpetration of an offence, nor present at its performance, but in some way accedes to or becomes concerned therein, either before or after the deed is committed." The law requires that an accessory should have a concealed knowledge of the crime either before or after its commission, or that he should give aid and comfort in some way to the criminal, or conceal his presence, or connive at his escape, or lay any obstacle in the way of the officers of justice; but Dr. Perpente, of Philadelphia, was tried and convicted and sentenced as an accessory after the fact, in a case of criminal abortion, where it was only proven against him that he did *not* notify the police authorities, and that he *did* take away the fœtus for the purpose of dissecting it, and with an implied view of concealing it from the officers of the law.

A physician who conceals his knowledge of the commission of a criminal abortion occupies a perilous position. He cannot tell what a day may bring forth in such a case, as the most promising of cases may take an unfavorable turn, and death may ensue; or in some other way the facts may come to the light, and he may be looked upon, and very properly, too, as *particeps criminis* in a case of murder.

Again, by taking this course, that of revealing the knowledge the physician has to the proper persons, the best measures are taken for procuring the arrest and conviction of those who make a business of abortion, and thus of breaking up their nefarious trade. Lawyers will tell you that it is a difficult matter to convict on the charge of criminal abortion, under ordinary circumstances, since so much must necessarily be proven; but the chances of conviction are greatly increased in cases where an early arrest of the accused person can be made. Abortionists, when they once know that physicians as a rule will take steps to secure their arrest whenever an opportunity presents, will be more cautious, and many of them will be driven from their damnable calling. And if physicians will do their duty in this direction, and at the same time lose no opportunity of impressing upon the minds of the people the right and true view of the whole subject, they will, at the same time, do their duty as good citizens of the state and as good physicians, and reduce criminal abortion to the minimum.

Physicians have said that if they were to act thus in some

cases they would lose their patients, and in others, where the woman has made a confession under fear of death, and the physician has notified the police and an arrest has been made, the woman, subsequently recovering, could not be got to testify against the abortionist, and might deny the whole matter, in order to screen herself. Much might be said on this point, such as that it would be an easy matter to make the woman's testimony non-essential to the case, etc., but I will only say this, that the physician knows his duty and should do it, without regard to what others may think, say or do; and if he does not, but allows his sense of duty to be benumbed by such excuses as the above, he is in a fair way of having it paralyzed completely and that very shortly.

A few words on the subject of what is called justifiable or necessary abortion, and I have done.

It is claimed that there are cases where it is absolutely necessary to procure an abortion, in order to save the life of the mother. I find myself almost unable to agree that there can be any case where it would be necessary to procure an abortion during the earlier months of pregnancy and prior to the time of viability when the child might be born alive. In England a medical man would lay himself open to a criminal prosecution if he procured the abortion of a woman at an early stage of pregnancy. "There could be no justification for this practice, since the child could not be born alive, and the life of the woman would be seriously endangered." If there be a case, however, where such an operation comes to be regarded as a necessity, then it should only be performed after the concurrent opinion of two or more reputable physicians has been obtained.

That there are cases where labor may be prematurely induced in the interest particularly of the mother, during the last months of pregnancy, when the child may be born alive, is a generally received opinion; and yet so great is the abhorrence of interference of this kind with the processes of nature, that many medical men urge very serious objections to it. Taylor says that "the grounds upon which many eminent authorities have objected to this are: 1. That there are few cases in which parturition, if left to itself, might not take place at the full period; 2. The toleration of the practice would lead to great criminal abuse; 3. It is attended with danger to the mother and child."

Dr. N. F. Cooke, of Chicago, Vice-President of the American Institute of Homœopathy, has written in severe and forcible terms against the production of criminal abortion or of premature labor at any time, and doubtless his is the correct view of the case. At all events if he errs, his error is on the right side, in my opinion.

I cannot close this paper without expressing my thanks to Henry S. Hagert, Esq., District Attorney for this city, for advice and counsel.

GOUT.

BY E. A. FARRINGTON, M.D., PHILADELPHIA, PA.

(Read before the Hahnemann Club of Philadelphia.)

Gout is a disease as obstinate as it is painful. It owes its origin usually to high living, although heredity has much to do with its development. Murchison, in his able lectures on functional diseases of the liver, traces gout to lithæmia; that is, to imperfect oxidation in the liver, with the consequent production of excreta less oxidized than normally—lithic acid and lithates, instead of urea. Now, Dr. Garrod determined that the gouty joint contained a concretion of lithate of soda. This salt accumulates in the blood by reason of its excessive production, which excess is favored by overindulgence in rich foods and by a functionally imperfect liver. The surcharged blood seeks to rid itself of the offender through the kidneys, and also by depositing it in various tissues removed from the central organs. This deposit would seem to be made first in the smaller joints, later in larger joints, and finally it encroaches on several of the viscera. If the kidneys are able to eliminate the lithates, the patient maintains comfortable health; but when these organs fail in their work or are overburdened, or, again, if, perchance, exposure start an articular inflammation, the joints become involved. As the disease progresses, the kidneys may become affected with morbus Brightii, the heart may suffer from inflammation, the stomach become deranged, and arthritic headache and ophthalmia complicate the case, rendering the torture intolerable. The Frenchman's diagnosis between rheumatism and gout is trite and painfully true: "Put ze finger in ze vice and screw him tight: zat is ze rheumatism; now give him one udder screw—zat is ze gout."

But why is it that all who indulge to excess in the pleasures of the table are not affected with gout? And, too, why is it that this lithic deposit so frequently selects the great toe for its punctum saliens?

The answer is involved in that great unanswered problem of *constitution*,—the soil in which disease is to grow, and by which disease is so materially modified. Hahnemann and Grauvogl gave us each three constitutions, but there must be many more. The physician who daily cauterizes the chancre or checks gonorrhœa with injections, is forming a "constitution" for his patient which will last him through life and seriously impress his offspring. *No disease is ever cured except it be removed to the periphery.* When we begin to treat our patients according to their several tendencies to disease, rather than according to the acute symptoms only, we will attain an amount of success never yet even dreamed of. Until then let each physician endeavor to make his prescription as accurately as his materia medica will permit, always valuing symptoms from the centre to the circumference; from mind to body; from more to less vital parts; from function to organ.

The treatment of gout may be divided into that of the acute paroxysm and that of the general symptoms.

In an acute attack the following have been most succsssfully used:

Colchicum.—In the evening fretful, cannot tolerate any annoyances; any external impression, noise, odor, touch or bright light makes him irritable. Toe joint becomes inflamed, dark red, hot and intensely painful; he is beside himself with agony. The foot becomes œdematous. Urine scanty and dark red. The smell of food makes him sick at the stomach. Greatly prostrated.

Ledum Palustre.—After abuse of alcoholic drinks; pimples on the forehead; face bloated; awakened with a hot, tensive swelling of the toe and foot, with tearing, shooting, grinding pains; cannot bear the least covering or the warmth of the bed; foot becomes œdematous, and yet the urine is copious and frequently passed. Old nodes, the sequelæ of former attacks, become excessively painful.

Arnica.—Inflamed joint is shining, red and hard. He dreads the proximity of any one, having a constant fear that they will touch him. Pains unbearable during the night; the bed feels too hard.

Sulphur.—Especially for drunkards or those who indulge in too rich food and take but little exercise; face blotched red; nose red habitually; as soon as he drops into a sleep the affected limb jerks and arouses him with excruciating pains. Pains are erratic and leave a sensation of numbness. Often indicated.

Eupatorium Perf.—In some cases, when the big toe is

swollen, the foot œdematous, the urine profuse and the body aches all over as if the "bones were broken."

Sabina.—Probably more for women; great toe hot, swollen, paining at night, worse warm in bed; high fever.

Antimonium Crudum.—Especially when the stomach is involved; tongue white, bowels costive; vomiting and retching.

Bryonia.—Joint swollen, tense, not very red; if he raises his head he feels deathly sick; tongue white down the centre; patient unbearably cross.

Nux Vom.—The patient is irritable, overbearing; leads a sedentary life, and yet eats to excess; habitually costive; face sallow, but often also a flushing of the cheeks; aroused at 3 A.M. with pains in the great toe. Useful for drunkards

Rhus Tox.—After exposure to wet; must move, though it intensifies the pains.

1 *Benzoic Acid.*—Usually his urine has an offensive odor and deposits a reddish, clouded sediment, but now it is nearly clear and he complains of tearing in the joints; old nodes become painful. As these pains abate, palpitation of the heart sets in, ceasing only when they increase.

1 *Berberis Vulgaris.*—Tearing, burning, stinging pains; patient subject to the formation of biliary calculi; darting, sharp pains radiate from the kidneys, usually downwards and along the ureters; urine cloudy, grayish, depositing a sediment; fistula in ano.

2 *Manganum.*—Toe or other joint dark red in spots; tendo Achillis shortened; pains shift, seem to be in the periosteum, and are worse at night.

1 *Cinchona.*—Painful; oversensitive to pain; great weakness; pains worse at night.

For subacute and chronic cases, choose from the following:

1 Causticum, nodes on the joints; joints stiff, toes or fingers contracted; pains relieved by the warmth of the bed.

1 Guaiacum, similar to the above and following it well. Limbs drawn up and curved; worse from motion.

1 Colocynth, stiffness of the joints, with boring pains.

2 Lycopodium, nodes; fingers and toes pain more at night; swelling of the dorsa of the feet; numbness; flatulence; rumbling in the splenic flexure; full feeling after a mouthful or two of food; lithic acid deposit in the urine. Must rise often at night to pass water.

2 Calc. carb., especially when the well-known "lime-constitution" exists. Useful for drunkards, who feel worse at

every change of weather. Also, when standing or working in water aggravates the disease.

1 Graphites, tearing in the toes; awakens at night and springs out of bed suffocating; eating relieves; gastralgia. Fleshy, bloated; nose red; skin rough, herpetic.

2 Rhododendron, always worse at the approach of a storm, especially of a thunderstorm.

1 Staphisagria, pain from the eyes to the teeth; eyes burn and feel dry despite the profuse lachrymation; patient weak, exhausted by dissipation; face sallow; eyes sunken.

Kali hyd., periosteum affected; distressing pains at night, preventing sleep; limbs contracted; morbus Brightii. Abuse of mercury.

2 Kali bich., pains in the fingers alternate with gastric ailments.

Natrum phos. caused pain about the heart, which ceased when pains returned in the toe.

1 Lith. carb., heart affected; worse stooping; tearing down the limbs; urination relieves the heart. Deposits on the valves of the heart; pain from heart to head; burning in the great toe.

1 Iodium, inveterate nocturnal pains, but not much swelling of the joints.

1 Ammon. phos., to remove deposit in the joints.

Aurum-mur., gnawing deep in the joints, which were recently inflamed.

Gout affecting the head or eyes—Bryonia, sharp pains, worse on motion, neck stiff, eyes sore when moved, sclerotica red; glaucoma. 1 Coloc., boring pains in head or eyes, better from firm pressure. 1 Ipecac., pains from head into tongue, with nausea. 1 Nux Vom., headache with persistent retching. 1 Kali hyd., lumps on the cranium; chemosis of the conjunctiva. Colchic. 2 Spigelia, severe pains in and around the eyes. 2 Sulphur, persistent headache; eyes inflamed, feel as if sticks or splinters were piercing the eyes. Lycopod. 2 Rhus tox., tearing about the head; iritis, glaucoma, piercing, tearing pains through the eye to the occiput, worse at night; lids spasmodically closed, scalding tears. 2 Staphis., eyes feel dry, yet there is lachrymation; pains from eye to teeth. 1 Sepia, pains shooting upwards, with nausea and sour vomiting.

Stomach or abdomen—2 Antim. crud., white tongue, vomiting and retching. 1 Bryonia, tongue feels dry, is coated, especially down its centre; deathly sick on sitting up; pains worse from any motion of the body. 2 Nux vom. 2 Nux moschata. 1 Sulphur. 1 Lycopod. 1 Arsenic. 1 Coloc.

Heart—1 Benzoic acid. 1 Lith. carb. 1 Kalmia. 2 Colchic. Phosp., arsenic.

Kidneys—2 Benzoic acid. 1 Berberis. 2 Lycopod. 1 Sarsap. 1 Sulph. 1 Kali hyd., contracted kidney. 2 Arsenic. 2 Colchic. Phosp. Phos. acid. 2 Zinc, can pass water only while bending backwards; yellow sediment. 1 Terebinth., urine dark, cloudy, depositing a dirty pink sediment. 1 Plumbum, contracted kidney. 1 Aurum.

BORAX IN MEMBRANOUS DYSMENORRHŒA.

BY C. S. MIDDLETON, M.D.

(Read before the Hahnemann Club of Philadelphia.)

SOME years since I read an article on the use of Borax in Membranous Dysmenorrhœa, since which time I have made frequent use of this remedy for cases of that character, and in almost all cases with curative results.

In Hahnemann's *Chronic Diseases*, vol. ii, p. 243, he says, "Easy conception observed during the use of Borax in five women."

I have prescribed Borax for newly married ladies for the double purpose of curing the dysmenorrhœa, and for the purpose of having them conceive "easily," which seems to have occurred in several cases.

How far the conception may be due to the use of *this* particular remedy, may be questioned, except in so far as it removes the barrier to impregnation, which membranous dysmenorrhœa is generally conceded to be.

Suffice it to say, as we all know, pregnancy is not always desired by husband or wife, but in spite of preventives, women conceive when using Borax, when they seemed quite safe against it before.

Hahnemann also mentions the case of a woman who had been sterile for fourteen years: "on account of a chronic acrid leucorrhœa, she received, among other remedies, Borax, *after which she became pregnant* and the leucorrhœa improved."

It may be advisable to quote a few cases:

I. Mrs. G., newly married, had dysmenorrhœa before marriage, which continued to grow worse. Prescribed Borax gr. j, night and morning, between menstrual periods.

This improved her condition at once and a pregnancy occurred in a short time and she was delivered of a fine boy.

II. Miss M., was relieved entirely by the same prescription in a short time, and remained well for a year or two, but has had trouble again within a few months in consequence of having taken cold.

III. Miss D., relieved but not cured.

IV. Mrs. S., a newly married lady, had suffered intensely at her monthly period during all of her menstrual life; had been treated by various physicians of both schools, but without relief. The above course of treatment relieved her in one month and she has had no return of the trouble.

V. Mrs. P., newly married lady, had been a great sufferer, was treated same way, and relieved at once, became pregnant immediately afterwards and has been delivered of a fine boy.

VI. A sister of the last named has been cured by same remedy, time of treatment two or three months.

Another case. A young lady, unmarried, who had become much reduced in strength and health, has been greatly relieved, but she neglects the treatment and I cannot report her well.

I had hoped to get a report from a case of long standing, of undoubted membranous variety, a married lady, but have failed to do so. This case is of so much interest that if I can ascertain anything definite in reference to it I shall be pleased to report.

An attempt to get like results from the 6th potency failed in my hands, and has been abandoned for the present.

CHRONIC HÆMATURIA CURED BY PETROLEUM.

BY JOHN G. HOUARD, M D.

(Read before the Hahnemann Club of Philadelphia, October, 1877.)

About twelve or thirteen months ago I reported to our club a case of hæmaturia of nineteen years' standing, in a lady seventy-two years old. You will remember that I reported the case as cured after three weeks' treatment with Petroleum. Dr. Dudley observed at the time that it would be well to wait and see whether there was any recurrence of the disease before deciding whether a cure had been accomplished. I am gratified to state that on the 11th inst. I called on the lady in question, and she informed me that she considered herself perfectly cured, as she had not experienced any inconvenience since I had attended her thirteen months ago, that her health had steadily improved, her appetite was good, and she attends to her domestic affairs better than she has done for many years past.

She had been treated allopathically for a long time, and had also been treated homœopathically by a physician in this city, without receiving any benefit from either treatment.

I have every reason to believe that the hæmorrhages proceeded from the kidneys, if I may judge from the symptoms in her case. Dr. Watson mentions in his work that there is one phenomenon, which, whenever it occurs, is very characteristic of hæmorrhage from the kidneys, viz., the expulsion with the urine of slender cylindrical pieces of fibrin, which have evidently been moulded in the ureter and subsequently washed down into the bladder by the descending urine. These little coagula are commonly of a whitish color; the red particles of blood having been removed, they look like slim maggots or small worms. They denote with much certainty that the hæmorrhage which they accompany is renal. In this case these little coagula were often observed by the patient. Moreover the following symptoms point to the fact that it was a renal hæmorrhage: Constant pain in the back, extending down on both sides of the abdomen to the groins; the pain was sharp and heavy and pressing downwards to the bladder; during the attacks of hæmorrhage a great deal of fulness and pressure in the bladder, with constant desire to urinate, voiding about a cupful at a time, after a great deal of exertion, causing a trembling of the whole body, with a creeping chill. She experienced frequent violent headache, mostly on the top of the head, as if it would burst. There was also œdema of the feet. Every exertion like walking, lifting, riding or mental emotions, would bring on an attack of hæmorrhage. The hæmorrhage would intervene sometimes about four to six weeks. She was excessively nervous, especially when in the act of urinating.

I had tried several remedies, such as Cantharis, Terebinthina, Hamamelis, etc., with no benefit, and finally gave Petroleum; cured this case radically. I consider this case a very interesting one, from the fact that she had suffered for nineteen years.

NEPHRALGIA.

BY M. M. WALKER, M.D.

(Read before the Hahnemann Club of Philadelphia.)

"SEVERE pain in the kidney, unconnected with inflammation of the organ, is ordinarily caused by the passage of a calculus."—DA COSTA.

The most painful diseases may be differentiated from nephritis, colic, abortion, lumbago, neuralgia of the kidneys, or the passage of a biliary calculus by the description of these different ailments found in textbooks on practice, in which the *treatment* of nephralgia is but imperfectly given.

We know that small calculi pass from the kidney to the bladder, producing the most intense agony, in consequence of their angular and roughened surfaces irritating and lacerating the walls of the ureter, while on other occasions calculi as large as small white beans pass with so little pain that their presence is not suspected till they are heard rattling against some object during urination.

"In composition there are three forms of urinary calculi of common occurrence, the *uric acid, oxalate of lime,* and *mixed phosphates.*

"1. Uric acid calculi are the most common. They are either red or some shade of red, usually smooth, and leave only a mere trace of residue after ignition.

"2. Oxalate of lime calculi are frequently met with. They are generally of a dark-brown or dark-gray color, and from their frequently tuberculated surface have been called mulberry calculi.

"They may, however, be smooth, and are soluble in mineral acids without effervescence. Considerable residue will remain after ignition.

"3. Calculi of mixed phosphates or fusible calculi are composed of the phosphate of lime and triple phosphate of ammonia and magnesia. They form the external layer of many calculi, but seldom form the nuclei of others; are exceedingly brittle, soluble in acids, but not in alkalies."—Tyson *On the Urine.*

TREATMENT.

Among the remedies of our Materia Medica we will give in detail the following:

Belladonna.—Spasmodic crampy straining along the ureter, through which the calculus makes its way.

Bryonia.—Rheumatic and gouty pains in the limbs, with tension, worse from motion and contact.

Lycopodium.—Colicky pain in the right side of the abdomen extending into the bladder, with frequent urging to urinate. Urine incrusts the vessel with red sand. Rumbling and bloated feeling in the abdomen.

Merc. Viv.—Frequent violent desire to urinate, with scanty discharge in a feeble stream. Bruised sensation in the back and limbs. Rheumatic pains worse at night.

Nux. Vom.—Pain, especially in right kidney, extending to the genitals and anterior crural nerve; nausea; vomiting; constant urging to urinate; insufficient urging to stool; inability to lie on the right side; better while lying on the back; rising and walking about increases the pain.

Opium.—Where large doses have been given by "our worthy opponents" the patient may require Bell. or Nux v. as an antidote.

Is indicated by pressive squeezing pains, as though something had to force its way through a narrow space. Shooting pains from different places into the bladder and testicles. Vomiting of slime and bile. Dysuria, face hot, pulse slow.

Ocimum Canum.—Turbid urine, depositing a white and albuminous sediment. Urine of saffron color. Cramp pain in the kidneys. Renal colic, with vomiting. Moans, cries, wrings the hands. After the attack red urine, with brickdust sediment, or discharge of large quantities of blood with the urine.

Thick purulent urine, with an intolerable smell of musk.

Pareira Brava.—Micturition difficult, with much pressing and straining, only in drops, with the sensation as if the urine should be emitted in large quantities. Violent pains in the bladder, and at times in the back. The left testicle is painfully drawn up, pain in the thighs, shooting down into the toes and soles of the feet. Paroxysms of violent pain with strangury: he cries out loud, and can only emit urine when on his knees, pressing his head firmly against the floor, remaining in this position for ten to twenty minutes; perspiration breaks out, and finally the urine begins to drop off with interruptions, accompanied by tearing burning-pain in point of penis.

Urine smells of ammonia, and contains a large quantity of viscid, thick, white mucus. The paroxysms appear generally from three to six A.M.; better through the day.

Similar to Berberis, the symptoms of which seem to correspond with those of nephritis and vesical catarrh.

I have condensed this paper for the purpose of eliciting a discussion on treatment, which may be the means of enabling us to relieve the occasional cases which present themselves, in the shortest possible time without the use of anodynes or anæsthetics.

PSEUDOCYESIS: A CLINICAL CASE.

BY B. F. BETTS, M.D.

(Read before the Hahnemann Club of Philadelphia.)

In September, 1878, Mrs. H. J., 36 years of age, the mother of five children and the subject of three miscarriages, consulted me to ascertain why she had not been delivered of a child, the movements of which she believed herself to have experienced for over nine months, and gave the following history: About a year ago her friends first called her attention to her enlarged abdomen, and suggested to her that she must be pregnant. Very soon after this she felt very distinct movements in the abdomen like those of the fœtus. She experienced the same degree of "morning sickness" for the next month or two that she had experienced upon former occasions of pregnancy. She had the longing and craving for unnatural articles of food. The abdomen kept on enlarging. The breasts became heavier and were found to contain milk, and in fact the symptoms attending her former pregnancies were all present, except that she now had a regular menstrual flow, which was not the case during the other pregnancies.

This flow lasted three or four days, was rather scanty, painless, and paler than natural. There was no leucorrhœal discharge. As the patient was seated, very decided movements in the abdomen, like those of a fœtus, could be seen, even through the clothing. The symptoms suggested extra-uterine fœtation or prolonged gestation, but she had experienced no labor pains.

Upon making a vaginal examination the uterus was found *unimpregnated*, and in a healthy condition. The abdomen was tympanitic, and found to contain no hard body like a fœtus.

By means of the hands applied to the abdominal parietes, the muscles, especially the recti, were found to be irregularly contracting, so as to appear as though they were pressed out by the movements of a child in utero, at intervals.

From an inspection it seemed almost impossible to distinguish these contractions from the movements of a fœtus, but by palpation the tendinous attachments of the muscles to the brim of the pelvis were felt to be put upon the stretch whenever the muscular contractions occurred.

Upon auscultating the abdomen, no fœtal heart-sounds could be heard; indeed, the vigorous movements of the muscles would have rendered it impossible to have heard them distinctly had they been present.

The patient was informed of the strong probability of her *not being pregnant*, but was requested to report at my clinic for diseases of women and have a further examination made under anæsthesia.

As soon as she was completely under the influence of the anæsthetic, the movements all ceased as if by magic. The tympanites disappeared, so that the abdominal walls sank back to their normal position again. Palpation and percussion both confirmed the previously expressed belief in the absence of a fœtus. No heart-sounds were heard upon auscultation. As soon as the effect of the anæsthetic passed off the movements commenced again as vigorously as ever. On account of the mental condition of the patient and the nature of the menstrual flow, etc., Pulsatilla in the 30th potency was prescribed, to be taken every three hours. In two days the movements had entirely ceased, and the abdomen gradually returned to its normal dimensions again.

REMARKS.

False pregnancy, to which the term pseudocyesis has been applied, is to be distinguished in literature from false conception, which is a term used to indicate the formation of a mole, hydatid, etc., resulting from an imperfect development of an impregnated ovum. Pseudocyesis is "a mental delusion resulting in a false interpretation of bodily sensations, experienced for the most part in the abdomen." A similar mental condition sometimes leads to a belief in the actual presence of a tumor in the abdomen when no real tumor exists, such as are known by the name of phantom tumors.

Air moving about in the intestines, twitching or clonic contractions of the abdominal muscles, or distension of the abdomen by gases or ascitic fluid, may all give rise to mental impressions of this kind, and are liable to be developed in women occupying the most varied social positions in life, either in youth or in old age, whether married or single, but especially when approaching the climacteric period.

In the unmarried the fact of having incurred the risk of pregnancy may be sufficient to incite the delusion. It may exist without any disease or disturbance in the functional action of the uterus.

For the purposes of diagnosis we are required to employ:

1st. Digital examination per vaginam to ascertain the condition of the uterus.

2d. Palpation externally.

3d. Percussion.

4th. Auscultation.

5th, and most important in difficult cases, Anæsthesia.

Under anæsthesia the movements cease and the inflation disappears, with or without an escape of flatus.

The concomitant symptoms, especially the mental symptoms, and character of the menstrual flow, if it is present regularly, will indicate the remedy.

Sometimes pseudocyesis terminates in a false labor attended by all the appearances of true labor pains, which may persist for several hours or even days, and then cease as suddenly as they came, with only a slight flow of menstrual blood, perhaps, to show for all the suffering endured. As soon as the mind becomes convinced of the spuriousness of the sensations experienced, the symptoms may vanish, hence the necessity in some cases for making a positive diagnosis as soon as possible.

The remedies to be studied for this affection are Crocus, Bell., Ratanhia, Lachesis, Ignat., Spongia, Pulsa., Sepia., Calc. c., Canth., Kreas., Tabac., Mag. Carb., Lyc., Nux. Mos., and Nitric acid.

CLINICAL CASES.

BY P. G. CLARK, M.D., UNADILLA, N. Y.

May 15, 1879, was called at 5 P.M. to see Miss ——. About three weeks previous she was taken with her catamenia, the discharge being quite profuse. When nearly through she got her feet wet, which was followed by severe pain in her right ovary. An allopathist treated her for two weeks with anodynes, cathartics, and external applications to the abdomen. When summoned I found extreme tenderness over the uterus and both ovaries, but most severe over the left. Pain constant over the lower part of the abdomen, with frequent spasmodic attacks of pain, especially in the left ovarian region. The pain was so severe that she could not refrain from crying out. Pain all over the head; could bear no noise, but was not disturbed by light. She was very pale and had a pinched expression. She could eat or drink but little, as it caused a full sensation in the stomach; had noticed for many days red sand in the urine; no sleep for three nights; bowels constipated; pulse 120; temperature 104¾° F. Gave Lyco^{30}, a dose every two hours.

May 16. The headache continued for two hours after taking the first dose of medicine. She then went to sleep and slept all night; pain in the ovaries and uterus had entirely stopped; tenderness much less; could take quite a quantity of food without distress. Said she felt well excepting the tenderness and weakness. Pulse 90, temperature 100¾°. Gave Sac. lac.

May 17, 9 A.M.—Still better, no return of pains; was in good spirits, had had a good night's sleep; pulse 82, temperature 99½°. Gave Sac. lac.

May 19.—Found her sitting up and feeling quite well, except a slight return of the stomach symptoms. Temperature 98½°. Gave one dose of Lyco[30] and left Sac. lac. In about one week she called at my office to report. Had steadily improved, was able to attend to her duties about house, and felt perfectly well.

July 28, 1879.—Mr. H—— consulted me with the following symptoms: He had been suffering for several days with sharp cutting pains, commencing just in front of the ear on the right side of the face, and extending down to the lower jaw and teeth. Not being able to obtain any more symptoms, I gave Bell[30], and requested him to call the next day. July 29, reported that for a few hours he was better, but that then the pain returned, and was more severe than before. He had had no sleep. He was now very much excited; could not keep still, must walk constantly; temporary relief from hard pressure, and by *holding ice-cold water in the mouth.* Gave Coff.[30]. July 30th called to report that he was entirely relieved; he had slept all night, and had no return of pain. The mental symptoms and relief from ice water suggested Coff., which acted promptly.

A CASE OF VALVULAR CARDIAC DISEASE, WITH DROPSY.

BY L. HOOPES, M.D., DOWNINGTOWN, PA.

(Read before the Homœopathic Medical Society of Chester, Delaware and Montgomery Counties.)

WAS called June 29th, 1879, to see Mary S——, aged 87; found her sitting up in bed, leaning well forward, gasping for breath. Examination revealed great irregularity in the heart's action, with some deficiency of both mitral and aortic valves. Hydropericardium and general dropsy, except of the upper extremities; great anguish and restlessness. Upon my approach to her bedside she remarked, "Doctor, I guess you can't do much for me this time," and I really thought there was little hope myself. I gave Ars.[30] in water, frequently repeated until better. She gradually improved for three or four days, when erysipelas set in in the right foot and leg, and the foot was soon threatened with gangrene. The parts turned purple, became covered with green watery blisters, and she suffered from terrible burning pains in the parts. Rhus[cm] was given, but without benefit; China[2c] also failed. I regarded the case as almost hopeless, but as a last resort I returned to Ars.[2c] in water, a teaspoonful every hour or two, and enveloped the affected limb in a boiled starch poultice. In the course of thirty-six hours I was surprised to find all her symptoms improving. The remedy was continued for several days. The erysipelas disappeared entirely and the dropsy greatly diminished, though at present writing it has returned, owing to the fact that she is suffering from incurable heart disease.

This patient cannot take Ars.^{2c} for any length of time, as it invariably produces diarrhœa.

N. B.—Since writing the above, the patient has died suddenly of heart disease. She retired in the evening, feeling as comfortable as usual. At 2 A.M., when one of the family entered her room, she remarked that she felt quite well, but at 6 A.M. she was found dead.

CLINICAL CASES—DIARRHŒA.

BY C. PRESTON, M.D., CHESTER, PA.

(Read before the Homœopathic Medical Society of Chester, Delaware and Montgomery Counties.)

I. On November 19th, 1879, I prescribed for the son of T. L., aged 5 years, who had chronic diarrhœa of six months' standing. Stools of a yellowish-brown color, containing much undigested food; sudden expulsion of stool with some straining and passage of much flatus; aggravations in the morning and always after eating, frequently having to leave the table to go to stool; cutting pains in the bowels just before stool; fruit and sweetmeats always increase the trouble. Gave *China* for two days without improvement; then *Nat. sulph.* six days, at first with some improvement, but after the third or fourth day the passages became as frequent as ever; still I persisted with this remedy till the eighth day, when I gave Crot. tig.^{2c} in water every three hours. On the following day the passages were reduced from twelve to two, and on the succeeding day, to a single, well-formed stool.

II. On October 26th, 1879, I was called to the son of D. N., aged four years, who had had diarrhœa for three weeks; stools yellowish brown, semi-liquid, containing undigested food; straining at stool with passage of flatus. Aggravations were in the morning hours, during and after eating, and from fruit and sugar. Prolapsus recti at every stool. *China* 30th was given for twenty-four hours, then *Nux-vom.*^{2c} for four days, but without improvement. November 4th, gave *Podophyl.* till the 6th, then *Nat. sulph.* till the 8th, but with no success; then *Ruta grav.* till the 10th, with much improvement as to the number of passages, but no change as to the prolapsus. This was followed by *Sulph.*^{6m} on November 12th, with great improvement, reducing the number of passages from seven or eight in twenty-four hours to one or two, without prolapsus. This improvement continued three days, when a change for the worse took place, and I found my patient no better than at the beginning of treatment. I returned to *Ruta grav.*, followed by *Natrum sulph.* on the 29th, which was continued till the 3d of December without apparent benefit.

After an arduous study of the case I found in the very last volume of Allen, page 29, under *Trombidium*, a number of very strongly marked symptoms of prolapsus ani, brown liquid stool and much straining, which seemed to cover the case much better than anything I had used. I gave the thirtieth potency, a powder after each stool. In three days my patient was apparently well, but in less than a week the trouble returned again. The symptoms seemed much as before taking the remedy, so I renewed the Trombidium in water and ordered a teaspoonful every three hours. In four days my patient was well and has remained so to the present time.

A PECULIAR CASE OF RECTO-VAGINAL FISTULA.

BY J. C. MORGAN, M.D., PHILADELPHIA.

LAST winter, at the request of Dr. L. A. Smith, I visited in consultation, Mrs. O. K., aged 33, who had suffered from inflammation of the connective tract between the rectum and vagina. This condition was consequent upon multiple protruding hæmorrhoids. An abscess formed, which discharged by rectum and vagina within their respective orifices. I passed a probe into the rectum, and thence out into the vagina. The overlying tissue was about an inch in thickness. To have operated by the usual method of division, would have amounted to the formation of a complete rupture of the perinæum. And, further, the patient was unprepared for surgical interference at that time. I accordingly advised rest, a replacement of the piles after defecation, and the internal administration of calc. sulph.

A few weeks later a cutaneous opening formed at the left of the vulva, whereupon the vaginal opening healed.

Being again summoned some time later, I operated in the usual way for recto-cutaneous fistula, and tied the hæmorrhoids. Both procedures were eminently successful, greatly to the satisfaction of all parties.

The raw surfaces were daily treated with the "mild caustic" of the eclectics (a so-called sesquioxide of potash, which, however, is only a mechanical combination of the carbonate and bicarbonate of potassa). The object of this cauterization was to destroy callous tissue and promote free granulation. The ordinary lint and bandage completed the dressing. The cure was radical.

THE DIFFERENTIAL DIAGNOSIS OF SOME DISEASES OF THE EYE, ATTENDED WITH HYPERÆMIA OF THE CONJUNCTIVA.

BY W. H. BIGLER, M D.

(Read before the Philadelphia County Homœopathic Medical Society.)

I PROPOSE in the following paper to draw attention to some diagnostic points, by which may be distinguished certain comparatively harmless eye affections from others of more serious import.

I have taken as my starting-point a condition of *hyperæmia of the conjunctiva*, the simplest and most readily recognized of all symptoms of the eye. This condition seldom occurs alone, but often accompanies a great variety of eye diseases, and, on account of its striking appearance, is quite likely to attract the physician's attention, and this too often forms the only object of his examination.

Objectively considered, we have here the white of the eye flushed and injected, looking watery and bloodshot from the swollen condition of the conjunctival vessels. On everting the eyelids we find the conjunctival lining red and velvety from the swelling of the papillæ, the Meibomian glands somewhat obscured by meshes of fine bloodvessels. Subjectively we have itching and smarting of the eyes, as from sand or dust, heaviness of the lids; sensations worse in the evening and from artificial light.

Since this condition occurs as a concomitant of so many other diseases of the eye, many of them most serious in their consequences, we must seek to discover some means by which to judge of its relative importance. We will find that the absence of certain symptoms, both objective and subjective, is the surest indication by which to diagnose a simple hyperæmia of the conjunctiva. We have objectively *no discharge*, unless it be a very trifling lachrymation, *no subconjunctival injection*, and *no change in tension;* subjectively, *no pain*, *no photophobia*, and *no impairment of vision.*

This hyperæmic condition may be produced by long-continued work on small objects, especially by strong artificial light. It is often a reflex symptom of hyperæmia of the choroid and retina, as in myopses with posterior staphyloma; also in hypermetropic persons who use no spectacles, or those of insufficient strength, by which their accommodative power is too severely taxed.

After the removal of a foreign body we usually have the symptoms of hyperæmia resulting.

As the absence of the symptoms mentioned above serves to

diagnose simple hyperæmia of the conjunctiva, their presence will serve as the most convenient guides in directing our examination, provided we use them according to their relative prominence.

We will therefore examine:

I. *Those diseases that are characterized by a discharge of tears, of mucus, of muco-pus, or of pus.*

If we have the hyperæmia attended principally by a discharge of tears, without any real pain, photophobia, or impairment of vision, we will be led in the first place to think of the presence of a foreign body. Under this we include not only larger or smaller substances from without, but eyelashes, either loose or as constituting trichiasis or entropium. This latter condition has been mistaken for and unsuccessfully treated as conjunctivitis dependent upon a cold or upon an error of refraction. Hairs have also been found protruding from the puncta lachrymalia, causing constant irritation by their friction on the ball of the eye.

Ectropium or some affection of the lachrymal apparatus, stricture, or blennorrhœa may also be the cause of hyperæmia with lachrymation. These conditions if slight may escape notice, but may readily be diagnosed by noticing that the lower lid seems to fall away from the globe of the eye and form a sulcus or gutter, which is constantly filled with tears. This is not seen in the lachrymation attending acute catarrhal conjunctivitis. Again, the cheek under the eye affected presents a glazed appearance, attended sometimes with swelling. The mere overflow of tears will not be cause enough for diagnosing an obstruction of the lachrymal apparatus, for it may result from a hypersecretion, and that the reflex of serious affections of the cornea, iris, or deeper structures.

If we find the injection of the conjunctiva confined to a segment of the surface of the globe, generally triangular in shape, we will also find at its apex, at or near the corneal margin, one or more phlyctenulæ in some stage of their growth, either as mere elevations or vesicles, or small ulcers. The formation of each vesicle in this phlyctenular conjunctivitis is attended with some lachrymation, burning or stinging pain, succeeded by itching and uneasiness, due to the conjunctivitis caused, but very little if any photophobia. If the phlyctenulæ form on the cornea we have much more serious symptoms. They occasion small ulcers, each with a leash of vessels running from the conjunctiva, clearly discernible on the cornea, constituting what is often called "recurrent vascular ulcer," or *phlyctenular corneitis.* These phlyctenulæ tend to recur with great obstinacy. They are accompanied with the great photophobia characteristic of all affections of the cornea. They frequently leave flattened facets or turbid dots on the surface of the cornea, occasioning irregular refraction, and seriously impairing vision.

Recurring phlyctenulæ, either of the conjunctiva or of the cornea, always point to some fault, either of constitution, mode of life, or condition under which the eyes are exercised, and will frequently find in carefuly selected spectacles their cure, when other remedies have signally failed.

In catarrhal conjunctivitis we find the vascularity well marked, especially toward the circumference of the globe, but according to the severity of the attack the whole of the eye may become of a uniform redness. There is a discharge first of tears, then very speedily of mucus, and then muco-pus, which often causes agglutination of the lids in the morning, leaving characteristic scabs adhering to the lashes, often mistaken for signs of blepharitis marginalis. There may be a varying amount of swelling of the lids. There is no pain and no photophobia, and the only impairment of vision is distinguishable as due to mucus floating over the cornea. When the discharge is puriform and very profuse, gushing out when the lids are separated, and renewing itself in an incredibly short time, with chemosis of the injected conjunctiva, and a red, shining, œdematous condition of the lids, we have purulent ophthalmia, or ophthalmia neonatorum.

Even here we do not find any decided pain, photophobia, nor impairment of vision, unless we are not successful in preventing the involvement of the cornea. The tendency is to produce corneitis with ulceration and the resulting nebula, leucoma or staphyloma of the cornea. A constant watch over the state of the cornea cannot be too emphatically enjoined, if we would preserve vision. The antecedents of the case, the history, rapidity, and severity of the attack, the pain in the eye and around the orbit, and the fact that but one eye is affected, will help us to recognize the purulent yellow discharge of gonorrhœal ophthalmia.

In granular ophthalmia there is nothing characteristic, either in the lachrymation or the muco-purulent discharge, in the chronic irritability of old cases, or in the excessive photophobia of the acute, to distinguish it as such. On everting the lids, however, the vascular projections or the vesicular sago-grain-like granulations will settle the diagnosis of acute, while the cicatricial appearance of the lid, with the paleness of the cornea, which almost invariably results, will decide the diagnosis of chronic forms.

In blepharitis marginalis the hyperæmia of the conjunctiva, and the consequent mucous discharge, are rather secondary to the irritation set up by the swelling of the lids, the eversion of the puncta lachrymalia, and the resulting epiphora. The scabs or crusts, which properly belong to this disease, differ from those adhering to the lashes in catarrhal conjunctivitis in that they are found at the base of the lashes, and consist of a watery secretion from the inflamed hair-follicles, mixed with a greasy secretion from the neighboring Meibomian and sebaceous glands. The red lids and scabs sufficiently mark the early stage of this affection, and the watery, bleared eyes, the red, shining, swollen palpebral margins, with their scanty and distorted lashes, present a picture of the chronic state of lippitudo easily recognized.

II. *Those diseases that are marked by subconjunctival or pericorneal injection.*

The vascularity of the conjunctiva is characterized by a superficial redness, produced by a larged-meshed network of brick-red or scarlet vessels, which run off to the edge of the cornea, are movable on the sclerotic, and can readily be emptied by pressure through the lids. In subconjunctival injection we notice fine parallel vessels of a bluish or rosy tint, radiating toward the cornea, around which they form a pinkish zone, the so-called ciliary, or better, pericorneal injection.

When this condition is present a deeper seated trouble is indicated, and we should at once proceed to examine the condition of the iris. In iritis the circle of pericorneal injection is one of the earliest and most constant symptoms. The iris has a prominent appearance, from the effusion of lymph on its surface, or into its texture. From the same cause it has lost its striated appearance and brilliancy, and is often changed in color. The pupil is sluggish and generally contracted. Later on the aqueous may become yellow and serous, or turbid with lymph or pus, which will sink to the bottom of the anterior chamber and constitute hypopyon.

The pain varies in degree, in some cases, especially of rheumatic iritis, being most intense in the eye, around the brow, and down the side of the nose (ciliary neuralgia), worse at night, and generally better from warmth.

The photophobia is not usually very marked, and seldom equals that attending affections of the cornea. The impairment of vision is considerable, depending upon the turbidity of the aqueous, the contracted pupil or limited power of accommodation. The tension is normal. Slow or unsymmetrical dilatation of the pupil under the action of Atropin will confirm our diagnosis.

In irido-choroiditis we find the early symptoms those of iritis. Then we have a pupil contracted and rendered immovable by posterior synechiæ (exclusion of the pupil), an iris convex, bulging forward, with a discolored hazy surface. Vision greatly impaired by contracted pupil, opacity of pupillary portion of lens capsule, and haziness of the vitreous. Tension in the early stages is increased, later diminished, from atrophic changes. In choroido-iritis the symptoms are reversed. The early stage is marked by failing sight, dilated and sluggish pupil and turbidity of the vitreous, without any very marked symptoms in the external appearance of the eye. The disease gradually extends to the iris, and has the symptoms of a low form of iritis.

Sympathetic ophthalmia is a peculiar form of irido-cyelitis, occurring in one eye, after an injury to the other. It is characterized by great degeneration of the iris, which becomes of a yellowish-red tint; total exclusion of the pupil, the area of which is covered with a film of exudation or even filled up by a dense yellow nodule. The ciliary region is generally acutely sensitive to touch, and we have more or less photophobia, lachrymation, and ciliary neuralgia. In the early stage the tension is increased, later it sinks below the normal.

Sympathetic irritation differs from this in the absence of fibrinous exudations. Hence there is no impairment of vision, although the eye may be practically useless from its extreme irritability. The power of accommodation is markedly diminished and every exertion of it is at once productive of hyperæmia of the conjunctiva, pericorneal injection, photophobia, lachrymation, and more or less ciliary neuralgia.

III. *Diseases marked by changes in the tension.*

We have already mentioned the changes in the degree of tension in the diseases of the iris and choroid, and will here only notice one disease, for the other symptoms of which we must ever be on the alert where we find decidedly increased tension, viz., glaucoma. The characteristic and almost constant premonitory symptoms of this disease are rapid increase of pre-existing presbyopia, a colored ring or rainbow when looking at a candle or gas flame, periodic dimness of vision, dilatation and sluggishness of the pupil, cloudiness of the aqueous and vitreous, more or less acute ciliary neuralgia, and a contracted field of vision, principally on the nasal side. In the sudden attack of acute glaucoma we have all the external signs of internal congestion and acute inflammation. There is a distension of the veins, which emerge through the sclerotic near the equator of the globe, and whose tortuous course when strikingly apparent always indicates increased intra-ocular pressure. Pericorneal injection is marked. The anterior chamber is shallow, the pupil dilated and sluggish, inactive, cornea clouded, and the eyelids puffy and red. The patient sees bright-colored halos around the light. Vision is rapidly impaired. The tension is greatly increased, even to stony hardness, while pain, usually very intense, is present and often referred to the back of the head. The presence of constitutional symptoms, fever, nausea, and vomiting, often obscure the diagnosis.

IV. *Diseases with marked Photophobia.*

As we have seen, photophobia accompanies many diseases of the eye, but in none (with the exception, perhaps, of sympathetic irritation) does it form so prominent a symptom as in hyperæsthesia of the retina and in diseases of the cornea.

Hyperæsthesia of the retina (formerly often mistaken for retinitis, which presents no external signs of irritability) can be diagnosed by the intense photophobia, lachrymation, and neuralgia, and the annoyance resulting from photopsies, either spontaneous or produced by slight pressure. The refracting media are clear, and the fundus perfectly healthy. The sight is always greatly improved by dark-blue glasses. The field of vision is sometimes concentrically contracted. This affection occurs most frequently in excitable, nervous, hysterical females.

In diseases of the cornea our attention is usually attracted by the intense photophobia present. We will then at once look for pericorneal injection, and either vascularity or loss of transparency of the cornea.

The diffuse superficial haziness, like a window-pane breathed upon, with regular reflection of objects, will enable us to diagnose corneitis.

Dots of opacity on the corneal tissue, especially in subjects of hereditary syphilis, will lead us to *chronic interstitial* corneitis. Signs of acute inflammation with a dull steamy-looking cornea; pus between its lamellæ (onyx); or, later, bursting through into the anterior chamber (hypopyon); or externally forming an ulcer, will point to suppurative corneitis or abscess of the cornea.

The various forms of ulcers of the cornea will be diagnosed

according to their depth, their shape, and the course they run. Of the phlyctenular corneæ I have already spoken.

The loss of substance, and consequent irregularity in the surface of the cornea, can be best recognized from the irregular distorted reflection of the image of some object caused to fall upon it.

Of the remaining diseases of the eye I am not called upon to speak, since their diagnosis can generally only be made out by the use of the ophthalmoscope. What I have given will be enough, I trust, to serve as a guide in the examination of the eye, and to enable any one to pass an approximately correct judgment on those of its diseases which occur most frequently in general practice.

MICROSCOPICAL EXAMINATION OF FECAL AND OTHER DISCHARGES.

BY J. C. MORGAN, M D.

(Read before the Philadelphia County Homœopathic Medical Society.)

THE contents and evacuations of the alimentary canal are not particularly inviting objects of microscopic study; yet none are of such daily, even hourly, interest to the practical physician. Numerous anomalies challenge him even to name them, and a sense of ignorance comes home to him who, from day to day inspecting, can return no answer. We will consider some of these.

First.—*Fragments of food* which have escaped digestion. Frey remarks that sometimes astonishing and even alarming fecal formations turn out to be composed merely of food. The common forms are merely starch grains and vegetable and animal tissues, as cellular membranes, spiral vegetable fibres, muscular fibre, fatty tissue, epidermoidal tissues, cartilage, bony tissue, fatty granules and oil-drops, condimentary substances, etc.

Second.—*Secretions* of the alimentary canal itself and of its dependencies, normal and abnormal, amorphous and crystalline.

Third.—*Anatomical elements* of the intestinal tissues, and products of diapedesis, or cell-migration from the blood-vessels.

Fourth.—*Parasites,* vegetable and animal.

Fifth.—*Foreign substances,* drugs, poisons, etc.

Each of these should, *a priori,* be familiar to the physician or student who employs the microscope, and they afford a practical series of studies for beginners; obtained, of course, directly from their original sources, or from the dining-table.

Passing mere aliments and condiments, as well as foreign substances, the other objects, which may appear in microscopic examination, may be briefly alluded to. It is sufficient to say in passing that usually only a very minute portion of material should or can be brought into the field of the microscope, hence the usual disgust is quite unnecessary. This minute portion is to be placed on an ordinary slide with a drop of water (or, in rare cases, of some preservative fluid), and a thin glass cover somewhat firmly laid upon it. It may be transported between two bits of window glass.

Among the commonest and most interesting elements are cells, and these are mainly of two kinds, viz., epithelial and lymphoid. Both may be easily studied in the saliva, a drop of which will be found rich in them. The large, flat, nucleated, pavement epithelial cells here abounding, are one of the commonest of microscopic sights, and once known will be readily recognized in fæces, in catarrhal discharges, etc. These cells, and also those of columnar shape appear in the fæces.

Very different are the small, round or oval, mono- or polynucleated lymphoid cells, also found in the saliva, in the fæces, catarrhal and croupous discharges. They can not be distinguished from the white corpuscles of the blood, or from pus-globules, except from the fact that the last-named are excessive in number, and granular from incipient fatty degeneration. These receive a confusing variety of names, according to locality, number, etc. In the saliva they are called "salivary corpuscles;" in the intestinal tube, "mucous corpuscles;" in inflammatory exudates, "lymph-corpuscles," "pus-corpuscles," etc.; in tumors they are simply called by the name, "small round cells." According to Frey, since they cannot be differentiated, they are considered as identical, whether, as some believe (Virchow), they be derived from connective-tissue cell-proliferation, or, as others say (Cohnheim), from direct migration of colorless blood-corpuscles through the walls of the small vessels. Under the name of "mucous corpuscles" these appear in the fæces.

Blood, fibrinous formations, etc., appear as in other cases, sometimes altered by the intestinal juices.

The secretion of the liver, also altered at times, shows biliary pigment, tablets of cholesterin, etc. Absence of bile greatly multiplies the normal number of fatty particles in the fæces; so also does absence of the pancreatic juice. In icterus, with pale (fatty) stools, the former secretion is proverbially at fault; in diabetes, however, similar stools may mean degeneration of the pancreas, so often found with that disorder.

Besides the intestinal worms and their ova, there are two important parasites of vegetable origin found in the evacuations; one mainly in the vomited matters of dyspepsia, viz., the *sarcini ventriculi*, looking like cubical hooped bales of merchandise, the other is always found in the human fæces; and this again best studied beforehand in the secretions of the mouth, particularly in *tartar* from the back teeth. This is the *Leptothrix*, a filamentous fungus, sometimes spoken of as an advanced quiescent bacterial development (Wagner).

I have made some observations of intestinal discharges, and preserved drawings, which are herewith submitted. The first is from a case of false membrane, with chronic intestinal irritation of the lower bowel. Fibrillated fibrinous exudation is the leading character. Lymphoid cells are not recognizable. Neither do the cells of flat epithelium appear.

The second is from a recent case of membranous dysmenorrhœa. Flat epithelial cells are but few; mono-nucleated lymphoid cells are very numerous; but in the drawing only a few are found detached. The fibrinous fibrillation is but feeble. In a case of membranous croup, precisely similar appearances existed in a specimen of the membrane, with the single reservation that the nuclei of the abundant lymphoid corpuscles were wholly hidden by the granular obscuration of the cell-protoplasm; becoming, however, instantly evident on permitting a drop of acetic acid to pass under the thin cover glass of the microscopic slide.

This dysmenorrhœal patient is also the subject of greenish, purulent leucorrhœal discharge, which consists of masses of flat epithelium and of lymphoid cells.

The latter, in her false membrane, have their nuclei apparently red-stained by the accompanying blood; looking, therefore, like incipient red blood-corpuscles (a new observation, if I mistake not).

The third drawing relates to a case under the care of Dr. M. M. Walker; a little child who has suffered with disordered bowels, along with rectal pain. The passages, for weeks together, consisted of a dark sandy material. I prepared a microscopic slide, by placing some of the little grains upon it, adding a little acetic acid (to dissolve it, if it were blood-pigment), and boiled it over an argand burner, by which, however, it was unaltered. The microscopic examination, before and after, gave the same result, as shown in the drawing, viz., roundish, united, mutually flattened, more rarely single, isolated and conoidal dark bodies, feebly translucent. When strongly illuminated by transmitted light they exhibit a deep-red color. Their size is quite various, appearing under a $\frac{1}{4}$ objective and No. 2 eyepiece, from about $\frac{1}{4}$ to 1 in. in diameter. From their resistance to acetic acid, their formation in chains, by mutual flattening, and the ensemble of the child's symptoms, I infer that they are of the nature of biliary calculi, and amenable to the same treatment. From the absence of plates of cholesterin they must be composed of biliary pigment only; from their color, probably of bilirubin. Chemical analysis is yet wanting.

CLINICAL CASES.

BY J. SPERRY THOMAS, M D.

(Read before the Philadelphia County Homœopathic Medical Society)

ELLWOOD G., age twenty months, had paralysis of the extensors of the left forearm and hand, and of the flexors of the left foot. The forearm, hand and fingers were flexed and perfectly useless. The foot was affected with talipes equinus. He had been under allopathic treatment for more than six months, and gradually, but persistently, grew worse, which fact was admitted by the attending allopath. The child was placed under my charge June 14th, 1879. He was of a leucophlegmatic temperament, and had herpes circinatus spreading over nearly the entire right side of the face, in addition to the paralysis referred to. *Calcarea ostrearum*[30] was prescribed, to be taken in water every four hours for three or four successive days. Patient commenced to improve during the first week. The prescription was renewed on an average of about every three weeks, some of the symptoms reappearing in their more aggravated form. In connection with the remedy I applied electricity, using the Flemming and Talbot ※3 Faradic battery, giving two applications per week of from seven to ten minutes each. The paralysis of the foot, which was the most recent symptom, was the first to yield to treatment, the little one being able to walk, and having perfect control of the leg and foot, in about six weeks from the day it was placed under treatment. The same treatment was continued for the forearm and hand, using the battery once a week. In applying electricity to the forearm the positive sponge-electrode was placed beneath the occiput and along the line of the cervical vertebræ, the negative on the affected parts. When treating the leg and foot, the positive electrode was placed along the lower extremity of the spinal column and in the region of the sacral plexus, following the course of the great sciatic; the negative to the leg. At each sitting both electrodes were applied the entire length of the spinal column, using the primary current for the arm and leg, and the secondary when applying the two electrodes to the spinal column; in this way bringing into action the two currents. The ringworm disappeared in about eight weeks, the paralysis of the forearm and hand being the last to yield to treatment. Patient discharged cured November 22d, 1879.

Pulsatilla in Intermittent Fever.—Thomas S. and Alfred G. applied for treatment October, 1879. Both had been under allopathic treatment, suffering for several weeks, and in each case quinine in massive doses had been persisted in without any benefit. They were emaciated and were steadily growing worse. In each case the chill came about 4 P.M., accompanied with nausea and vomiting, loss of appetite, but little thirst; and in the case of Alfred G., chill of a wandering character, coming in spots in different parts of the body. Both cases were of the quotidian variety. *Pulsatilla* 3^d in water was prescribed; the one prescription for each case radically effecting a cure.

Coto Bark in Colliquative Diarrhœa of Phthisis.—I beg leave to call attention to a certain drug, not yet having had any homœopathic proving, but which may be of great value to us, namely, *Coto bark.*

It is known to possess certain curative properties, not manifested in the crude physiological action of the drug, which have been especially noted in colliquative diarrhœa, in the exhaustive and later stages of disease.

In the *Medical News* of January, 1880, Dr. J. Burney Yeo writes that he is satisfied from his experience of more than two years in the use of the drug that it is a valuable remedy, which will control the grave and exhausting attacks of diarrhœa, occurring in the advanced stages of phthisis. He says I have given it in many cases of apparently uncontrollable diarrhœa, which would not yield to the ordinary remedies, such as Opium, Bismuth and Tannin, and have found it almost invariably to arrest the intestinal flux, and to relieve intestinal pain and irritation in a very short time. Dr. Yeo prescribed the drug in a case of "exhaustive and uncontrollable diarrhœa, in one of the graver forms of exophthalmic goitre, which not only arrested the diarrhœa, but had a remarkable influence in allaying the distressing nervous phenomena associated with the case."

Coto bark is imported from Bolivia, South America, and

has been but recently introduced as an article of commerce.* Dose given by Dr. Yeo, five to eight minims of the fluid extract.

I had hoped to present to the society this evening a proving of the bark, but owing to my being unable to procure it in this market, am disappointed in doing so. I have written to New York, ordering a small quantity, expecting to receive it in a day or two. If the allopathic fraternity *can* find in a drug a useful remedy, what can't we do as homœopaths through our provings and in the application of the great law of cure?

TARENTULA IN EPILEPTOID.

BY CLARENCE BARTLETT, M D.

(Read before the Philadelphia County Homœopathic Medical Society.)

SAMUEL W., æt. eleven years, has for five years been subject to peculiar fits, which begin with a sensation as of a cloud before the left eye, gradually increasing to complete blindness on that side. Then follows a numbness of the left arm and right leg, gradually increasing until the former becomes powerless. After this, drowsiness supervenes, followed by a deep sleep, from which he awakens with a throbbing frontal headache and blindness in the left eye, these two symptoms gradually disappearing together. Urine normal. Fundus oculi normal. The longest interval between any two of these attacks was five months. Of late the attacks have been coming at intervals of one week. His parents have never placed him under treatment for this trouble, as they had been told that he would outgrow it. He received Sac. lac. for two weeks, during which time he had one fit, which occurred on June 13th, 1879. *Tarentula* was then prescribed; two grains of the third decimal trituration dissolved in eight tablespoonfuls of water, of which the patient took one tablespoonful every three hours. The medicine was renewed from time to time until September 5th, 1879, when it was discontinued. In the latter part of September he suffered from an attack of otitis media, for which he was treated by Dr. Bigler. Belladonna[30] and Mercurius[30] were the remedies employed. On February 9th, 1880, he reports himself as well, not having had an attack since the 13th of June, 1879.

---

* According to Stille and Maisch this bark is of uncertain origin, but is probably derived from a lauraceous tree. It has been clinically studied, especially by the Germans. It has proved useful in cholera infantum, diarrhœa of typhoid, of phthisis, and also in profuse sweating. Its smell is aromatic and its taste acrid. It is not astringent. Compare Œnothera biennis.—EDS.

HOMŒOPATHIC MEDICAL SOCIETY OF THE COUNTY OF PHILADELPHIA.

REPORTED BY CHARLES MOHR, M.D., SECRETARY.

THE regular meeting was held at the Hahnemann Medical College, on Thursday evening, February 12th, Dr. E. A. Farrington presiding. After routine business, the Censors reported favorably on applications of Drs. S. M. Trinkle, W. P. Sharkey, L. F. Smiley, and G. T. Parke, and these gentlemen were duly elected to membership. Drs. T. S. Dunning and J. O. H. Banks then applied, and under the rules their names were referred to the Censors. Under new business, the Secretary read a communication from Dr. R. E. Caruthers, Corresponding Secretary of the Homœopathic Medical Society of Pennsylvania, asking the Philadelphia County Society to prepare a paper to be presented to the State Society at the annual meeting, to convene at Easton in September, 1880. Referred to a committee (Dr. C. Mohr, chairman) to report at the March meeting.

Dr. A. R. Thomas, in a few well-chosen words, announced the death of Dr. W. H. Smith, who departed this life February 12th, 1880. The doctor's health had been poor for a year past, but the immediate cause of death was pneumonia. Dr. Smith was born in England in 1811. He studied physic under Sir Astley Cooper and Abernethy in the Old World, and after arriving in this country placed himself under the tutorage of Dr. George McClellan, graduating from the University of Pennsylvania. A decided taste for horses and horsemanship led Dr. Smith to study the veterinary art, and he was the first veterinary surgeon to apply homœopathic treatment to animals. This was about 1840. Later he became more interested in general medicine, and graduated from the Hahnemann College of Philadelphia, and practiced for many years at 919 Pine Street. Dr. Smith was little known to the younger men of to-day, but those who knew him best appreciated his merits as a physician and remembered him as a kindly gentleman.

The Bureau of Clinical Medicine, Diagnosis, General and Special Therapeutics, A. Korndœrfer, M.D., chairman, then made a report, the following papers being presented: 1. Microscopical Examination of Fecal and other Discharges, by J. C. Morgan, M.D.; 2. The Differential Diagnosis of some Diseases of the Eye, attended with Hyperæmia of the Conjunctiva, by W. H. Bigler, M.D.; 3. Tarentula in Epileptoid, by C. Bartlett, M.D.; 4. Calcarea ost. and Electricity in Paralysis, etc., by J. Sperry Thomas, M.D.; 5. Clinical

Gleanings, by H. L. Stambach, M.D.; 6. Clinical Studies, by C. Mohr, M.D.; 7. Bryonia in Anasarca, by A. Korndœrfer, M.D. (For Nos. 1 to 4, see present number; the others will appear in April number.) The papers were accepted and ordered to be published, and then the following short discussion ensued:

Dr. Mohr desired to know whether the otitis media in Dr. Bartlett's case could be traced to any cause, or if it was the result of the prolonged use of *Tarentula*. The late Dr. Nunez in his provings of this drug has reported all the symptoms of otitis media.

Dr. Bartlett believed the otitis media in his patient was the result of exposure to cold.

Dr. Morgan thought such questions should be answered with mathematical accuracy. He referred to the provings of *Hydrastis* made some years ago, and said Dr. Korndœrfer could say something on that subject. He said if a drug is capable of producing a dynamic impression, which may be represented by a horizontal line, and, on the other hand, there is exposure to cold weather, which may be represented by a perpendicular line, then the resulting catarrh will be represented by a diagonal between the two forces. As clinicians we must observe what effects different kinds of weather produce while a patient is under drug-action.

Dr. Bigler thought Dr. Bartlett had answered Dr. Mohr's question as mathematically as possible. It is difficult to tell often, whether symptoms are due to the action of a drug or not, as many other influences are at work capable of producing them.

Dr. Korndœrfer made some remarks on the provings of *Hydrastis* in 1866. For twenty years prior to that time he never had a cold in any form, but during the proving he was seized with a violent coryza, and believed the attack was due to *Hydrastis*, about twenty other provers suffering similarly.

Dr. Lee did not believe the question could be reduced to mathematical rules, as there were too many causes at work. Certain results are due to certain causes other than drug-action, and this fact has been instrumental in having our Materia Medica filled by a great deal of trash. Mere coincidences are recorded as facts having great therapeutic value.

Dr. Morgan agreed that we must be cautious and not run into extremes, and yet there ought to be some belief in the "*post hoc, propter hoc.*" Judging from our present method of talking and writing, one would suppose that if a symptom follows the use of a certain drug, that fact must be taken as evidence that it was *not* caused by the drug, and that symptoms are never produced, diseases never *cured*, by drug-action.

Dr. Dudley believed that the sooner physicians learned that there were uncertainties in medical science the better. He thought mistakes were made on both sides in ascribing to drug-action phenomena occurring after the administration of medicines. Frequently the cure under homœopathic treatment is due, not so much to the medicine prescribed, as to the discontinuance of allopathic drugging.

Dr. A. Korndœrfer was continued as chairman of the bureau for another year, and the Society then adjourned.

VINDICATION OF THE BUREAU OF MATERIA MEDICA.

BY J. P. DAKE, M.D., NASHVILLE.

In the February number of the *North American Journal of Homœopathy*, the editor, in an article styled, "What is Homœopathy?" makes use of the following language:

"*The Bureau of Materia Medica, on the other side, tries to stifle all clinical experience won by high potencies as unworthy of scientific men. The scheme proposed by this one-sided bureau reads thus.*"

After presenting a copy of the prospectus of the bureau, as issued some weks ago in our various journals, he goes on to say: "*If Dr. Dake tries to overthrow the facts gained from cures made by potencies higher than the sixth decimal, by experiments furnished by analogy from the field of impalpable morbific agencies, we fear that the proof of their efficacy will be on the other side.*"

And again: "*Is a Dunham's assurance of less weight than that of Dr. H. M. Paine, whose standing at Albany shows him to be prejudiced against high potencies?*

"*Dr. Lawton is to us personally unknown; but could not the chairman of that bureau select on that third point of that second series one member of the Institute who had personal skill and experience in the use of the attenuations above the thirtieth, without being a fanatic?*

"*Have we not a Holcombe, a Joslin, a Neidhard, Thayer, Wells, and others among our seniors who would be an honor to any committee, and whose impartial expressions would carry so much weight?*

"We cannot help seeing partiality in the selec-

TION OF THE MEMBERS OF THE BUREAU; AND SHALL WE THEREFORE CRY OUT WITH HILBERT, IS HOMŒOPATHY GOING TO THE DOGS?"

The appearance of these extraordinary comments, these grave charges, in a reputable journal, against the most important bureau of the American Institute of Homœopathy, in advance of its report of work done and conclusions reached, calls for some attention on the part of those so roughly arraigned.

As the chairman of the bureau in question I address myself to the members of the Institute, and to the profession generally, not in any spirit of anger or retaliation toward the editor of the *North American*, in view of his strange misrepresentation of the purposes and methods set forth in our bureau circular, and his very disparaging estimate of the character and qualifications of the medical men whom I have appointed as my associates, but to make known more fully the real objects of the bureau, and the benefits likely to be derived from its investigations.

1. As to the subject selected for inquiry, and upon which we shall report at the next meeting of the Institute, I may explain, that for the first time in the history of the Bureau of Materia Medica, Pharmacy, and Provings, attention has been directed, this year and last, to the important department of pharmacy in an official and earnest manner.

Last year we investigated and reported upon the history of drug attenuation, as practiced by Hahnemann and his followers, setting forth its objects, as explained by them, together with the methods and means adopted. I do not hesitate to vouch for the entire honesty and thoroughness of the efforts made to arrive at the truth on the part of the bureau. No preconceived opinions influenced the investigation, certainly not adversely to the interests of homœopathy. When our report appears in print it will bear the closest scrutiny and most rigorous criticism.

It was our purpose, at Lake George, further to present the subject, in reports upon the probable limits of drug attenuation and power, as determined by the *scientist* and the *therapeutist*, but our time being exhausted we could not read our papers upon those important topics.

Regarding my reappointment to the chairmanship of the Bureau of Materia Medica as an indication of the wish to have the questions of drug attenuation and the persistence of drug power, continued as matter for investigation, I organized my bureau accordingly, and proposed as our special subject, "*The Limits of Drug Attenuation and of Medicinal Power in Homœopathic Posology.*"

The members of the bureau accepted the subject and the divisions assigned to each in our published circular, which reads as follows:

"*The Limits of Drug Attenuation and Medicinal Power in Homœopathic Posology.*

"I. The Proofs of Drug Presence and Power in Attenuations above the Sixth Decimal:

"1. As furnished by the tests of Chemistry, W. L. Breyfogle, M.D. 2. As furnished by the Spectroscope and Microscope, C. Wesselhœft, M.D.; J. Edwards Smith, M.D. 3. As furnished by the tests of Physiology, T. F. Allen, M.D.; Lewis Sherman, M.D. 4. As furnished by analogy from the field of Impalpable Morbific Agencies, J. P. Dake, M.D.

"II. The Proofs of Medicinal Presence and Efficacy in Attenuations above the Sixth Decimal:

"1. As furnished by the tests of Clinical Experience, in the use of attenuations, ranging from the sixth to the fifteenth decimal, J. F. Cooper, M.D. 2. As furnished by Clinical Experience, in the use of attenuations, ranging from the fifteenth to the thirtieth decimal, A. C. Cowperthwaite, M.D. 3. As furnished by Clinical Experience, in the use of attenuations above the thirtieth decimal, C. H. Lawton, M.D.; H. M. Paine, M.D.

"At the last meeting of the Institute this bureau reported upon the 'History, Methods and Means of Drug Attenuation,' in an exhaustive manner. The reports of the current year, passing from the domain of pharmacy somewhat into that of posology, will complete a work of vast importance for homœopathy.

"The bureau will be pleased to receive items of information and experimental aid from members of the profession, and also from scientific persons outside, who may be interested in any division of our subject. J. P. Dake,

"Nashville, Tenn." Chairman.

If there is anything in this statement of our subject, or in the divisions made, indicating "one-sidedness," or an effort to "stifle all clinical experience, even by high potencies," on the part of the bureau, no one but Dr. Lilienthal has yet made the discovery.

As a very sufficient offset to his unfavorable opinion, I must here quote a paragraph from a letter lately received from an ex-president of the Institute, a man of great culture and long experience with attenuations, high and low. He says: "*The special subject you propose for discussion is important, the divisions first-class, while the recognized ability of those composing the bureau is sufficient guarantee that the various topics presented will be thoroughly handled.*"

Were I to here give the name of the author of these cheering words, I am sure nine-tenths of our physicians would, on sight, exclaim: "That testimonial fully repairs all the damage attempted by Dr. Lilienthal." But I have a number of similar expressions from other good men.

2. Regarding the character of those placed on the bureau by me, I hardly need say a word. They seem to be well and favorably known, as honest and capable investigators, to the American homœopathic profession, with the single exception that has manifested itself in the editorial sanctum of the *North American.*

Who questions the ability and honesty of Breyfogle, of Louisville?

Moulded at the old Hahnemann in Philadelphia, well acquainted practically with attenuations, high as well as low, and second to no man in our ranks as a successful practitioner, what possible object has he to "stifle clinical experience won by high potencies?"

Conrad Wesselhœft, of Boston, taking homœopathy almost by inheritance, trained to love and practice it from very boyhood, what inducement can there be for him to shut his eyes to the truth and bear false witness?

J. Edwards Smith, of Cleveland, without a rival in this country as an expert microscopist, knows no such feeling as *a fear of facts* in matters of science. He can see medicinal particles as far up the scale of attenuations as any living man, and seeing them will not shun to declare their presence.

Who questions the capability and earnestness of Allen, of New York?

Surely Dr. Lilienthal should not thus accuse his brother professor before the public. If his scholarship, and industry, and good-will toward homœopathy are not sufficient to save him from the charge of trying to "stifle clinical experience won by high potencies," there is little hope for the enlightenment of the medical fraternity.

Sherman, of Milwaukee, educated, systematic, thorough, so

afraid of error that he puts a double sentry at the door to challenge every incoming candidate for his belief,—loving truth more than the creeds of parties, and facts more than the dicta of men,—he is not of the kind likely to send homœopathy "to the dogs."

Who questions the ability and honesty of Cooper, of Allegheny City?

His has been a long and careful experience in the use of attenuations, high and low. Distinguished for his practical success, his conservatism and unvarying fairness, he is one of the last men now to show himself "one-sided" as an investigator, or disposed to "stifle clinical experience" for any purpose whatever.

Cowperthwaite, Professor of Materia Medica in the University of Iowa, and author of an excellent textbook on materia medica, placed upon the bureau by request of President Wilson, is he to be turned aside as unable or unwilling to deal fairly with any questions relating to the efficacy of attenuated drugs?

If I am not mistaken the doctor excels the traducer of our bureau in the use of high attenuations.

Lawton, of Wilmington, Delaware, against whom especial objection is made, was put upon the bureau last year by request of a strong advocate of high potencies. At Lake George he had an excellent paper ready for presentation to the Institute, which time did not allow him to read. From my knowledge of the qualifications of Dr. Lawton, I am persuaded that he will do ample justice to the claims of "all clinical experience won by high potencies;" and that his paper to be presented at Milwaukee will prove highly satisfactory to the advocates of drug dynamization.

And as for Paine, of Albany, against whom Dr. Lilienthal uses strong language, he is a man of most thorough education, and of long experience in the practice of homœopathy. He has accomplished much for the cause in the Empire State, and won much of distinction and honor for himself. He has every reason to labor for the soundness and success of homœopathy that can possibly actuate his accuser; and I am persuaded that his report will not be wanting in thoroughness, candor, and courtesy.

Thus I have felt compelled to speak in behalf of the medical gentlemen whom I have had the honor of associating with me in the organization of the body which Dr. Lilienthal characterizes as "this one-sided bureau," trying "to stifle all clinical experience won by high potencies."

In regard to the appointment of some of the excellent members of the Institute named by Dr. Lilienthal, in place of Dr. Lawton and others now on my bureau, I should mention that the rules of the Institute require the chairman of a bureau to hand a list of his appointments to the President, for announcement to the Institute before adjournment; and, further, to call a meeting of those appointed for the selection of the special subject, and the laying out of work for the year. But one of the persons so named was present at Lake George.

3. As to my own opinion and purposes regarding the subject in the hands of the bureau, Dr. Lilienthal has endeavored to lead the profession to believe that I will "try to overthrow the facts gained from cures made by potencies higher than the sixth decimal."

Perhaps it would have been quite as well for him to wait for the report which I shall submit at Milwaukee before thus sounding his notes of alarm.

I have never uttered a word against the acknowledged efficacy of attenuations above the sixth decimal; nor have I any intention or wish so to do.

I seek the "overthrow" of no *facts*, but simply the most effective exposure of the fruits of imagination and fraud palmed off *as facts*.

As the chairman of the Bureau of Materia Medica, it has been my aim to develop every kind and all of the proofs of drug power and efficacy in our attenuations, not simply up to the sixth decimal, but up to the thirtieth, and on as far as any species of test can go. Chemistry and the microscope and spectroscope have, by no means, been the only resorts for information. Physiology, or provings upon the healthy, and clinical experience, or provings upon the sick, are called upon for all their facts.

No relevant testimony will be ruled out; no facts neglected. No previously formed opinions, on my part or on the part of any member of the bureau, will be allowed to hinder a full and faithful presentation of the truth as we find it in the field of our research and experimentation.

It may be some relief to Dr. Lilienthal for me to say that, each member of my bureau is informed that *he is at liberty, besides the elaboration of his allotted portion of the special subject, to investigate and report upon any other portion he may desire to discuss.* The papers thus presented, out of the appointed order, if not allowed a hearing for want of time, will be published along with the papers read.

And to show how the anxious critic himself may come to the rescue and make up for deficiencies in the bureau, I will repeat a clause, some time ago printed in our circular, viz.:

"*The bureau will be pleased to receive items of information and experimental aid from members of the profession, and also from scientific persons outside, who may be interested in any division of our subject.*"

Do all these liberal provisions look like "one-sided" work?

Can we be justly charged with "partiality" and unfairness.

Is ours the spirit to "send homœopathy to the dogs?"

Have we not left the witness-box wide enough open?

Whose fault will it be if "all the clinical experience won by high potencies" is not properly set forth and defended at Milwaukee?

Let us be MEN, endeavoring to get above the quarrels of children.

Let all who regard what is proper and fair, who value truth more than party or faction, who have self-respect and a real desire for good feeling among the members of our school, frown upon all attempts to personally malign and forestall and injure the work of an individual or of a bureau commissioned to Investigate and report upon an important subject.

Homœopathy will, indeed, "go to the dogs" when its friends shrink from the light, and grumble and groan and howl whenever an attempt is made to display, in proper order, the foundation facts upon which it rests.

LETTER FROM DR. H. N. GUERNSEY.

PARIS, FRANCE, January, 1880.

CHARLES MOHR, M.D.

MY DEAR DOCTOR: As the representative of that portion of the profession which so kindly tendered me an honorary banquet, just before my departure for Europe, I deem you the proper one to whom I should address a short sketch of my tour.

After bidding adieu to children and friends, we embarked on the good steamer *Illinois*. When, on the following day, we were steaming out upon the high seas, symptoms of that annoying attendant of a sea-voyage, seasickness, became prevalent. My first patient was a young lady. Regardless of the *name* of the disease, I applied most rigidly our law of cure. She complained of a constant and painful empty sensation at the pit of the stomach, and increase of nausea at the smell of food. Sepia 55^{m} a few doses, cured, and she remained well the rest of the voyage. An elderly lady was my next charge. Her tongue was coated white, she had nausea with empty retching and gagging and a severe pain in the hollow of the right knee, worse evening and night; could not lie in bed on account of the pain. Bell 40^{m} cured her speedily and permanently. Your humble servant thought himself safe, but soon found the necessity for Cocculus. A gentleman, who was sick during every voyage, sought advice. He craved cool food and drink; but so soon as these became warm in his stomach, nausea and vomiting were increased. Phosph. 70^{m} relieved promptly. Ars. 40^{m} cured some cases, Bry. 70^{m} others. Some could not be induced to try homœopathy and were sick all the way over. I am fully convinced, from what I have seen, that seasickness is amenable to the similimum, given in the smallest dose that will cure. Our voyage was the most tempestuous that some old travellers had ever seen.

The harbor at Queenstown is very extensive and beautiful. We landed at 2 A.M., June 24th, having completed our passage in a little less than ten days. In this northern latitude daylight during summer lasts from 2 A.M., until 9 P.M.

We left Queenstown and journeyed to Cork, thence to Blarney Castle, and thence to the Lakes of Killarney. The scenery was charming. The broad, smooth roads, with massive walls on either side, the green fields, the ruins of Ross Castle, Lord Brandon's Cottage, etc.,—all serve to lend a peculiar fascination to the journey. After we reached Dublin, one of the earliest places we visited was Trinity College. The buildings are massive and surrounded by lovely grounds, set with blooming hawthorn hedges and adorned with every variety of shrub and flower. In the medical museum is a skeleton of one James Magrath, whose height is 8 feet 4 inches! I could but little more than reach the top of his head with my upstretched umbrella.

Our journey to England was by way of Holyhead, a route which affords fine views of the Welsh coast. Chester, which we reached by a delightful journey from Holyhead through a part of neat, thrifty Wales, was an old Roman stronghold. It is surrounded by a wall, upon which were erected watchtowers. Here stood King Charles, September 24th, 1645, and witnessed the defeat of his army on Roman Moor. We visited in turn

Edinburgh, every part of which denotes the great mental culture and wealth of its inhabitants—Liverpool, that wonderful city, with its two hundred acres of docks and fifteen miles of wide quays—Glasgow, rather dismal, with its buildings of granite—the Highlands—and then London, the interesting sights of which claimed a month's stay and will demand another four weeks on our return. I am glad to say that homœopathy is rapidly increasing here, and that the pharmacies present an imposing appearance. We dined with our well-known friends, Wilson, Wilkinson, and Berridge, and learned that Hahnemann's Organon is growing in favor with the most thoughtful of the profession.

While in London we saw Queen Victoria, for whom I have always entertained great respect, because, although a queen, she was so devoted a wife and fond mother of a large family.

At Antwerp we noticed that the homœopathic pharmacies are merely separate apartments of the allopathic drug stores, as is the case pretty generally on the Continent. We spent several pleasant days here and were much amused with the dog carts, led by women, and with the ceaseless clatter of the wooden clog shoes. Brussels, that beautiful city, with its wide thoroughfares and long rows of Linden trees, was next visited. The road thence to Cologne is charming. We hurried past beautiful farms and fields, threaded with broad white limestone carriage-ways, with not a fence to mar the extended view. At Cologne we of course paid our respects to the great Cathedral, the grandest Gothic edifice in the world.

"Up the Rhine" was our next endeavor, and well were we repaid. As we sailed along we observed the fields on either side covered with heavy-laden grapevines, ruined castles looming up above the hills, whose summits they crown. Even these old castles are surrounded with the richest vineyards. At Ems we landed and stood on a slab which marks the identical spot where the Emperor William and the French Ambassador held their unsatisfactory council, which was followed by the late Franco-German war.

At Heidelberg we visited the renowned University, its chemical and medical departments, and its hospital. The buildings are all very plain and considerably separated from each other. It was exceedingly interesting to see the sanctums in which great men had toiled and thought to astonish the world. Here, for instance, is Bunsen's, in which he brought out his famous battery.

Munich was next in order. Its fine buildings are so embellished with gold and display such perfect art that one imagines at times that nature herself is here arrayed in her gayest attire.

We journeyed south to Switzerland and feasted our eyes on its ever-varying scenery. Towns, lakes, mountain views, many of which are memorized in painting and poem, or recorded on the hard, cruel pages of history, passed by, like a living panorama.

At Lake Geneva we visited Chillon Castle, of historic and Byronic renown. Geneva itself is a very interesting place, and here I made the acquaintance of Dr. Edward Dupresne, a most skilful and learned homœopathist. From our hotel window we could see Mont Blanc, and in the evening were charmed with the Alpine glow upon the whole mountain.

After an extended tour through Turin, Milan, and the Italian lakes, we repaired to Florence, a city whose beauty is unique and wholly indescribable. It is worth the visit to see Galileo's room, in the centre of which he sits, sculptured in purest marble and surrounded by his astronomical instruments. We visited the studio of our late countryman, Hiram Powers. The mantle of the gifted father has fallen upon his son, who promises to rival him in reputation.

Prejudiced by reports of the unhealthiness of Rome, we approached the "Eternal City" with fear and trembling. My surprise was great, then, when I found my health improving more than it had in any place since leaving home.

Homœopathy has a foothold here that nothing can dislodge. Dr. G. Pompili is a host in himself. He is certainly a true disciple of Hahnemann. This is a grand field for some good and true physician, and Dr. Pompili is very anxious to see such, with whom he might enter into copartnership.

The Romans, I find, are a liberal, wholesouled people. I was several times consulted professionally, and although in no instance did I make any charge, I received, in each case, a good honorarium. Several Catholic priests, who, of course, could hardly be charged, were on the grateful list. Were I a young man, I would unhesitatingly locate here, with every expectation of a brilliant and successful future, both for myself and for the cause.

Naples is an enchanting city. What with its beautiful bay and grand surroundings, we were loath to leave it. A little south of the city is Pompeii. Of course we saw that terrible offender, Vesuvius. We commenced its ascent, and as we rode through the immense lava beds, we had some demonstration of its fearful power. Finally we stood upon the edge of the crater and gazed down into the hot bed below. We felt its intense heat and also the quaking, undulating motion of the ground beneath us, as it vomited its molten lava hundreds of feet into the air. As a familiar illustration, imagine millions of locomotives combined into one. There is the puffing, the pouring out of dense smoke and the scattering of sparks—such is Vesuvius to-day.

Naples has four pharmacies, which are exceptionally distinct from the allopathic stores. Twenty physicians practice here, one of whom is the author of several medical works. Those here who practice our art, in its simple purity, are very successful in the management of the fever prevailing in the locality.

We visited Pisa and were anxious to hasten on to Genoa, the birthplace of Columbus. At length, however, we bent our way towards France, passing through Nice, Marseilles, Avignon, Lyons, Dijon, etc., arriving at Paris on the 19th of December, 1879.

And now I am very happy to state that my health has greatly improved. If you or any of our mutual friends are careworn and weary, I can confidently recommend a tour similar to the one I am taking. If age is a prominent cause of the weariness, let your journey be not too short. Nine or ten months or even more may be needed.

Fraternally yours,

H. N. Guernsey.

Do Cold Winters Make Healthy Summers?

"Unreflecting people argue in this wise: First. A cold winter kills all the vegetation and makes a succeeding summer healthy. Second. A warm winter fails to kill all (or so much of) the vegetation, and makes the succeeding summer unhealthy.

"Now the real fact is that when the cold weather kills the vegetation so extensively, there is more dead vegetation; and if the mere *quantity* of *dead vegetation* controlled the ratio of its disease-producing influence, then the summer following an extremely cold winter ought to excel in unhealthiness.

"For the opposite reason, the mild winter, leaving a large proportion of the vegetation in a condition of life instead of death, ought to be followed by a healthy summer.

"Neither of these conditions, however, are the real factors governing our climatic sanitation, but *cleanliness and dryness* govern the whole. Thus, for instance, in our own city of Savannah, proper sanitary government in the city itself and proper drainage of the adjacent low grounds, not allowing moist or stagnant or putrid accumulations or surfaces, will insure our general good health, whether a summer succeeds a moderate or a cold winter, the moisture, putridity, and consequent poisonous evaporative capacity being the elements of its dangerous nature, and these elements being removable by proper hygienic treatment."—Dr. L. A. Falligant in *Savannah Morning News.*

THE

HAHNEMANNIAN MONTHLY.

A HOMŒOPATHIC JOURNAL OF

MEDICINE AND SURGERY.

Editors,

E. A. Farrington, M.D. Pemberton Dudley, M.D.

Business Manager,

Bushrod W. James, M.D.

Vol. II. Philadelphia, Pa., March, 1880. No. 3.

☞ The Editors consider themselves responsible for the maintenance of the dignity and courtesy of the journal, but *not* for the opinions expressed by its contributors.

Editorial Department.

Wanted, a Hospital Superintendent for the Pennsylvania State Hospital for the Insane, at Norristown, Pa. A graduate of the Rip Van Winkle school preferred. No homœopathist need apply.

The above advertisement indicates the completion of another —the fifth—step in the work of supplying a certain favored portion of the citizens of Pennsylvania with hospital accommodations for their insane, from the benefits of which the remaining portion of her people are rigidly excluded. The work of furnishing like accommodation for these less favored citizens has not yet been begun, and the authorities have not the slightest intention of making such a beginning. It may be, however, that our Solons at Harrisburg think that people who employ homœopathic methods of medication never become insane, and that all the crazy people are allopaths; if so, we have nothing more to say in the matter.

It may be well to state, however, that the new hospital at Norristown is partly homœopathic. That is to say, about one-third of the cost of its construction was paid by homœopathists, and a similar proportion of its maintenance fund will be drawn from the same source. Some of these homœopathic contributors are unreasonable enough to think they ought to be admitted to a share in the benefits of said hospital, simply because they furnish the money to build and run the institution, as if any American legislator could listen for a moment to such an absurd reason as that. Cannot any one see that the thing is about equally divided? The homœopath pays the bills, and the allopath attends to the other little matter of reaping the benefits. Nobody ever heard the allopath complain of *his* part of the business, and why should the homœopath raise such a howl about it? But these homœopaths are an insatiable set of people all around. The more they don't get, the more they want.

Seriously, is it not about time that this long lane should have a turn? The idea that a whole community of from one to two millions of people should be left utterly without hospital accommodations for even a single insane patient, while at the same time they are pouring out their money to build and maintain hospitals for a neighboring community,—hospitals to whose shelter they would not be admitted for a single hour except at the sacrifice of their therapeutic preferences,—involves a servility so deep and degrading that we wonder the men of Pennsylvania can tolerate its continuance for a single year. How long would an allopathic community of equal size submit to be taxed for the support of other people's hospitals, whose doors they could not enter? How long would *they* pour their millions into the lap of a government which did not even offer a pretence of using these funds for the benefit of those who furnished them? Not very long, we warrant. Such governmental indifference to the just claims of a body of people not already familiarized with outrage and wrong, would evoke a spirit which would shake this old Keystone State to its rocky foundations. We, it seems, have been so long accustomed to wear the yoke of bondage that we forget its galling humiliation. We see magnificent hospitals rising all around us; we know that our money has paid for some of them; their doors are slammed in our faces, and we have not even the manhood left to feel that we are both robbed and insulted.

Homœopathists of Pennsylvania, we can put an effectual quietus upon this infamous and persistent outrage if we will, and we can do it speedily. It is idle to suppose a million of people cannot besiege our legislative halls and back up their demands with a power that will brook neither refusal, nor evasion, nor delay. We can call to our aid the influence of petitions, of personal and organized effort, of public meetings all over the State, and of the whole unsubsidized newspaper press.

And our demands should be of a wholesale character. They should include, first, the immediate erection and the maintenance of two homœopathic hospitals for the insane, with a homœopathic board of management for each of them,—one in the eastern and the other in the western portion of the State,—and the setting apart of portions of all the others for homœopathic patients and under homœopathic management until the construction of the two new hospitals can be completed. Second, the appropriation of money to our already existing hospitals in sums as liberal as those already appropriated to allopathic institutions. Third, the immediate and permanent discontinuance of the favoritism now practiced towards one particular school of medicine in appropriations and in appointments to places of professional trust or honor. We can get all this. We *cannot* get it without effort, nor without well-organized, persistent, determined effort; and the sooner we begin the better. We know that we have the power; the only question is, shall we make our power felt? We suggest an early consideration of this subject by our local societies and by physicians generally, and the adoption by the State Society of a well-prepared plan of action to be put into immediate operation, and persisted in until complete success is attained.

A SLIGHT MISTAKE.—The Cincinnati *Medical Advance* is somewhat in error in the supposition that when the HAHNEMANNIAN MONTHLY came under its present management it was nearly or quite moribund. In fact there was not about the journal the slightest symptom of approaching dissolution. All the indications, on the contrary, pointed to a robust and vigorous future. The sharpest criticism of its editorial management came nearly always from those who disagreed with its administration on purely medical questions, while its rapidly growing subscription list gave pretty solid evidence that a large proportion of the American profession were more or less in sympathy with its opinions and its policy. Whatever else may have been said of it during our predecessor's editorship, no one could deny that it was a *live* journal in the full sense of that term. We desire here to express our grateful appreciation of the kind wishes of the *Advance* for the success of the HAHNEMANNIAN under its new management.

Book Department.

Brainwork and Overwork. By Dr. H. C. Wood. Published by Presley Blakiston. Philadelphia, 1880.

This little brochure is one of a series called the *The American Health Primers.* The object of this series of primers is to diffuse as widely and as cheaply as possible a knowledge of the elementary facts of preventive medicine. The books are neatly printed, handsomely bound in cloth, and sold for the moderate price of fifty cents each. The volume before us, on brain-work, discusses a subject of vital importance to the sanitary welfare of the community. Unfortunately, patients suffering from brain-fag seek professional advice when it is too late to entirely avert the consequences of overwork. Should these patients early seek such hygienic information as this little primer affords, they might reap the full benefit of the proverbial ounce of prevention.

The book passes under review many of the general causes of nervous troubles, such as exposure, sexual excesses, dissipation, abuse of tea, coffee, etc. We are glad to see that the author deals justly with the much-disputed question of teetotalism. While deploring the baneful effects of abuse of alcohol he is candid enough to acknowledge its beneficent effects when given to the weary, the care-worn and the illy-fed.

Concerning tobacco the author says, after treating of it as a deadly poison:

"In the busy mart of the city, . . . in the exposure of a sailor's life, wherever men strive and endure, the nervous system craves something that shall soothe it into quiet."

This he thinks tobacco tends to do. Excellent, indeed, is the advice to parents as to their duty in the instruction of children concerning the relations of the sexes. The language here is plain but well chosen, and the information given may tend to prevent some of those social and private vices which undermine the health of our youth of both sexes.

The chapters on Work and Rest are teeming with sound advice, while that on Recreation is really a masterpiece of thought. The nicest discrimination is drawn between dissipation, "constitutional walks," overstrained Sunday-school teaching, idleness, and misdirected exercise on the one hand, and genuine recreation, rest, and pleasant mental diversion on the other.

We commend the book to our readers, and urge that they recommend it to those for whom it is written, the laity who seek to know how to live. F.

An Elementary Textbook of Materia Medica. By A. C. Cowperthwaite, M.D., Ph.D. Duncan Brothers, Chicago, 1880.

The object of the author of this new textbook is, as he expresses it in his preface, to "furnish the beginner with a systematic basis of knowledge, that may facilitate his study of the complete Materia Medica, and enable him the more readily to comprehend the wider application of drug-action as there afforded."

To effect so desirable an end, Dr. Cowperthwaite has arranged the characteristics of over one hundred and forty drugs, with frequent references to drugs having similar symptoms. Each remedy begins with its technical name, followed by its common name and the place in the natural kingdom to which it belongs. Next is given a short "General Analysis." Then follow "Characteristic Symptoms," arranged in a very readable form, according to locality, etc.

In addition to the usual schedule of Hahnemann, embracing such headings as MIND, HEAD, etc., our author has interposed what he calls "THERAPEUTIC RANGE." The difficulties which encompass this last "heading" are anticipated by the doctor, for he remarks in reference to this subject, page 9 of the Preface, "Yet it must be remembered that diseases are not treated by name, and that it is only when the totality of the symptoms presented by the patient correspond to those of the drug that its use becomes homœopathic." Thus he shows the inutility of this portion of his own work. Still, there are some valuable hints included under this heading, which might have been differently classified with great advantage.

Of the value of the work as a whole there can be no question. Professor Cowperthwaite has shown in his selections great ability and a most excellent analytic knowledge of the Materia Medica. The work has the appearance of more than a mere compilation. It is a labor which shows careful study and a nice discrimination in the choice of such material as is absolutely needed by the student during a collegiate course.

Not the least useful feature of the work is the distinction in the value of symptoms by means of italics. While it is true that homœopathy is a rational science, which will not admit of arbitrary arrangement, it is also a fact that the student needs to know which symptoms of a remedy have been most frequently confirmed or used. Hence in his elementary studies they necessarily take the foreground in his memory. As his knowledge ripens with experience he learns to weigh symptoms more relatively, and he soon finds that a very characteristic indication in one relation may become of minor importance in another.

The author very properly, we think, prefers Calc. ost. to Calc. carb., Cinch. to China, Ailantus to Ailanthus. We would, however, rather see Staphis. than Staphys., which is a misspelling of our early writers.

Though the type is not always as clear as it should be, the book is nevertheless convenient in size and readable. Typographical errors seem to be few.

We miss several characteristics which have been of service to us, the omission of which rather weakens one or two of the remedies. For instance, Calc. phos. would be much more usefully presented if mention had been made of the cool cheeks and nose, sunken abdomen, and craving for bacon—all so valuable in its selection in cholera infantum, etc. But this is hypercriticism, and neither can or should detract from the value of a book which is the best effort of the kind in our literature. F.

Gleanings.

SUGAR AND TEETH.—A tooth soaked in sugar-water becomes jellylike from a combination with the lime. Refined sugar injures the teeth, either by immediate contact or by gas developed in the stomach.—*Chemist and Druggist*, January, 1880.

TREPHINING.—It is not uncommon to find sinuses of considerable size in the region of the pacchionian bodies, opening into the longitudinal sinus. This fact should be remembered in connection with the operation of trephining.—*N. Y. Medical Record*, February, 1880.

INTERNAL USE OF TAR.—Professor Reclam, of Leipzig, gave Tar in the form of pills or capsules, and noticed that the urine of patients so treated did not decompose for five or six days. He employs Tar for chronic catarrhal inflammation of the mucous passages of respiratory or urinary organs.—*Chemist and Druggist*, January, 1880.

CALOMEL.—For the benefit of those who persist in the local application of Calomel to the eye, we quote the following from the *Archives of Medicine*, February, 1880: "Calomel causes severe superficial inflammation in the eyes of those who are taking Potas. iod. The latter, when taken into the system, is widely diffused, appearing in the tears in a very few minutes after ingestion. If it meets the Calomel here, it is at once attacked by the Mercury, with the resultant formation of the Iodide and Iodate of Mercury, both of which act as caustics."

LACERATED PERINÆUM.—Dr. Thad. A. Reamy proposes immediate operation. He uses No. 28 silver wire, and insists on numerous sutures, as many as three or four to the inch. He believes that more perfect coaptation is thus insured, and that consequently the lochial discharges cannot readily insinuate themselves into the wound. The urine is to be drawn by the catheter during the first two or three days; he does not insist on bandaging the limbs, but simply directs the patient not to separate the legs widely. —*Obstetric Gazette*, January, 1880.

TRANSITORY ALBUMINURIA, without the existence of renal disease, has been noticed as follows: After extensive injury of the skull; from external applications of Iodine in children; from inhalation of Turpentine; one physician could produce albuminuria in his own person, lasting eight to ten hours, by drinking a pint of milk.—*N. Y. Medical Record*, February, 1880. *Per contra*, Dr. George Johnson considers every case of even transient albuminuria as always pathological. Traces of albumen in the urine after food, exercise, etc., will, he thinks, lead to persistent albuminuria if not systematically and promptly treated.—*Medical Record*, February, 1880.

THE FILIARIA SANGUINIS HOMINIS is a parasite common in India, China, and other countries, and quite likely to visit us, with our motley and changing population. It inhabits, as the name implies, the blood, migrating to the lymphatics, but seldom infesting outside tissues, like the trichina. Its length is $\frac{1}{76}$th and its diameter $\frac{1}{3500}$th of an inch—just about the diameter of a blood-corpuscle. Among the diseases attributed to its presence is chyluria. This affection, however, may also, doubtless, arise from other causes, as from a diseased kidney, which eliminates granular fat, just as it does abnormally sugar or albumen.—*N. Y. Medical Journal*, February, 1880.

SCLEROTIC ACID exists in Ergot of rye in the proportion of four or five per cent. It is a very feeble acid. It is so rapidly eliminated by warm-blooded animals that no trace of it can be found in the system after twenty-four to forty-eight hours. Very large doses produce death by general paralysis. The temperature is from the first reduced from 1° to 3° Cent. In frogs the reflex irritability of the cord is entirely destroyed; but in warm-blooded animals it is not entirely removed until shortly before death. Respiration ceases before the heart-beat. It excites contractions in the pregnant and non-pregnant uterus, and is considered by Ziemssen superior to Ergot, because less likely to induce inflammation at the point of entrance.—*Med. Times and Gazette*, Dec. 6th, 1879. Dr. J. Williams states that two uterine fibroids have been successfully treated with this acid.—*Trans. Hom. Med. Soc.*, New York, 1879.

HINTS FROM ALLOPATHIC SOURCES.—Manganese produces, according to allopathic investigators, progressive wasting and feebleness, staggering gait, and paralysis, very much as does Zinc. These two drugs should be studied together. *Manganese* has been used successfully in high potencies for lumbar backache, with languor of the legs, heaviness of the feet, trembling; feet (right) go to sleep when he stands; tension and drawing in various parts of the body.

To our remedies for duodenal catarrh, namely, MERC., *Podo.*, *Ars.*, *Iris*, *Kali bich.*, and LYCOPOD., we may add, from allopathic provings, *Argentum nitricum.*

Cinchona is recommended in cholera infantum; after much straining the child voids a transparent mucus, streaked with blood; no fever; cases, it is added, which resist every possible combination of astringent and laxative. Thus, we see, it is suitable to cases rendered more atonic by drug abuse. It might be well to remember this hint as a parallel to our use of Nux.

Among the pathogenetic effects of *Cocculus*, *Picrotoxin*, allopathists speak of paralysis of the sphincters. This should receive a place along with Gelsemium, CAUSTICUM, Arsenic, Hyosc., etc., for trial.

Duboisia myoporoides (not the weaker, Pituri) ought to be thoroughly tested as a mydriatic. It promises to act more advantageously than Atropin.

Hammond advises Picrotoxin in epilepsy, especially in the anæmic; spasms worse at night. We already know its use in convulsions, caused by the weakness following prolonged sleeplessness.

Xanthoxylon is proposed for chronic pharyngitis, with great dryness. The mucous membrane is glossy, shining, and dry. This recommendation is by no means foreign to the provings as recorded in Allen, and should claim our attention. Popular practice has given this drug considerable reputation in paralysis of the tongue. As to this symptom our provings are wholly silent.

BELLADONNA IN CHOLERA INFANTUM.—One of the editors of the *Anglo-American Organon* publishes in the last number of that journal a case of cholera infantum which came under his care in Philadelphia, July 19th, 1879. The child was "eighteen months old; had been very sick all night; had very frequently vomited; his bowels had been moved every hour; stools of thin green mucus; at times he would cry very loudly and violently for five or ten minutes, but was lying most of the time in heavy stupor, out of which he started with a face very much flushed and red; pulse full, hard, 120 in a minute; had not passed any urine since the previous evening; had no appetite, and refused his usual food, but drank as much water as was offered him. Gave him one dose of Belladona^{cm} at noon. The starting from sleep and the crying ceased before morning, when I found him paler, sleeping better, had not vomited any more, stools less frequent, pulse 96. The improvement continued for five days, when he had more pain in the abdomen, stools not frequent, but consisted of very deep-green mucus; his thirst had entirely ceased. A few doses of Pulsatilla fully restored him. I learned that the boy had fallen out of his little carriage about nine months before, injured his tibia, and was almost entirely deprived of the use of his leg; he walked seldom and only with apparently great pain. The upper part of the tibia was very much inflamed, and pus was discharged from two openings. Silicea^{cm}, three doses, was given, and the child is (October 20th, 1879) progressing rapidly towards recovery without local treatment." The writer further says that "the very fact that the boy was so promptly cured of so very grave a disease as cholera infantum has always proved to be in this locality (Philadelphia) and at that season, proved that the apparently carious condition of the tibia did not depend on a deepseated diseased condition of the organism (scrofula or psora, etc.), but was merely the result of neglect. A child taken at that age with cholera infantum in this place at that season, suffering at the same time from other deepseated diseases, such as scrofula, hardly ever recovers, and then only after long tedious treatment."

The acute symptoms of the above case were similar to those presented in an unusual proportion of the cases of cholera infantum and other gastro-intestinal disorders occurring in this city during the summer of 1879, and for which Belladonna was largely prescribed. We think, however, that the doctor must be somewhat unfortunate as regards his cases of cholera infantum complicated with scrofula and other deepseated disorders. Such cases occurring in our own practice do not justify the statement that they "hardly ever recover," or that they get well "only after long tedious treatment," and we feel warranted therefore in holding the efficacy of homœopathic treatment in these disorders at a much higher estimate than he evidently does. It may be proper to state that in treating cholera infantum, either simple or complicated with "scrofula or psora," we use only the *lower and lowest* preparations. D.

News and Comments.

ANTI-VACCINATION.—The "First Anti-vaccination League of America" has been formed in New York. The prime mover in the matter is Mr. William Lebb, an Englishman, who has resisted thirteen prosecutions for refusing to have his children vaccinated. He believes it makes people liable to take inoculable disease, and does not insure them against smallpox.—*Exc.*

IMPORTANT TO THE PROFESSION.—Dr. James B. Bell, of Augusta, Me., author of *Bell on Diarrhœa,* writes us that he is preparing a new edition of his book. He asks that physicians having valuable clinical observations on diarrhœa will forward them immediately to him for use in his revision. Compliance with this request will, of course, be of service to the whole profession by adding to the value of an already indispensable book.

THE GERMANTOWN HOMŒOPATHIC SOCIETY.—This is the title of an association of the physicians of Germantown and vicinity, organized in October, 1879. The names thus far enrolled in its list of members are, John Malin, M.D., W. H. Malin, M.D., Horace Homer, M,D., J. R. Mansfield, M.D., Daniel Karsner, M.D., C. Van Artsdalen, M.D., M. M. Walker, M.D. The meetings will be held monthly, and will be of a social as well as scientific character. We shall be disagreeably surprised if the new society does not achieve success.

LOCATIONS FOR HOMŒOPATHIC PHYSICIANS.—E. Hadley Greene, M.D., of Charlotte, North Carolina, writes that he thinks "a real good, live, well-posted man could soon build up a fair practice in almost any of the thriving towns of the 'Old North State.' The idea that men from the North would not be well received is a great mistake. If they do not come for political purposes, to get office, they will be warmly welcomed, and will secure the respect of the citizens." We believe there are no homœopathic physicians in any of the chief towns of the State except Charlotte, and Dr. Greene will gladly furnish information respecting these places.

THE TRANSACTIONS OF THE HOMŒOPATHIC MEDICAL SOCIETY OF PENNSYLVANIA are at last under way with the certain promise of their early issue. Dr. J. C. Guernsey has taken charge, and is pushing the work through the press with his usual energy and dispatch. We are informed that the printers are returning to the doctor sixteen pages of proof daily. At this rate we shall, barring accidents, have the pleasure of giving the volume a review in our April or May number, as over 200 pages are now in type.

The book will comprise the proceedings of the Society for the five years from 1874–1878 inclusive, will be well printed and substantially bound in cloth, and will contain from 600 to 700 pages octavo.

All members in arrears must at once forward their dues to the treasurer, if they desire a copy of these *Transactions.*—EDS.

THE HAHNEMANN MEDICAL COLLEGE OF PHILADELPHIA.—The Thirty-second Annual Commencement of this institution will be held in the Academy of Music on Wednesday, March 10th, at 12 o'clock, M. The valedictory to the graduating class will be delivered by Professor McClatchey. Any physician can obtain a stage ticket by addressing Professor J. E. James, N. W. corner Tenth and Green streets.

The spring course will open on Monday, March 15th, and continue ten weeks. It will embrace lectures upon the following subjects:

Physical Diagnosis, by Professor A. R. Thomas, M.D.
Diseases of Children, by Professor O. B. Gause, M.D.
Hygiene, by Professor B. F. Betts, M.D.
Normal Histology, by Professor Pemberton Dudley, M.D.
Neurology and Dermatology, by Professor R. J. McClatchey, M.D.
Materia Medica and Pharmacy, by Charles Mohr, M.D.
Surgical Anatomy and Osteology, by R. B. Weaver, M.D.
Morbid Anatomy, by W. C. Goodno, M.D.
Chemistry, by W. S. Roney, A.M.
Venereal Diseases, by W. B. Trites, M.D.
Diseases of the Eye and Ear, by W. H. Bigler, M.D.
Medical Clinics, by Professor A. Korndœrfer, M.D.
Surgical Clinics, by Professor C. M. Thomas, M.D.
Gynæcological Clinics, by Professor B. Frank Betts, M.D.
Practical Anatomy, by R. B. Weaver, M.D.
Practical Surgery, by W. C. Goodno, M.D., and W. H. Keim, M.D.
Practical Obstetrics, by J. N. Mitchell, M.D.
Practical Chemistry, by W. S. Roney, A.M.
Practical Microscopy, by J. N. Mitchell, M D.

Tickets for the course, $15, which can be obtained of the Dean, Professor A. R. Thomas, No. 1733 Chestnut Street. Tickets for the practical courses, $10 each; optional.

MARRIED.—WILLIAMSON—WOODWARD.—On the 5th of February, 1880, by the Rev. William Suddards, Matthew S. Williamson, M.D., to Mary B., daughter of the late William Woodward, both of Philadelphia, Pa.

DECEASED.—Among a large number of distinguished physicians who have recently died we may mention the following:

THOMAS HUNT, F.R.C.S., author of treatises on diseases of the skin, died November 26th, 1879, aged 81 years.

J. SOLLBERG WELLS, M.D., F.R.C.S., Professor of Ophthalmology at King's College, and Ophthalmic Surgeon to King's College Hospital, died December 2d, 1879. In his early years he was assistant to Von Graefe. He was but 43 years old.

WILLIAM H. SMITH, M.D., of Philadelphia, died February 11th, 1880. Some years ago, and previous to engaging in general practice, he was more or less occupied in treating diseases of the horse, and is believed to have been the first physician to apply homœopathy in veterinary practice, having adopted that system so early as 1840.

M. FRIESE, M.D., of Harrisburg, Pa., died recently in Philadelphia. We hope to present a somewhat extended notice of his life and services to the cause of homœopathy in our next issue.

W. H. WOODYATT, M.D., Professor of Ophthalmology and Otology in the Chicago Homœopathic College, died January 31st, 1880, of malignant diphtheria. Professor Woodyatt settled in Chicago in 1871, and was the first homœopathic physician who adopted his specialty in that city. Both as a practitioner and as a teacher he was regarded as one of the very best in our profession. Both of the Chicago colleges, and also the medical societies of that city, have adopted resolutions of respect to his memory.

OBITUARY.

DR. JOSÉ NUÑEZ.

A FEW lines in a recent issue of the *Belgian Homœopathic Review* announced the sudden death of that very distinguished homœopathist, Dr. José Nuñez, Marquis de Nuñez, of Spain, and the November number of *El Criterio Medico* comes to us in mourning for him, the oldest and most distinguished of the Spanish physicians of our school. On its title-page we find the following announcement:

"The Most Illustrious JOSÉ NUÑEZ,

MARQUIS OF NUÑEZ; Doctor of Medicine; Honorary President of the Hahnemannian Society of Madrid; Founder and Director of the Hospital of San José and of the Homœopathic Institute of Madrid; Grand Cross of the Royal and Distinguished Order of Carlos III; Member of the Legion of Honor; Ex-Senator of the Kingdom, and corresponding member of various learned societies both foreign and domestic, died on November 10th, 1879.

"The Hahnemannian Society and the editors of the *Criterio Medico* entreat their friends to commend his soul to God."

At an extra session of the Hahnemannian Society of Madrid, held November 24th, 1879, convened to do honor to the memory of their deceased brother and leader, addresses were delivered by Dr. Garcia Lopes, the President, by Dr. Lopez de la Vega, by Dr. Thomas Pellicer, and by various other members, and several poetic tributes were read. All show the profound love and veneration which this veteran inspired in his followers; and from them we translate a brief sketch of his career.

The Marquis of Nuñez was born April 27th, 1805, in Benaventi, in the Province of Zamora, and was consequently in his seventy-fifth year at the time of his death. He was of a distinguished family, which bore the title of Marquis de la Salados, and was liberally educated. In 1825, when scarcely twenty years old, he began the study of law in the University of Valladolid, winning golden opinions by his zeal and acuteness.

Yielding to the example and persuasions of his comrades, young Nuñez decided to adopt an ecclesiastical career, and actually received orders. In 1830 he moved to Astaga, where for some years he acted as Secretary of the Ecclesiastical Council, at the same time that he practiced law with great success. The large clientage which he then acquired, and his personal qualifications, stood him in such good stead that in 1837 he was appointed Deputy Superintendent of the Province of Leon.

About this time the Civil War for the Succession broke out in Spain, in consequence of the death of King Ferdinand VII, and Nuñez, following his convictions, took part in favor of Don Carlos, not as a military man, but as one of the Assembly of Notables, who under the title of Counsellors, surrounded the Pretender. But speedily disgusted by the bad management of Don Carlos, he soon left him, and emigrated to France, abandoning politics, and seeking another field for his talents.

During his university course he had a strong inclination for the study of medicine, to which he now yielded. He matriculated at the College of Bordeaux, and pursued his studies with great assiduity, under the professors of the Hospital of Saint Andrew, in that city. About this time the new method of treatment discovered by Hahnemann began to penetrate into France. Nuñez threw himself heartily into the cause of this great reform; read and carefully studied all the works published on the subject, and put himself in correspondence with the principal homœopathic physicians of the country.

To his most brilliant talents Nuñez united a prodigious memory, which enabled him to overcome the difficulties of Hahnemann's Materia Medica, which he mastered to an extent rarely equalled. Thus prepared he could not avoid putting this new theory to the test of actual practice, and successfully treated many serious cases, especially among the Spanish residents of Bordeaux. These triumphs so exasperated the practitioners of the old school that they accused him of practicing illegally; and nothing shows more clearly the reality of the remarkable cures he made (without accepting any fee or honorarium) than the sentence of the tribunal that he should pay a fine of one franc, because he practiced without a regular license. This was the lowest penalty which the code could impose for a violation of its laws, and was a virtual confession of the merit of the cures for which he was arraigned.

His great success induced various influential Spaniards whom he had cured in Bordeaux to petition the Government to allow him to return to Spain, take his degree, and practice homœopathy. This request was granted; and in 1844 Nuñez returned to his native country, graduated as Bachelor of Medicine at the College in Madrid, and the same year stood an examination at the University of Barcelona, from which he received the degree of Doctor of Medicine.

In Madrid, where he lived and practiced for the remainder of his life, a period of thirty-five years, in spite of the unceasing hostility of the "regular" practitioners, he soon acquired an extraordinary reputation; and his fame spread year by year, not only throughout all Spain, but throughout the civilized world.

Although homœopathy was known in Spain before this time, and as far back as 1830 some few practitioners had embraced it and had translated some works upon that subject, Nuñez, by reason of his high position, his great ability, his untiring activity, his indomitable zeal and his wondrous cures, may justly be termed the apostle of homœopathy in Spain. So potent was his influence that he soon gathered around him, as a centre, all the physicians of the new school, and formed an association for the propagation of the new method of cure. This association was by royal edict, in 1846, erected into the Hahnemannian Society of Madrid, of which Dr. Nuñez was President for many years, and until increasing years and infirmity compelled his withdrawal. In the same year (1846) under his inspiration and active co-operation a journal was started called the *Bulletin of the Hahnemannian Society*, which, in 1851, was merged in the *Annals of Homœopathic Medicine*, which again was in 1860 replaced by *El Criterio Medico*, which still remains the official organ of the Society, composing in all a collection of thirty-one volumes. Herein are to be found the numerous and valuable contributions of Dr. Nuñez to medical science, which space fails us to mention. Besides many clinical reports, and essays upon various acute and chronic diseases, which are of great practical value and show the indefatigable industry as well as the profound learning of this great man, we find a monograph upon the pathogenetic effects of the poison of the *Tarentula*—a most valuable addition to our Materia Medica, and one which has of late come into extensive use in the West Indies and United States.

In 1849 he was President of the Homœopathic Congress at Paris, and in 1851 presided, in conjunction with Drs. Staple and Bœnninghausen, at the inauguration of the statue of Hahnemann in the city of Leipsic. In 1847 he obtained royal authorization to practice medicine in France, and in a few years later the Emperor Napoleon conferred upon him the diploma of the Legion of Honor in recognition of his medical eminence, all of which amply compensated him for the persecution he had undergone at Bordeaux.

But while thus honored abroad he was equally honored at home. For several years he was Special Physician to Queen Isabella II, and also had charge of the Infanta D. Sebastian. He was successively graced with the grand crosses of several royal orders, and in 1865 he received the lofty title of Marquis de Nuñez. He was also elected a Senator in the next to the last Legislature.

But all these distinctions both public and private were always used by him to strengthen and extend the homœopathic school.

He ardently desired to establish a college and hospital in Madrid, and was unceasing in his efforts to do so. But though ably seconded by several of his colleagues, the various attempts did not succeed until quite recently. It is now only two years since the Hospital of St. Joseph was formally opened. Its existence is due to his indefatigable efforts, aided by the Hahnemannian Society, and homœopathy is now taught in Madrid, both theoretically and practically, in a public institution under a management composed of some of the most prominent citizens of that city.

When this hospital and institute was opened to the public, Dr. Nuñez took up his residence there, living in very modest apartments, and giving all his time and labor to its firm establishment, fearful that if he should die before its success was assured all the hopes and labors of his life would come to naught. He himself visited the wards and directed the treatment of the more serious cases; and who can say that he did not offer up his life to the cause he so loved? for had he not taken up his abode within these walls he would probably be living to bless us this day by his presence.

To this institution, the child of his old age, dearer than all else to his heart, he gave $30,000 during his life; and in his will he has bequeathed the magnificent sum of $375,000 for its perpetual maintenance as a homœopathic hospital and college. And still more touching proof of his love, in accordance with his express wish, for which he obtained governmental sanction a year ago, all that was mortal of the Marquis de Nuñez now lies buried in the garden of his beloved hospital. To him no ground so sacred as that upon which stands the charity, the embodied realization of that medical reform to which he consecrated his life. R. J. McC.

THE

HAHNEMANNIAN MONTHLY.

Vol. II., New Series } Philadelphia, April, 1880. No. 4.

Original Department.

SILICEA IN ENCHONDROMA.

BY W. T. LAIRD, M.D., WATERTOWN, N. Y.

On March 18th, 1876, I was called in consultation by Dr. Knickerbocker, in the case of E. B., a delicate but comparatively healthy child, two years old. About four weeks before, his parents first noticed a morbid growth, involving the second joints of the index and middle fingers of the left hand. The tumors were oval, hard, smooth, painless, and evidently were growing from the bone. The affected parts were now twice their natural size. We readily agreed upon the diagnosis of enchondroma, and, as the child had been under treatment nearly a month, and had taken Silicea, Fluoric acid and the much-vaunted Hecla lava, without appreciable benefit, we advised an immediate amputation. To this the parents were unwilling to consent without first consulting a New York surgeon. They were accordingly sent, with a letter of introduction, to Professor Helmuth, who confirmed the diagnosis, and appointed the following day for the operation. At this stage of the proceedings, the family received a telegram from a relative, requesting them to defer all active treatment until the case could be seen by his friend, Dr. G., an old-school physician. He agreed in the diagnosis, but vehemently opposed any operation, assuring the parents that the tumors had attained the limit of their growth, would cause no inconvenience, and would prove less of a deformity than the removal of the fingers. In this view he was sustained by Professor Hood, of Bellevue, whom he called in consultation. This advice, coinciding as it did with the wishes of the family, was eagerly accepted, and the patient was brought home on the following day. In spite of these positive and comforting assurances, the perverse tumors continued to grow, and on the 12th of April I was again summoned to see the case. The fingers were now four times their natural size; the skin, stretched to its utmost tension, had begun to ulcerate; the morbid growth had extended to the first metacarpal bone; and a third tumor was found on the little toe of the left foot. The parents were frankly informed that immediate removal of the fingers afforded the only chance of saving the hand, and to this they at last reluctantly consented. At 2 P.M., assisted by Dr. Knickerbocker, I etherized the patient, and after applying an Esmarch bandage, removed the index finger with one-half of the metacarpal bone, and disarticulated the middle finger at the metacarpo-phalangeal articulation. It was decided not to amputate the toe, but to await developments and remove it later, if the tumor should become large enough to be troublesome. The child reacted well from the operation, and a few doses of Aconite^{30} were given to control the inevitable surgical fever. On the following day, the hand was considerably swollen, and showed an erysipelatous redness around the wound; the tongue was dry, with red tip and edges; the patient feverish and restless. These symptoms were readily subdued by Rhus tox 2^{c}. The larger part of the incision united by first intention and the wound was practically healed in ten days.

Meanwhile the tumor on the toe had been rapidly growing, and was now as large as a small walnut. My attention had recently been called to an article in the *Medical Investigator*, by Grauvogl, on "Silicea in Enchrondroma;" and as this remedy had already been given in various potencies, from the 3d to the 200th, it was decided to try the very highest that could be obtained, simply as an experiment, without any hope of effecting a cure. April 22d, a single dose of Silicea 71^{m} was given dry on the tongue. Two days later the tumor suppurated, discharged for a few days, and then the opening closed. It steadily decreased in size for a week, and afterwards remained stationary until May 10th, when Silicea 71^{m} was repeated. The second dose was again followed by suppuration and discharge of part of the contents of the tumor. A third dose was given June 6th; a fourth, July 14th; and a fifth, November 12th. Each repetition of the remedy was followed by the same phenomena as at first. The only external application used was a bread-and-milk poultice. By December the growth had entirely disappeared, and the only trace of it that now remains is a small, hardly perceptible scar.

All surgical authorities agree in pronouncing enchondroma incurable by medical treatment. Professor Gross says: "The only remedy for this tumor is early and efficient extirpation." Professor Miller states, in his *Principles of Surgery*: "Discussion is impossible, and therefore extirpation is expedient." Paget, Druitt, Erichsen, and Markoe, use substantially the same language; and Billroth emphatically declares that "The only *treatment* is removal of the tumor if it can be done without endangering life." The only apparent exception is Professor Hamilton, who claims that he has "occasionally seen these growths, especially when occurring in early life upon the fingers, delayed and finally arrested by air, exercise, nutritious food, and tonics;" yet he nowhere speaks of ever witnessing a *cure*. In view of this unanimous and positive testimony, the skeptical may naturally inquire: Was the tumor cured by Silicea an enchondroma? It exactly resembled in every respect those removed from the hand, which were pronounced enchondromatous by five different physicians, including no less competent authorities than Professor Helmuth, of the New York Homœopathic College, and Professor James Wood, of Bellevue. It would seem, therefore, that there could be no reasonable doubt about the diagnosis. Was not the suppuration a natural process, and the cure a spontaneous one? Upon this point Professor Markoe, in his classical work on *Diseases of the Bones*, uses the following language: "There may be rapid softening to which inflammation is afterward superadded. . . The products of inflammation collect in a focus, forming a sort of abscess, which breaks and discharges its contents. Ulceration now begins, sometimes with sloughing, and we have imitated in all respects the behavior of the most malignant growths, an imitation which is carried out unfortunately through all the worst and most destructive phases of malignant disorganization. I do not pretend to say that such a process may not, in some cases, terminate in simple destruction of the growth, and be followed by a proper healing process; but it must be confessed that when such action is observed in a cartilaginous tumor, the reasonable apprehension is that the ill behavior is indicative of ill character, and that the originally benign tumor has assumed the nature as well as the behavior of a malignant growth, and will probably vindicate its claims to be so considered by ultimately destroying the patient." Surely no one will claim that the healthy suppuration, by which this tumor was cured, without pain, fever, or constitutional disturbance, bears any resemblance to the sloughing, ulcerated, malignant-looking degeneration described by Markoe. Besides, if this had been a case of "spontaneous enucleation," the whole morbid growth would have been eliminated *en masse*, not destroyed piecemeal by several distinct suppurative processes. The series of phenomena which followed each dose of the medicine were too regular and recurred too frequently to be explained on this theory or on that of coincidences. It certainly was not a "faith cure," for the child was too young to have either belief or disbelief, and neither the family nor the attending physician expected a successful issue. Whether the high potency of Silicea would have cured the tumors which were removed, cannot now be determined; but reasoning from analogy, we should be justified in answering in the affirmative; and it will always be a matter of regret that the experiment was not tried before resorting to operative measures.

FOUR ONE-LUNG CASES.

BY M. M. WALKER, M.D., GERMANTOWN, PA.

(Read before the Hahnemann Club of Philadelphia.)

Frank H——, six years and seven months old.

When four years of age he had a severe attack of bronchial catarrh which merged into an abscess of the left lung. For several weeks he was very ill, but as the abscess formed he gradually recovered, walked about, but could not lie down. There was a pointing of the whole chest toward the base of the sternum, until one day, about three months subsequent to the attack of bronchial catarrh, the abscess opened, discharging over a pint of pus, and left an opening between the cartilages of the sixth and seventh ribs, somewhat to the left of the sternum, which continued to discharge pus till the time of his death. He generally slept in a sitting posture, with his head resting on a table or pillow in front of him.

In height he was equal to most boys of his age, very thin, delicate, subject to colds, coughed a great deal, with considerable expectoration, cough always loose and very rattling. The left lung was gradually destroyed, the ribs compressed, the spine curved to the right, and the heart pushed over to the right side.

In January, 1879, owing to rapid and severe changes in the weather, he, like many others, had an attack of bronchial catarrh, followed by pneumonia, and terminating in his death, on February 12th.

The post-mortem, made by Dr. Horace Homer and myself, in addition to the above description, revealed the following conditions: Pneumonia of right lung, which was hepatized throughout, except a small portion of the middle lobe.

Left lung entirely destroyed. Heart considerably enlarged, and pushed to the right of sternum.

The cavity for the left lung so compressed as to permit of the introduction of but one finger between the flattened ribs and the spine.

Scapula, clavicle, and head of humerus of the left shoulder, very prominent. The inferior surface of the pericardium was thickened and rough, as well as the tissues of the pleura and diaphragm. From these roughened surfaces pus had evidently been secreted for months. No tubercles were found.

I learn a brother of this boy's mother died two years ago from abscess of the right kidney, at about thirty-six years of age. This boy's father died in January, 1880, from phthisis.

This case seems to confirm Dr. Hutchinson's assertion, that in ordinary respiration we use but one-sixteenth of our lung capacity.

In treating this case for three years, I took a great deal of time to study out the exact similimum, using from the 6th to 50^{m} dilutions. *Tar. em.*, *Ipecac.*, and *Sticta pul.*, seemed to relieve him more than other remedies.

He had good motherly care at home. I was anxious to see him grow up, but the struggle for existence was too great for him.

Mrs. Ann M. F——, in her seventieth year. Has been an invalid over forty years, has coughed daily during that length of time, and during the first thirteen years of her married life gave birth to nine children. It was the prayer of her life to see her youngest child grow up, and she feels her prayer answered, that child being now thirty-two years of age.

There were two curvatures in her spine, one in the dorsal and one in the lumbar vertebræ. Whenever she was ill, lying in bed aggravated the irritation produced by these curvatures, causing sleeplessness and pain. Many of her nights were passed in a sitting posture. Her heart and lungs had been more or less affected for nearly twoscore years; had been auscultated and percussed by many physicians, and various opinions given concerning them. During the three and a half years I attended her she required one or more visits every week, principally for attention to her loose, harassing cough and palpitation of the heart. She finally succumbed with pneumonia, January 2d, 1879. The autopsy exhibited the following conditions:

Chronic bronchitis, with enlargement of the calibre of the bronchial tubes of the left lung to twice their normal size.

The bronchial tubes white, leathery, double their normal thickness, and from their inner surface had been secreted quantities of ropy mucus, which, during life, she frequently drew to a cup or basin in her lap.

The left lung adherent throughout its posterior extent, thickened, black, compressed, and had been of no use for years.

Right lung hepatized in both lower lobes, less than one-fifth of her lung capacity being available. No tubercles found.

Heart. Suffered during life with frequent palpitations, would almost suffocate at times, her lips and fingers turning blue. The heart was fifty per cent. larger than it should have been. Along three-fourths of its median posterior line an adhesion had formed, interfering with its free action. A white fibrinous clot, six inches long, tapering from the middle to either end, had formed in each of the two cavities. Dilatation of the right auricle and ventricle, with thickening of the walls of the left. One ounce of serum in the pericardium. Ossification of aortic valves, the ossific points varying from size of a pin's head to that of a pea, and five or six in number. She had had an intermittent pulse for many years.

She requested a post-mortem on several occasions when she thought her last day had come, that her children might profit by the result should any of them be similarly afflicted.

ANNIE B. F——, aged sixty years, of a bilious temperament, a slender woman, probably five feet three inches in height; had not exceeded ninety-eight pounds in weight since her youth. Thirty-one years ago had pneumonia, which left a permanent thickening of the middle lobe of the right lung, for which affection she was advised a year later to remove to this suburb of Philadelphia for her health, her physician adding "he did not think she would live a year."

She drank tea three times a day for many years, and several years ago had an attack of congestion, with enlargement of the liver, but of late years there has been a diminution in the size of that organ.

She had terrible headaches at regular and irregular intervals, and a few years ago an attack of sciatica prevented her from sitting for several weeks. A sojourn at Cape May relieved that. She was very delicate, yet attended to the management of her house, took great interest in church affairs, and every summer enjoyed extended tours to the monntains or seaside resorts, Atlantic City being her place of recuperation the last three years.

In August, 1874, after a shopping excursion to Philadelphia, and while hurrying to the train, she spat up a tablespoonful of blood; she kept quiet a few days and recovered. At irregular intervals after that she spat up the same quantity; by November, streaks of pus came with the clotted blood. The pus gradually increased, irregular chills and fevers supervened, till a gill of pus would be expectorated in twenty-four hours. She became thinner and more emaciated every month till, eighteen months prior to her death, she weighed but seventy-three pounds. No case of phthisis could be traced among her long-lived ancestors, although we could trace them back to Francis Daniel Pastorius, who located in Germantown in 1693.

Auscultation indicated clearness of the left lung to the last week of her life.

Diagnosis.—Abscess of the right lung, the result of pneumonia over thirty years before.

I often queried whether this abscess extended to the liver. She was frequently constipated, but the expectoration, although of a pale-greenish or bluish cast, never showed the characteristic yellowness or green color of bile, or small particles of bile, it was more the color we find in some cases of phthisis. Any enlargement or unusual hardness of the liver, indicative of abscess of that organ, could have been very easily detected upon her emaciated body. Occasionally, during the last two weeks of her life, an effort, like contraction of the diaphragm, sometimes voluntarily, at others involuntarily, took place; a tablespoonful or more of dark, congealed blood would come into her mouth or gush down her clothing before she could signal aid. This congealed blood was odorless, except when it occurred immediately after taking food or drink, when it partook of the odor of the ingesta, particles of which came with it. It frequently came with pus after coughing, but generally when she was quiet.

Was there perforation of the stomach or œsophagus, or a *cul-de-sac* somewhere in the diseased lung, which irregularly ejected its contents?

Rheumatic paralysis of her right arm increased as destruction of the lung progressed, till at times she could not hold anything in her hand or control its shaking.

She suffered intensely with intercostal neuralgia and neuralgia through the right lung and down the arm. Many remedies were studied over and given, one at a time, in frequent or long-repeated doses, and in potencies from the 3d decimal to 70^{m}, generally from 200th up. *Bry.*, *Phos.*, *Arnica*, *Asclepias tuberosa*, *Rhus tox.*, *Nux vom.*, *Hepar s.*, *Silicea*, *Secale cor.*, and some of Scheussler's remedies, were given, but none gave more than temporary relief, not even the mixtures the family *would* give, aided her much in her downhill journey of life.

She died February 6th, 1879. No autopsy permitted.

LIZZIE G., nine years old in January, 1880. In March, 1878, had a very severe attack of bronchial catarrh while visiting in the country, and was under the care of a good homœopathic physician. She came home May 9th, in poor health, took another cold, had an attack of pneumonia, followed by rigors and fever, occurring at different times nearly every day, great rattling in the right lung, the child being very ill, an abscess also formed, and began to point, in the lower part of the lung, to the right of the spine.

On July 14th, Dr. M. Macfarlan, assisted by Mr. A. S. Mattson, student, and myself, aspirated the abscess by plunging the needle into the side of the lung, between the sixth and seventh ribs. We took about one pint of pus out, then, by reversing the action of the aspirator, we rinsed the lung thoroughly with carbolized water. The little girl, during the operation, stood half-reclining between her father's knees. No anæsthetic was used. In a few minutes she exclaimed, "Oh! I taste that horrid medicine in my mouth," gave a slight cough, and spit two tablespoonfuls of blood and carbolized water into her father's vest pocket, showing we had not only rinsed the diseased lung, but had punctured one of the lesser bronchial tubes, establishing a circuit from the basin on the floor through our patient thence to a cup held by her father.

About August 1st the abscess opened, not at the point of puncture, but below the tenth rib and three inches to the right of the spine. Curvature of the spine to the left gradually took place as the lung became displaced and lost by suppuration, which continued till October 22d, 1879, when the abscess ceased to discharge and the opening healed.

Hepar sulph. did her more good than any other remedy, although *Tart. em.*, *Stan.*, *Arsen.*, *Silicea*, *Phos.* had been given, while many other remedies were consulted. I kept her on Hepar for a month, when she went to the Children's Seashore Home, Atlantic City (old school), where Dr. Bennett had her carefully looked after, although very little medicine was administered. She improved very much during a stay of four weeks, gaining flesh and strength.

The parents of this child are in very moderate circumstances, the father intemperate, the mother delicate, suffering from hysteria and uterine troubles. Dr. Macfarlan, in 1875, I think, removed an ovarian tumor weighing twenty-six pounds, from the abdomen of the child's mother's sister. The patient recovered from the operation and in three years died from three similar tumors arising from the other ovary.

Occasionally during the last two years I have examined this child carefully. A year ago there seemed to be a destruction of the two lower lobes of the affected lung. The spinal curvature deformed the child, yet she grew, was as fleshy as many children of her age, enjoyed life, and part of the time attended school.

To-day, February 20th, 1880, she is in fine spirits; her spine is perfectly straight. There is quite a flattening of the chest, especially below the seventh rib; down to the sixth rib the respiratory murmur is very clear; below that point it can be heard but gets fainter and fainter till lost. The lung has expanded, and now there seems to be a loss of not more than one-third of the lung capacity. She had measles last month, from which she recovered in a few days. She coughs only when she takes cold, then spits up thick phlegm; is very happy, and thinks her doctor must attend her, although she is about moving twelve miles away.

KEEP YOUR MOUTH SHUT.

BY W. H. WINSLOW, M D., PITTSBURG, PA.

NOTWITHSTANDING the general good sense of the people, the time devoted to the study of hygiene, in schools and out, and the great amount of space occupied by articles upon health in all our journals, we are exceedingly careless. No one is happy who is unhealthy, for the discomfort and suffering occasioned by lesions of the organism depress mental action and remind us too often that we are mortal.

We are opposed to contemplating Charon's duties, and not in such a hurry to cross his ferry as Brooklynites to get to business over the East River, yet carelessly and unconsciously we do suicidal acts as calmly as we eat our breakfast. Either hygiene is not properly taught, or the pursuit of pleasure and business crowd it out of consideration. Though the average of life has been increased by improvements in food, cooking, clothing, and habitations, and some of the evils of barbarism have been abolished, yet in individual personal care we are behind the Romans. We look in vain amongst our modern cities for one equal to Rome, with her perfect system of drainage and splendid free marble baths. Paris has been made magnificent by imperial squanderings, but her people live over the festering, foul corpses of her massacres, and the sewers meander through her catacombs to pollute the Seine, from the waters of which the people make their soup, and which they must drink when they are too poor to buy wine.

Proper ventilation of dwellings is hardly thought of by our builders, and the primitive, health-conservative, open fireplaces of our fathers have given place to stuffy-stoves and lung-desiccating furnaces. Our mucous membranes creak and crumble like parchment, and noxious gases permeate our capillaries and rob our hæmatin of ruddy colors. Our doorsteps and pavements are deluged with water, and Bridget wears out a broom weekly, while from byways and alleys pour noxious streams of dish-water, floating away the debris of the kitchen and the slop-bucket. It makes one sick to go out in the still hours of the night in one of our large cities and inhale the air of freedom. As if we could not remedy the evil if we choose. Let us wage war against the enemies of life, and protect ourselves from their stealthy treachery.

There is one evil that I wish to call attention to now more particularly. The weather has been severe during the last few days, and overcoats and wraps have come from the pegs where the foolish belief in the groundhog superstition consigned them. Old Boreas has sharpened his northwesters, and sent their lances against our teeth and into every rent and gap in our habiliments. Diseases of the throat, ears, and lungs have become alarmingly prevalent, and in many cases they are the heritage of ignorance. To caution and to enlighten would be more useful than to scold. A cold man generally stands with his back to the fire. This instinctive action results from his anatomy. The great blood-currents flow forwards, and the nervous system which regulates it is at the back, along the spine. The thin sheets of muscle and fascia over the back soon give up their heat, but those of the abdomen and chest, warmer from their blood-currents, possess reservoirs of heat in the richly vascular underlying viscera. The back first shivers at low temperatures, and a chill is followed by a lumbago or a renal disorder; but chilling the interior surface of the body—

depressing the temperature of all the blood—causes most formidable and dangerous diseases.

In accordance with fashion and feelings we cover the back with layer upon layer of woollen, and leave the chest and abdomen with buttonless gaps and a triangular exhibition of linen. Death comes through the brain, the heart, or the lungs, the tripod of life. The anterior chest-wall is on an average about an inch thick. Just beneath and behind the collar-bone the apex of the lung comes very near the surface. These apices are generally covered by but two thicknesses of clothing, and women frequently don't cover them at all. It is a significant fact that this is the part usually first filled with tubercles when consumption begins; the disease that kills about thirty-three per cent. of the human race. Very few Friends (Quakers) have consumption. They shield the upper lobes, by solid gray woollens, from treacherous drafts and icy blasts. Fashion opposes this dress and offers flannel pads, buckskin breast protectors, and other abominations. The lungs should be covered even above the root of the neck if we would escape destruction.

Now I have noticed, during the last cold snap, that many persons hurrying through the streets were puffing like locomotives. To get over the ground and through business rapidly they overexerted their muscles; these required more oxygen, hence more respirations; the cold air stinging the nose in many cases could not be drawn through the turbinated passages fast enough, and so the mouth was opened, the watery vapor of the exhaled breath was condensed into visible molecules by the cold air, and hence the locomotive appearances of locomotion. More than half the persons I met were steaming along in this reckless fashion, with mouths wide open to the wintry blasts. Did any one have neuralgia, toothache, inflammation of the ears, sore throat, and pulmonary trouble from this insanity? Ask our jaded and nightly-disturbed doctors. Did I chuckle at the prospect of a harvest of ear diseases? No! I was indignant that people of this intelligent age should be such fools, and yet I found myself doing the same thing one day rushing for a train.

There are few acts so dangerous as breathing with the mouth open in cold weather. The nose warns one of the presence of filth, delights with agreeable odors, and warms the air for the capillary tubes and racemose groups of air-cells in the lungs. God has so impressed these differences of function upon the organ as to leave no doubt of their duality. The part devoted to smelling is high above where the air passes, and its surface is covered by flat epithelium, like the tiles of a floor; while the respiratory tract below has the mucous membrane covered by thousands of little whips, or cilia, which move ceaselessly in life, like a field of ripe grain in summer breezes. These catch particles of dust and vegetable and animal products, and discharge them periodically with inspissated excretions, so that they cannot produce disease of the lungs by their mechanical irritation, nor carry into the circulation those nondescript germs which are thought to produce epidemic disease.

The interior of the nose is a complex of cavities, channels, curves, and scrolls, to present as much warm vascular membrane to the incoming currents of air as possible, and thus prepare it for the more delicate structures in the lobules and lobes of the lungs.

When cold air, loaded with deleterious particles, rushes through the mouth, down the devious passages, there is great peril to the integrity of the ears, pharynx, larynx, and pulmonary structures. Diseases of the respiratory tract are most common amongst us, and they are due in a great measure to our careless manner of breathing.

Deafness among our North American Indian tribes is very rare, and has been explained by the care which is exercised from infancy to keep the mouth shut during respiration.

Let us take a hint from the Friends and cover our lungs with warm clothing; and learn wisdom even from barbarous Indians, and keep our mouths shut. Thus may we contribute to our health and happiness, and diminish the rate of mortality.

CLINICAL GLEANINGS.

BY H. L. STAMBACH, M D, PHILADELPHIA.

(Read before the Homœopathic Medical Society of Philadelphia)

A PART of the prescribed work of the Bureau of Clinical Medicine, etc., is the collation of clinical cases that illustrate the principles of homœopathy. This task (or pleasant duty shall I say?), as a member of said bureau, has devolved upon me, and I herewith present for your consideration the following clinical gleanings made from such of the journals as it was my privilege to examine. Many more cases might have been cited, but I selected those that, in my judgment, most clearly illustrated the working of the single remedy chosen by the rule *similia*.

ARNICA.—Dr. J. F. Edgar reports his observation of a

probable characteristic of *Arnica*, viz., "A cold, clammy sweat on the forearms, from elbows to ends of fingers." His attention was particularly attracted to it, in treating acute hydrocephalus, with a history of several severe blows on the head, and found corroboration in a half dozen more recent cases, when the 30x and preferably the 200th of *Arnica* cured. Allen gives Jörg's proving, "skin more moist than usual on chest and inner surface of arms."—*The Medical Counselor*, January, 1880.

CARBO VEG.—Dr. H. N. Guernsey says that sometimes after delivery, pains producing the utmost suffering appear in parts distant from the pelvic region. In the shinbone, for instance, the exacerbations and remissions occur as regularly as if in the uterus. When appearing in the shinbones *Carbo veg.* cures.—*The Medical Counselor*, April, 1879.

IPOMŒA.—Dr. E. A. Farrington reports the following case: "Intense soreness over left kidney, with paroxysms of pain along course of ureter, as well as in the back; *pain always accompanied with nausea*, and occasionally vomiting. *Ipomœa*^{30} promptly relieved, and in five days a calculus was passed without pain.—*The Medical Counselor*, August, 1879.

PICRIC ACID.—Dr. H. C. Allen reports two cases cured by *Picric acid:* (1.) Brain-fag in the principal of a school; complete exhaustion caused by her daily duties; so tired that she can scarcely reach home; headache, completely incapacitating her for work; begins in the morning on waking; increases as the day advances; always relieved by sleep at night; chiefly affects forehead, extending gradually to vertex, and involving entire cerebrum, with constant vertigo; worse from motion and mental exertion, especially her school-work; much worse on going upstairs; sometimes an intense throbbing, at other times a dull pressing; always better from quiet; pain in eyes; worse on moving them; with the headache, sense of *terrible prostration, she feels so tired;* feels better in the open air, but is too tired and exhausted to walk; after walking a few yards, thinks she will never reach the next block, as it seems so far away; sometimes unrefreshed by sleep. (Compare Allen, 387-97.) *Picric acid*^{30} and ^{6} cured.

(2.) After a severe mental shock from a *death, languor, exhaustion, "feels so tired;"* wants to lie down and sleep all the time, which she would do if not aroused. (Compare Allen, 400–10.) *Picric acid*^{3} cured.—*The Medical Counselor*, August, 1879.

CINA.—Dr. A. McNeil reports success with *Cina*, the epidemic remedy for the prevalent intermittents and remittents of the children of his region. The 200th at the close of a paroxysm prevented a return of the former, or the latter were cured in two or three days. Last summer he found *Cina* frequently indicated in the so-called malarial diseases of children and again promptly cured with the 200th. Intermittents of children, when the paroxysms are attended with convulsions, are almost invariably cured by *Cina*, given during or *immediately after* the attack.

Symptoms.—Boring at the nose; exceedingly unamiable; short hacking cough; frequent swallowing, as if to swallow down something; the urine turns milky; tossing during sleep; often sullen and unwilling to play during the day. Vermiculous symptoms, with him, never require Santonin or vermifuges of any kind.—*Cincinnati Medical Advance*, January, 1880.

CANTHARIS.—Dr. Claude, of Paris, reports the following case: Miss C., after exposure to a strong current of air while walking, had frequent attacks, at irregular intervals, of pain, like red-hot iron in right zygomatic process, causing the most piercing screams, coming and going suddenly, and lasting twenty to thirty minutes. During attack, pallor, right face contracted and completely distorted by sudden jerkings of muscles, and pupils greatly dilated. *Cantharis*^{3} cured.—*N. E. Medical Gazette*, September, 1879.

THUJA.—The same French physician also reports the following: Almost constant terrible neuralgia in *left* face, on a level with zygomatic process and malar bone. *Thuja*^{3} cured. —*N. E. Medical Gazette*, November, 1879.

LACHESIS.—In the *Homœopathic Journal of Obstetrics and Diseases of Women and Children* Dr. Bahrenberg reports the case of a lady who was nervous, ached all over, with hysterical spells of trembling; could not move, work, or sleep; dark foreboding of the future; any news, excitement, or harsh words aggravated her troubles; worse after sleep. Cured by *Lachesis* 2^m.

COLOCYNTHIS.—The *British Journal of Homœopathy* reports a case of renal calculus in which the pain was relieved by Colocynthis^3 *before* the expulsion of the stone, again demonstrating the non-necessity of resorting to opiates " to deaden the pain until the calculus has passed." (See Dr. Farrington's case cured by *Ipomœa.*)

BARYTA MUR.—To the *Monthly Homœopathic Review* (London) Dr. Flint contributes a case of aneurism of the abdominal aorta greatly relieved by *Baryta mur* 1^x or 2^x.

LYCOPODIUM.—Through the *London Homœopathic World* Dr. Loosvelt suggests "half-open eyes during sleep" as a characteristic of *Lycopodium.*

PODOPHYLLUM.—Dr. Ussher, in the same journal, states that *Podophyllum* causes stools of garlicky carrion smell, and one or two patients have observed the odor on their bodies.

RUTA.—Dr. Ussher also says that *Ruta*° applied to a sprained wrist caused bearing-down pains in the uterus.

PHOSPHORUS.—Dr. George Gale, of Quebec, reports a case of a woman suffering with rush of blood to head, heat of face, scalp sensitive to touch, sudden shooting pains in the head, especially in the vertex, induced by and always aggravated when *washing clothes* or *walking fast.* Must go to bed with the attack. Small ulcer on left foot. Cured with *Phosphorus*^{cm}. —*The Organon,* January, 1880.

TARENTULA.—Dr. Swan reports two cases of pruritus vulvæ:

1. A widow, æt. 45, had for sixteen years sensation of motion in the uterus like a fœtus; singing like a teakettle in left ear; constipation profound unless she takes pills; occasional stoppage of urine, which is high-colored, with red sediment; pain in region of the kidneys; occasional palpitation without particular cause; sensation of something crawling up the legs under the skin from the feet until it reaches the uterus; this causes great sexual desire, which is aggravated by intense pruritus, and rubbing, which it is impossible to resist, makes her nearly crazy. Gave four powders of *Tarentula*^{m}. A few days later she reported herself "relieved of all the symptoms except the singing in the ear and constipation." Gave six powders of *Tarentula*^{m} and cured the case.

2. Young lady complains of intense unbearable pruritus vulvæ, extending into the vagina, with dryness and heat of the parts; worse at night; white, thin leucorrhœa; thick, white sediment in urine; pain in right side of abdomen; nausea; accumulation of mucus in the throat; mouth parched and dry; thirst often and for large quantities; very restless at night. Gave *Tarentula*^{m}, at 11 A.M. She was not troubled with pruritus next night, and the other symptoms also disappeared the next day.—*The Organon,* October, 1879.

LAC. V. DEFLOR.—Dr. Swan also reports in *The Organon,* October, 1879, the following: A woman had been suffering all the afternoon from sudden suppression of menses, caused by putting her hands in cold water to rinse out some clothes;

pain all over, especially in the head. Gave *Lac. vaccinum defloratum*^{m} in water. The first dose put her to sleep, free from pain; slept all night; in the morning had slight flow. A second dose brought on the flow profusely, and at 11 A.M. she was able to attend to her duties, feeling entirely well. The flow continued the usual time. (The pain ceasing before the restoration of the flow proves this case a homœopathic cure and not merely a "get well.")

LAC CANINUM.—Dr. George H. Carr contributes to *The Organon*, April, 1879, a case of diphtheritic sore throat, always occurring before the menses. A woman, æt. 28, dark hair and eyes, full person, has suffered as above noted ever since she had diphtheria. At present right side of throat is worse, but sometimes one side will be affected and sometimes the other. Small yellowish-white patches of exudation on the tonsils of the affected side, with great difficulty in swallowing and sharp pains moving up into the ear. Patches also present on back part of throat and on uvula; some are quite yellow and some white. Scraping them off makes them bleed. *Lac caninum*^{cm}, one dose dry, completely cured the whole difficulty in twelve hours, and she has since had no trouble with her throat at the menstrual period.

CLINICAL STUDIES.

BY CHARLES MOHR, M.D., PHILADELPHIA.

(Read before the Homœopathic Medical Society of Philadelphia.)

1. NASAL CATARRH AFTER MEASLES.—On May 2d, 1875, was consulted on behalf of G., a well-developed girl, aged seven years, who for a long time had been troubled with a peculiar *sensation in the left nostril, high up, as of some foreign body there, which must be blown down.* This sensation, noticed most by the parents at mealtime, when efforts were frequently made to detach the offending substance, was considered only a bad habit, for which the child was frequently reproved or punished. An inquiry into other conditions revealed the fact that she had frequent attacks of catarrhal croup, occurring usually after midnight, generally attended during the decline of an attack with the expectoration of *tough stringy mucus* after a *strangling cough.* She often returned from school with a severe headache, a great deal of pain being felt in two spots, which could be covered with the point of the fingers, directly over the frontal protuberances. The patient being a stout,

chubby, light-complexioned child, I decided without hesitation to prescribe *Kali bich.*²⁰⁰, one powder, dry, night and morning, the wisdom of the choice being shown by the development on the fourth day after beginning the medicine of an eruption on the face, and subsequently over the body, of a papular character. The father thought this strange, as he informed me she had had measles about a year before, and the present eruption looked just like them. I visited the girl and found an eruption as near resembling measles as anything I ever saw, but there was an absence of fever, and the catarrhal irritation was very slight. A further inquiry into the history of the former attack of measles revealed the cause of the persistent nasal catarrh. Before desquamation had well begun she had been allowed to go out into the street to play, the weather being warm and pleasant, this imprudence resulting, as the mother remembered, in a severe coryza, croupy cough, and following the subsidence of the more acute symptoms, leaving the child subject to the attacks of catarrhal headache (pain in frontal sinuses), and the disagreeable sensation compelling the expulsive efforts to dislodge some imaginary body from the left nostril.

Now what was to be done? A subject for study presented itself. The symptoms had changed; was a change of medicine necessary? Just in such cases mistakes are often made. The phenomena occurring after the administration of a *similimum*, in chronic affections at least, should be carefully studied, and no hasty new line of treatment decided on if symptoms different from those for which it was prescribed should arise. A study of every feature of the case is demanded; a study of the pathogenesis of the given drug should be carefully made, for a switching off at such a time may lead one away into a little wilderness of medicines, one after another being vainly tried, until the heterogeneous mass of resulting symptoms brings the physician to a dead halt in the search for another *similimum*. I made such a study of the case before me, and decided to treat it as an ordinary first attack of measles in all respects save the administration of medicine. Of that enough had been taken; its discontinuance was therefore ordered, believing that the *Kali bich.*, in its curative effects, had brought out a suppressed exanthem. I therefore advised the child to be kept from all drafts or exposure to changes of temperature; had the room well ventilated, kept moderately dark, and ordered a light, nourishing diet, and of cold water as much as she wanted. My expectations of a cure were realized. Desquamation progressed to its termination, and every symptom—headache, sensation in nostril, and croup—never reappeared. It is just possible that the second eruptive attack was rubeola (German measles), because there was an absence of fever, and no new exposure to measles could be traced; but, taking into consideration the fact of the papular character and crescentic form of the eruption, and later the branlike desquamation, continuing several days before the epidermis was clean, I believe this was one of the anomalous cases sometimes met with in practice.

2. GASTRO-DUODENAL CATARRH.—In the first days of December, 1879, H——, a little girl, aged six years, generally enjoying good health, seemed to have an abnormal craving for pickles (gherkins), of which she would surreptitiously obtain some, and eat them with an addition of salt, of which she was also fond. After midnight of December 7th she was suddenly awakened by a spell of severe vomiting, consisting mostly of undigested food and a sour, watery fluid, succeeded by some prostration; bowels unaffected. Face, particularly nose, felt cold; rest of body cool; pulse accelerated and weak. Desired cold water, but was worse therefrom. Remedies that occurred to me as useful in such cases had to be compared mentally before selecting the *similimum*. *Belladonna* for the suddenness and sour vomiting, and *Ipecac.* for the vomiting of sour fluid without diarrhœa, received a passing notice, but my mind dwelt more on medicines found in repertories under the following heads:

DESIRE FOR ACIDS: *Ant. crud.*, *Arsen.*, *Phosph.*, *Veratrum.*

DESIRE FOR PICKLES: *Ant. crud.*, *Veratrum.*

DESIRE FOR SALT THINGS; *Calc. ost.*, *Phosph.*, *Veratrum.*

DESIRE FOR COLD WATER: *Arsenic*, *Calc. ost.*, *Phosph.*, *Veratrum.*

Which of these shall be given? The case threatened to be one of cholera morbus, and I must make no mistake. The child lacked the "whitewashed" tongue and the excessive crossness of *Ant. crud.*, the anxious restlessness of *Arsen.*, any of the pinching pains and obstinacy of *Calc. ost.*, and so the choice lay between *Phosph.* and *Veratrum.* The patient wanted cold water; "I want it *very* cold, mamma;" but after remaining in the stomach long enough to become warm, it would be vomited. This looked more like *Phosph.*, but *Verat.* has vomiting after drink, too, and the latter has the desire for gherkins (Bœnninghausen), which *Phosph.* lacks altogether. My recipe, therefore, was *Veratrum*^{3}, of which one dose was sufficient to prevent any recurrence of symptoms, until the night of December 11th, when much the same symptoms occurred, the attack being renewed by eating fried calf's liver at the preceding evening meal. *Veratrum* changed the condition of thirst and vomit, but the child did not recover. She remained dull and languid, had some fever in evening, and seemed generally worse from 4 to 9 P.M. During her brighter moments she would ask, "Mamma, can I eat a whole lot after awhile, when I am better?" At these times nourishment was offered, but a mouthful or two completely satisfied her. *Lycopod.* here suggested itself, but a further analysis of symptoms revealed the fact that *everything, even water, tasted bitter, but there was no bitter taste except when eating or drinking.* I now remembered a note to *Pulsatilla*, by that master-observer Hahnemann, who says: "Pulsatilla seldom (and mostly only in the evening or morning) causes a *persistent* bitter taste in the mouth; the most frequent condition is, no bitter taste by itself, but only while eating or drinking, or only after swallowing food or drink." December 14th I gave one dose of *Pulsatilla*^{30}, with entire relief in twenty-four hours, and on December 16th she seemed well enough to "see Grant." This however disagreed. She was brought home very sick. Had quite a severe chill, followed by fever; pain in stomach with nausea and vomiting. It will be remembered that the day, though bright, was cold, the air sharp and penetrating. *Aconite* did no good. She grew worse hourly, next day (December 17th) complaining of tenderness to pressure over stomach and in right hypochondrium. Persistent nausea, and vomiting after any eating or drinking. Appetite poor, could not be coaxed to eat. Tongue was dry, coated white anteriorly, slightly yellowish at base, tip and edges somewhat red. Headache, with dizziness, if she moved. Skin hot, but very slightly moist, decidedly icteric; some itching on back. Pulse 132. Very drowsy, and desired perfect quiet. Wanted to be covered, complaining of chilliness on uncovering. Urine contained bile. Stools were clay-colored while formed, but cream-colored whilst diarrhœic; a foam, like whipped-up cream, floated on urine voided with stool, while the bottom of the vessel contained white, fatty lumps. Conjunctivæ very yellow. The child was certainly very sick, my diagnosis being gastro-duodenal catarrh. The fresh cold contracted on December 16th reawakened the catarrh of the stomach, and by extension soon invaded the duodenum, the consequent swelling of the ductus choledochus and occlusion of its orifice giving rise to the marked jaundice. But the name of the disease, or any theory as to the production of symptoms, avail little. A medicine is wanted, and that medicine must be the *similimum*. Very easy here to give *Calomel*, but the result would be questionable. A comparison of *similar* remedies was again necessary. Shall it be *Bellad.*, *Bryon.*, *Magn. carb.*, *Mercur.*, *Sulphur*, or what? Guided by the unerring rule for the selection of the remedy, what could be indicated as well as *Gelsemium*, which has all the symptoms enumerated, and is the only remedy, so far as known, having a *cream-colored stool*. A few doses of *Gelsemium*³ in water were followed by prompt relief; next day convalescence began, and by Christmas Day she was well enough to enjoy the festivities without let or hindrance, except as to sweetmeats or other indigestible food.

A CASE OF PUERPERAL CONVULSIONS.

BY J. N. MITCHELL, M.D., PHILADELPHIA.

(Read before the Homœopathic Medical Society of Philadelphia.)

In the evening of October 21st, 1878, I was called to see Maggie —, aged about 25 years, and found her pregnant with her first child, the pregnancy advanced to the middle of the 7th month. When I first saw her she was lying in a deep coma, with flushed face and stertorous breathing. I was informed that she had been in convulsions all that day and had shown no consciousness since morning. The physicians who had preceded me in the case, two allopathic physicians, had drugged her pretty thoroughly, and had also bled her very freely. I made an examination of the os uteri, and found no more than the normal dilatation of that far-advanced pregnancy, and on auscultating could hear the fœtal heart. While making my examinations she was taken with a very severe convulsion. I sent for my uterine dilators, and with the assistance of Messrs. William Barnes and J. C. McClelland, students at the Hahnemann Medical College, I rapidly etherized and dilated. At the end of about three hours I delivered my patient of her child, which gave a gasp or two and then died. Before proceeding to the dilation I had emptied the bladder of about a teacup of urine, which I was informed was all that she had voided during the entire day. Unfortunately this urine was emptied by mistake before I could test it. During the entire time of my operating there were no convulsions, and when the os was well opened and the bag of waters broken, the woman bore down with great energy during each pain, although thoroughly under the effect of the ether.

On the following morning when I called to see my patient I found her conscious but very much exhausted, and totally unconscious that her baby had been born or that anything unusual had occurred to her. She had passed no urine, and on passing the catheter I could find but a few drachms, which, when tested by heat and Nitric acid, became almost entirely solid. Her temperature I have forgotten exactly but remember that it was somewhat below the normal. In the evening when I called I found her wild and delirious. She could scarcely be restrained, so great was her horror at the sights that she saw; one minute it would be the devil that she would be shrinking from and the next the entire wall would be lined with ghastly figures. She would at times break into prayers to God and then sing parts of hymns of praise. She had passed no urine all day, and I could scarcely find any with the catheter. I prescribed Stramonium in the 3d decimal, a dose every hour.

The following morning I found her somewhat quieter, and with a greater quantity of urine, which she had passed voluntarily, and which was still full of albumen. I continued the Stramonium for several days until she became entirely rational, and her urine, day by day, became more in quantity and less albuminous. It was fully one month before the albumen disappeared entirely under the action of different remedies given at different times according to their special indications.

Thirteen months after the delivery I attended her in her second labor, which was natural in all respects.

ATRESIA OF THE VAGINA.

BY HARRIET J. SARTAIN, M.D.

(Read before the Homœopathic Medical Society of Philadelphia.)

March 27th, 1879.—Mrs. C., aged 31years, fair complexion, prominent blue eyes, light-brown hair, five feet seven inches high, weight 199 pounds, called at my office for examination and treatment.

The history of the case was as follows: The patient all through her childhood was troubled with shortness of breath on going upstairs, walking rapidly, or making any slight exertion, which had gradually increased until the time of her visit; the walking from one room to another caused panting and almost gasping breathing.

At ten years of age commenced to have nosebleed, and the attacks had continued at frequent intervals up to the time of her visit. At about the age of seventeen the menstrual effort began, with pain every month, but *no flow*. During that year she had violent cough, with frequent attacks of spitting of blood, when the lungs were supposed to be affected; but on reaching her eighteenth year a bloody discharge appeared, relieving the lung symptoms somewhat, but not returning for another year, when it came on at intervals of from one to four months, but never amounted to more than a slight show.

For the succeeding six years she was most of the time under homœopathic treatment for supposed diseases of the heart, kidneys, liver, falling of the womb, and suppression of the menses.

Was married at twenty-four, and up to that time had been slight in figure, excepting a large abdomen, so large as to cause unpleasant remarks, which annoyed her very much. After her marriage she went to the country to live, and gained flesh and strength, but had many attacks of severe illness, in which she was attended by the homœopathic doctor from the town nearest her country home, who at one time visited her daily for three months, and occasionally for five months longer, for disease of the liver. She also, during the years that followed, came occasionally to the city and remained for weeks at a time, under the care of her old physician, in whom she had great confidence. At one period, after having chills daily for two months, an allopathic physician was called in, who treated her with no better result than her homœopathic physicians.

During the year 1876 she had three attacks, pronounced by her medical attendant, rush of blood to the head. Several times she was supposed to be pregnant, on account of her increasing size and the absence of the menses.

During all these years there had been no local examination made to ascertain the cause of the suppression.

I found, on examination, the vagina an inch and a half in length, terminating in a smooth cul-de-sac, which, when fully distended with a quadrivalve speculum, revealed no opening. The abdominal walls were so fatty and tense, that nothing could be defined through them, and only through the rectum could be felt a large and indurated uterus.

After satisfying myself that she *had* a uterus, I sent her home to come back to me when the menstrual show appeared.

On the third of April she came, when I introduced the speculum, and by distending the parts, and waiting for some minutes, I saw at the extreme right *a faint bloody line, like a very fine thread, running down.* By long-continued pressure, and as much force as I dared use, I succeeded in introducing a small silver wire about half an inch, then a small hard rubber probe, after it a number one bougie; the withdrawal of which was followed by a drop of fluid, the color and consistence of tar. Thomas's dilator was then introduced, and with much difficulty opened sufficiently to allow of the escape of about three ounces of the same tarry-looking fluid, followed by a natural flow, which continued two or three days.

As the flow diminished I introduced a sponge-tent, which was removed with difficulty, owing to the undilatable character of the tissues. On the following days I used a second and a third, which, although they made little improvement in dilating the opening, caused a profuse discharge.

On the 9th of April, Dr. E. H. Lang assisting, I carefully divided the septum, making an incision an inch and a half in depth and two inches in length, disclosing an enlarged, indurated, and fearfully congested uterus.

The sound passed without difficulty; length of cavity seven inches. The hæmorrhage, which was quite profuse, was controlled by Hamamelis dressings, with which it was daily packed for two weeks. The divided tissues retracted in small knots, on an otherwise natural-looking vagina, and healed rapidly. A soft rubber ring was then introduced to prevent any contraction of the parts, and she returned to her home to wait for the menses, which appeared on the twenty-eighth day without any pain.

The flow was normal, lasting several days. The ring was worn most of the time for several weeks, when the parts showing no disposition to contract, it was dispensed with. In one week after the operation the difficulty of breathing had ceased, and has never returned, nor has she since had an attack of bleeding at the nose.

Mrs. C. has had three serious falls since the operation. In the early summer she fell backward from a chair, on which she was standing; at another time fell downstairs, and in August had a fall from a carriage, striking the lower part of the abdomen on the carriage block, causing a serious retroversion, with ovarian inflammation, from which she is now recovering. Her many diseases are fast becoming things of the past; the uterus is softening, the vagina is natural and healthy, the knotted remains of the divided septum having at this time almost disappeared. Her weight is now 240 pounds, but with her general increase the abdomen has decreased, until it is proportionate to the rest of the body. The remedies used were Arnica for several days after the operation, followed by Cimicifuga, Conium, Helonias, and since her fall Lilium and Apis.

DIABETES MELLITUS, WITH PRURITUS VULVÆ.

BY MARY BRANSON, M.D., PHILADELPHIA.

(Read before the Homœopathic Medical Society of Philadelphia.)

November 27th, 1877.—Mrs. L., aged 47, mother of five healthy children, youngest nine years old, dark hair, florid complexion, very intelligent, lives in great luxury. For the past ten years has increased greatly in flesh, weighing over 200 pounds; generally excellent health, though occasional attacks of indigestion, during which eyes become sore, smart, and burn; conjunctiva red; sees sparks and black spots before eyes. She says blue pill always clears away these symptoms.

For six weeks she had been suffering intensely with pruritus vulvæ. The labiæ were swollen to twice their natural size, and fiery red. This redness extended up on the abdomen almost to the umbilicus, down the inside of the thighs half way to the knees and around the anus. Inside the vulva the inflammation was intense. The surface was broken in thousands of points the size of a mustard seed, yet each point distinct from the rest.

The burning, stinging, and scalding were violent, and anything touching the abraded surface would feel to her like a "coal of fire." She said she would have a few minutes' rest at times, then there would come a violent dart, like a very fine, long needle, or the sting of an insect deep into the flesh, then another, until she would feel thousands of them.

Her condition was deplorable; she could neither sit nor stand, and yet lying down was almost as bad, for the heat of the bed aggravated all her sufferings. Her nights were almost sleepless, and she would many times have to get up and walk about, the distress was so great. Hot water or ice gave momentary relief, followed quickly by an aggravation. Urination increased the suffering so that for an hour afterward she would cry and ring her hands in agony, though she carefully bathed the vulva with tepid water after micturition. She always had been troubled with constipation, partially owing to atony of the rectum.

A local examination revealed the vagina highly inflamed and slight ulceration of the cervix.

As the case came to me while I was in the allopathic practice, I depended on pretty active medication, mostly anodyne, antiphlogistic, and cathartic remedies. She had applied to the vulva numerous ointments, Pulv. calomel, Bismuth subnitrate, Ung. zinc. oxid., Cosmoline, solutions and ointments of Morphia, etc. Some of above were used on her own responsibility, unknown to me at the time. They never appeared to relieve nor permanently aggravate the condition.

Having been for a year studying homœopathy, and being on the eve of changing my practice, I persuaded her to try the new school, only consenting to continue to prescribe for her on this condition.

On December 24th, 1877, we made the change. At that time the pruritus was raging unabated, her condition being much the same as a month ago. In addition she was suffering from a sharp attack of indigestion, with flushed face, eyes inflamed, and objects appearing blurred. She said her liver was affected and she wished she could have blue pill. Dryness and itching of the skin, with an appearance of hives when scratching. Upper lip much swollen; puffiness of eyelids, especially the *lower* lid. She had been losing flesh for several months. She always inclined to drink water in large quantity, but thirst was increased at this time. Gave Apis^{3} in water every three hours.

December 27th.—Slight improvement in all her symptoms.

December 29th.—Local suffering increased. Changed to Arsenic^{6}.

December 31st.—No better; gave Canth.^{30}.

She had never consented to a consultation, but I talked with Dr. Sartain about the case, who reminded me that diabetes sometimes gave rise to serious pruritus.

I examined the urine, found the quantity increased, specific gravity 1030, and sugar in abundance.

January 6th, 1878.—Called hurriedly to Mrs. L. About 10 A.M. she was seized with rush of blood to the head, nausea, and vertigo, ending in unconsciousness for a few moments.

She said she had had such attacks before, only lighter; often about the time of the menses (which occur regularly). Attacks generally between 10 A.M. and 11 A.M. They are always relieved and often prevented by eating. Gave Sulph.^{6} in water.

January 10*th*, 1878.—No improvement in pruritus; general health about the same; no return of fainting.

January 12*th*.—Gave Sulph.^{200} in water.

January 19*th*.—No return of paroxysm since the 6th; irritation of vulva less; much itching of skin, which is dry and scaly (especially arms and hands), and nettlerash marked.

January 28*th*.—Careful analysis of urine in college laboratory revealed specific gravity1021; sugar, 19.68 gr. per f℥.

February 4*th*.—Called in haste to Mrs. L.; found her unconscious. She had four attacks in one day. Commenced with nausea and retching, faintness, loss of vision, hot flushes surging up over body; must have head high and hold of some one's hand, or she will die (she thinks); dizziness and a sinking down until consciousness is lost. Face purple red, with yellow ring around the mouth; lips drawn; perspiration after each attack; numbness in hands all the time, most in left hand.

On inquiry, finding she had taken Sulphur^{200} much more freely than directed, I gave no medicine, but watched her closely. She had no more paroxysms, was weak as after a long sickness, for two or three days, then steadily improved.

February 12*th*.—Local irritation slight; feels quite well.

February 15*th*.—Urine again carefully examined (in laboratory); quantity normal; specific gravity 1014; sugar, mere trace.

March 19*th*.—Felt perfectly well; no medicine since February 4th.

Late in summer of 1878 Mrs. L. had a serious illness, commencing suddenly when feeling perfectly well. Temporary loss of power on right side. Attended by a noted allopathic physician, who attributed her sickness mostly to approaching menopause. A member of the family told the doctor of her previous diabetic trouble. He examined the urine, said there was no abnormal condition, and laughed at the idea of diabetes ever having existed.

During this illness there was no return of pruritus.

SOME PRACTICAL POINTS IN OBSTETRICS.

BY J. C. GUERNSEY, M.D., PHILADELPHIA.

(Read before the Homœopathic Medical Society of Philadelphia.)

UNDERSTANDING from the worthy chairman of the Bureau of Obstetrics and Gynæcology, Dr. Mitchell, that this is to be a "go-as-you-please" report, I have chosen to go on some practical points in obstetrics, and these practical points are, how to manage cases with bad records of parturition, overcome the dyscrasia, and bring about a natural and easy delivery. My rule for this, and it will bring success to the faithful applicant thereof, is to *carefully collate all the symptoms of the patient, even the slightest departures from the normal standard of health, and prescribe the similimum.* The earlier the stage of pregnancy you are called upon for advice the better chance you have for success at the parturition. By persistently applying the proper remedy for every ailment during the pregnant term, the final act in the grand chain of reproduction will be performed, no matter what the previous record may be of instrumental delivery, post-partum hæmorrhage, adherent placenta, long and tedious labor; all these will vanish under the sway of that magic wand, the *similimum.* Allow me to illustrate by some of my own experiences in this direction, and first I would call attention to Case 1, an article of mine published in the HAHNEMANNIAN MONTHLY, September, 1877, under the title of "Pregnancy to Full Term after Four Miscarriages." When first called to see her she had been married over five years; had had four miscarriages, the first occurring three months after marriage; a year later another miscarriage at six months; in something over a year she miscarried again at seven months; seventeen months later she miscarried for the fourth time. When I was called to see her she was still childless and pregnant three months, for the fifth time. Her treatment in the foregoing had been entirely allopathic, and each of her several doctors told her she could not ever possibly go to full term. By carefully watching her symptoms and prescribing accordingly she went to full term and was happily delivered of a fine boy. My main remedies were *Nux vomica, Kali carb., Sepia.*

CASE 2. Had one child; labor long-lasting, severe; pain irregular and insufficient; instrumental delivery. Family history bad; all the females have difficult labors on her father's and mother's sides—sisters, cousins, aunts, etc. Took charge of second confinement, and about two months before parturition, which was dreaded by the patient with horror. Gave, in harmony with her symptoms, *Cimic. rac.* Result, labor only three hours; not severe; birth natural.

CASE 3. I reported in the January number of the HAHNEMANNIAN MONTHLY a case with unfavorable record, whose labor terminated happily under the influence of Gelsemium.

CASE 4. A lady with a serious umbilical hernia; mother of two children; hernia produced by the severity of her first labor. In her second labor the protruding bowel had to be grasped by the hands, and as well as possible held in place by her attending physicians, and finally Chloroform was administered *ad libitum* to relax muscular resistance as well as to deaden susceptibility to the horrible pain. Forceps were used both times to effect delivery; hæmorrhage followed, etc. This lady had an easy delivery, after only a few hours of labor, under the influence of *Belladonna*, which was given because her symptoms demanded it.

CASE 5. A few months ago I was engaged to attend a lady in her seventh confinement. Her record indeed made me tremble and loath to take the case. Her recounted experience was: post-partum flooding after one or two confinements; adherent placenta, which had to be peeled off by her attendant physician after another confinement; a baby weighing only three pounds had to be taken by the forceps another time; and still another time, in a breech presentation, the baby was born with both its arms broken. On this occasion our worthy colleague, Dr. M. Macfarlan, was summoned, and three hours after birth he had both arms "set" so skilfully that the fractures united perfectly. All her labors had been long-lasting and abounding with useless pains, and some serious abnormal incident had occurred at every delivery. Further, she had always suffered greatly from after-pains. What wonder then that I looked forward to the denouement of this case with dread and foreboding, particularly as she had in each case previously been under careful homœopathic treatment. However, I carefully worked up her *symptoms*, those trusty signposts which, with unerring finger, point to the proper remedy. She had rheumatism of wrist-joints, pain in back, headache, etc., all of which I found mirrored in *Cimicif. rac.* In due time I was summoned to attend her. Found her sitting up, very jolly, and sure she had called me uselessly. An examination showed that labor had set in, and I started her husband for the nurse. In an hour's time they came in together, and just fancy their surprise to hear the baby, which had arrived, loudly calling for them! She only had *three* severe pains. After-birth came away easily, and, during her lying-in, for the first time in her experience, she had *no after-pains!*

But now I must describe that baby. It was normal in size and weighed about seven pounds, but upon each hand was a supernumerary finger to the ulnar side of the little finger; and upon each foot, between the fourth and fifth toes, a supernumerary toe, resembling the fourth; double harelip; palate cleft clear through from front to back; on the right of the septum, with the intermaxillary bone attached, containing the germs of two central incisor teeth, a corresponding segment of the upper lip was thrust downward and forward and to the left, completely flattening the nose upon the face, and presenting the appearance of an unsightly tumor below the nose. The eyes were so small and so deeply located, and the opening in the lids so extremely small, that it is doubtful whether they would have given useful vision had the child lived. An examination by means of a hairpin, bent in the form of a hook, revealed a clear cornea and an ordinary-looking infantile iris, but the whole ball was exceedingly small. The umbilical cord measured but twelve inches. The child (a female) died on the third day.

I could narrate many more cases similar to those just given where I have always found the application of the law of similars to work out the most satisfactory results. But the expiration of my limited time warns me to desist.

AN UNUSUAL CASE OF LABOR—CONGENITAL OVARIAN CYSTS.

BY CHARLES M. BROOKS, M.D., OF PHILADELPHIA.

(Read before the Homœopathic Medical Society of Philadelphia.)

I WAS called at 3 o'clock on the morning of December 26th, 1879, to see Mrs. A., then said to be in labor. She is the mother of four healthy children, and this was her fifth pregnancy, in which she had advanced about seven and a half months. I found she had been aroused from sleep a short time before I had been sent for, by large quantities of water coming from her, but that she had very little if any pain. I at once made an examination, and found the os dilated to about the size of a quarter-dollar piece; but I could not make out the presentation at that time, although I made every effort to do so, and could only feel, through the abdominal wall and high up on the right side, what I made out to be the child's head.

She continued losing comparatively large quantities of water from time to time, so that the napkins had to be frequently changed, the water coming most freely whenever pain occurred; or if she happened to be standing in an erect posture the water would come in such gushes that a puddle would be left upon the floor.

The pains seemed to be very slight, and continued so throughout the day and the evening, the os all the while slowly dilating. I should judge that during this time there must have drained off not less than a bucketful of the waters. At about 11 o'clock P.M. the pains became more frequent, and were very severe although of very short duration. At this time upon examination I found the os well dilated, with a soft body presenting, which gave to the sense of touch the same sensation as is conveyed by the bag of waters; but for all this I was still unable to make out the presentation. Persisting, however, I was enabled to feel the left hand and arm of the child. A few minutes after this, upon making another examination, I found the umbilical cord in the vagina, and upon following the cord up I found that the umbilicus presented centre for centre, with the head of the child to the right side of the mother. I now endeavored to effect version, but upon introducing the hand I was unable to find the feet, and could not distingush any part of the lower extremities, the whole mass feeling like a bladder full of water, and receding from the hand upon the slightest pressure.

Feeling that I needed help, a messenger was sent for another physician, but before he arrived the child was born, dead, at half-past 1 o'clock in the morning, having been born spontaneously, the umbilicus presenting and coming first, the child doubled up, the head extended far back upon the spinal column.

There was a lack of development of one of the legs from the knee down, only the bones being present, without flesh upon them. The parents of the child were both healthy, the mother being well formed, and having a large well-shaped pelvis. During this pregnancy she was in great distress from the weight of the uterine load, and during a part of the time she was hardly able to be about on her feet, owing to the swelling of her limbs, which, however, passed away before she was taken in labor.

The expulsion of the child *en masse* caused a slight laceration of the perinæum; but the woman made a rapid and good recovery, and is now enjoying very good health.

I present this case, first, on account of the unusual presentation, and the unusual circumstance attending the expulsion of the child; and, second, on account of the curious results of a post-mortem examination, performed by Dr. J. N. Mitchell at my request. Dr. Mitchell found two ovarian cysts, and at the seat of the ovaries a calcareous deposit. These cysts contained about a pint of fluid each, and another pint of fluid was found in the abdominal cavity. All the other organs appeared to be in a healthy condition.

ABDOMINAL INCUBATION IN THE COMMON FOWL.

BY A. R. THOMAS, M D., PHILADELPHIA.

(Read before the Philadelphia County Homœopathic Medical Society.)

In the month of January last I received by mail from Dr. S. E. Anderson, of Dover, Delaware, a remarkable object with the only explanation that it was found in the abdominal cavity of a chicken. The specimen consisted of an oval mass of the size and color of the yolk of a hen's egg. The density was more that of a slightly boiled egg. The body was flattened in form, while from one end sprang a knotted mass, of about the size of a small cherry, upon which appeared several small imperfectly formed feathers. From the lower border of the flattened oval there sprang two tufts of feathers, nearly two inches in length, and strongly suggestive of a pair of legs.

In seeking for an explanation of this curious case, we are first reminded of the fact that in the mammalia, including man, it occasionally happens that the impregnated ovum, failing to be caught by the Fallopian tubes, as it drops from the ruptured Graafian vesicle, falls into the abdominal cavity, and there, forming attachments, becomes more or less perfectly developed, such cases being known as abdominal pregnancies.

Again, we are to remember that in birds, the ovum, as it drops from the ovary, consists of the yolk alone. This yolk is caught in the oviduct, and, while passing through that tube, receives first its albuminous, and lastly its calcareous covering, these being secreted from the lining membrane of that passage.

Notwithstanding the large size of the ovum of the bird, we

may readily conceive that it might sometimes fail to be taken up by the oviduct, and thus lodge in the peritoneal cavity, any development of the ovum in this situation being fairly denominated "abdominal incubation."

Admitting this explanation to be the correct one, why should we find such an imperfect development of the chicken's ovum under these circumstances, while in abdominal pregnancy in the human being the development is so much more complete? This will not appear so remarkable, when we remember how essential is the presence of oxygen in all embryonic growth. The mammal obtains this supply from the arterial blood of the mother through the placental attachment; the bird obtains the same directly from the atmosphere, through the pores of the shell and moistened inclosing membrane. In this case, however, the egg being confined within the peritoneal cavity, must have been quite excluded from the necessary supply of oxygen.

Why there should have been developed feathers only in this case, without any growth of other tissues or organs, may not be so easily explained. A solution might, perhaps, be found, however, in the well-known tendency to the development of dermal appendages,—hair and teeth,—in certain ovarian and other cysts found in human beings.

HOMŒOPATHIC MEDICAL SOCIETY OF THE COUNTY OF PHILADELPHIA.

REPORTED BY C. MOHR, M.D., SECRETARY.

THE regular meeting was held at the Hahnemann Medical College, on Thursday evening, March 11th; the President, Dr. E. A. Farrington, in the chair. After transaction of routine business, the following committee report was made: "Your committee, appointed at the February meeting, to consider and report on the communication of Dr. R. E. Caruthers, Corresponding Secretary of the State Society, in reference to the preparation of a paper by the Philadelphia County Society for presentation to the Homœopathic Medical Society of the State of Pennsylvania at the annual meeting, in September, 1880, at Easton, Pa., beg leave to report, that they have duly considered the subject, and recommend the Society to prepare a paper as requested, and, further, that they have selected as a topic "The Pancreas and its Diseases," to be elaborated as follows, viz.:

Anatomy and Physiology, by A. R. Thomas, M.D.
General and Special Pathology, by J. C. Morgan, M.D.
Etiology, by B. F. Betts, M.D.
Diagnosis and Prognosis, by A. Korndœrfer, M.D.
Medical and Dietetic Treatment, by E. A. Farrington, M.D.

Your committee cannot too strongly urge the Society to favor this subject with the attention demanded by its importance. The time allotted for the preparation of the paper is sufficient to guarantee the production of an article that will reflect credit upon our Society, and prove highly interesting, the subject being one of the few not too much written up, and one that will doubtless elicit profitable discussion, in which many facts relative to diseases of the pancreas may be presented, which have not hitherto been published.

Respectfully submitted by

C. Mohr, M.D., Chairman,
H. L. Stambach, M.D.,
Clarence Bartlett, M.D.,
Committee.

The report was accepted, and by vote, the recommendations were adopted.

The censors reported favorably on applications of Drs. J. O. H. Banks and Thomas S. Dunning, and these gentlemen were elected to membership. Applications for membership were then submitted by Drs. Edward M. Gramm and Anna M. Marshall. Referred.

Nominations for officers, to be elected in April, were made as follows:

President: Dr. E. A. Farrington.
Vice-Presidents: Drs. W. B. Trites and J. N. Mitchell.
Treasurer: Dr. A. H. Ashton.
Secretary: Dr. Charles Mohr.
Censors: Drs. W. H. Bigler, J. K. Lee, and A. Korndœrfer.

J. N. Mitchell, M.D., Chairman of the Bureau of Obstetrics and Gynæcology, presented the following papers: 1. Congenital Double Ovarian Cysts, by C. M. Brooks, M.D.; 2. Atresia of the Vagina, by H. J. Sartain, M.D.; 3. Diabetes Mellitus, with Pruritus Vulvæ, by M. Branson, M.D.; 4. Obstetric Hints, by J. C. Guernsey, M.D.; 5. Puerperal Convulsions, by J. N. Mitchell, M.D. (See present number.) The papers were read, accepted, and ordered to be published, and the following discussion ensued:

Dr. Bigler desired to know if, in Dr. Sartain's case, peritonitis followed the operation. He asked the question because several years ago he had a similar case in a young lady, nineteen years of age. Dr. C. M. Thomas performed the operation, and delivered a pint of black tarry blood. Immediately afterwards she was attacked with peritonitis which was subdued promptly by the use of Opium 1^x. Since that time the young lady has menstruated regularly. Dr. Sartain replied that there had been no peritonitis nor any bad symptoms whatever. Dr. Bigler, continuing, said that the fact of Dr. Sartain's patients having been treated by so many physicians without any of them arriving at a correct diagnosis, should teach physicians to insist upon being allowed to make an examination, or else refuse to treat the case.

Dr. Lee agreed with Dr. Bigler. When a patient refused to permit him to make an examination, he always referred her to a reputable lady physician. In regard to Dr. Mitchell's paper, he thought that the doctor maintained the right position, to evacuate the uterus as soon as possible. He thought that if all cases were treated homœopathically, convulsions would be of rare occurrence. He had had a case in which the lady was very dropsical, marked albuminuria was present, and yet under the use of the proper remedy, her labor took place so speedily that she was safely delivered before he could reach her.

Dr. Mitchell had had cases of convulsions in which there were no premonitory symptoms whatever. What he desired to bring out in his paper was the necessity for evacuating the uterus in cases of convulsions occurring before delivery. He had also had cases in which the urine contained large quantities of albumen, yet convulsions did not follow. In regard to Dr. Guernsey's paper, while being a firm believer in *similia similibus curantur*, he did not believe that the fact of a woman's having three or four difficult labors, and then under homœopathic treatment had an easy delivery, proved anything. He had had just such cases in which no treatment had been pursued prior to the easy labor.

Dr. Guernsey believed that the similimum would in *every* case bring about an easy labor unless the cause of dystocia was abnormal development in the mother or child. In the case of the lady whom he delivered of the deformed child, the only cause the mother could give for the deformity, was a fall on the face which she had in the third month of her pregnancy.

Dr. Toothaker said that he had had in his practice many cases which would confirm Dr. Guernsey's method of treatment.

Dr. Dudley said that cases were frequently met with in which ladies say that physicians who had attended them in their first labors had told them that they could never be delivered of a living child, and yet such cases were frequently delivered safely, without any aid whatever from the obstetrician. He remembered a case in which he believed that it would be impossible for the woman to have a child without the use of forceps; yet the child was delivered before the physician could reach her. He agreed with Dr. Guernsey that where disorders of parturition are due to deeply seated constitutional or functional disturbance, the homœopathic remedy would relieve this condition, and render more certain a normal and easy labor. He had given Actea racemosa to one patient subject to difficult labor. In that case the woman was delivered with scarcely a pain.

Dr. A. R. Thomas, at this point, offered a report of an interesting case of what he said might be termed "Abdominal Incubation," and exhibited the specimen. (This report will also be found in our present number.)

Dr. Lee suggested that the pruritis in Dr. Branson's case might have been caused by an eczematous eruption.

Dr. Sartain did not believe the pruritus to be due to any other cause than the saccharine urine, for whenever the quantity of sugar in the urine increased or diminished, the pruritus increased or diminished with it.

Dr. Korndœrfer said that he had corroborated the symptoms given by Dr. Mitchell for Stramonium in a case of threatening convulsions. He had once been called to a case, arriving just as the patient was breathing her last. In that case the patient at just about the full development of the second stage of labor, was taken with convulsions. Labor was so rapid that instruments were useless. The convulsions became worse and worse, and the woman died an hour or two after the birth of the child. He believed that while dilatation and rapid delivery are desirable in some cases, the results are not always good.

Dr. Farrington remarked that Stramonium is not always sufficient for that form of mania, for which it is so often prescribed, when reflex from uterine irritation.

Dr. H. Gross has reported a case of retained placenta with

mania, in which the patient clapped her hands over her head, alternately laughing and crying, in which Stramonium failed him and he gave Secale, and cured her. Dr. Farrington said that he had attended a similar case,—in which the patient had had every gas-burner lighted,—with mania, and Stramonium failed him utterly. He then gave Secale^{30}, which relieved the mental symptoms. In the morning the placenta was delivered spontaneously.

Dr. Korndœrfer did not think that the laughing and silly humor were the important points in the indications for Stramonium, but the singing, etc.

Dr. Dudley referred to three cases of Stramonium poisoning which he saw at the Pennsylvania Hospital Clinics many years ago. The patients were laughing, crying, swearing, praying, singing, etc., the character of the delirium being subject to constant variations.

Dr. Mitchell advocated dilatation and rapid delivery in cases of convulsions occurring before delivery, because experience had taught him that such treatment was attended with good results. Out of seven cases thus treated six recovered. He thought that in the case of Dr. Guernsey, in which it was necessary to use instruments to deliver a three-pound baby, there must have been some inflammatory trouble present. In such cases the causes of miscarriage or dystocia should always be reported.

Dr. Guernsey spoke of the case of a lady, who gave a bad family history as regards confinements. She had had several bad labors. In her last the pain set in badly. That night she went to sleep, and slept peacefully. The next morning the pains came on, but were weak and irregular, with considerable backache, and very tired feeling. He gave her Caulophyllum 5^{m}, and in a short time the child was born.

The meeting then adjourned.

FINAL REPORT ON THE MILWAUKEE TEST OF THE THIRTIETH DILUTION.

The Milwaukee Academy of Medicine, in completing the pathogenetic and therapeutic test of the thirtieth Hahnemannian dilution, makes the following report:

That the unavoidable delay in making the report was due

to the removal of the depositary, Rev. G. T. Ladd, from this city to Brunswick, Maine; to his absence from home, caused by the illness and death of his father; and to the tardiness of the reports from the experimenters.

That in carrying out the provisions of the test, we have adhered strictly to the details of the plan for a scientific test of the pathogenetic and therapeutic action of the thirtieth Hahnemannian dilution, full particulars of which were published in the circular issued by this society in December, 1878. The *object* of the test and the modus operandi were announced as follows:

. . . "The object of this test is to determine whether or not this preparation can produce any medicinal action on the human organism in health or disease.

"A vial of pure sugar pellets, moistened with the thirtieth Hahnemannian dilution of Aconite, and nine similar vials, moistened with pure alcohol, so as to make them resemble the test pellets, shall be given to the prover. The vials are to be numbered 1, 2, 3, 4, 5, 6, 7, 8, 9, and 10. The number given to the Aconite vial shall be unknown to the prover, and it shall be his task to determine which of the ten vials contains Aconite.

"These preparations are to be put up with the greatest care, in the presence of the members of the Milwaukee Academy of Medicine, and then placed in the hands of an unprejudiced layman of unimpeachable honor, who shall number and dispense the vials as they are called for by the provers.

"The provers must be physicians of acknowledged ability, who possess a good knowledge of the recorded symptomatology of Aconite, and who have faith in the efficacy of the thirtieth dilution. . . .

"Preparations of *Arsenicum album*, *Aurum metallicum*, *Carbo vegetabilis*, *Natrum muriaticum*, and *Sulphur* in the thirtieth Hahnemannian dilution, made with the same precautions and care as this of *Aconitum*, shall be used as a test of the *therapeutic* powers of the thirtieth dilutions. In consideration of the inconvenience of experimenting on the sick, arising from popular prejudices, the number of vials of "unmedicated" pellets may be limited to one for each remedy, and the experiments tried mostly in chronic diseases. The real gain to the healing art, which will be accomplished by the establishment of the truth or falsity of the theory of "potentization," will amply compensate for the risk of delaying a few cures.

"The experimenters must be physicians of acknowledged ability, who possess a good knowledge of the therapeutic indications of the remedies tried, and who profess faith in the efficacy of the thirtieth dilution." . . .

The committee appointed by the Milwaukee Academy of Medicine, for the purpose of making arrangements to prepare a scientific test of the efficacy of the thirtieth Hahnemannian dilutions, reported as follows:

"MR. PRESIDENT: Your committee have carefully considered the plan proposed in Dr. Lewis Sherman's paper, for testing the efficacy of the thirtieth Hahnemannian dilution, and we are unanimously of the opinion that the test proposed in that paper is fair and honorable, and that the interests of science demand that it should be made.

"We recommend,

"That our society undertake to carry out the provisions of this test, and that to this end the essential features and the practical details of the test be given for publication as soon as practicable to every regular homœopathic periodical printed in the English language; and that translations of the same be sent to every known regular homœopathic periodical printed in foreign languages; and that all other appropriate and accessible means be employed to give the test publicity.

"That the directions given by Hahnemann for the preparation of the thirtieth dilution be followed with the most scrupulous exactness; that the alcohol used be of the purest quality obtainable, and that to this end, a quantity of the best so-called 'Homœopathic Alcohol' be redistilled in glass for the purposes of this test.

"That the Rev. George T. Ladd, of Milwaukee, be selected to number and dispense the vials of test pellets as they are called for by the provers and experimenters; and that he give a solemn pledge that he will not, in any manner, reveal to any person which of the preparations coming from his hands have been medicated with the thirtieth dilution until he shall have been called upon to do so by this society, and that he will use every means in his power to preserve the purity of the materials intrusted to his care, and to make the test fair and honorable.

"That all provers and experimenters be required to send their reports to the secretary, Dr. Albert Schlœmilch, before the first day of December, 1879; and that the result be published in full about the 1st of January, 1880.

"And, finally, that this society appropriate a sufficient sum of money to defray the expenses of furnishing and delivering the test pellets of Aconite to one hundred provers—these being selected from the first who apply,—and that the other provers and experimenters be required to pay in advance to the secretary of the society the sum of thirty cents for each set of test pellets sent them.

"EUGENE F. STORKE, M.D.,
ROBERT MARTIN, M.D.,
E. M. ROSENKRANS, M.D.,
JULIA FORD, M.D.,
ALBERT SCHLŒMILCH, M.D.,
G. C. MCDERMOTT, M.D.,
O. W. CARLSON, M.D.

"MILWAUKEE, December 3d, 1878."

The society unanimously adopted the report, and has used every possible means to give the test publicity.

We would further report,

That the medicines used in making the dilutions for the *therapeutic* test were obtained from the pharmacy of Messrs. Boericke & Tafel, and the *Aconite* tincture was tested by several members of this society, and found to produce its pathogenetic effects.

That the dilutions were made by this society in accordance with the Hahnemannian directions for the preparation of the thirtieth dilution.

That at a regular meeting of the society, held April 1st, 1879, the following resolution was unanimously adopted:

"Upon application by any professor in a medical college, or any other public advocate of the high potencies, the Academy will prepare and furnish the thirtieth Hahnemannian dilution of *any remedy* in common use, for the purpose, and in accordance with the terms, heretofore published in the pamphlet entitled, 'A Test of the Thirtieth Dilution.'"

That in accordance with various requests of the provers we have prepared, in addition to the dilutions mentioned in the pamphlet, *pathogenetic tests* of *Nux vomica*, *Belladonna*, and *Arsenicum album*, and *therapeutic tests* of *Sulphur* and *Digitalis*.

That the bottles containing the thirtieth dilutions, thus prepared, together with a bottle of the alcohol used in their preparation, were given directly into the custody of the depositary.

That he was also supplied with pure sugar pellets, vials, and mailing boxes, and that he was requested to medicate the pellets and dispense them according to orders which he might receive from the secretary.

That the applications for the test cases were given directly to the depositary as soon after their receipt as possible, that all cases given out were sent by him in response to applications received by this society from the provers, and that in answer to our request we received from him a thoroughly sealed envelope, containing the subjoined report:

BOWDOIN COLLEGE, BRUNSWICK, MAINE, January 26th, 1880.

TO THE MILWAUKEE ACADEMY OF MEDICINE.

GENTLEMEN: The report which is herewith submitted to you I beg leave to preface with the following statements: The work which you did me the honor to intrust to me has been most carefully and scrupulously done; the record has been accurately kept, and secluded from all eyes but my own.

Great pains has been taken to exclude entirely the possibility of guessing the medicated vials, instead of discovering them by scientific experiment.

Nothing has been permitted to indicate a difference in the vials tested, or to make it possible for any experimenter to detect in any way the reasons for choosing one number rather than another of all the vials numbered to contain the medicated pellets.

So far as the test has been made, it has been made under the fairest conditions possible for me to secure.

With these remarks I invite your attention to the appended itemized statement of the tests sent, the time of sending, the persons to whom sent, and the numbers in each test of the medicated vials.

These, gentlemen, are all the vials sent out by me in accordance with the instructions received from your committee.

I am, very respectfully, yours,

GEORGE T. LADD,
Professor of Mental and Moral Philosophy.

In the tabular statement, the number of the medicated vial in the cases not tested or not reported has been withheld by the society for obvious reasons. The last column, giving the report of the experimenter, has been added to make the report complete.

Date.	Number of case.	Name of experimenter.	Residence of experimenter.	Test.	No. of tests.	No. of med. vial.	Report of experimenter.
1879.							
Jan. 13	1	Dr. J W. Thompson	Greenfield, Mass.	Path.	1		No report.
" "	2	Prof. C. B Gatchell.	Ann Arbor, Mich.	Ther.	5		" "
Feb. 26	3	Dr H. L. Waldo.	West Troy, N Y.	Path.	1		" "
" "	4	Dr. W. S. Gillett.	Fox Lake, Wis.	Ther.	5		" "
" "	5	Dr. E. Lippincott.	Bowling Green, Ky.	Path.	1		" "
March 1	6	Dr. W. H. Blakely.	Bowling Green, Ky.	"	1	10	Number 5.
" 31	7	Dr. W. B. Trites.	Manayunk, Pa.	"	1		No report.
" "	8	Dr G R. Mitchell.	Richland Centre, Wis.	"	1	2	Number 4.
" "	9	Dr. C. R. Muzzey.	Watertown, Wis.	"	1	7	Number 1.
" "	10	Dr. A.W. Woodward	Chicago, Ill.	"	1	1	Number 2.
" "	11	Dr. J. H Thompson.	New York, N. Y.	"	1		No symptoms.
" "	12	Dr. N. S. Pennoyer	Kenosha, Wis.	"	1	10	Number 4.
June 18	13	Dr. N. S. Pennoyer.	Kenosha, Wis.	Ther*	1		No report.
March 31	14, 15	Dr. C. H. Hall.	Madison, Wis.	Path.	2		" "
May 5	16	Dr. M. A. Reis.	Milwaukee, Wis.	"	1	2	Number 10.
" "	17	Dr. O. W. Smith.	Union Springs, N. Y.	"	1		No report.
" "	18	Dr. O. W Smith.	Union Springs, N. Y.	Ther.	5		" "
" "	19	Prof. A. Uhlemeyer.	St. Louis, Mo.	Path.	1	3	Number 5.
" "	20	Prof. A. Uhlemeyer.	St. Louis, Mo.	Ther.	5	Ars. 1	Arsenicum 1.
" "	21	Dr. W. F. Morgan.	Leavenworth, Kan.	Path.	1		No symptoms.
" "	22	Dr. W. F. Morgan.	Leavenworth, Kan.	Ther.	5		No report.
" "	23	Dr. O. S. Childs.	Beaver Dam, Wis.	"	5		" "
June 18	24	Dr. Collesson.	St. Louis, Mo.	Path.	1		" "
" "	25	Dr. Collesson.	St. Louis, Mo.	Ther.	5		" "
" "	26	Dr. Wm Eggert.	Indianapolis, Ind.	Path.	1		" "
" 27	27	Dr. P. Nelson.	Minneapolis, Minn.	Ther.	5		" "
July 25	28, 29	Dr. H. A. Foster.	Buffalo, N. Y.	"	2		" "
" 28	30	Dr T. L. Brown.	Binghamton, N. Y.	"	1		" "
" "	31	Dr. E. C. Morrill.	Norwalk, Ohio.	"	1		" "
" "	32	Dr. C. W. Mohr.	Philadelphia, Pa.	"	1		" "
" "	33, 34	Dr. W. M. Butler.	Middletown, N. Y.	Ther.	2		" "
" "	35 to 39	Dr. L. A. Campbell.	Attleboro, Mass.	"	5		" "
" "	40	Dr. J. A. Pearsall.	Saratoga Spring, N. Y.	Path.	1		" "
" "	41	Dr. T. A. Martin.	Delavan, Wis.	"	1		" "

* Five vials, one containing *Arsen.* 30*th*.

NOTE.—Beside the above an application was received from Dr. Adams, of Toronto, Canada, for Lyc.[30], in a ten-vial test. The material was prepared at a special meeting of the Academy, and sent by express to Professor Ladd. Dr. Adams's name not appearing in Professor Ladd's report, we infer that the package did not reach him after his removal from this city.

RECAPITULATION.

Ten-vial or Pathogenetic Test.

Number of tests applied for and sent out, ... 25
Number of tests on which reports have been received, . 9
Number of tests in which the medicated vial was found, 0

Two-vial or Therapeutic Test.

Number of tests applied for and sent out, ... 47
Number of tests on which reports have been received, . 1
Number of tests in which the medicated vial was found, 1

Five-vial Test of Dr. Pennoyer.

Number of tests applied for and sent out, ... 1
Number of tests on which reports have been received, . 0
Number of tests in which the medicated vial was found, 0

The thanks of this society are due to Professor George T. Ladd, of Bowdoin College, Maine, for his disinterested work in the interests of medical science; to the HAHNEMANNIAN MONTHLY, the *St. Louis Clinical Review*, and the *U. S. Medical Investigator*, for publishing the plan of the test; and, above all, to the persons who have magnanimously taken part in the experiment.

By order of the Milwaukee Academy of Medicine.

SAMUEL POTTER, M.D.,
President.
EUGENE F. STORKE,
Secretary.

MILWAUKEE, WISCONSIN, February 16th, 1880.

MATERIALISMUS VERSUS LIVING DYNAMIC FORCES.

A REPLY TO DR. DAKE, OF NASHVILLE.

EDITORS HAHNEMANNIAN: In the March number of your journal, page 170, Dr. J. P. Dake tries to vindicate himself as chairman of the Bureau of Materia Medica from partiality in selecting the members of his bureau, but facts speak louder than mere assertions, and any one present at the meeting at Lake George could plainly see that the materialists, with their microscopes, their probabilities in relation to the now famous Milwaukee Test, intended to have it all their own way, and had it their own way. Dr. Dake knows it, as well as all the members of the Institute, that the chairman of any committee has perfect liberty to add members to his bureau, whether such members were present at the meeting or not. In fact, very often this is the case, in order to get the best work done, as many a valuable co-worker might be accidentally prevented from attending the meeting.

I would request Dr. Dake to point out in my article, "What is Homœopathy?" the name of any physician I mentioned, except that of Dr. Horace M. Payne, and in putting Dr. Payne as judge of the clinical experience in the use of attenuations above the thirtieth decimal the cloven foot is shown, as his hostility to high potencies is too well known, and he would be recreant to his whole life and to all his writings if he should bring in a defence of the use of high potencies. Why not put Dr. Cooper or Cowperthwaite as judge of these high potencies and leave Dr. Payne to his low attenuations. I never objected to any of these valuable members, but I do object to see an enemy to high potencies sit in judgment about them. Dr. Lawton is to me personally unknown; if this is an offence I plead guilty, but it is my fault and certainly no disparagement to the doctor was meant by it, and if an apology is needed I hereby freely offer it to Dr. Lawton.

In my whole article neither Dr. Breyfogle, C. Wesselhoeft, or T. F. Allen are mentioned, men whom I have known and esteemed for years for their private as well as for their public virtues. It has been my misfortune to know less of Drs. J. E. Smith and Lewis Sherman, but where can you show me that I accused them of partiality? Be careful how you make accusations which can be disproved by any reader. I only said and reiterate it now: "Gentlemen of the bureau! clinical experience does not care a straw about the negative proofs of Nos. 1 and 2 (chemistry, microscopy, and spectroscopy)." Dr. Dake shows his animus when he says: "I seek to overthrow no facts, but simply the most effective exposure of the fruits of *imagination and fraud* palmed off as facts." FRAUD!!! a severe accusation towards a brother practitioner, and if proven, deserving not only the highest condemnation, but also expulsion from any honorable medical society. And who shall be the judges? Dr. Paul Sick (*Die Homœopathie am Krankenbette erprobt*, Stuttgart, 1879) considers in all natural sciences, and therefore also in homœopathy, not the exploration of a principle the *sine qua non*, but the question, *are the facts true, do they correspond with constantly repeated observation, with experience?*

It is, I believe, considered a *homœopathic cure* where the symptoms of a diseased person are removed by a drug showing similar symptoms in its provings; and where such observations are constantly repeated they become *undeniable facts*, though it may be in full opposition to all "so-called" scientific theories. Our great expert, Edison, only lately replied to a scientist, who opposed his facts on account of their being against all preconceived theory, that it is so much the worse for the theory, but the fact remains victor. *The law of similarity can be only the sole judge, for it is a law of nature.* To this judge we bow in all simplicity, and we will not, we cannot, accept any other.

Suppose there should be only one case, cured by the millionth potency, for example, but that case should stand the strictest application of the law of similarity, though it would be a puzzle to many, the fact would be neither the fruit of imagination nor of fraud. It may be totally impossible to show any drug presence by any of these fine scientific tests; clinical experience of a host of materialists may oppose it on account of its being in contradiction to all common-sense, but still the fact stands; *e pur el muove*, the world does move though all priesthood was opposed to it.

But a cure by a high potency is not a puzzle; constantly repeated observations in all climes and by many observers have stamped such cures as the clinical experience of the best men in our school.

Homœopathy, pure and simple, is true and does not shrink from the light. Its working, being dynamical, we may yet be unable to explain, but we say with Edison, "first, facts;" let us accumulate them by thousands and they may be acknowledged as true facts, whenever they stand the touchstone of the law of similarity. Is the chairman of the Bureau of Materia Medica willing to accept these true facts?

SAMUEL LILIENTHAL.

ALUMINIUM PROBE.

BY JOHN C. MORGAN, M.D., PHILADELPHIA, PA.

I DESIRE to call attention to my device of the Aluminium Probe, as a substitute for the old-fashioned silver instrument. Its superiority will speedily appear in the exploration of parts requiring exact differentiation of fascia, bone, foreign bodies, etc. The texture of the metal gives great extension of the sensitiveness of the fingers, clears up diagnosis, and guides the forceps, etc., admirably.

INDUCED ABORTION.

CHICAGO, March 24th, 1880.

TO THE EDITOR: Let me correct a misstatement of my position, inadvertently made by Professor McClatchey in his admirable article, as published in your March issue: I am an opponent of *induced abortion*, under any conceivable circumstances, but I am an advocate of *premature labor* in cases requiring the operation. The one is done to kill, the other is done to save!

Respectfully, N. F. COOKE.

THE

HAHNEMANNIAN MONTHLY.

A HOMŒOPATHIC JOURNAL OF

MEDICINE AND SURGERY.

Editors,

E. A. FARRINGTON, M.D. PEMBERTON DUDLEY, M.D.

Business Manager,

BUSHROD W. JAMES, M.D.

Vol. II. Philadelphia, Pa., April, 1880. No. 4.

☞ The Editors consider themselves responsible for the maintenance of the dignity and courtesy of the journal, but *not* for the opinions expressed by its contributors.

Editorial Department.

THE PROVING OF DRUGS.—Drug-proving demands the fullest exercise of the powers of observation, together with a faithful record of every circumstance noticed. To complete the work, the physician conducting the provings should review all the symptoms, elicit their full meaning by questions, and employ every means for determining their accuracy.

Physicians are not always the most desirable drug-provers, because they forget that their duty is to record rather than to judge. Especially unfortunate is the exclusion of symptoms merely because they have been often experienced before. True, such symptoms are frequently of no importance; but sometimes they are of the highest value. Why not preserve them, then, with a cautionary word of explanation?

Nearly half a century ago, when Dr. Hering instituted his Lachesis provings, he was conscientiously particular in recording every circumstance, new or old. For years he had not been annoyed by any snugly fitting clothing. While under the influence of the snake poison he noticed that the pressure of his collar was more than usually annoying. He thought that this could hardly be attributed to the drug; nevertheless, it was faithfully written down, explained, and left for the unfailing test of experience. And what tyro in medicine to-day does not know the value of this cutaneous susceptibility of Lachesis?—a symptom so characteristic, that it determines the choice of the remedy, even in cases in which the patient lies in a stupor.

Quite recently we read in Dr. Pope's excellent journal, a record of "heart cases" treated with Lycopus virg. (See *Monthly Homœopathic Review*, January, 1880.) Now, two-thirds of the cardiac symptoms of this plant were the results of a personal proving of a Dr. Morrisson, who had, for nine years, been subject to rheumatic pains, depressed cardiac action, faintness in a crowded room, systolic basic murmur at the second left interspace, thought to be hæmic, etc. (See Allen, vol. vi, p. 69).

The worthy prover published his symptoms, qualified their meaning with a statement of his condition, and as a result, we read of their successful test in practice.

The lesson to be drawn from these facts is manifold. Never discard as useless any condition which develops or redevelops during a drug-proving. Never discard a proving because it was made upon a comparatively unhealthy person. And, lastly, never discard new symptoms which may arise while treating the sick. Keep a record of all such questionable items, test them repeatedly, and then give them publicity through the journals.

THE MILWAUKEE TEST AND ITS RESULTS.—The *experimentum crucis*, proposed by Dr. Lewis Sherman, and carried out by the Milwaukee Academy of Medicine, for the purpose of demonstrating the potency or impotency of the thirtieth dilution of drugs, has been completed in accordance with the published programme (see vol. xiv, p. 169), and the final report is before the profession (see current number). And now, all classes of homœopathists may congratulate themselves,—the "low dilutionists" because the test has not proven them to be in error, and the "high potentists," because it has not proven anything else; the experiment having been too limited in its application to establish either the presence or the absence of drug power in the preparations used. We can imagine the sigh of profound relief with which the report is received. We all love science and desire to learn the truth,—of course we do; but we all interpret the proverb, "*Magna est veritas et prevalebit,*" as meaning that our side is bound to win. The possibility therefore of being forced to change our opinions on short notice, is not pleasant to contemplate, and to have the foundation-stones of our belief unceremoniously jerked out from under us, and feel the superstructure come tumbling about our ears, while our neighbors stand looking on with Christian sympathy in their faces and a big unchristian laugh in their sleeves, hurts our feelings dreadfully. If it is all the same to the Milwaukee people, we each prefer that they should get up their little earthquake on some other man's premises.

Looking at the report of the Milwaukee test, the first thought is one of regret that so few physicians were willing to engage in so important and necessary a work, and that so many were found ready to denounce it, and to prejudge its results, without giving, so far as we can see, good and sufficient reasons for occupying so strange an attitude. If it had been shown that such a test is not needed, or that this particular test is unfair in its management or otherwise unreliable in its character, no one could be surprised at the opposition it encountered, and the harsh criticism measured out to it and to its managers, would be sufficiently explained.

Notwithstanding the unfavorable auspices under which the test has been conducted, it has accomplished some good. It has brought the profession face to face with the proposition, that if any crucial test can demonstrate, beyond possible doubt, that there is, or is not, curative and pathogenetic power in the high dilutions, it is our duty to make such a test. It has set numbers of practitioners to thinking upon the subject, with the result of convincing them that the making of such an experiment is a duty which we owe to ourselves as a profession, to medicine as a science, to physical science aside from its relation to medicine, to the allopathic profession, and to a disease-stricken race.

It seems that of the twenty-five pathogenetic tests sent out, only nine reported. Of these nine attempts to distinguish the one medicated from among the nine unmedicated vials, no one succeeded. It is known that some of the remaining sixteen tests were not experimented with at all, but it is presumable that some of them were used, and that the results were not considered valuable by the experimenters, else they also would have been reported. It is probable, therefore, that there were more than nine failures without any successes to record against them. This certainly is not sufficient to satisfy any reasonable physician that the thirtieth dilutions are destitute of pathogenetic properties; it does, however, make out a *prima facie* case against these dilutions, and throws upon them the burden of proving their symptom-producing power, and of doing it in such a manner as to explain away the nine failures of the Milwaukee experimenters.

It must not be forgotten that many physicians doubt the pathogenetic power of high dilutions even while believing implicitly in their *curative* virtues. These physicians will be naturally disposed to regard the Milwaukee experiment as confirming their doubts on the one hand, without in the least weakening their faith on the other. It is to be greatly regretted that but a single report was received from those who experimented with the therapeutic test. In this case the reporter succeeded in distinguishing between the medicated vial and its unmedicated companion, but this one curative success, like the nine pathogenetic failures, is of little value in enabling us to decide the interesting question under consideration.

There are but few physicians,—at least we hope there are,—who would like to have the profession abandon the task of crucially testing our dilutions of drugs, until the demonstration, one way or the other, is complete and incontrovertible. This work should be taken in hand by that authoritative body, the American Institute of Homœopathy. It should be so hedged about with safeguards, undertaken by such competent hands, and conducted with such scrupulous care and consummate skill, as that nobody but an idiot or a knave could ever doubt the correctness of its conclusions. It is unreasonable to expect that such a work can be done in a year. It ought to require that length of time merely to perfect the details of a plan, such as would be entirely satisfactory to the great mass of the profession, and two or three years, perhaps even more, to execute it. As physicians engaged in controversy with the doctrines of allopathy, we shall never be quite content until we know that all our lines of defence are safe lines, and fortify ourselves with this inductive bulwark. Meanwhile let us not waste precious time in idle boastings. As the matter now stands, no prediction of the results of a thorough test can be quite sure of fulfilment, and the man most certain of the stability of his position may find his dominion wrested from him. Of one thing, however, we may be sure, that whatever the future may develop in reference to the potency question, homœopathy has nothing to lose and everything to gain by any experiment that honest men may make. Founded on eternal truth, *she* will stand secure, though the wisest of men may fall.

"THE REGENERATION OF MATERIA MEDICA."—This is the title of a paper by Dr. J. P. Dake, published in the January number of the *British Journal of Homœopathy*, in which the author asks the questions: "Is it possible that we must sit down content with the 'text' of Materia Medica we now have? Is there nothing attainable that may be more perfect, more reliable, more useful? Can we do nothing but 'illuminate,' comment upon, compare and classify, or perhaps, extend, the symptoms now recorded? Shall we have no correction, no purification, except as brought by the 'side-lights' of toxicology, and the slow, halting, stumbling advances of clinical experience? In short is it not possible for us to have a *pure* Materia Medica, such as was at first contemplated by Hahnemann and always demanded by the law *similia?*" Then recounting the opportunities and facilities we possess for securing so essential an object, our "thousands of physicians with millions of clients; our well-appointed and well-managed medical schools, with hundreds of medical students, male and female, qualified and ready to act as drug provers; scores of experts capable of applying every necessary test or means in the diagnosis of drug affections;" he asks, "what has kept the Homœopathic school so long from the realizations of its greatest *desideratum*, a pure Materia Medica?"

A more practical question than the one last quoted, would be, what shall longer prevent us from acquiring a pure Materia Medica? Perhaps the chief obstacles will be; first, the fact that there are so many physicians who do not yet fully realize our crying need for something better than we have. Very few of us are sufficiently dissatisfied with our failures; we think that so long as we are more successful than our allopathic neighbor, we are doing well enough. Our standard of success is not high enough. We have no right to be satisfied with our scientific knowledge so long as the apparently indicated remedy ever fails to cure. Secondly, we shall find an obstacle to the realization of our hopes for a pure Materia Medica, in the fact that the ways and means thus far proposed have not as yet impressed the profession as being in all respects practicable and satisfactory. Yet the suggestions made, not only by Dr. Dake, but also by Dudgeon, Hughes, Dunham, and others, have had and will continue to have their desired effect upon professional thought, and must sooner or later work out practical results. Indeed we already see their effects in the demand for more thorough observations of drug effects and especially objective effects; a more careful scrutiny of the symptoms themselves, a more thorough comprehension of their significance, their relation to each other and to co-existing pathological states and processes, and a vastly more careful and exact notation or description of symptoms. The American Ophthalmological and Otological Society is even now urging upon the profession a reproving of our remedies for the purpose of studying their objective effects upon the more deeply seated structures of the eye and ear, a necessity forced upon us by the rapid development of these specialties, and which cannot and must not remain long unsupplied.

That there are in drug symptomatology such things as absolute certainties, is sufficiently obvious. That there can be no certainty in therapeutic art except upon the basis of certainty in our knowledge of drug effects, is equally unquestionable. And that many of our failures in endeavoring to apply the law of similars in the treatment of disease are due to incorrectly described and even to false symptoms incorporated in our provings, is not a matter of doubt. Let the advocates of a pure Materia Medica, then, one and all, continue to "cry aloud and spare not."

A NEW TEST.—We publish this month, the final report of the Milwaukee Academy on the subject of the "Test." So far as a scientific answer to the test-question is concerned, the report is too meagre to be conclusive on any one point. Dr. Greenleaf proposes a very ingenious test, which, if faithfully and honestly carried out, will add many valuable facts, serviceable in the solution of the vexed question of potencies. He suggests the appointing of trustworthy judges, to whom will be referred all the particulars requisite for the successful carrying out of the project. Physicians who have been eminently successful with certain remedies in certain potencies, are to send such facts to the judges. The latter in return will remit the drugs, prepared in both high and low potencies, but marked so as not to be deciphered by the physicians who are to use them. After a suitable period reports are to be made to the judges, stating which bottle or bottles acted most promptly. If, for example, a doctor has been accustomed to the use of Bellad. 1^x, let him receive the 1^x, 30th, and 200th, marked, perhaps Bellad., a, b, c. After repeated trials he writes:

"I was most successful with Bellad. b, or a, or c, as the case may be."

Who will assist Dr. Greenleaf in this good work?

OUR CONTRIBUTORS.—The physicians of Philadelphia are furnishing, through their County Society and the Hahnemann Club, some excellent papers for this journal, and we are also receiving first-class articles from more distant friends. The comparative infrequency of these latter, however, leads us to say that we should be glad to have many more of them. It is held that a medical journal is just what its subscribers make it, and this being true, *we* can publish as good a journal as any in the land, and with the kindly help of our readers and friends we mean to do it.

☞ SUBSCRIBERS upon paying their subscriptions will find their receipts in the next succeeding number of the journal. If otherwise, please notify the Business Manager at once. We learn that a few subscribers are receiving two copies,—one direct from this office, and one from some one of our agencies. It is causing us and them a good deal of annoyance. Will such subscribers please inform us of all the facts, so that we may get our lists straightened out? Also please write us, if any of your numbers fail to reach you. We are very anxious that our patrons should have as few occasions of complaint as possible.

ERRATA.—On page 164, March number, in description of microscopic appearances of false membrane from the rectum, the absence of lymphoid and epithelial cells should be ascribed to washing the membrane in water after it had been passed with the stool.

Page 155, 6th line from bottom, for "sesquioxide" read "sesquicarbonate."

Book Department.

THERAPEUTICAL MATERIA MEDICA. By A. C. Jessen, M.D. Published by Halsey Bros., Chicago, 1880.

Dr. Jessen has arranged after a novel plan two hundred and sixteen of our remedies. They are printed in columns of two, three, and even four remedies on a page. The objects of the author "are to place such remedies together as are naturally related, to bring as many remedies as possible before the eyes at once, and to enumerate the most important diseases to which the pathogenetic symptoms of the remedies correspond." Such a plan, he thinks, will greatly aid in "making the treasures in our remedies more readily attainable."

The weary student will heartily welcome any plan which promises to make his labors less arduous and, at the same time, more productive; but we question if the method here adopted will fully suffice. The system is too broad. The association of drugs, merely because they belong to the same kingdom, only aids the mind in a very general way. The mere fact that Aconite and Bryonia are plants, Apis, Cantharis, and Lachesis are animals, or, Kali bich. and Silica are minerals, is of little moment therapeutically. If the doctor had compared remedies of similar origin, such as Ignatia and Nux, Apis and Vespa, Sepia and Murex, Calc. ost. and Calc. phos., the practical value of his book would have been greatly enhanced. But even when two or more similar drugs chance to come together they are not compared. The author especially disclaims any such intention (see Preface). Aside from a possible advantage in viewing two or more drugs at the same time, the arrangement of the book does nothing more than put on one page what is usually printed on several.

The author, in arranging the drugs, has endeavored to present their symptoms in connection with corresponding diseases. This method, he thinks, "entitles his book to be called A Therapeutical Materia Medica." But at what sacrifice he has completed his design is evident when we glance over the symptoms. Characteristics are numerous, but they are often so worded that the novice in Materia Medica would fail to recognize them. And, again, they are frequently robbed of those nice qualifications which make them so valuable. Thus, the neuralgias of Spigelia are dismissed with the following: "Sticking, tearing, burning pains, ... neuralgic affections of the fifth pair of nerves." The unique vomiting of Kreasote is dismissed in the most commonplace terms, "nausea, vomiting;" "vomiting of pregnancy." Sambucus has its laryngeal spasms omitted, while its famous sweat is merely set down as "profuse and debilitating." Kali bich. is honored with its "stringy mucus," but is deprived of another of its great characteristics, "ulcers as if punched out." Rhododendron is referred to as worse in rough, stormy weather; but its equally valuable modality, worse in a thunderstorm, is forgotten. Podophyllum is acknowledged as of use in diarrhœa; but how is the practitioner to discriminate if the concomitants as to time, etc., are not made known? So we might multiply examples from almost every page.

In the division of the respective remedies, the author has adopted quite an original plan. He begins with leading therapeutics. This he follows with mind and sensorium. Next he introduces cutaneous system and trunk and extremities, before he considers head, eyes, ears, and nose. After the special senses follow nervous, circulatory, respiratory, digestive, urinary, and generative systems, and, lastly, special remarks. The carrying out of his pathological plans would require an alteration of Hahnemann's schedule; but it seems to us that the symmetry of a remedy is sadly marred by crowding symptoms of the skin, trunk, and limbs, between those of the mind and the head.

The book is bound in stiff cover, is clearly and neatly printed, and so well spaced as to admit of easy reading.

THE MICROSCOPE AND MICROSCOPICAL TECHNOLOGY. A textbook for Physicians and Students. By Heinrich Frey, Professor of Medicine, University of Zurich. Translated and edited by George R. Cutter, M.D. Second edition. Octavo, 660 pp. William Wood & Co., New York.

At the present day when it has become necessary for every physician to have some acquaintance with the use of the microscope, when it is as indispensable to him for purposes of diagnosis and prognosis as many of his older aids, a new addition of such a standard work as the above cannot but be received with welcome.

There was a time when the physician was satisfied with guesswork, but that time has passed. It is now requisite for him to be to a degree positive, and he has to bring to his aid all the discoveries that science and inventive genius can give him. The boundary line between health and disease is in some situations so indistinct that man's senses unaided cannot distinguish it. The study of histology is necessary to the thoroughly educated and progressive physician, and any author who has fully investigated this field of research, and who gives the results of his labor and the method by which such investigations may be made by others is deserving of the hearty thanks of his co-laborers in the profession of medicine.

Such a work is now before us, and so heartily has it been appreciated in the past that a second edition has been called for.

It begins with the theory of the microscope, and in successive chapters explains the different instruments in use, and much of the accessory apparatus used with them. Then follow the method of preparing tissues for examination, the different chemical reagents used, the methods of staining and of injecting, and finally, full directions for mounting for permanent preservation.

This comprises the first half of the book, the first eleven chapters. The final eleven chapters describe and illustrate with numerous plates the different histological preparations. We notice many new things in this edition which serve to bring the work up to date in every respect. We have not space to note all of these, but will point out a few, to show how thorough our author has been in his researches. On page 51, we find mention of the comparatively recent use of the microscope in spectral analysis. On page 108, section cutters are fully explained, and the translator gives due prominence to that most useful of section cutters, the mechanical one of Dr. C. Seiler, of this city. On page 114, we find transparent soap spoken of as a valuable agent for imbedding certain tissues for section cutting. On page 119, carbolic acid is recommended as useful to prevent decomposition of animal fluids when used as media of delicate changeable tissues. As new chemical reagents we notice Phosphoric, Boric, Lactic, Formic, and Tar-

taric acids among the acids, and Hypochlorate of soda and Cyanide of potash amongst the alkalies.

In the section on staining we find mention of picro-carmine tinging, purpurine tinging, erosine tinging, tinging with aniline iodine violet, and with chinolin blue, and a full description of different methods of double staining.

In section 9, on the methods of injecting, we find mention of Heidenhain's method of using Indigo-carmine in the study of the kidneys, and a description and plate of a new apparatus for injecting with compressed air and Mercury.

In the section on mounting the author gives the results of his experiments with Dammar resin in turpentine, mastic in chloroform, and sandarac. He also recommends dissolving Canada balsam in benzin in preference frequently to the older and more troublesome way of heating the slide and the balsam. In every respect this edition shows what has been discovered in microscopy since the first edition was published, and it should be in the library of every physician. To any one wishing to become a finished microscopist we feel confident in recommending this book, as any one who studies this work thoroughly from the beginning to the end and carefully follows the directions laid down in it cannot fail to completely grasp the subject. With regard to the printing and binding we can give no higher praise than to say that it is on a par with all the books published by the same firm. Finally, we would congratulate the translator on the faithful manner in which he has done his work and for the useful additions he has made to the book. J. N. M.

THE GUIDING SYMPTOMS OF OUR MATERIA MEDICA. By C. Hering, M D. Published by the American Homœopathic Publishing Society, Philadelphia, 1879, 1880.

Volume II of this valuable work is just issued, and contains over forty remedies, from Arnica to Bromine.

Having had something to do with the manufacture of this book we feel somewhat qualified to pass judgment upon it. We discontinued our labors before the MSS. of Volume I went to press; but two years of work previous to that time initiated us into the mysteries of the vast storehouse whence Dr. Hering draws his material for this gigantic work. We recall especially our task of "boiling down" Aconite. We were presented with a stack of symptoms, which, without exaggeration, was six or seven inches thick, fourteen inches long, and eight or nine wide! This was the industrious accumulation of nearly half a century, and it was to be condensed into twenty-four printed pages.

Let the reader imagine a proportionate amount of work for each remedy, and he will be able to comprehend how many arduous hours Dr. H. and his co-laborers have spent in preparing these volumes.

Concerning the make-up of the books several matters of vital importance present themselves. In the first place, Dr. Hering's mode of arranging drugs is the most searching of any yet devised. It lays bare every quality of the drug, the most subtle as well as the most palpable. When, however, we come to synthetic study, when we desire to comprehend a remedy as an individual whole, we miss the constructive method, such as that of Dunham. Nevertheless, it is a comparatively easy task for the reader to institute this synthesis for himself, because the books before us present him with every part of the remedy, nicely and definitely described, like well-hewn building stones, orderly disposed.

The chief use of Dr. Hering's book is, as he expresses it himself, to furnish the profession with a reliable collection of "cured symptoms" in addition to confirmed provings. Thus the work becomes complementary to Allen. The latter is the treasury whence we draw forth material for confirmation. The former is designed to be a systematic arrangement of confirmations themselves. Hering's book assumes to deal with certainties; Allen's both with certainties and probabilities. We think that those members of the profession who utterly discard cured symptoms deprive themselves of at least thirty per cent. of the possibility of healing the sick. Indeed, clinical additions are so essential a part of positive materia medica that no one can avoid using them, whether he admits them theoretically or not. Who, for instance, can do without Hepar in abscess, Hypericum in wounded nerves, Arnica in bruises, Gelsemium in serous effusion in the eye, Natrum mur. as antidotal to lunar caustic?—and yet these are purely clinical. But, it may be said again, as it often has been before, what proof have we that such indications are genuine? And, further, what becomes of our law if drugs cure what they have not produced on the healthy? Such questions are really nothing but a jumble of fallacies. Health is a relative word and weighs nothing against susceptibility. Let the prover be sick or well, his record is valuable only so far as he is susceptible to drug-action. And always during sickness susceptibility is greatly increased. The value of clinical symptoms depends upon their selection; and the proof of their genuineness is included in this selection. It is not every symptom which disappears after an administered drug that is genuine. Remove the supports of a building and it falls; remove the characteristics of a disease and all its other symptoms fall. Cured symptoms, then, demand a most careful examination before adoption. They must agree with the provings; they must express the same kind of action. They must be observed *over and over again.* Sometimes they will be found to be amplifications of obscurely recorded symptoms in provings. Then they are gems indeed. Cyclamen, for instance, produced amblyopia. Clinical test amplified this symptom into blindness *with* gastric disturbances.

How far, then, has Dr. Hering adhered to strict rules in compiling his book? And in the answer to this question lies the true estimate of the value of the guiding symptoms.

In Volume I we fear the erasing pen was not used often enough. Indications appear which are not clear and unmistakable. They are not "guiding symptoms." But Volume II shines in highly finished polish.

We notice but few rough places which need polishing anew. Under Bellad., page 401, "pains gradually increase and gradually decrease" should be added, because although exceptional it has been confirmed. On page 400, "typhus" is only a useless repetition of "typhoid," which follows. And, further, we think it hardly in keeping with the action of Bellad. to relieve "sliding down in bed." At least the characteristic mark should be removed from the symptom.

The Belladonna headaches are generally better from sitting up. This should have been included in lines 19 to 21, p. 363. We are of the opinion that the Bellad. patient is relieved by holding the head in the opposite direction to the part of the head affected. Thus, if the forehead aches, he is better holding the head backwards, and vice versa. The generally diffused headache is better sitting up.

The symptom which begins on line 11, p. 361, is but a repetition of lines 14 to 16 from foot of page 363. We cannot see, therefore, why only one is marked as verified; or, indeed, why both are inserted.

On page 463 a symptom from Schreter—fretful, indolent before stool; contented, cheerful, after—is, for convenience, divided into two. As the whole has been confirmed, why is only one part marked? This is evidently an oversight; for under "mind," where the entire symptom is recorded, it is correctly characterized.

We know from experience that it is a very difficult task to correctly arrange the various grades of symptoms; but for accuracy's sake we would urge a careful review of Volumes I and II, the results to be incorporated as a page of errata in the next issue.

Near the top of page 465 we read: "Prolapsus by increased heat of vagina." Surely this is not a "guiding" symptom. Such vagaries are few and far between, however.

But apropos of care in introducing cured symptoms, we notice an instructive illustration under Borax.

On page 461 we read: "Rapidly forming ulcers in the mouth; gangrenous." Now no proving of Borax affords such a symptom, and yet who may dispute it? Most allopathic works are silent on the toxic effects of this salt of soda; but Stillé and Maisch ascribe to it the same consequences as follow the prolonged use of other salts of sodium, viz., liquefaction of the blood, scorbutic symptoms, etc. And, further, they credit it with antiseptic properties, and advise it in ulcerative stomatitis. But such a hint as Hering has given may be justly called "guiding," since, if other symptoms concur, as the emaciation, diarrhœa, or fear of downward motion, we would feel confident in its use, even if the case were one of gangrenous stomatitis. And we would feel more assured than without this bit of clinical information.

In type, quality of paper, and general style, the book is everything that could be desired. F.

Gleanings.

COLD CREAM WITHOUT FATS: Mucilage of quince, 4; almond soap, 1; stearic acid, 10; glycerin, 2 parts.—See *Chemist and Druggist*, February 14th, 1880.

CHEAP AUDIPHONE.—Dr. Turnbull makes a cheap audiphone out of well-calendered binder's-board. It costs but a few cents, and is quite as good as those made of rubber.

ANÆMIA, without apparent cause, is generally hepatic. In such cases the alkalies and not iron are needed. Potash acts better than soda.—*N. Y. Medical Journal*, March, 1880.

CEDRON, says Dr. St. Pève, is more powerful than Sulphate of quinine. The bean is cut into bits as large as a pea, several of which are given in the interval between the paroxysms of fever.—*Medical Record*, Feb. 28th, 1880.

MODIFICATION OF POLITZER'S METHOD.—Dr. J. O. Tansley causes the patient to pucker up his lips and blow from the mouth while he forces air into the nasal cavity with the bag.—*Medical Record*, Feb. 14th, 1880.

A NEW DISEASE, somewhat resembling anthrax in its lesions, and attended with continuous fever, has appeared in Japan.—*Medical Record*, February 28th, 1880.

SAPO VIRIDIS.—To avoid the impure green soap of the market, Dr. Fox employs a soft olive soap, made from cold-pressed olive oil. It owes its green color entirely to the chlorophyl of the olive.—*The Medical Record*, Feb. 14th, 1880.

MOVABLE KIDNEY has been noticed in children. When a swelling appears beneath the border of the rib, especially on the right side, and of the consistence and shape of the kidney, which can easily be pushed upwards, it is doubtless a movable kidney.—*N. Y. Medical Journal*, March, 1880.

RENAL INADEQUACY is a condition which offers no characteristic symptoms; but may be surmised when the urine is deficient in urinary solids, and the patient is always made worse by anything that adds to the amount of solids to be excreted.—*N. Y. Medical Journal*, March, 1880.

CHRYSAROBIN AND PYROGALLIC ACID have been tested in Helva's clinic in psoriasis. The latter works well; the former often fails. The acid locally applied produces little or no irritation, and discolors less than the Chrysarobin.—*Medical Record*, February 28th, 1880.

NITRITE OF AMYL, according to Dr. Gaspey, of Heidelberg, causes dilatation of the bloodvessels. This was demonstrated on the web of the frog's foot and on the tongue of curarized frogs. The degree of dilatation was, at the utmost, one-third the original diameter of the vessels.—*Medical Record*, February 28th, 1880.

REST IN TYPHOID.—Dr. R. P. Howard considers that the fatality in typhoid depends largely upon neglect in regard to proper early treatment, especially with reference to confinement of patients in bed. Many cases of death are traceable to the effects of prolonged high temperature, and especially cardiac weakness.—*N. Y. Medical Journal*, March, 1880.

SUBSTITUTE FOR SIMS'S SPECULUM.—In an emergency, place the patient in Sims's latero-prone position, and with the index and middle fingers of the right hand retract the perinæum just as Sims's speculum is used. The cervix and vagina will be almost as well exposed as when the instrument is employed.—*Chicago Medical Gazette.*

SALICYLATE OF SODA IN URTICARIA.—Although Heinlein has stated that urticaria is sometimes produced by Salicylate of soda, Pietrzycki reports three cases cured with this drug.—*Medical Record,* Feb. 28th, 1880.

We would have worded this for accuracy's sake: *Because* Salicylate of soda has produced urticaria, *therefore* it has, when tried, cured three cases!—EDS.

MALTIN is said to be identical with ptyalin. A cold water infusion of the former is an active diastatic agent. To prepare it take of malt, 3 oz.; mix with half a pint of cold water. Let this stand from twelve to fifteen hours; filter until perfectly bright. Malt should not be used *after* meals, but during their progress.—*N. Y. Medical Journal,* March, 1880.

HIGH TEMPERATURE.—Dr. W. Scott Marshall reports a case of pneumonia in which the thermometer recorded 110° F. The case, however, recovered.—*The Medical Record,* Feb. 14th, 1880. A patient suffered with a temperature of 117° F., and yet he recovered. There seems to be no importance in the rise of temperature *per se.*—*N. Y. Medical Journal,* March, 1880.

BILHARZIA IN THE URINE.—Patient, while travelling in Arabia, was annoyed by severe pains in the bladder; frequent desire to urinate; urine red and bloody. Urine exhibited the ova and embryos of the bilharzia. The full-developed worms are about half an inch or more in length. Dr. Harley found their eggs in the urine of patients from the Cape of Good Hope, who were suffering from hæmaturia.—*N. Y. Medical Journal,* March, 1880.

RECTAL ALIMENTATION.—Desiccated, defibrinated blood is recommended as an agent adapted for rectal alimentation. No heat above 110° F. must be used in drying the blood, and the process must be as instantaneous as possible, and without agitation. Blood thus prepared is readily soluble in water below 160°, and contains all the elements of blood, except water and fibrin. Use a drachm to an ounce of water.—*N. Y. Medical Journal,* March, 1880.

TYPHOID FEVER is not rare in infancy. In the afternoon it may be noticed that the child is restless and has some flushing of the face. If, now, the temperature be taken each afternoon, it will be found typical of typhoid. As Peyer's patches are small, and other intestinal glands but slightly developed, abdominal symptoms will be few. Bronchial catarrh and broncho-pneumonia may be very severe, as may also a meningeal hyperæmia, which develops with a high temperature.—*N. Y. Medical Journal,* March, 1880.

WE commend Dr. Goodell's suggestion to remove the after-birth while the patient lies on the back, instead of on the side. The object of this change of position is to prevent the ingress of air into the uterine cavity, which might favor the onset of puerperal diseases. In the lateral position, and still more in the position for the application of Sims's speculum, air rushes into the vagina, and of course into the uterus, if its cervix is open. This may be of little or no moment in the various operations requiring a speculum, but it may be of serious concern in the parturient case.

REMOVING SUPERFLUOUS HAIRS.—Dr. Hardaway uses a No. 13 cambric needle. This he attaches to the negative wire of a galvanic battery; a moistened sponge electrode is connected with the positive pole. Guided by a strong magnifying lens the needle is entered into the hair-follicle; then the patient approaches the sponge (positive) to the palm. The needle is not withdrawn until a slight frothing shows around its stem. If the depilating forceps easily remove the hair. we know that the papilla has been destroyed.—*Medical Times*, Philadelphia, Feb. 14th, 1880.

Aural Disease Influenced by the Condition of the Teeth.—Dr. Sexton thinks that affections of the ear are frequently caused by decay of the teeth, by the eruption of the first teeth, amalgam fillings, imperfectly fitting plates, etc. He especially objects to vulcanite, because of the Sulphide of mercury used in its manufacture. Both furuncles and collections of cerumen, he claims, may be found in the external meatus in connection with carious teeth. Aural hyperæmia may arise during dentition by sympathetic irritation.—*The Medical Record*, Feb. 14th, 1880.

Nature of Malaria.—Professors Klebs and Crudelli, after an elaborate series of experiments, conclude: 1. That it is possible to reproduce malarial infection in rabbits. 2. That the malaria is generated by organisms existing in malarial soil at a time when the outbreak of the fever has not yet taken place. These organisms are true bacilli malariæ, and appear in small rods, .002 to .007 millimeter in length, graining into long-twisted threads. Dr. Marchiafava has found them in the spleen, marrow, and blood of three persons who had died of pernicious fever.—*Phil. Medical Times*, March 13th, 1880.

Substitute for Carbolic Acid.—In the employment of Lister's dressings the danger of Carbolic acid spray may be avoided by substituting Oil of eucalyptus, which is effective and harmless. The wound should be dressed with a mixture of 10 per cent. of Oil of eucalyptus in Olive oil. The spray may be made of the pure oil or its solution in alcohol. Siegen has shown that this oil abates septic fever in rabbits, and Binz has demonstrated that it prevents the migrations of white blood-corpuscles, and thus prevents suppuration. Further, Siegen has shown that it prevents, even to a greater degree than Quinine, the fermentation of meat-solutions.—*Phil. Medical Times*, March 13th, 1880.

Eruptions.—The prevailing type of the Quinine eruption is erythema, or exceptionally eczema or purpura. Copaiva rash has a preference for ankles and wrist; Iodide of potassium for face and back of neck and shoulders; Chloral, face and neck. The Quinine exanthem is essentially ephemeral. It is of a bright vivid hue, disappearing on pressure, and resembles scarlatinal rash. It first appears on face and neck, and thence spreads over the body. In some instances it comes in distinct spots and resembles measles; in others it is an urticaria, with some œdema, and distressing burning, tingling, and itching. Five cases of purpura are authentically reported.—*N. Y. Medical Journal*, March, 1880.

Mosquitos, those torments to man and beast, nevertheless have their uses. Before they are gifted with wings they live, in the larva-state, in stagnant pools, marshes, and wells. Here they bounce about with wonderful celerity, and do a great deal towards purifying the water. When they cast off their coverings they afford a mechanical means for clearing the water. Indeed, so useful are they, that it is supposed some marsh-lands would be too poisonous for animal life to endure, but for their presence.

Mr. J. J. Friedrich found that the larvæ of mosquitos consume the weaker micro-organisms and leave only the largest of the infusoria, such as Hypotrichous diliata, etc. Septic liquids containing putrid meat and decaying plants were purified of their odor by these wrigglers, who feasted upon their myriads of bacteria, flagellata, etc.—See *American Journal of Microscopy*, February, 1880.

News and Comments.

A Michigan Doctor informed a patient that "both his livers were affected."—*Exc.* Our colleagues at Ann Arbor should be more careful.

The Homœopathic Hospital of Michigan University was dedicated with appropriate ceremonies on Friday evening, March 12th. Addresses were delivered by Professors Jones, Franklin, and Wilson, and also by President Angell, Dr. Eldridge, of Flint, and Dr. Sawyer, of Monroe.

J. H. Buffum, M.D., has been elected Professor of Ophthalmology and Otology in the Chicago Homœopathic College, vice Dr. W. H. Woodyatt, deceased. Dr. Buffum's host of acquaintances in the East will consider this an excellent appointment, and their best wishes will follow him to his new field of usefulness. His residence is No. 90 E. Washington Street, Chicago.

G C McDermott, M.D., succeeds Professor T. P. Wilson as Ophthalmologist and Otologist of Pulte College, Cincinnati. Professor J. D. Buck has been elected Dean. At the session just closed, six of the students were ladies. These students report that "from the beginning to the end of the term they were treated with courtesy and respect."

The Medical Counselor has passed under the control of Dr. H. Arndt, of Grand Rapids, Mich. We are told that the journal will "carry water on both shoulders," whereat we greatly rejoice, presuming it to mean that its pages will be open to the presentation of both sides of all mooted questions in homœopathy, and that the editor will be impartial in his attentions to his contributors.

Transactions of the Homœopathic Medical Society of Pennsylvania, for the years 1874–78 inclusive, in one neatly bound volume, will be ready for distribution during the month of April. As there are not sufficient funds in the society's treasury to pay for the printing and distribution of the volume, members who are in arrears are requested to forward their dues *at once* to J. F. Cooper, M.D., Treasurer, 87 Arch Street, Alleghany City, Penna.

The Western Academy of Homœopathy holds its annual meeting this year at Minneapolis, Minn. Extensive preparations are being made for a session of substantial profit and enjoyment. Papers should be sent as early as possible to the chairman of the various bureaux, that they can report to the General Secretary for publication. We append the list:

R. L. Hill, M.D., Dubuque, Iowa; Statistics, Registration, Legislation, and Education.

B. Bell Andrews, M.D., Astoria, Ill.; Sanitary Science, Climatology, and Hygiene.

J. W. Hartshorne, M.D., Cincinnati, Ohio; Obstetrics.

A. T. Baker, M.D., Davenport, Iowa; Clinical Medicine.

D. T. Abell, M.D., Sedalia, Mo.; Provings.

H. B. Fellows, M.D., Chicago, Ill.; Pyschological Medicine, Anatomy, and Physiology.

L. Sherman, M.D., Milwaukee, Wis.; Pharmacy.

A. Uhlemeyer, M.D., St. Louis, Mo.; Materia Medica.

E. A. Guilbert, M.D., Dubuque, Iowa; Gynæcology.

W. A. Edmonds, M.D., St. Louis, Mo.; Pædology.

J. A. Campbell, M.D., St. Louis, Mo.; Ophthalmology and Otology.
A. E. Higbee, M.D., Minneapolis, Minn.; Surgery.
Letters of inquiry, applications for membership, etc., can be addressed to

C. H. GOODMAN, M.D., Gen. Sec.

2619 PINE STREET, ST. LOUIS MO

THE BABY ELEPHANT.—The birth of an elephant occurred at 2.30 o'clock, on the morning of March 10th, in the building occupied by Cooper & Bailey's Great London Circus, in Philadelphia. As it is the first event of the kind known to have occurred among elephants in captivity, and certainly the first on the Western continent, it has excited a good deal of interest among physicians and naturalists. Through the kindness of Mr. Cooper, one of the proprietors, and of Mr. Craven, the keeper, we had the privilege of visiting the little stranger, and learned that the period of utero-gestation was apparently 20 months and 19 days, counting from the last copulation; but there had been several copulations during the month which preceded it, thus leaving a doubt as to the exact period. As bearing on this question it may be stated that another elephant in the same collection is believed to be pregnant, and copulation is believed to have taken place in her case subsequent to conception. The term, however, is limited, in the case of the "baby" recently born, to 20 months and 19 days as the minimum, and 21 months and 19 days as the maximum. The time given by Aristotle is two years.

"Hebe," the mother, is a huge Ceylon elephant, weighing about 8000 pounds, and is 24 years old. The father is of about equal size, and is 26 years old. According to the statement of the keeper he first noticed Hebe standing with one hind foot on the top of the stake to which she was chained, and "straining." In a short time he "observed the trunk of the 'baby' protruding, and in a few moments the delivery was effected." He thought the whole period of labor could not have lasted more than a few minutes. The secundines followed in about half an hour, and the amount of hæmorrhage was probably about two quarts. Immediately after the delivery the mother became intensely excited, broke her chain, and then, turning her attention to her offspring, she "pushed and rolled it about thirty feet from where it was lying in the centre of the ring."

The elephantine stranger appears likely to do well. It is a female, of the same color as the mother, weighs 213½ lbs.; has already cut some of its teeth, as one officious individual learned in an experimental way; sucks with its mouth, and *not* (as the modern books tell us) with its trunk; has been christened "America," in honor of its native country, and "will not be exhibited until warm weather." The placenta was presented to Dr. Chapman, who will make a full report of the case to the Academy of Natural Sciences.

PULTE MEDICAL COLLEGE OF CINCINNATI.—The commencement exercises of Pulte College took place, March 4th, in College Hall. Twenty-three graduates composed the class who received diplomas on the occasion. An address was delivered by Rev. C. W. Wendt.

HOMŒOPATHIC MEDICAL COLLEGE OF MISSOURI.—This college held its annual commencement on Thursday evening, March 11th. Twenty-five members of the class received the degree, and the valedictory on behalf of the Faculty was delivered by Professor Parsons.

THE NEW YORK HOMŒOPATHIC MEDICAL COLLEGE.—This college sent out a class of thirty-one graduates, the commencement being held on Thursday, March 4th. The educational qualifications of the class, both preliminary and technical, we are told, are highly encouraging to the Faculty and to their friends.

HAHNEMANN MEDICAL COLLEGE OF CHICAGO.—The twentieth annual commencement of this institution came off February 26th. The degree was conferred upon eighty-seven candidates, seven of whom were ladies. Professor Hawks delivered the valedictory on behalf of the Faculty, and an address was also delivered by Professor A. E. Small, President of the College. The total number of students in attendance during the session was two hundred and five.

UNIVERSITY OF IOWA.—The first annual commencement of the Homœopathic Medical Department of Iowa University was held in the Opera House on Tuesday evening, March 2d. The degree of Doctor of Medicine was conferred upon Miss Joanna Disbro and Messrs. S. C. Delap, William G. Edmonds, J. B. Hitchcock, L. K. Hunter, Charles H. M. Schwartz, A. R. Van Sickle, and F. William Winter. Total, eight. The matriculation list shows the names of forty-five students in attendance, thirty of whom are from Iowa. A most encouraging exhibit.

BOSTON UNIVERSITY SCHOOL OF MEDICINE.—The seventh annual commencement took place on Wednesday, March 3d. The graduating class consisted of nineteen gentlemen and sixteen ladies. Total, thirty-five. His Excellency Governor Long, being called on for an address, spoke of the important place filled in the community by physicians, and the value of well-instructed, conscientious men and women in the profession. The valedictory was delivered by Professor C. Wesselhœft. We learn that the school is reaching out for an important addition to its clinical facilities, an effort in which we hope and expect to hear of a complete success.

THE HAHNEMANN MEDICAL COLLEGE OF PHILADELPHIA.—The thirty-second annual commencement of this institution was held in the Academy of Music, at noon of March 10th. The vast auditorium was packed in every part, there being fully three thousand people present to witness the ceremonies. Prayer was offered by Rev. Herman Jacobson, of the First Moravian Church. The valedictory to the graduates was delivered by R. J. McClatchey, M.D., Professor of Pathology and the Practice of Medicine. It was full of sound advice and practical suggestions, but was by no means one of the dry, tedious affairs for which "commencement day" has become noted. President William McGeorge, Jr., Esq., conferred the degree of the college upon the following named gentlemen: Adams, T. Louis, Media, Pa.; Anderson, Edwin O., Braddocks, Pa.; Baker, Alfred E., Philadelphia, Pa.; Baker, William H., Philadelphia, Pa.; Baldwin, Alva Morse, Groton, N. Y.; Balliet, Lorenzo D., Milton, Pa.; Boericke, William, San Francisco, Cal.; Boynton, John R., Boston, Mass.; Caldwell, Frank E., Minneapolis, Minn.; Castle, Asbury B., Pittsburg, Pa.; Chadwick, Sylvester, Wilmington, Del.; Challenger, Harry P., Wilmington, Del.; Clements, Thomas O., Marydel, Md.; Conlyn, Edward S., Carlisle, Pa.; Connor, D. Wilmot, Bloomsburg, Pa.; Conover, Charles H., Philadelphia, Pa.; Crowther, Isaac, Upland, Pa.; Curry, George H., Red Bank, N. J.; Curtis, Walter H., Moravia, N. Y.; Dean, S. Eugene, Rockford, Minn.; Dexter, Byron P., Newport, Me.; Douglass, M. Eugene, Liberty, Me.; Du Bois, William G., Clayton, N. J.; Du Four, William M., Williamsport, Pa.; Fair, Hezekiah W., Glen Rock, Pa.; Fornias, Edward, Trinidad, Cuba; French, Benjamin F., Indianapolis, Ind.; Gale, Charles A., Barre, Vt.; Gramm, Edward M., Philadelphia, Pa.; Griffith, Lewis B., Honeybrook, Pa.; Gross, Francis O., Philadelphia, Pa.; Helffrich, Calvin E., Fogelsville, Pa.; Herb, Charles K., Pitman, Pa.; Hoffman, Lewis A., Reading, Pa.; Hurd, S. Wright, Medina, N. Y.; Kehrer, Augustus B., Philadelphia, Pa.; Kemble, James, Philadelphia, Pa.; Kingsbury, Ed. N., Francestown, N. H.; Kirk, Enos L., Philadelphia, Pa.; Knerr, Levi J., Philadelphia, Pa.; Kunkel, William E., Williamsport, Pa.; Laird, Frank F., Ogdensburg, N. Y.; Macdonald, John, Philadelphia, Pa.; McGill, Edward K., Philadelphia, Pa.; Marsh, Franklin F., Claremont, N. H.; Mattson, Alfred S., Philadelphia, Pa.; Parker, T. Ellwood, Parkersville, Pa.; Pitcairn, Hugh, Altoona, Pa.; Proctor, Willis H., Claremont, N. H.; Reading, L. Willard, Hatboro, Pa.; Rice, Alfred, Marysville, Ohio; Richardson, F. C., M.D., Boston, Mass.; Sampson, Allen W., St. Albans, Me.; Sanders, Christian B., Houston, Texas; Saylor, Norman A., Waterloo, Iowa; Schwartz, Charles W., Littlestown, Pa.; Scott, Fremont W., Medina, N. Y.; Sharpless, Edward S., West Chester, Pa.; Shinkle, Horace J., Philadelphia, Pa.; Simon, Samuel H., Harrisburg, Pa.; Smedley, Isaac G., West Chester, Pa.; Smith, John M., Moorton, Del.; Smith, William Parker, Sunbury, Pa.; Stilson, Willard C., Palmyra, Me.; Stoddart, Alfred P., Philadelphia, Pa.; Tabor, John M., Burke, Vt.; Thompson, Charles S. W., Lebanon, Ohio; Van Baun, William W., Philadelphia, Pa.; Van Fleet, Walter, Williamsport, Pa.; Van Lennep, William B., Great Barrington, Mass.; Wall, Benjamin P., Oakland, Cal.; Wheeler, William A., Phelps, N. Y.; White, George E., Skowhegan, Me.; Wilberton, Lawrence G., Rochester, N. Y.; Wurtz, Charles B., Philadelphia, Pa.

The three college prizes, consisting of Hahnemann Medals of gold, silver, and bronze, respectively, were then conferred upon the three gentlemen who had exhibited the greatest proficiency in the final examination as follows:

First prize, Hahnemann Gold Medal, to William B. Van Lennep, of Massachusetts. Second prize, Hahnemann Silver Medal, to Frank F. Laird, of New York. Third prize, Hahnemann Bronze Medal, to William H. Baker, of Pennsylvania. Professor Gause, the Registrar, in awarding the prizes, announced that twenty-five members of the class had each a graduating average of ninety-five and upwards, and were, therefore, rated as "distinguished." A large number of floral gifts, as well as of more substantial tokens of friendship—books, medical and surgical cases, etc.—were distributed among the graduates. The occasion was enlivened with choice music by the Germania Orchestra.

The Hahnemann Medical Institute.—This organization, composed of students of Hahnemann College of Philadelphia, gave its annual banquet on the evening of March 8th at the Continental Hotel. The members of the Institute and their guests assembled at 8 o'clock in "Parlor C," and after an hour spent in social converse adjourned to the dining-hall, where a bountiful repast was served. Mr G. H. Curry acted as toast-master, and the following sentiments were offered:

1. The Memory of Samuel Hahnemann. 2. The Faculty and College, responded to by Professor A. R. Thomas. 3. To the Class, Mr. B. F. Wall. 4. To the Institute, A. M. Baldwin. 5. To the Undergraduates, J. K. Wade. 6. "My College Notes," Professor R. J. McClatchey. 7. The Ladies, A. E. Baker. 8. "Our Motto," Professor O. B. Gause. 9. Our Future, B. F. Dexter. The valedictory was delivered by Mr. Frank F. Laird. The occasion was a most enjoyable one, and will not soon be forgotten by any one of the hundred gentlemen who participated in it. We had hoped to give at least some extracts from the speeches of the evening, but find to our regret that the limit of our space forbids it.

Married.—Nowell—Cook. On the 17th of March, at the residence of the bride's mother, by Rev. H. S. Cook, assisted by Rev. A. S. Hartman, J. Fletcher Nowell, M.D., of Greencastle, to Miss R. Jennie Cook, of Chambersburg, Pa.

Deceased.—December 24th, 1879, Dr. May, of Grossrohrsdorf, Germany, and on January 28th, 1880, Dr Bonhoff, of Cassel, Germany.

Dr. J. Lockhart Clarke, well known as an able writer on the nervous system, died of phthisis on the 25th of January last.

OBITUARY.

MICHAEL FRIESE, M.D.

DR. MICHAEL FRIESE, of Harrisburg, Penna., a well-known physician, departed this life February 4th, 1880, at the St. Cloud Hotel, Philadelphia, after a lingering illness, which he bore with remarkable fortitude and Christian resignation. Dr. Friese was born near Carlisle, Cumberland County, Pa., on the 7th of February, 1832. His father, who was a practical farmer, was a man of strong literary tendencies, and recognized the importance of a good education for the future welfare of his children, and consequently the subject of this sketch was sent to a good school at an early age, and subsequently devoted the years of his youth and early manhood almost exclusively to the acquisition of knowledge and the obtaining of a good education.

In the year 1853 he commenced the study of medicine with his preceptor, Dr. J. K. Smith, of Carlisle, Pa., and matriculated at the Homœopathic Medical College of Pennsylvania in 1855, at which institution he pursued the studies, graduating with honor in the class of 1860. After graduating he located in Mechanicsburg, Pa., where he soon built up a good practice; but the work proving exceedingly laborious, necessitating long drives and much exposure, he removed to Harrisburg, Pa., where he continued to practice almost up to the time of his death, beloved and respected by a large clientèle.

Dr. Friese was well known to the writer as an amiable and exceedingly modest man, ready at all times to yield his place to others, and often to men of less merit than he. He was a man of considerable literary ability and a frequent contributor to the HAHNEMANNIAN MONTHLY and other journals of our school, and he prepared many valuable essays and papers for the Homœopathic Medical Society of Pennsylvania, of which society he was a member from the time of its organization, and at one time its Vice-President. He was also a member of the Dauphin County Homœopathic Medical Society and of the American Institute of Homœopathy. R. J. McC.

JOHN MICHAEL WEICK, M.D.

JOHN MICHAEL WEICK, M.D., of Philadelphia, died suddenly on the morning of the 17th of February, 1880, in the 78th year of his age. He was born in Rhodt, Rhenish Bavaria, January 6th, 1803. When about fifteen years of age he entered upon his medical studies under Dr. Kœnig, of Edenkoben, later continuing his studies at the University of Heidelberg, and completing the same at the Surgical School at Bamberg, from which he graduated in the year 1828, his medical studies having extended over about ten years. The first field of his professional labors was at Ohrenback, Middle Franconia, Bavaria, in which place he practiced about eighteen years. Toward the close of this period his attention was directed to homœopathy, which, after careful investigation, being thoroughly convinced of its great superiority, he was led to adopt. Soon after this he determined to settle in America, where we find him in July, 1847. Beginning practice in Philadelphia he soon became known, but was induced to remove to the West with a new colony. After a short season he returned to Philadelphia, where he continued in practice with unabated ardor until but a short time prior to his death.

Thus another of our older champions has been called home. He goes in the ripeness of old age, his life's work accomplished. Age and infirmity compelled him to lay down the armor which he so loved to bear, but death soon came that he might enter into rest.

A. K.

THE

HAHNEMANNIAN MONTHLY.

Vol. II., New Series } Philadelphia, May, 1880. No. 5.

Original Department.

MITRAL INSUFFICIENCY.

BY BUSHROD W. JAMES, M.D.

(Read before the Hahnemann Club of Philadelphia.)

IN America, the mitral valve appears to be the one most frequently affected. In England, the aortic is probably more subject to disorder than on this side of the water. The diseases to which the mitral valve is liable are arranged as follows:

1. Those which consist essentially of vegetations on their surfaces, and those which depend on ossification or thickening of their structure.

2. Those which affect the orifice, such on the one hand as *constriction*, either from a thickening of the margins or vegetations, or atheromatous growths; or on the other hand, *dilatation*.

They may be termed incurable cases, that is, pathologically considered, for the structures here, once thoroughly altered, do not regain their former normal condition, and yet remedies will remove many, and in some instances all of the uncomfortable sensations at or near the seat of the lesion.

A disease located in the valves, or in the orifices which they close, as a consequence produces some irregularity in the circulation, and the weaker structures or organs of any particular case will feel the influence of this irregularity, and a diseased state result at that point. Hence, we frequently meet with functional derangements in some distant part of the body, depending solely on valvular disease of the heart, and this is one reason that patients have so slight a hold upon life, independent of the probability of the cessation of the heart's action from the organic disease itself.

We will summarize the results and the induced conditions of mitral insufficiency, and then the diagnostic symptoms and the most useful remedies in the treatment.

In cases of inadequate closure of the valve we find the following general results:

1. A reflow of a part of the arterial blood back into the left ventricle causing a blowing sound at the seat of this valve, heard during the first sound of the heart at its apex.

2. The flow of blood coming from the lungs through the pulmonary vein is correspondingly impeded, and the additional pressure has a tendency to dilate this vein, and also in process of time to distend the left auricle. A louder second sound of the heart is now heard, and is a very diagnostic sign.

3. The next result is a damming back of the blood in the lungs, producing a liability to stagnation there, with such results as dyspnœa, pulmonary and bronchial congestions and inflammations, periodical hæmoptysis, bronchial catarrhs, etc. (Digitalis).

4. Tracing the effect further, we find that owing to the impeded circulation through the lungs, the pulmonary artery and right ventricle have greater labor to force the venous blood into the lungs, and they also in time become dilated. This extra work thrown upon the right ventricle induces hypertrophy, and where this is well pronounced, a dulness on percussion is noticeable over a larger area in the cardiac regions, than exist in the normal conditions.

5. The damage does not always stop here, for this surcharging likewise affects the right auricle, the vena cavæ, and the veins emptying thereinto, and the thoracic duct. The fluids thus pass along more sluggishly than in a healthy state, and cause the later abnormal conditions of hepatic, renal, enteric, gastric, splenic, pancreatic, cerebral and spinal congestions and inflammations, according to the greater or less resisting power that may exist in these parts.

6. Still later, we have anæmia, cyanosis, general debility, and finally hydrops in various situations, and a general giving way of the vital powers.

7. The direct and immediate local symptoms of mitral insufficiency are mainly these, modified, of course, by various temperaments and states of the system of the invalids affected. For diagnosis, however, they are not sufficient; we must have in addition the characteristic blowing murmur before deciding.

This sign is present from the beginning, and in some cases there is a distinct thrill, though this is not an invariable accompaniment.

Later in the progress of the valvular insufficiency, come the additional signs,—left ventricular dilatation and hypertrophy, left auricular dilatation and hypertrophy; then the more permanent pulmonary engorgements; then the right ventricular dilatation and hypertrophy, and the same right auricular states;—and finally heart failure, or possibly fatal organic obstruction, or diseases in remote parts of the body.

The first symptom is *palpitation*, but this is very uncertain, being frequently due to a nervous irritability, resulting especially from loss of blood, or from general debility, arising from other causes. The second is *debility* and sudden weak feeling, especially præcordial. Next we observe *breathlessness on movement*, which causes an undue action of the heart. This sign, however, is also unreliable, like the palpitation first mentioned. If, however, these three symptoms occur with other exciting causes absent, they possess some diagnostic value. Next, the *pulse becomes weakened*, and following this there may be *congestion of the lungs*, as the next noticeable symptom in the early stage of mitral insufficiency, and accompanying this, *a light tendency to cough*;—an annoying hacking, as if to clear away mucus, or relieve a fulness of the bronchia. This effort causes the expectoration of some thin mucus, perhaps tinted or streaked with blood at times, and which may later on prove to be the precursor of more serious complications,—a small clot,—a mouthful of blood, or even a violent hæmorrhage. These latter are more common, however, when the mitral orifice is narrowed. *Dyspnœa* comes on with the pulmonary congestion.

TREATMENT. *Rest.*—This is the prime remedy in all heart disorders, especially in their incipient stages, and it must include physical, mental, and emotional quiet, as far as possible.

As a general rule the more active in habits and excited a patient is after valvular insufficiency occurs, the more rapidly will the secondary diseased states above referred to be induced, and death hastened. The avoidance of all excitements, and all exciting and sympathetic causes of aggravation being first insisted upon, we then select the homœopathic medicinal agent.

Arsenicum alb. is frequently the first one thought of; it has the palpitation, debility, weakened pulse, and oppression as indicative symptoms.

Digitalis purp.—This remedy, in its primary action, has a

tonic effect upon the muscular structures of the heart and a beneficial action upon the engorgements of the lungs, head, and other organs which the disease of the heart produces.

Spigelia comes frequently in order, having even the very characteristic and diagnostic sign of systolic blowing at the apex.

Gelsemium, Cimicifuga, Lilium tigrinum, Anacardium, Cactus grand., Naja tripudians (especially where the nervous system is much involved, and where hypertrophy is going on), *Lycopus virginica, Aconitum nap.,* and *Sulphur.*

The order in which I have named these remedies is that in which I have found them most generally indicated in cardiac disease where the mitral valve or orifice has been involved. I will now give more fully the chest, heart, and pulse symptoms of each of these remedies.

ARSENICUM ALBUM. *Chest.*—Pains in the chest; burning in the chest; tightness of chest, as if bound by a hoop; *oppression of the chest when walking fast,* stitches under the ribs; headache, as if heat were in it during cough. In the chest a stitching, tearing, tensive, pressing and burning pain; stitching in the left chest during an inspiration, which is impeded by the stitching, obliging to cough; stitching pain in the sternum from below upwards, when coughing; very great præcordial anxiety; great oppression in the præcordial region.

Heart.—The heart-beats are irritable; feeble and hurried action of the heart; *palpitation of the heart.* When lying on the back, the heart beats much faster and stronger. *Irregular palpitation of the heart, but so violent at night that he imagines he hears it, accompanied with anguish;* palpitation of the heart and tremulous weakness after stool; absence of pulse, with frequent irritated beating of the heart.

Pulse.—Quick, weak, and irregular; unequal, occasional fluttering; scarcely noticeable.

DIGITALIS PURP. *Chest.*—Œdema of the lungs; weary sensations across the chest to the left side; tension in the chest and pressure in the pit of the stomach, frequently obliging the patient to take a deep breath; suffocative painful constriction of the chest, as if the internal parts were grown together, especially in the morning on waking; obliged to quickly sit upright; contractive pain in the sternum, aggravated by bending forward the head and upper portion of the body; tension in the left side of the chest, on becoming erect, as if the parts were contracted; violent drawing-pressive pain in the lower portion of the right side of the chest, in the evening, preventing sleep;

sharp stitches in the chest, on the right side above the pit of the stomach; fine stitches, corrosive, itching, sticking, rhythmical with the pulse, in the left side on a line with the pit of the stomach.

Heart.—Dull uneasiness in the various parts of the region of the heart, with a sensation of weakness of the forearm; *a sudden sensation as though the heart stood still, with great anxiety;* single, violent slow heart-beats, with sudden violent heat in the occiput, and transient unconsciousness, the whole lasting only a moment; oppressive sensation in the heart, and need to inspire deeper; action of the heart strong and energetic; this increased action extends over the entire left side; first sound dull and prolonged, the second clear; beats intermittent and irregular; congestion of the head, and roaring and ringing in the ears; action of the heart feeble and constantly accompanied by palpitations. *The heart's action loses its force, its beats are frequent and intermittent, and sometimes irregular;* scarcely perceptible beating of the heart; palpitation and uneasy feeling at the heart, readily excited by even moderate exercise; inflammation of the pericardium, with copious serous exudation.

Pulse.—Small, irregular; slow, particularly when at rest; becomes accelerated, full, and hard from every motion, intermitting the third, fifth, or seventh beat.

Spigelia anth. *Chest.*—Constriction in the chest, with anxiety and difficulty of breathing; stitches in the chest, worse from the least movement, or when breathing; sensation of tearing in the chest; trembling sensation in the chest, aggravated from the least movement; can lie only on the right side, with the head high; hydrothorax; dyspnœa and suffocating attacks on moving and raising the arms up; can only lie on the right side, or with the head very high; violent cough; stitches in the diaphragm, with dyspnœa.

Heart.—Stitches about the heart; sometimes synchronous with the pulse; with anxiety and oppression; often with commencing valvular disease, endocarditis, etc.; purring feeling over the heart; wavelike motion, not synchronous with the pulse; palpitation, violent, worse bending forward; high fever; stitching pains; when he sits down, after rising in the morning; from deep inspiration or holding the breath; from least motion; systolic blowing at the apex; burning at the heart.

Pulse.—Iregular; strong but slow; trembling.

Gelsemium semp. *Chest.*—Great weakness in the chest on

speaking; heaviness upon the chest; burning in the chest, with fulness, sighing, and anxiousness, going into the pit of the stomach, and radiating thence all over the whole abdomen like the branches of a tree; this burning is not in the intestines, but in the abdominal walls; constrictive pain round the lower part of the chest; short paroxysmal pain in the superior part of the right lung on taking a long breath; it strikes from above downward; this pain is one of the prominent symptoms; burning under the lower part of the sternum, with heaviness of the chest, stitches in the chest, drawing towards the place of the stitch in the left lower anterior side of the chest, which is repeated, and pain like ulceration, tender to touch; as soon as the burning passes to the left side, the chest feels easier; burning like fire where the patient lately had the stitch in the left lower anterior side of the chest, as large as a dollar, and painful to the touch, like an ulcer, and from the pressure of even a loose dress.

Heart.—Stitching sensation in the region of the heart; at every exertion, shocks at the heart, throbbing of the pulse through the whole body, tremulousness, weakness, and sweat; beating of the heart, irregular as to quantity and quality; excessive action of the heart; a peculiar action of the heart, as though it attempted its beat which it failed fully to accomplish, the pulse intermitting each time; worse when lying, especially on the left side; fears that unless constantly on the move, her heart will cease beating; nervous chill, yet skin is warm; wants to be held that she may not shake so; heart's action feeble, slow, depressed; hands and feet cold.

Pulse.—Frequent, soft, weak, almost imperceptible; slow and full; very rapid, small, and weak.

Cimicifuga. *Chest.*—Lancinating pain along the cartilages of the false ribs, increased by taking a long inspiration; very severe piercing pain, so as almost to prevent inspiration for a short time, immediately after retiring, between 10 and 11 P.M., and continuing for half an hour; a catching pain in the left side, "just where the heart is," which comes on when the patient bends the body forward, and sometimes when sitting still.

Heart.—Pain in region of the heart followed by slight palpitation; stitches in the region of the heart or in the heart; palpitation and faintness.

Pulse.—Quick and weak; full, hard, and irregular; slow, every third or fourth pulsation intermitting.

Lilium tigrinum. *Chest.*—Full feeling in the chest, with

distended abdomen; constricted sensation in left side of the chest, extending to right, with sharp pains running up to throat, clavicle, left axilla, and scapula; better from changing position.

Heart.—Heart feels as if squeezed in a vice, with pain and heaviness, extending from left mamma to scapula; heart feels as if violently grasped, then suddenly released; heaviness in region of heart; palpitation, worse from lying on either side; fluttering, general faint feeling, hurried and forced feeling about the apex; better sitting still; with cold hands and feet covered with cold sweat; sharp quick pain in left chest; conscious pulsations over whole body, and sensation in hands and arms as if blood would burst through the vessels.

Pulse.—Small and weak, as if the blood did not reach the radial artery in the usual quantity.

ANACARDIUM ORIENT. *Chest.*—Uneasiness in the chest, apparently about the heart, especially in the forenoon; pressure on chest, with fulness, especially when sitting; oppression of chest, during an expiration, with pressure upon the sternum; oppression of the chest, with weeping, which relieves it; drawing pain in the muscles of the chest; single sharp sititches in the chest; sharp pulsating stitches in the chest above the heart; sudden, quick pressure in the right side of the chest, close by the axilla; at the same time pressure felt on the opposite side of the back, without any influence upon breathing; *dull pressure, as from a plug, in the right side of the chest;* tearing, with some pressure, on the left side of the chest, reaching as high as the heart, as though the whole side were being crushed, especially when stooping; short breath; cutting in the præcordial region; sharp stitches in the præcordial region, extending thence to the small of the back; very faint on going up stairs.

Heart.—Short stitches piercing the heart, succeeding each other two by two.

Pulse.—Beating of the pulse perceived in the arms while sitting quietly, observed in the prover while the arms were loosely crossed; pulse observed in the whole body (after some bodily effort).

CACTUS GRAND. *Chest.*—*Sanguineous congestion in the chest,* which prevents him from lying down in bed; *painful sensation of constriction in the lower part of the chest, as if a cord was tightly bound around the false ribs, with obstruction of the breathing;* pressive pain in the chest, that impedes respiration and causes deep breathing; is worse in walking and going up stairs; is very troublesome on account of palpitation of the heart; *sensation of great constriction in the middle of the sternum, as if the parts were compressed by iron pincers,* which compression produces oppression of the respiration, aggravated by motion; oppression in the left subclavian region, as if a great weight prevented the free dilatation of the thorax.

Heart.—Increased action of the heart, and on walking, pulsation in the chest with anxiety. Rapid, short, irregular beats of the heart, on rapid motion. Beating of the heart and pulsation of the chest, worse when lying on the back, more perceptible and audible when lying on the side, together with anxiety and restlessness at night. *The palpitation* occurs very frequently during the day, and always at the commencement of any motion whatever, such as stooping, rising, turning around; but walking for some time does not bring it on; it is accompanied by an anxious sensation in the chest, rising into the throat. The palpitation of the heart consists of small, irregular beats, with necessity for deep inspiration. *Sensation of constriction in the heart, as if an iron band prevented its normal movement.* Very acute pain, and painful stitches in the heart.

Pulse.—Hard and sudden, without being frequent. Throbbing, intermitting, weak.

NAJA TRIPUDIANS. *Chest.*—Most acute pain and sense of oppression at the chest, as though a hot iron had been run in, and a hundred weight put on top of it. Dull heavy pain over the lower half of the right chest, with stabbing on taking a deep inspiration; chest not affected by movement, but intensely aggravated by inspiring deeply; the attempt to take a deep breath causes a sudden, short, puffing cough; a real cough is impossible, from the stabbing in the lower part of the right chest, in bed; cannot lie for a moment on the left side, but pain and breathing much relieved by lying on the affected side.

Heart.—Feeling of depression and lowness about the heart; a great pain near the heart. Fluttering of the heart attended by headache.

Pulse.—Regular in rhythm, but unequal in force, most of the beats, however, being tolerably full and strong. Weak and thready.

LYCOPUS VIRG. *Chest.*—Severe pain in right side of thorax, at insertion of pectoral muscles, becoming acute on inspiring deeply, before retiring; returning in the morning on awaking;

passing during the day to apex of heart, from heart to right axilla, down pectoral muscles to former spot, again to apex of heart, and passing off from right side of thorax. Intercostal pains, worse when lying on right side. Sensation of constriction across lower half of thorax, impeding respiration, with subacute pain, increased by lying on right side.

Heart.—The cardiac pains are of a rheumatic character. Constrictive pain and tenderness around the heart. On lying down, palpitation, with altered rhythm, the systole being shortened and the interval lengthened. Cardiac depression with intermittent pulse. Subacute pain over cardiac region, with cardiac distress. Heart-sound indistinct, systolic running into diastolic; basic murmur very slight; apex murmur not perceptible; action very feeble.

Pulse.—Diminished in force, with intermissions.

Aconitum nap. *Chest.*—Hæmoptysis; blood comes up with an easy hawking, hemming, or slight cough; expression of anxiety; great fear of death; palpitation, quick pulse; stitches in the chest, caused by mental excitement; exposure to dry, cold air; cannot lie on the right side; only on the back; dry, hacking cough; pleurisy. Lancinating through the chest, with dry heat, difficult breathing, often violent chill. Pressure, weight, and burning under the sternum. Stitches in the chest with cough.

Heart.—Oppression about the heart, burning flushes along the back. Anxiety about the præcordia, beats quicker and stronger; fear of death. Palpitation, with a feeling as if boiling water was poured into the chest. Anxiety, difficulty of breathing, flying heat in face, sensation of something rushing into the head. Feeling of fulness; stitches at the heart; lies on the back, with raised shoulders. Fainting, with tingling.

Pulse.—During three beats the apex strikes only one. Full, hard, and strong, contracted, febrile, exceeding one hundred beats per minute; slow, feeble, intermittent; feels as if blood does not fill artery.

Sulphur. *Chest.*—Congestion of blood to the chest. Feeling as if a lump of ice were in the right chest. Stitches in the chest, extending into the left scapula; worse when lying on the back and during the least motion. Burning in the chest rising to the face. Pain as if the chest would fly to pieces, when coughing or drawing a deep breath. Weakness in the chest, in the evening while lying down, when talking.

Heart.—Palpitation of the heart, worse when going up

stairs or when climbing a hill; sensation as if the heart were enlarged.

Pulse.—Full, hard, and accelerated, at times intermittent.

PROVING OF DAMIANA.

(Extract from Thesis, presented to the Faculty of the Hahnemann Medical College of Philadelphia, by Charles H. Conover, February, 1880. Published by permission of the Faculty.)

DAMIANA consists of the leaves of two or three Mexican plants, which E. M. Holmes ascertained to belong to the TURNERA MICROPHYLLA. *Nat. order*, Turneraceæ, and the Aplopappus Discoideus. *Nat. order*, Compositæ.

The leaves of the former are alternate obovate, entire at the base and above on each side, with three or four teeth, light green, rather rough, and covered with short, whitish hairs. They readily fall off and the much-branched stems, if present, have some resemblance to broom tops. The leaves have an aromatic taste, suggesting that of confection of Senna.

Of these two species, the one described as the Turnera Microphylla, was employed in the following provings.

June 6th, 1879.—Took 10 drops of the fluid extract, 4.30 P.M. and again at 7.30 P.M. Three hours after the second dose, sharp, darting, well-defined pain through the head, from a point a little to the right of the occipital protuberance to the right frontal eminence. Dull aching in the right eyeball, relieved temporarily by pressure with the hand. 11 P.M. again took 10 drops.

June 7th.—Pain in the eyeballs gone. Took 10 drops at 6, 9, and 11 A.M. and at 1.30 P.M. Sharp lancinating pains through the head from behind forwards, two hours after fourth dose, 4.30 P.M. 10 drops. Sensation of coldness in the eyeballs, relieved by closing the lids, two hours later. At 7.30 and 10.30 P.M. took 10 drops.

June 8th.—Cold sensation gone. Repeated doses at 7, 9.30, 1.30, 5.30, and 10.30; no symptoms.

June 9th.—Took seven doses, the last two of 20 drops each; no symptoms.

June 10th.—Dull, heavy, languid feeling on awaking; inability to raise the eyelids directly on waking; had to rub them and wash them. Took 5 doses of 20 or 30 drops; no further symptoms.

June 11th.—6 A.M., same heavy tired feeling as was felt yesterday on awaking; sharp, stitching pain in the right mastoid process; took medicine at 7, 9, 12, 2, and 4 o'clock; soon after 12 o'clock dose, burning pains in the stomach, slight nausea, worse from motion; 5 P.M., dull aching in region of apex of heart, lasting only a few minutes.

June 12th.—Heavy, dull, stupefying headache, worse from the least motion, morning; five doses, as usual.

June 13th.—At 10.30 A.M. took ʒj fluid extract; frequent desire to take a long deep breath, with a constricted feeling as though the lungs were only partially filled with air, which produced great restlessness and irritability; doses at 5.30 and 11 P.M.

June 14th.—At 10 A.M., and at 1, 6, and 11 P.M. took 80 drops. Same desire to draw a long breath as was noticed yesterday.

June 15th.—No symptoms.

June 16th.—Took three doses of 80 drops each. Sharp stitching pain in the region of the bladder, near its neck; aching and tired weak feeling in the lumbar region, relieved temporarily by lying down.

June 17th.—Heavy confused feeling in the head on waking; tired feeling in the limbs, as after a long walk, with aching like "growing pains;" desire to keep perfectly quiet, as the least movement requires great exertion; doses as before.

June 18th.—Aching of the limbs entirely relieved by sleep; on waking, dull gnawing pains all over the abdomen, relieved for a short time by eructations; slight nausea while riding in a car; aching between scapulæ (afternoon); cannot direct the limbs with precision; it requires great effort to walk straight, especially in the dark (for ten days); doses as before.

June 19th.—Great straining; stools offensive; pressing, suffocative pain in the heart; profuse bright-red hæmorrhage from the right nostril (time during the day); usual doses.

June 20th.—Irresistible drowsiness after dinner, with weary feeling in lower limbs.

June 21st.—Dull headache on waking, worse on motion, better sitting or lying perfectly quiet; indescribable pains in the abdomen, with urging to stool, early morning; no appetite for breakfast; two stools during forenoon, the first natural, the second loose, with pain in the abdomen.

June 22d.—Dull headache on awaking; stool natural; took 80 drops at 9 A.M.

June 23d.—Drowsy all the morning; no headache; doses, 1.30 and 4.30 P.M., each 80 drops.

June 24th.—Dull stupefying headache on awaking, worse from motion; passed off at about 10 o'clock; three doses.

June 25th.—Slept soundly; heavy, languid feeling on awaking, with dull gnawing pains in the abdomen, going off after getting up and moving about. (This was after an unusually long walk yesterday afternoon.) Sour eructations one hour after breakfast; very severe shooting pain from the region of the right kidney to the left side of the abdomen; same doses.

June 26th.—Stool so large and hard it seemed impossible for it to pass the sphincter; it caused the most intense pain, which continued for some hours after passage; 80 drops at 7 A.M.

June 27th.—Took 80 drops; no symptoms.

June 28th.—Medicine at 8 A.M. and 4 and 9 P.M.; stool at first hard and in lumps, then very watery, and attended with pain, which ceased after eructation.

June 29th.—No symptoms; 80 drops, 7 A.M.

June 30th.—On awaking in the morning, mouth and tongue dry; tongue heavily coated, dirty yellow. 4 and 6 P.M., 30 drops of 1st dilution. Very weak back during the whole proving thus far.

July 1st.—Flatulent colic; dull, heavy headache, principally on the left parietal region, increased when shaking the head, but almost entirely relieved after getting up and moving about (on awaking). Drug, same.

July 2d.—Little sores, resembling so-called fever blisters, on lower lip, at border of mucous membrane. Lips tend to crack. Lobe of right ear much swollen, with a hard lump in the centre about the size of a pea and sore to touch. Urging to urinate, 3 or 4 A.M., with pain at the neck of the bladder. This urging always causes an erection.

July 3d.—Very large dry stool, causing much pain in passing. Oversensitive; least noise startles; hearing excessively acute.

July 4th.—Oversensitiveness continues.

July 5th.—Awakened at 5 with urging to stool; at first formed, later watery, with pinching after, but not during a passage. Lasted off and on for two days, and worse from least movement (probably caused from getting overheated yesterday, and drinking what purported to be lemonade, but which was probably far from it).

July 6th.—Profuse gushing diarrhœa, early in the morning; griping pains in the abdomen at intervals of five or ten minutes through the day. Severe grinding pain in the abdomen while urinating; relieved immediately afterward.

July 7th.—Watery stool early in the morning, and several through the day; pinching less severe.

July 8th.—Stool natural; no pain. Urging to stool after dinner, but when attempt was made desire ceased. 10.30 P.M., 30 drops of 1^x.

July 9th.—Desire for stool earlier than usual. Puffiness of lower eyelids on awaking. 30 drops of 1^x at 9 A.M. and 1.30 P.M.

July 10th.—Medicine, but no symptoms.

July 11th.—Slept soundly; very lazy on awaking. Stool large and hard to pass. Two doses.

July 12th.—Very bitter taste in the mouth on awaking. Severe aching in the small of the back when first rising in the morning. Colicky pains in the abdomen, relieved by passing flatus. Two doses.

July 13th.—No symptoms.

July 14th.—Three doses. Stool so large it threatens the anus. Long-lasting pain after stool. Nausea while riding in a car.

July 15th.—Dull grinding pain in the abdomen, going off after breakfast. Three doses.

July 16th.—Continued medicine, but without any symptoms.

July 17th.—Took five doses of 2^x.

July 18th.—Very severe headache, mostly on top of head, relieved temporarily by firm pressure with the hand, and going off entirely after breakfast. Three doses of 2^x.

July 19th.—Three doses. Weak, gone feeling in pit of stomach, with ravenous appetite.

July 20th to 25th.—Medicine, but no symptoms. Changed to 12^x on the 24th.

July 25th.—Took four doses of 12^x. Sharp, lancinating periodical pain in the first phalanx of right middle finger. Muddled feeling in the head, with desire to press the vertex with the hand, which seemed to temporarily relieve. This was followed by intense splitting headache, deepseated; worse from shaking the head, and from any jarring in walking. Pains better by sleep, but on waking, a sore, bruised feeling all over the head.

July 26th.—Took five doses of 12^x. Urging to stool after the usual passage in the morning.

July 27th.—Pinching pain in the abdomen, with a feeling as if diarrhœa would set in.

July 28th.—Slept soundly and did not awaken at the usual time. Four doses.

July 29th.—Four doses. Uncomfortable feeling in the bowels, as if diarrhœa would come on. Indescribable sick feeling, with great oppression of breathing, all the afternoon. Want of expulsive power in the bladder; could not urinate without a great deal of straining and pressing on the abdominal muscles.

July 30th.—Constant desire to urinate, passing only a small quantity at a time. Urine turbid as it passes. Dull feeling in the head. Took 18^x, four doses.

July 31st.—Sleep full of dreams of rather a pleasant character; on waking, head dull and heavy; rather exhausted. Very irritable all the morning, did not want any one to speak to me; uncontrollable disgust for everybody and everything. General sick feeling, which was relieved after dinner. Usual doses.

Aug. 1st.—Urine has a strong odor, and after standing forms a white, quite thick pellicle on its surface. Small aphthous ulcers under the tongue, to the left of the frænum (disappeared on the second day).

Aug. 2d.—Urine still has a very strong odor. Dose, 20 drops 18^x, 9 A.M. and 3.30 P.M.

Aug. 3d.—Two very watery painless stools, between 8 and 9 P.M.

Aug. 4th.—Loose stools, with creeping chills up the back. 20 drops 18^x, 9.30 A.M., 3.30 P.M.

Aug. 5th.—No symptoms; two doses.

Aug. 6th.—No symptoms; two doses.

Aug. 7th.—Very profuse watery stool, with pain in the abdomen, relieved immediately *after* stool (after a sudden change in the temperature during the night).

Aug. 8th.—On awaking, dull gnawing pain in the abdomen, worse after rising, better from eating. Dull headache.

Aug. 9th, 1 P.M.—Very violent urging to stool, followed by profuse mushy stool, unattended with pain, but with an empty, weak feeling in the abdomen, relieved by pressure with the hands. Abdominal walls seem to be relaxed. Feeling as though diarrhœa would come on, all the afternoon. Burning pain just above the umbilicus.

Aug. 10th.—Very severe, dull, aching pains in the legs, with dull headache and general feeling of lassitude; complete loss of energy, desire to keep perfectly quiet (came on two hours after last dose and remained all the evening).

Aug. 11th.—Aching of legs is somewhat better, headache

the same; pains more in vertex and occiput. Headache relieved after breakfast. Urine very pale (after eating watermelon).

Aug. 12*th.*—Very weary feeling on awaking, with dull, heavy, deepseated headache. Very heavy and drowsy after dinner, lasting until near evening; energy all gone; feel as though I had "spring fever."

Aug. 13*th.*—Drowsy after dinner, with great confusion in the head.

Aug. 14*th.*—Severe griping pain in the region of the transverse colon; somewhat relieved by bending double.

Aug. 15*th.*—Respiration difficult, with constant desire to take a long deep breath.

Aug. 16*th*, 4 A.M.—Excessive sneezing (awaking me from sleep), and followed by a profuse discharge of a bland mucus from the nose; later, titillation in the right nostril as though a fit of sneezing would come on. Voice rough and hoarse. 8 A.M., stool at first natural, then very watery and profuse, without pain. Urine alternately turbid and clear while passing from the urethra. 3 P.M., vertigo on rising suddenly; everything turns black before the eyes. No sneezing and no discharge from the nose through the day.

Up to August 13th the 18^x was taken; on August 14th the 30^x was substituted.

Aug. 17*th.*—On awaking, severe itching of the internal canthi. Rumbling in the abdomen with discharge of flatus, early in the morning.

Aug. 18th.—Irresistible drowsiness after dinner.

Aug. 19*th.*—No symptoms, except a constant desire for more air.

Aug. 20*th*, 5 P.M.—Sudden urging to stool.

Aug. 21*st.*—Peculiar stuffed or stopped-up sensation in the left auditory meatus. Immoderate appetite, especially for dinner; hasty eating.

Aug. 22*d.*—Same stuffed feeling.

Aug. 23*d*, 6.30 A.M.—Feels very languid and drowsy after eight hours and a half sound sleep. No appetite for breakfast.

Aug. 24*th.*—Sudden and violent urging to stool after breakfast. Very short and labored respiration, which became so annoying that I had to discontinue the use of the drug. Weak and trembling as though convalescing from some severe sickness. No desire for mental or physical work.

Aug. 25*th.*—Weak feeling continues. Dark-brown, watery

stool, 10 A.M., without pain but with a great deal of flatus. Confused feeling with pressure in the head (all the afternoon).

Aug. 26*th.*—Again took the 30ˣ.

Aug. 27*th.*—The confusion and muddled feeling in the head is greatly aggravated by whistling (have noticed this repeatedly). 9.30 A.M., took 20 drops of the 30ˣ.

Aug. 28*th.*—Two doses.

Aug. 29*th.* Painful stye on the upper lid of the left eye, near the outer canthus (lasted thirty-six hours). At 11.30 A.M. and 1.30 P.M. took 20 drops of the 30ˣ. Very drowsy two hours after dinner. Suddenly hard sneezing followed by watery discharge, with a stopped-up feeling in the nose. Violent itching of the end of the nose while at supper.

Aug. 30*th.*—All the catarrhal symptoms have disappeared. A peculiar crackling in the temporo-maxillary articulation, left side, while eating breakfast.

Aug. 31*st.*—Burning pain in the region of the neck of the bladder, aggravated by expiration, but entirely relieved by inspiration.

Sept. 1*st,* 6 A.M.—Violent fits of sneezing, with mucous discharge from the nose. Dose, 20 drops of the 30ˣ.

Sept. 10*th,* 1 P.M.—Sudden dimness of vision, followed by the most violent bursting headache, lasting all the afternoon. This headache suddenly appeared while eating dinner, after I had felt well all the morning. It was worse from the slightest motion, noise, or bright light, and somewhat relieved by a short sleep.

Sept. 11*th.*—While at stool feeling as though something gave way in the left iliac region.

[The eclectics claim that Damiana is a powerful aphrodisiac. Dr. Conover, in his Thesis, quotes from Stillé and Maisch to the effect that there is not the slightest reason for confiding in this statement of its virtues. "Still less can it be credited with the restoration of an atrophied testis to its normal size and function, which has been set to its account."—EDS.]

GYNÆCOLOGICAL CLINIC.

BY PROFESSOR B. FRANK. BETTS, M.D.

(Hahnemann Medical College of Philadelphia, Thursday, November 20th, 1879.)

ANTEFLEXION.—Gentlemen: The patient before you on the couch has been under treatment for anteflexion of the uterus. She suffered from the pelvic pains usually attributed to such displacements; became very nervous and hysterical, but felt better in every way from "holding herself with her hands," or applying a support to the external genitals. Lilium tig. was indicated, and has afforded her great relief. The flexion has been treated by the introduction of a cotton wad into the vagina, so as to press the cervix back until the long axis of the uterus was straightened. To this wad a string was attached, by which it was removed by the patient herself within thirty-six hours after each application. I consider this treatment applicable for those forms of anteflexion caused by the cervix being flexed forward, with the body in its normal position, or when both body and cervix point forward. Now those of you who will now examine this case will find that this treatment has resulted in permanently straightening the cervix. The atrophied tissue at the point of flexion has been enabled to receive its proper nutritive supply, and is now firm enough to resist a bending of the fundus upon the cervix, so that we have an *anteversion* of the uterus instead of the original *anteflexion*. An anteverted uterus is much more readily kept in place by a pessary than one anteflexed. We shall therefore apply this anteversion pessary, and rely upon its keeping the uterus in its normal position.

TERTIARY SYPHILIS—HEPAR.—This patient is fifty-two years of age, and contracted the disease she is suffering from nearly twenty years ago. For the past seven years it has manifested itself as you see it here. The nates, the under part of the thighs, and the external genitals, are involved in an extensive suppurating mass, discharging yellowish or bloody fluid through numerous sinuses. Into one of these I introduce the probe, and find it quite tortuous and passing in the direction of the ischio-rectal fossa. The inner surface of the right tibia is sensitive, and the cutaneous covering is red, swollen, and very painful.

She suffers from aching pains in different parts of the body, worse at night. Throbbing, boring, and pressing pains in the head, with great mental depression amounting almost to a suicidal tendency.

She came to us after having used Mercury for a long time, and Hepar[30] was administered. To-day she reports great improvement, and we find the number of the sinuses diminishing.

PELVIC HÆMATOCELE.—This patient is sterile. She suffers from profuse, thick, offensive, excoriating leucorrhœal discharges. The menses are scanty, and the flow dark in color, attended with pain in the back and bearing down in the pelvis, as though the uterus would protrude. The hands, feet, and face are œdematous. Urination is painful and interrupted, more especially during the menses. She has alternate attacks of diarrhœa and constipation, and complains of a constant bruised feeling in the occiput, extending to the forehead. By a vaginal examination I detect a hard, immovable mass, about the size of a man's fist, in the left side of the pelvis, encroaching upon the vagina, quite sensitive to touch. I pass the uterine sound into the cavity of the uterus 2¾ inches, and find the organ in its normal condition. The location of this mass is below that usually occupied by fibroid tumors; it is quite sensitive and evidently disconnected with the uterus. Fibroid tumors are not sensitive; they are attached to the uterus, and movable with it, unless pedunculated or attached to neighboring structures by inflammatory adhesions.

Perhaps a further inquiry into the patient's history will throw light upon this case. She informs us that she lifted a heavy weight during a former menstrual period, and felt a severe pain in the left side, became weak and faint, and had to be carried to bed. From that time until the present she has suffered as I have just told you. That was the origin of her trouble. She is a large and healthy-looking woman; but from the rupture of one of the pelvic veins at the time she mentioned, an effusion of blood took place into the connective tissue space alongside of the vagina, constituting that variety of hæmatocele or bloody tumor of the pelvis known as *subperitoneal,* to distinguish it from a hæmorrhage occurring *into* the peritoneal cavity, which gravitates into the *cul de sac* of Douglass, because this is the most dependent part, and known as *introperitoneal.* The effusion in this case has become organized by consolidation of the fibrin of the blood, and will have to disappear by gradual absorption or perhaps by suppuration; in the latter case it will become softer than at present. You will remember that *pelvic cellulitis* is characterized by fever, sensitiveness, and hardness, due to infiltration, in the parts attacked, followed by softening of the mass, as suppuration develops an abscess; whilst the *hæmatocele* comes on suddenly, without fever, is soft at first, then gets hard, to soften again if suppuration takes place.

This patient should have rest in the recumbent posture, so as to promote absorption. And I have advised her to go into the hospital, but she cannot leave home. We will, therefore, have to rely entirely upon the indicated remedy, which seems to be *Sepia.*

Amenorrhœa.—This patient is eighteen years old. The menses were regular from puberty, until within the past five months; they have ceased entirely, and she complains of backache, vertigo, and full feeling in the head. She has a thick yellow leucorrhœa, always very profuse at the time the menses should appear. This perverted functional action we can correct with our remedies. We give no Emmenagogues, but aim to restore the patient to health. When this has been accomplished she will menstruate regularly and at the proper time. From temperament and symptoms we find *Pulsa.* indicated.

Retroflexion—Labial Abscess.—This patient came to us in a very nervous condition, suffering from frequent attacks of sick headache, great weakness from nursing, and retroversion of the uterus. She has worn a Smith's pessary, and taken the remedies indicated, with great relief. She is subject to the recurrence of an abscess in the right labium. These abscesses often originate from an occlusion of the small duct leading from the vulvo-vaginal gland and the imprisonment of its contents. After the abscess has once developed it is very apt to recur from time to time, because it does not become completely evacuated by the suppurative process, consequently it is considered best to dissect out the whole gland through an incision into the labium.

NUX MOSCHATA—A CRITICISM.

BY JOSEPHINE VAN DEUSEN, M.D., PHILADELPHIA, PA.

In the February number of this Journal is published an article, written by Dr. E. M. Howard, entitled: "An Accidental Proving of Nux Moschata." I would like to ask the doctor if he will please separate the whiskey symptoms from those of the drug in question. He says the young lady placed one ounce of nutmeg in a half-pint of whiskey, and on retiring drank off the liquid. In the morning he found her in a semi-unconscious condition. Would it not have been marvellous, had he found her perfectly conscious, after so large a dose of any powerful alcoholic stimulant? Rapid pulse, oppressed respiration, loss of memory for a time, want of concentration, are all primary effects of over-stimulation, and many a man can testify to the large size of his head, and to the multiplicity of bureaus, tables, etc., in his apartment, after a proving of whiskey. Altogether it is quite apparent that the article of Dr. Howard is not properly titled.

SPASMUS GLOTTIDIS.

BY E. A. FARRINGTON, M.D., PHILADELPHIA, PA.

(Read before the Hahnemann Club of Philadelphia.)

Spasmus glottidis, whether considered as a symptom or as an idiopathic disease, possesses considerable interest, since it occasions much alarm and distress.

As a symptom, it causes the croupy cough and dyspnœic paroxysms incident to laryngitis. It also constitutes the main symptom of spasmodic croup. It is produced, too, during hysterical attacks, and as a reflex effect of tumors, which press upon the par vaga or their branches, especially upon the superior or inferior laryngeal. It forms an alarming complication in some cases, of the convulsive stage of tubercular meningitis.

As a distinct disease,—as a neurosis,—it appears independently of inflammation, tumor, or any organic affection, although it may be complicated with such affections. It appears usually between the fourth and eleventh months, more rarely after the first year of life, and very exceptionally among adults.

Of exciting causes the principal are: Dentition, rachitis, excess of food or improper diet, intestinal irritation, emotions. Enlarged glands, especially the thymus, have been considered an exciting cause; but of this pathologists are uncertain. Possibly goitre, by pressure on the larynx, may act as an exciting cause; still, bronchocele is rare in infancy.

The disease is unattended by fever, cough, or catarrh, and the intervals between spasms, except in far-advanced cases, are free from all symptoms. The general health, however, is below par. Its essential phenomenon is difficult breathing, caused by a spasmodic closure of the rima glottidis. In mild cases the child suddenly stops breathing, as if "holding its breath." The paroxysm soon ceases, and with it, of course, the mingled expression on the child's face of astonishment and fear. In severer forms the crowing inspiration is very decided. Every little excitement, even a sudden awaking from sleep, induces an attack. In the worst cases, the paroxysms are frequent and alarmingly severe. During the attack the child kicks and struggles, clutches at its throat, throws back its head, and exhibits a very characteristic flexion of fingers and toes; the face becomes livid, the eyes project, and general convulsions or asphyxia may follow. Sometimes the spells terminate in coughing or crying; in other instances a distressing convulsive action of the diaphragm ensues.

When the affection tends to recovery, which, by the way, is always tardy, the paroxysms grow less frequent or less severe, and the child seems less annoyed by them. Death may result either from convulsions brought on by cerebral hyperæmia, or from asphyxia, or, again, from secondary affections.

Complicating diseases are rachitis; scrofula, with its swollen glands and delayed dentition, favoring reflex spasm; marasmus; intertrigo, possibly because of the attendant swollen glands, etc.

DIAGNOSIS.—From croup, it differs in the absence of a harsh barking cough, fever, etc.; from œdema glottidis it is distinguished by the absence of the serous infiltration about the rima, and by the breathing, which, in the dropsy, is very easy during *expiration*, the outgoing air pushing up the sacs of water, and so obtaining easy exit. From asthma it is diagnosed by the seat of the dyspnœa, and by the sonorous râles of asthma. Spasm of the respiratory muscles may indeed complicate spasm of the glottis, but as a distinct symptom, it is plainly separable. If tonic, the spasm holds the thorax in the position of forced inspiration, the diaphragm conducting the breathing. If clonic, inspiration and expiration are both rapid and noisy.

SYNONYMS.—Laryngismus stridulus, crowing spasm, asthma Millari, asthma Wigandi, asthma spasmodicum, asthma Thymicum. Only the first two are correct.

TREATMENT may be divided into preventive, palliative, and curative. Avoid all excitement, overfeeding, or improperly selected diet. If the mother's milk does not agree, substitute cow's milk mixed with sweetened barley-water; or, milk with Ridge's food. So-called table-food must be proscribed until the child shall have cut the majority of its teeth. Even oatmeal is injurious to children under six months old. If worms excite the disease, administer honey twice daily. If constipation acts as a provoking cause, use enemata or suppositories of castile soap or cocoa-butter.

As palliative, instruct mother or nurse to instantly warm the hands or feet when they become cold. Pat the child on the back or the nates, plunge the hands into warm water, press down the tongue, titillate the fauces; and, in extreme cases, employ artificial respiration, as in asphyxia.

Remedies to cure the disease must always be selected according to the rules of the *Organon;* but the following hints may be useful and instructive.

Drugs causing more or less spasm of the glottis: ACONITE, *Arsenic*, *Asafœtida*, Atropine, BELLADONNA, BROMINE, Calc. phos., Camphor, Chamom., *Cicuta*, CHLORINE, Coral. rub., CUPRUM, FLUORINE, GELSEMIUM, *Hepar*, *Hyoscy.*, *Ignatia*, IODINE, Ipecac., (Kaolin), Lauroc., LACHESIS, Lobelia inflata, Lycopod., *Mephitis*, MOSCHUS, Naja, Nux vomica, Oleum animale, *Opium*, *Phosphorus*, *Phytolacca*, (Physostigma), PLUMBUM, *Sambucus*, Silica, SPONGIA, STRAMONIUM, Strychnine, *Sulphur*, Verat. album, Zinc. 41.

These may be divided into three classes. 1st. For the acute paroxysm: CHLORINE, *Iodine*, BELLADONNA, SPONGIA, *Mephitis*, LACHESIS, CUPRUM, *Sambucus*, STRAMON., *Arsenic*, *Hyoscy.*, *Phytolacca*, *Opium*, Veratrum album, Fluorine, Oleum animale (Naja), MOSCHUS.

2d. Chronic forms: PLUMBUM, *Iodine*, *Arsenic*, Calc. phos., *Phosph.*, Silica, Lycopod., Sulph., Hepar.

3d. Diseases with the spasm as a symptom; as croup: ACONITE, SPONGIA, BROMINE, IODINE, HEPAR, LACHESIS, (Kaolin); hysteria and other similar nervous affections: *Asafœtida*, IGNATIA, MOSCHUS, Strychnine, Zinc, Physostigma, GELSEMIUM; asthma: IPECAC., Lobelia, Camphor, SAMBUCUS, etc.; brain affections: BELLADONNA, HYOSCY., STRAMONIUM, Cicuta, CUPRUM, OPIUM, Atropine, etc.; spinal affections: Nux vomica, Zinc, Physostigma, Strychnine, Belladonna, Veratrum album, etc.; affections of the par vagum: LOBELIA, GELSEMIUM, LAUROCERASUS, Naja, LACHESIS, *Arsenic*, etc.; suppressed hives: ARSENIC.

It is here necessary to give only the symptoms of classes 1 and 2.

CHLORINE, recommended by Dr. Dunham, quite typifies the disease. Inspiration crowing, expiration impossible. Face livid; lungs fearfully distended; partial coma, followed by cessation of the spasm. Similar to mephitis.

IODINE, tightness and constriction about the larynx, soreness, hoarseness. Glands enlarged. Tendency to marasmus. Appetite excellent, yet emaciation; or, indifference to food, clayey stools, high-colored urine. Skin yellow. Child irritable, especially with enlarged mesenteric glands.

BELLADONNA, the least fluid drank excites the spasm; larynx painfully dry, yet averse to water. Interrupted breathing. Awakes startled, affrighted. Sleep restless, tossing, talking, or crying out; quarrels in sleep. Brain excited; strabismus; enlarged pupils, injected eyes; red face. Convulsions; skin hot, dry, or bathed in hot sweat, especially the head. Oversensitive to external impressions; hence worse from light, noise, cross words, irritation from dentition, or the presence of undigested substances in the alimentary tract. Urine scanty, and stains yellow, or suppressed.

SPONGIA, starts from sleep with contraction of the larynx; whistling inspiration; head bent backwards; convulsions; *Mephitis,* when drinking or talking, gets substances into the larynx; expiration all but impossible. Convulsions, see Chlorine.

LACHESIS, spasms during sleep or on awaking. Neck sensitive to slight touch. Symptoms of asphyxia. Naja is similar.

CUPRUM, convulsive stage. On taking a deep breath, stridulous inspiration. Face bluish, sometimes covered with cold sweat. Body stiff, spasmodic twitchings; or, violent flexor spasms, thumbs clenched. Gurgling down the œsophagus.

Sambucus, used by Hahnemann, but seemingly more adapted to asthma. Suffocative paroxysms after 12 P.M.; aroused with anxiety, trembling, shortness of breath to suffocation; wheezing in the chest, difficult inspiration; face blue, eyes and mouth half-open; profuse hot sweat.

STRAMONIUM, aroused frightened, knows no one, clings to those around. Face blue; muscles of the chest spasmodically affected; convulsions.

Arsenic, attacks sudden, at night, threatening suffocation. Child breathes freely between spells, but is weak, restless, and irritable. Face pale, waxen, or sallow; convulsions; body hot, sweating, and pale.

Phytolacca, frequent spasmodic closure of the larynx, drawing the thumbs into the palms, toes flexed, face distorted, one eye moves independently of the other.

Opium, after fright. Recent cases.

Veratrum album, spasmus glottidis with protruded eyes; great weakness, cold sweat on the forehead; great debility.

Oleum animale, larynx feels as if it would be closed by outward pressure when lying on the back with the head bent forward.

MOSCHUS, excellent in hysteria; also recommended in children with spasm of throat, larynx, and lungs. Sudden sensation as if larynx closed, as from inhaling vapor of sulphur.

CLASS 2.—PLUMBUM, sudden difficulty of breathing and asphyxia; convulsions; expiration suddenly arrested, as if a valve closed the glottis; emaciation; constipation, with much straining, the stool passing in hard balls.

PHOSPHORUS, child unusually tall and slender; skin clear, transparent. Easily catches cold on the chest. Stridulous inspiration evenings on falling asleep. Tuberculous parents.

Silica, rachitis. Head large, body small and emaciated; head and feet sweat, toes sore; nervous, excitable; external impressions readily arouse convulsions; delayed dentition.

Calc. phos., delayed dentition; child sweats easily, especially during sleep; emaciated; abdomen flabby; child gets suffocative attacks when lifted from the crib; rachitis; diarrhœa, green, hot, watery; craves bacon. Compare Calc. ostr.

SULPHUR, suddenly attacked when dropping off to sleep. Jerks the limbs in going to sleep; slow dentition; predisposed to fever, etc.

LAUROCERASUS, heart affected. Child blue, gasps for breath; face even livid, pulse thready.

THE QUARANTINE POWERS OF THE NATIONAL BOARD OF HEALTH.

BY LOUIS A. FALLIGANT, M.D., SAVANNAH, GA.

[THE following paper, which appeared in the Savannah *Morning News* of April 5th, 1880, is from the pen of one of our most distinguished Southern homœopathists, and will be read with interest, not only because of the views set forth in relation to the origin of yellow fever, but also as bearing upon the now much-discussed question of national quarantine.—EDS.]

AN ADDRESS.

FELLOW-CITIZENS OF THE SOUTH: In venturing to come before you in the character of a student of your commercial welfare, I trust I shall not be thought presumptive if from a medical standpoint I indicate to you certain facts connected with your commercial interests and certain dangers looming up in the horizon of ambitious and consolidative legislation.

When the Board of Experts was organized under authority of Congress it was supposed to be a board intended for the ascertainment of all possible information concerning certain epidemic diseases—more especially yellow fever; but in the inscrutable accidents of individual selection, under human instead of divine guidance, its *personnel* was made up almost exclusively of gentlemen whose opinions leaned towards the germ theory and the exotic origin of that disease. Naturally its conclusions merged into a comprehensive necessity for a grand national quarantine; and the exercisable powers of the National Board of Health, the outgrowth from the Board of Experts, have been confined by Congressional legislation chiefly to the quarantine aspect of the public service. In my individual capacity as a member of the Board of Experts, I entered my solemn protest against this dwarfing of a great creation into the mere representative of a faction of medical theorists, since grown smaller by degrees and beautifully less in numbers; and claimed in behalf of the great, intelligent body of the opposition that *local hygiene* deserved at least as much study and as extensive governmental assistance as any possible quarantine service. This was in January, 1879.

What have we seen since? The frost-bitten "germs" in the woodwork of the Plymouth defying the Arctic ice-freezing experiments, and the snow-clad "germs" in Memphis defiantly "hibernating" through a season of almost unparalleled coldness and "budding into renewed vitality," as the germists would have us believe, after a season of suspended animation! Yet in New Orleans, in 1879, as in Savannah in 1877, we find that careful previous sanitation and prompt local hygienic measures applied to the outcropping cases from separate special exhibitions of the disease prevented any epidemic development of the disease, whilst in Memphis the incomprehensible filthiness that fouled her atmosphere again furnished a bed for epidemic devastation. The lesson is too plain for mistake: a wayfaring man though a fool may run and yet read.

Now let us see how these facts concern our commercial welfare. If it proves (and it has already been proven in New Orleans in 1879, and in Savannah in 1877) that in the mere sporadic outburst of cases from *special local foci*, the prompt application of local hygienic measures will arrest epidemic growth of the poison where the general atmosphere is not foul, then our remedy is not by quarantining our cities, crippling and driving away our commerce, and reducing our people to poverty because of our ignorant and scarecrow method of dealing with the disease, but by prompt isolation and disinfection, so that it cannot spread; always presupposing that we have already prudently avoided permitting our general municipal atmosphere to become putrid by means of internal or surrounding noxious elements. Thus much for our sanitation.

Now look at the dangers confronting us. Being personally acquainted with several members of the present National Board of Health, I but do them justice in saying that I fear no wrong at their hands; but when we have seen fraud triumphant in government, the Supreme Court packed to change opinions, immense powers and privileges conferred at the bidding of corporations and sections, the vast machinery of the government wielded for partisan purposes, and constitutional safeguards set at defiance whenever in the way of higher law theories, *we but court corruption* when we place our whole commercial transportation and welfare under the control of a central body which may be changed at any time in the interests of corporative or sectional interests having temporary control of the appointing power.

I have little doubt that the purpose of the National Board of Health in seeking certain additional powers in quarantine matters is a commendable one in itself, originating in a desire to prevent irregular local shotgun quarantines, often doing more inconsiderate injury than more responsible officers are likely to inflict. If its actions should be confined to objects of this kind we would have more reason for approval than censure. But the proposed deprivation of all right of subsequent jurisdiction by State or municipal authority may work serious harm in forbidding that scrutiny which subsequent information may make desirable, even though a national inspector may have already given his certificate to a clean bill of health.

Now, what are we to gain? A few minor "sops to Cerberus," a few sub-inspectorships for needy doctors, a few thousands of dollars expended on quarantine stations, and the nominal "paternal interest of the central government in our welfare," whilst our ports may be shut up whenever "the Executive Committee of the National Board of Health so direct," whether our far more experienced physicians think such extreme measures necessary or not; our interior towns cut off from commerce by unadvisable quarantines, and our commerce driven for exit to ports having no interest in our local welfare. Is this at last of any real value to us? Let us see:

The more powers and duties are *distributed* in a country like ours, the more effectually are they applied. Whenever we put upon the General Government the vast responsibility of looking after the diseases of every hole and corner of the country, just so far we educate the people of these holes and corners to a neglect of their own welfare; and there will be a universal system of abusing the government for every trouble growing out of our own ignorance and neglect. This National Board of Health is not the paternal or maternal nurse of our infirmities. It is simply a quarantine bureau, without the power to help us in our needs, but with the proposed power to shut us within the walls of distress and poverty. It needs new powers, but not new quarantine powers. It needs the powers necessary to assist our poverty-stricken cities in improving their sanitary conditions; and these powers, properly and judiciously exercised, will bring us blessings instead of woes.

ANGINA MEMBRANACEA.

BY C. S. MIDDLETON, M.D.

(Read before the Hahnemann Club of Philadelphia.)

THE too limited knowledge possessed by the profession upon the subject of angina membranacea, and the desire to add something to that knowledge, has led to the preparation of this paper. The passive treatment laid down in most of the textbooks often leaves us under the greatest embarrassment if we adhere to this teaching and fail to recognize the necessity for prompt and energetic treatment. We do not purpose to enter into any discussion on the pathological nature of croup, as that is well understood, but we wish to direct attention rather to the treatment of the malady.

Croup is generally divided into two varieties, spasmodic and membranous. From the first variety but little danger need be anticipated, this form being generally relieved with *Spongia*, Aconite, or some other well-indicated remedy in a short time, often as suddenly as it has appeared; but with the latter variety we are less fortunate. Catarrhal croup, inflammatory croup, and chronic croup are sometimes used as synonymous with membranous croup. Although this form often sets in suddenly, it does not yield as readily, for obvious reasons; still, if it be taken in hand without delay, very much may be reasonably hoped for under careful homœopathic treatment.

Probably no disease in the whole catalogue presents so constantly the same local pathology and the same unvarying symptoms as croup does during its first and second stage. We have, of course, varying trains of mental symptoms, and some others dependent upon the different nervous temperaments or idiosyncrasies of the patients, but these in a case of croup are but reflex, and usually secondary in importance.

Homœopathy is necessarily a system of individual specifics, and we are naturally obliged to seek for each one as occasion may require; but, as before remarked, croup is so nearly constant in its local effects and symptomatic manifestations, that it seems almost possible to say that a specific exists for all cases.

We were taught from the earlier works on practice that *Aconite* and *Spongia* are the grand remedies for croup; yet modern experience shows that these two remedies, valuable as they are when their own peculiar indications are present, will not serve us except in a small minority of the graver and more malignant cases. Ipecac., Tart. em., Bry. alb., Phos. are of no greater service during the first stage, and are to be used only as intercurrent or adjunctive remedies.

It remains for two substances to have almost exclusive control over this disease in its most formidable stage, viz., Bromine and Iodine. Of these the first named is exceedingly volatile, and as the latter possesses medicinal qualities very similar to those of the former without its inconveniences, it may be said that IODINE is one of our grandest specifics for membranous croup.

If it be thought that this seems like general specific medication, we have simply to keep in mind the facts referred to in a former paragraph, and compare the pathology and the characteristic symptoms of the disease with the pathogenesis of Iodine, in order to satisfy ourselves that the value of this drug in the treatment of membranous croup has not been overrated.

With these facts in view, and with many cases in verification, I always furnish to my families having "croupy" children a vial of the first decimal of Iodine, in liquid, to be used immediately the "bark" is heard, and many times they are thus enabled to control the trouble at once, and while the incipient croup is yet in the form of a laryngitis.

When high fever is present, with soreness and pain in the larynx, and other indications of general cold, *Aconite* should be given occasionally until relief is obtained. It may be preferred by some, even to use it in alternation with Iodine. The use of the latter should be continued so long as the larynx is sore and painful on coughing, the membrane remains vigorous and organized, and the cough croupy.

When the "bark" is heard only at night, other remedies, such as may be indicated, can be administered through the day, and the Iodine be given again at night. I find it not difficult to obtain the effects of the medicine upon light-complexioned children equally as well as upon the dark.

When the inflammation has subsided, and the peculiar bark is no longer heard, the cough is loosened, either from mucous secretion or softening of the membrane, discharge from the nose sets in, etc., *Hepar sulph.* is often applicable, and when the expectoration is stringy, *Kal. bich.*, as recommended by Bæhr. In this stage, when a catarrhal condition has spread throughout the smaller bronchia, some of the remedies previously mentioned, *Ipec.*, *Tart. em.*, *Bry.*, etc., will be required; but the case is now no longer croup, and the danger is nearly passed, except in the cases of very young children, or when catarrhal fever has supervened. Since adopting this general course of treatment, about ten years ago, I have lost but one case of croup. In that case, which had been neglected in the earlier stages, the operation of tracheotomy was resorted to, but without avail.

It is, of course, essential that children suffering with croup should be kept in one room, of an even temperature, at about 70°, and that they be kept away from the windows and out of drafts.

OUR MATERIA MEDICA.

BY E. B. NASH, M.D., CORTLAND, N. Y.

SOME physicians want only one Materia Medica, and want that condensed. The mere mention of Allen's *Encyclopedia* seems to terrify the great majority of our school. "Too many symptoms," is the cry. Hering's *Guiding Symptoms*, though the best work in our literature, will no doubt find its ready opponents in our ranks, who are either too indolent or too ignorant of the true principles of the art of medicine to recognize its indispensableness.

Several years ago I treated a child suffering from an obstinate attack of dysentery. The remedies which are usually successful failed utterly. Counsel was summoned, but our combined efforts were equally unsuccessful. At one of my visits the mother chanced to be changing the child's diaper. I noticed that the anus was wide open. I could have inserted my little finger to the depth of two inches without touching the bloody, mucus-lined walls. Neither Jahr's *Manual*, Snelling, Bell *On Diarrhœa*, nor Hering's *Condensed*, contain this important symptom. Finally I discovered this under Phosphorus in Lippe's *Textbook:* "Discharge of mucus out of the wide-open anus." Three days after the use of the remedy, nought remained of the troublesome disease, except the resulting weakness.

A lady after her confinement suffered from a severe pain,

which lasted for hours after a stool. Here again, failing to select the strictly indicated drug, the case continued unabated for several days. This time neither Hering, Lippe, nor Jahr, helped me out. A diligent search, however, was rewarded with the similimum, Nitric acid, which I found among Raue's *Therapeutic Hints* in his *Pathology*. Relief, following its employment, was speedy and complete.

Now I know that these two symptoms are characteristic of their respective remedies; but some young practitioner may not possess such knowledge. How, then, is he to obtain it, if complete works on that vital subject, Materia Medica, are withheld?

We never can possess a surfeit of Materia Medica—at least until that time has arrived, when we shall have a remedy for every symptom which is in the least characteristic of a diseased state.

No one man, however skilful and energetic, can prove all drugs, or verify all those already proved. Consequently no author, however industrious, can collate everything that is verified in our school. Still, so elaborate a work as Hering's *Guiding Symptoms* promises more than any of its predecessors, and the profession should welcome it accordingly. And we shall be able to accomplish such good results that we shall demonstrate beyond peradventure, the pre-eminence of the homœopathic healing art.

OBSERVATIONS ON THE INORGANIC ELEMENTS OF NUTRITION.

BY PEMBERTON DUDLEY, M.D.

(Read before the Hahnemann Club of Philadelphia.)

It has long been a custom among allopathic writers to attribute a large proportion of the recoveries occurring under homœopathic treatment to a careful regulation of the diet and of the sanitary environment of the patients. To us such a statement always seems to be merely a pretext for refusing to accord any beneficial results to the medicinal treatment. In other words, if so-called homœopathic cures can be ascribed to hygienic precautions, it relieves our opponents of the unpleasant necessity of acknowledging the efficacy of our system of therapeutics.

We have but to look over the literature of our school to see how utterly baseless such an assumption is. To be sure our surgeons are not behind their allopathic contemporaries in this respect, and our homœopathic surgical textbooks lay down full and explicit directions regarding diet, rest, exercise, ventilation, dress, and other hygienic measures; but how few of our more strictly medical works give to these subjects a tithe of the attention which their importance merits! In the directions for the treatment of many diseases,—sometimes even of developmental diseases,—the subject of diet may be almost entirely ignored, and where it is introduced at all, it is too often for the sole purpose of cautioning the practitioner against the use of certain articles considered incompatible with the remedies prescribed, with never a word as to the special dietetic needs of the cases under treatment. We are carefully told what the patient must *not* eat; but are left in the dark as to what he *must* eat.

The evident cause of this defect in our literature, and the consequent imperfection of our clinical practice, is to be found, at least in some measure, in the view held by many homœopathic physicians, that defective nutrition is generally the result of some pre-existing morbid condition; that, when this condition is once corrected by proper medication, nature will soon restore her wasted, perhaps even her degenerated tissues, and that it is almost useless to prescribe nutritives until after the successful use of the homœopathic remedy.

It is not enough that this homœopathic fact (if it be a fact) overthrows a false allopathic assumption. These things ought not so to be. For while it may be true that a defective nutrition is frequently the consequent of some morbid action or state, it is equally true that it frequently becomes the cause of very grave and far-reaching disease, and, further, that even when such is not the case it is extremely probable that the action of medicines is always facilitated, and to some extent insured, by that vigorous condition of all the tissues and organs which can exist only in connection with a healthy and well-sustained nutrition.

It is necessary to remind ourselves that in the nourishment of the animal tissues, the three classes of elements, viz., the albuminoids, the hydrocarbons, and the inorganic elements, are all equally essential. We are too much disposed to regard the first-named group as holding a sort of pre-eminence, because of the histogenic value of the principles composing it. The hydrocarbons we assign to the second place, because of their manifest calorific properties; while the inorganic or third group is kept almost out of sight, unless, peradventure, rachitis or anæmia should force us to a recognition of the claims of Lime or of Iron. In this particular disregard of the essential value of the inorganic elements of nutrition, the average allopathist is not far, if any, in advance of his unrecognized homœopathic brother. Buck's *Hygiene*, with its two portly volumes, devotes just two pages to their consideration,—two pages of glittering generalities, with nothing of special value or force in relation to any one of these elements.

There is one feature of the inorganic group of alimentary principles which makes it a necessary subject of special consideration, namely, that its principles cannot be substituted one for another in the animal economy, except possibly in a very few instances. The albumen, the gluten, the casein, and the legumin may, one or all, be converted into the albuminoid elements of animal composition; the oil, the starch, and the sugar be alike used in the maintenance of animal temperature or the production of animal fats; but the *in*organic elements of nutrition stand, each by itself. No one of them can take the place of any other one, or be a substitute therefor. Hence, the physiological relations of each member of this group must be an object of separate and special study, and each one of them must be supplied to the organism in due proportion, else the nutrition of some part will be impaired.

It seems fortunate that in devising a diet which shall nearly or quite meet the requirements of the nutritive process, as it goes on in all the tissues, we have a perfect standard in milk. This substance we know to be adapted to all the necessities of the rapid growth of the infant and young child, though we are not so clear as to its adaptedness to the highest needs of the organism in a state of energetic muscular, mental and reproductive activity. Taking milk, however, as the best standard within our reach, we find its inorganic elements to consist of the two chlorides of Sodium and Potassium, the two carbonates of Soda and Lime, the two sulphates of Soda and Potassa, and the four phosphates of Soda, Magnesia, Lime, and Iron. To the question sometimes asked, whether mineral matters can enter directly into the constitution of animal tissues, it ought to be sufficient to remember that in infancy the nervous tissue partakes of the same rapid development that we observe in the bones and muscles, that one of the essential elements of nerve-tissue is Phosphorus, and that this substance exists in the infant's normal food only in the form of a mineral combination. The value of Potassium chloride as an element in muscular development must be sufficiently obvious when we observe the large proportion of this salt found in the expressed muscular juice. Here let us remark, that when from any cause milk cannot be used for the nourishment of the infant before the commencement of dentition, muscular flesh furnishes perhaps the only good and sufficient source of supply. It seems no longer questionable that the substance named is an actual and essential element of composition, and not a product of retrogressive metamorphosis, for the reasons that we find none of it in the lymph, but little of it in the urine, and a comparatively large proportion of it in the infant's food. How is it possible, then, to withhold this element even for a few days, from the growing infant, without inducing serious and even fatal muscular atrophy? There is in the writer's mind little doubt that many instances of this malady could be traced directly to neglect of proper precaution in this particular.

It seems well to call special attention also to another inorganic principle of nutrition, which is entirely too much neglected by the great majority of homœopathic physicians. The necessity for a free exhibition of Iron in combination with a well-selected albuminoid and carbonaceous diet, as an essential to the rapid restoration of the blood from a condition of impoverishment, arising either from anæmia, as we ordinarily use that term, or from the effects of exhausting diseases or hæmorrhage, cannot be too strongly insisted on. The universal experience of the whole allopathic profession, for more than a hundred years past, has furnished confirmations of the essential value of this agent as a blood-food, that we cannot ignore without injury to ourselves and detriment to our patients. And we think that just about in the same proportion as our underestimate of the value of Iron as an article of special diet has been our over-estimate of its deleterious effects. To this statement, however, we must make one exception: the hurtful effects of the administration of Iron in material doses, in cases of menorrhagia and metrorrhagia, and perhaps in other forms of hæmorrhage, can never be lost sight of by the observant homœopathist. Aside from this, the ill effects arising from its judicious administration as a food, bear no respectable comparison with the benefits derived from its employment,—benefits which cannot be so rapidly obtained by any other method. A careful observation will show that the aggravated condition of those cases of anæmia which come to us from allopathic hands, is due, not to the action of the Iron administered, so much as to the complete neglect and consequent increase of the morbid processes which have caused and maintained the anæmia, and which, of course, manifest their effects in a still more marked degree whenever the use of iron in quantity is discontinued. One of the reasons why we become dissatisfied with the use of iron is, because we are unwilling to allow sufficient time for its action. The absorbent and assimilative power of the organism enables it to appropriate this element only in very small quantity and by slow processes, and weeks are required in many cases before we can expect its effects to be visible.

We have thus briefly considered some two or three of the members of the inorganic group of nutritive principles. Not less important, however, are each and all of the others. It may be accepted as an axiom in physiology that all the elements of composition must be supplied to the organism in due quantity, otherwise atrophy or other evidence of malnutrition will speedily supervene, and when this has advanced beyond a certain point, the nutritive powers will have become so enfeebled that a return to a judicious diet will not then avail to prevent a fatal result.

THE VOMITING OF PREGNANCY—WHAT IS ITS EXPLANATION AND WHAT ITS BEST TREATMENT?

BY ROBERT J. M'CLATCHEY, M.D.

(Read before the Hahnemann Club of Philadelphia).

THE causation of the vomiting which occurs in the earlier months of pregnancy is by no means well defined, even at this day of advancement in the studies of physiology and pathology. Authors speak of it as "reflex nervous irritation," induced in consequence of the changes going on in the system, and especially in the uterus; and, doubtless, this definition, although somewhat vague, is correct.

When we consider the insignificant part played by the stomach itself in the production of nausea and in the act of vomiting, and regard the intimate relations existing between its nerves and all other parts of the organism, we can readily understand how so great a systemic disturbance as occurs during pregnancy can bring about such curious results.

The causes of nausea may be divided into two classes, viz., those which act directly upon the stomach, and, second, those which act primarily upon the system at large. As examples of the first, we have the nausea and vomiting produced by such drugs as are termed emetics, the overloading of the stomach with food, or the taking of certain kinds of food or drink which, sooner or later, act on the stomach and produce nausea and vomiting. In the second class we have numerous causes, which, acting upon parts of the body often quite remote from the stomach, yet produce phenomena similar to those of the first class of causes. A notable example will be found in the motion of a vessel at sea, producing the horrible nausea and vomiting known as seasickness. The vomiting also which occurs with some forms of cerebral diseases affords another example of remote causation; and numerous other examples may be cited, such as the smelling of certain odors, the passage of renal and biliary calculi, hernia, or intussusception; and, again, causes which act entirely through the medium of the mind or imagination. These various circumstances, although presenting such wide differences in their origin and nature, are all capable of producing similar effects upon the stomach, such as induce nausea and vomiting; and this is explainable only upon taking into consideration the intimate nervous connections which exist between the stomach and every other part of the system, and particularly between the stomach and the other abdominal viscera. And upon this basis the explanation of the phenomena known as the vomiting of pregnancy must rest.

The vomiting of pregnancy is usually termed "morning sickness," but inappropriately so, inasmuch as it may come on at any hour of the day or night, is often brought on by eating, and in bad cases invariably so. Almost all pregnant women suffer from this distressing symptom, although I have known many who have declared that in certain of their pregnancies they were exempt from it, while in others they suffered more or less; and again I have known multipara to declare that they were never troubled with this sickness at all.

In some cases it amounts to a simple vomiting in the morning, either before or after breakfast, often with little or no nausea, and then immunity until about the same hour of the next day; and from this mild form there are infinite gradations up to those alarming cases where neither food nor drink of any kind is retained by the stomach, and the patient is in danger of dying from inanition. In these very severe cases it is my opinion that there is a dependence upon some uterine lesion or displacement, and, indeed, so far as my own experience goes I have found in these cases of severe vomiting, lesion or displacements of the uterus invariably.

In some cases the morning sickness, which commences about the end of the first month and usually ends about the third or fourth, is renewed about the end of the eighth month. In these cases it is probable that the vomiting is produced by direct pressure of the gravid uterus.

Therapeutics.—The remedies for this condition are numerous, and, in fact, any remedy may be the curative one, if indicated by the symptoms of the case. In my own experience Ipecacuanha has been more frequently called for than any other remedy. I have given it merely because of its prominence as an emetic, and without reference to the symptom so often mentioned as indicative of it, viz., "one continuous nausea," which is rarely the condition in the vomiting of pregnancy. It has rarely failed to relieve the cases for which I have prescribed it, and when it has, I have generally obtained success with either Pulsatilla or Nux vomica, given in accordance with the symptoms of these two important drugs; their several indications, especially in the matter of temperament, disposition, and mental and moral status, being clean-cut and well-defined. Other remedies are: Ant. crudum, Ars., Bry., Bismuth, Conium, Nitric acid, Kreosote and Carbolic acid, Lycopodium, Phosph., Sepia, Tabacum, Lobelia inflata, Oxalate of cerium., etc.

In regard to the value of the Oxalate of cerium, I have had occasion to change my opinion several times. I now scarcely ever resort to it.

I have found Calomel, in the third decimal trituration, three or four times a day, relieve a number of cases where there was much salivation.

These means will be sufficient in almost every case, especially if carefulness in regard to diet is observed. It is a good idea to not allow the patient to get up in the morning, or even to sit up in bed until she has taken something into the stomach, such as a cup of tea, coffee, or cocoa, or, in bad cases, a glass of cold milk with lime-water added.

If the patient vomits always after a meal, she should eat at irregular intervals, according to her desire, or take food, usually in liquid form, often and but little at a time. Beef-tea and broths may be used in this way, and so, too, may iced milk, with or without lime-water. Johnson's beef, Liebig's extract, Valentine's meat-juice, or home-made beef, mutton or chicken teas, are all of service here. Some stomachs will tolerate these but when they are hot, others when they are cold. Home-made beef-tea or "essence" may be frozen and taken into the stomach in the shape of pellets or little blocks of ice, piece after piece, without exciting the rejecting powers of that viscus. There are, in fact, many ways of feeding an irritable stomach without exciting its irritability.

Iced champagne is one of the best quieters of a sick stomach in the whole category of remedial means, and very often proves of great service in the vomiting of pregnancy.

Ice may be given freely in bad cases, as it has a strong tendency to settle the stomach.

In very bad cases, when almost every particle of food taken is vomited, recourse must be had to injections of nutritious foods per rectum, such as beef-tea, broths, gruel, milk or cream, or defibrinated bullock's blood, as recommended by Dr. Seguin, of New York.

Very minute doses of Morphia sulph., $\frac{1}{32}$ or $\frac{1}{64}$, given in ice or in ice-water, has done good service formerly. It has been recommended that in the most severe cases, where apparently nothing is retained by the stomach, and there appears to be danger of death from starvation, *an abortion may be procured.* There could not possibly be a more humiliating confession of the failure of medical science and art than to admit the truth of this proposition. I am not able, however, to conceive of a case where such a procedure would be justifiable or necessary. The stomach never rejects all of its contents, and enough may be retained to carry on the business of life. Then there is to be taken into consideration the possibilities of cure by medicinal means, the probable removal of the cause of the vomiting by the progress of gestation, and the certainty of being able to feed per rectum; and with these in view there can be no reason why labor should be brought about. Indeed, to admit its necessity under such circumstances is only to open the door to the commission of the crime of abortion yet more widely; whereas the labors of the medical profession should be directed towards so closing that door that the most ingenious tools that can be devised by wicked man as suggested by the devil shall fail to open it.

QUEBRACHO.

TRANSLATED BY S. LILIENTHAL, M.D., NEW YORK.

PROFESSOR PRIBRAM, of Prague, used this remedy in six cases of emphysema and chronic bronchial catarrh. The patients took daily two teaspoonfuls of Extr. quebracho aquosum (10 of the pulverized bark with 100 Alcohol, extracted, filtered, evaporated, dissolved in water, again evaporated to dryness, and dissolved in 20 water). He finds it a most valuable palliative in emphysema, bronchial catarrh, and dyspnœa from pleuritis. Though given for several days it never disturbs digestion or the beats of the heart, nor does it produce motory paralysis or weakness.

Dr. J. Krauth employed it in two cases of cardiac hypertrophy in its last stage, with dropsical exudations in the cavities and general œdema, severe dyspnœa, and great debility; in three cases of morbus Brightii after scarlatina; in one case of tuberculosis with œdematous dyspnœa; in a traumatic case, where the lung was punctured, with bloody or serous exudation in the pleura and excessive dyspnœa. All received Extr. quebracho aquosum 5 grams with 25 aqua dest., and its rapid action on the breathing was wonderful. The dyspnœa disappeared rapidly, respiration became quiet and easy, so that I consider it my duty to lead the attention of my colleagues to this drug. Though it cannot change tuberculosis or cardiac defects, the relief thus given to the tortured patient is a benefit to the sufferer as well as to the attending physician. He uses the solutio Aquosa 1 to 25, or a tincture, 1 to 10 Alcohol, a teaspoonful every three hours.—*Allg. Med. Central Zeitung*, No. 12, 1880.

NOTE BY THE TRANSLATOR.—How often have we all witnessed this want of breath, which Hufeland so beautifully describes, when he listened to the patient's cry for air: "Give me air, only a little more air," and for which he knew no other remedy than Opium, the sweet deceiver, lulling the sufferer to his doom. Many a good homœopathic physician stands equally lost at the bedside of his patient, and when his Antimonium tart., Arsen. iod., Stannum, Carb. veg., Digitalis, Moschus, or any other remedy, not apparently, but well indicated, leaves him in the lurch, should he not feel justified, as an honest and conscientious physician, to take refuge in a promising palliative. Where a cure is out of the question, relief is a duty commanded by mere humanity. Liberty, but not licentiousness.

[A writer in the *Berliner Klin. Wochenschrift*, 10, March 8th, 1880, has produced dyspnœa in animals by administering Quebracho in large doses; thus indicating that the remarkable curative effects, above referred to, were homœopathic.—EDS.]

SEPIA IN PLEURITIS.

BY DR. KUNKLE, IN KIEL.

(Translated by S. LILIENTHAL, M.D., New York.)

MANY physicians acknowledge that Aconite, Bryonia, Rhus,

etc., leave us frequently in the lurch in the treatment of pleurisy, and we find it often difficult to choose the remedy from the symptoms alone. We have to look then to the anamnesis, and compare past and present symptoms of the patient. Anamnesis is of great value and has a good pathological basis.

We are in the habit of considering a case acute or chronic according to the intensity of the morbid symptoms, the rise of temperature, frequency and other modifications of the pulse, etc. This is all wrong, for even in acute diseases the present symptoms, though caused by a transient accident, may be based on a constitutional ailment. Such diseases are often sporadic pneumonia (symptoms of psora, malaria, etc.), articular rheumatismus, pleuritis. The apparently acute invasions are only symptoms of a morbid disposition, and have to be treated accordingly.

About ten years ago I treated the wife of a farmer, whose chronic headache had been greatly relieved by Sepia, and which for some time had troubled her again. With the appearance of pleuritis the headache suddenly vanished. I considered Sepia^{30} again indicated, which acted rapidly and favorably, so that no other remedy was needed. Since then I frequently used Sepia in pleuritis, and no other remedy enjoys with me the same reputation in this disease.

Eight years ago I treated at the same time two aged men, suffering from a severe attack of pleurisy, and both rapidly recovered under the use of Sepia. I am convinced that both would have died without it.

Last year I treated a boy of six years, where the exudation had spread over the whole left chest. After using Sepia^{200} (Lehrman) for five days, I could only discover in the chest a small remnant of the exudation. Only a few days ago I cured a severe attack in a young woman with Sepia, where Phosphorus, though apparently indicated, failed.

I might give more cases, but this suffices, as I only desire to lead the attention of other physicians to this reproving. May they compare symptoms 1005 to 1190 in Hahnemann's *Chronic Diseases*, and they will find full justification for the use of Sepia in pleurisy. In regard to the doses, I use the thirtieth and two hundredth potency, especially as the latter acts very quickly and intensive. In some cases I give daily one or two doses for three or four days and stop, or I give one dose and wait. In chronic cases, threatening phthisis, I use one or two doses daily for some time. I do not doubt that low potencies of Sepia may also act well, and perhaps more favorably, where we have to deal especially with the product of the disease, just as Sulphur[3] does in the latter stages of pneumonia. *Only I have no experience about it.* Individuality and age must be recognized as factors in the selection of high or low potencies, and general rules cannot be given.

That the symptom pleuritis may need other constitutional remedies I know from experience. Thus, I treated a young man of 17 years, whose left thorax was so overfilled with pleuritic exudations that not a trace of respiratory murmur could be detected. Vertebral column strongly bent towards the right side, wall of thorax perforated near left nipple; decided fluctuation and formation of abscess, which broke and discharged a large quantity of pus. After a week cannot get a trace of respiratory murmurs, and everywhere dull sound on percussion. Perfect restoration under the use of Sulphur[200], and after years I examined the chest repeatedly and found it perfectly sound. He belonged to a family where Sulphur always acted favorably.

Last year I treated a girl of 13, suffering from abundant pleuritic exudation in the right chest with high-graded dyspnœa. Allopathy had failed. All her symptoms pointed to Phosphorus, which was given steadily for two months in the second potency. All exudation vanished, and she felt well for about nine months, when her old dyspnœa returned and was again relieved by Phosphorus. (Would Phosphorus high have more radically cured the case?—S. L.).—*Allg. Hom. Zeitung*, No. 9, 1880.

THE PHILADELPHIA COUNTY HOMŒOPATHIC MEDICAL SOCIETY.

REPORTED BY CHARLES MOHR, M.D., SECRETARY.

THE annual meeting of the Society was held on the evening of April 8th, 1880, at the Hahnemann Medical College. Dr. E. A. Farrington presided. Section I, article III, of the Constitution, was amended, so as to read as follows:

"The officers of this Society shall consist of a President, a Vice-President, a Treasurer, a Secretary, and three Censors, to be chosen by ballot, at the annual meeting of the Society, and to continue in office until the meeting following the election of their successors."

The Censors reported favorably on applications for membership of Drs. Edward M. Gramm and Anna M. Marshall, who were thereupon elected.

The Committee on Organization, Medical Education, Statistics, and Legislation, then made a report as follows:

"The Committee refers with pleasure to the increased and increasing interest manifested in our Society by its members. Since our last annual meeting, 24 new members have been added to the roll, which now numbers 86. All our meetings have been characterized by 'good feeling.' There has been no lack of papers for discussion, and the bureau plan, put into operation in December last, promises to be all that was expected of it. The papers written since number nineteen, presented by four different bureaux. It is recommended that the chairman of the various bureaux, as soon as appointed, should choose their associates, call meetings, and be ready at the following Society meeting to report the composition of the bureaux, and, if possible, an outline of the work expected to be accomplished. Perhaps it would be well for each bureau to choose but one topic for elaboration, and thus invite a *direct* discussion. It is recommended that our Society take a lively interest in all public medical matters. We should, individually and collectively, through our legislators, try to secure recognition in all public institutions, hospitals, and asylums. There is no reason why we should be excluded therefrom, any more than our more favored allopathic brethren. So far as possible, we should endeavor to have our State create a properly organized Board of Health. We call attention to the request of the Department of the Interior (through Hon. F. A. Walker, Superintendent of the Census, who supplies free of cost, the necessary blanks) that every physician of the United States furnish a proper return of every death occurring in his or her practice. Vital statistics are important, and we trust the members of our Society will give due heed to Mr. Walker's plan for collecting them.

The Secretary of our Society is preparing a directory of the Homœopathic Physicians of the County, which he desires to make as complete as possible, and we recommend those concerned to give him all needed assistance.

This report was accepted, and after some discussion, at the request of the secretary, it was decided to place the compilation of the directory in the hands of the Committee on Organization, etc., inasmuch as a question arose as to the exclusion of certain names on professionally moral grounds.

The treasurer made his usual annual report, which was accepted after audit by the censors.

The annual election was held at 9 P.M., resulting as follows:

President, Dr. E. A. Farrington; *Vice-President,* Dr. W. B. Trites; *Treasurer,* Dr. A. H. Ashton; *Secretary,* Dr. Charles

Mohr; *Censors*, Dr. W. H. Bigler, Dr. J. K. Lee, and Dr. A. Korndœrfer.

The president elect then delivered the following address:

REMARKS OF THE PRESIDENT ELECT.

When I saw on the notice of this meeting, "Address by the President elect," it occurred to me that, although there was but one nominee for the presidency, still as any member of the Society is eligible to the office, it behooves every one to come to our annual meetings prepared to make an address in the event of his possible election. Either this becomes necessary, or else our secretary has so exalted an idea of our extemporaneons ability, that he considers preparation not at all necessary.

Since, however, you have decided to reappoint me to the office I now hold, it relieves you of all anxiety on the subject of an address, and throws the onerous duty upon me. But I am not prepared with any written address, and prefer, if you will permit, to forego the conventional forms, and present to you extemporaneously a few thoughts, which may lead to interesting and profitable discussion. I will select for my topic,

THE PRIORITY AND SUPREMACY OF THE NERVOUS SYSTEM.

It is a shame that physiologists forget that man is a living being, possessed of a soul, and that his whole physical life is but the soul's manifestation in a material body. They are wont to describe the marvellous functions of the brain as mere activities of matter, making the brain nothing more than an exalted gland. Intellectual force is thought to be produced by changes of the gray matter of the brain, resulting in the development of heat, ideation, and tissue waste in the form of phosphates.

If we recall the development of man in utero, or rather in the egg, we shall see that after the vitellus segmentates and produces the blastoderm, the soul from the father, through the fecundating semen, begins at once to operate upon these membranes. This segmentation in itself is not wholly the effect of the semen, for it is attempted, though never completed, in the unimpregnated ovum. The first appreciable change is the folding of the blastoderm into the form of a brain and spine, with derivative fibres. Thus we see the priority of the nervous system. Almost immediately follow other parts, of which the heart is the earliest. This organ does not exist at first as a formed viscus, but as a tube, which soon twists itself into normal shape. It is my conviction that the heart is produced from and by derivative nerve-fibres; for its primary structure is very similar to the fibres projecting from the cortex cerebri. And the same applies to the remaining portions of the body.

Now, the idea which I wish to convey to you is that each organ and function of the body, having been produced from the brain and spine, resembles its parent in action and derives power thence. The cortex cerebri is composed of myriads of minute glands, each of which, I believe, has its efferent nerve-fibre, which is distributed to the respective organs of the body. Hence every bodily organ is subservient to the brain and through the brain, to the soul.

There have been experiments made within the last ten years or so, which tend to disprove many of the absurd notions of histologists. Among these I may refer you to those of Hitzig, Ferrier, and others. Quite recently Dr. Amidon made some extended experiments, which you will find recorded in Seguin's *Archives of Medicine*, April, 1880. This ingenious physician thought that if the muscles had their cerebral centres, and if exercise develops heat, there ought to be an increase of temperature over that portion of the brain which was called into activity. He arranged thermometers over the calvarium, and then instructed the subject to exert his will and exercise a certain set of muscles, say those of the hand. Very soon he noticed a decided rise in one of the thermometers, the others remaining unaltered; and by changing the group of muscles exercised, he could mark out definite regions on the skull, varying for each set of muscles. What is remarkable, too, his regions, as you will see by comparing these plates in the *Archives*, correspond quite accurately with those of Ferrier, made by electrizing the exposed brain.

If these facts are confirmed in relation to the muscles, who may deny cerebral centres also to other structures of the body?

In all experimentation, then, we should keep before us the supremacy of the brain and spine. When we attempt the proving of drugs, we should record with the greatest care each mental symptom *plus* the part or parts of the body affected at the same time; and thus we see the wisdom of Hahnemann's advice to treat mental symptoms as of the highest importance in the choice of a remedy.

I commend these few facts to your consideration, and hope that if they embrace matters of interest the Society will proceed to a discussion of them.

The following discussion then ensued:

Dr. Charles M. Thomas did not see how the surface temperature could be so suddenly affected by changes in the circulation of the brain, on account of the great thickness of bone tissue between the brain mass and integument, together with the hair. Again, placing the body as much at rest as is possible, there will always be a certain amount of motion going on, if not in the muscles certainly in the internal organs. He should not therefore think that the results would be positive.

Dr. Farrington said that the thermometer variations, and of course the motions, would be uniform. Thermometers placed at symmetrical points would register the same temperature. In regard to the motions of the viscera exciting an increase of temperature, Dr. Amidon in his experiments had evidently taken that into account.

Dr. Dudley.—Twenty years ago Professor Charles D. Meigs used to say that man might be defined as "a brain and spinal marrow," because every other part of the body was designed to minister to the wants and welfare of the nervous system. But Professor Meigs would not apply the same definition to the inferior animals, for he did not believe that they were created for anything else than to minister to man. He (Dr. Dudley) thought that all physiologists and histologists recognize the important relation of the brain and spinal cord to all the other structures in regard not only to their functions but to their development also. Disorders of nutrition, depending on disease of the cerebral hemispheres, are known to exist. A paralyzed condition of the spinal cord has resulted in a rapid gangrene of distant parts. The excitement of contraction in definite groups of muscles by galvanization of certain portions of the gray matter of the convolutions, is a well-observed phenomenon; and all these indicate a close physiological relation between certain ganglionic cells in the cerebrum and certain of the voluntary muscles. It has been observed, however, that the more intense the excitement of the ganglionic centre, the more widely does the excitement spread throughout that centre, a fact illustrated in the galvanization of the convolutions, and in the irritation of the decapitated frog. Conversely it seems probable that the more energetic the will power which excites muscular action, the larger the amount of gray matter involved in the increased functional activity. These circumstances, one would suppose, must materially affect the accuracy of the thermometric experiments mentioned. He thought the objections raised by Dr. Thomas against accepting Dr. Amidon's observations were well taken; for, admitting that certain parts of the cerebrum undergo increased nutrition and consequently exhibit an increase of temperature under the stimulus of the will power, still it seems improbable that this increased heat could make itself perceptible through the dura mater, the cranial bones, the muscular and fibrous layer, and the integument. Moreover, the blood circulating through the gray matter would receive the increased heat, and carrying it directly further away from the thermometer bulbs would distribute the increased quantity of heat throughout portions of the brain which had not been at all concerned in the original excitation, thus impairing the accuracy of the thermometric results. We may, of course, accept Dr. Amidon's observations as such, but the observer may have been mistaken as to the cause of the effects noted.

DR. FARRINGTON.—In the first place the pre-eminence of the brain is not really acknowledged by physiologists, although it is apparently so. I do not call that pre-eminence, which debases the functions of the brain to mere molecular activity, with resulting ideation and phosphatic debris. If we practically acknowledge the brain's supremacy we will admit its charge over every part of the body below it, giving each organ its activity, just as primally it gave to it existence. Thus, and thus only, can the mind be supreme. And to be supreme, the brain must have the most intimate association with the body, each part of the body receiving its own nervous fibres. It is known that there is such a thing as supplementary action in the body; when one organ is impaired another takes up its function. The action of the cerebrum can be as a whole or as to its parts. Maudsley, in his work on the mind, speaks of ideation, emotion and all other exercises of the mind as due to changes in the state or form of the parts. Heat is very intense when developed by nervous action, and this may account for the rapid spread of the heat from the nervous centres to the surface of the scalp. These experiments should be tried repeatedly before they can be considered conclusive.

DR. KORNDŒRFER would not like to reject the facts in the paper unless he had thoroughly experimented and proved them conclusively to be in error.

A short discussion ensued relative to the treatment of the croupous inflammation and bronchitis connected with the epidemic of measles now prevailing in Philadelphia. The discussion was participated in by Drs. H. N. Martin, Korndœrfer, Mohr, and Dudley. The remedies mentioned as having been most frequently indicated were Bryonia, Scilla, Drosera, Sulphur, and Tartar emetic.

Drs. H. H. Groth, Alfred E. Baker, F. T. Price, and C. F. Goodno were proposed for membership, and the meeting then adjourned.

DR. LILIENTHAL'S CRITICISM OF THE BUREAU OF MATERIA MEDICA.

EDS. HAHNEMANNIAN:—I have neither the wish nor the time to bandy words of contradiction with Dr. Lilienthal, as to what he said and what implied in his singular attack upon my bureau, in the *North American* of February, and to what I said, in defence, in the March number of the HAHNEMANNIAN.

I am quite willing to leave all that to the judgment of those who have read both articles.

If the members of the bureau are satisfied with the doctor's explanations and apologies, I am quite ready to excuse his attempted reflections upon my choice of associates, and my status in the work which we have undertaken to perform in the name and in behalf of the Institute.

I have clearly shown how any member of the profession, including your anxious critic, may furnish data and proofs with regard to drug attenuation, for presentation at Milwaukee.

I have shown how wide open is left the witness-box, and how the advocates, on either side of the cause, are qualified and ready for the handling of testimony.

I should little appreciate the dignity of the American Institute, and the excellent character of those associated with me on the Bureau of Materia Medica, did I not promptly and firmly repel an assault like that made by Dr. Lilienthal, and indignantly deny the right of any man, be he editor or correspondent, *to forestall and belittle an important official work, in advance of its consummation.*

I cannot allow myself, here, to notice the issues thrust before me in the caption of the critic's communication, and in various remarks appearing in his reply. I must leave him with his "*living* dynamic forces," developed from drugs, and his notions of "homœopathy, pure and *simple*," while I attend to other work of greater moment.

J. P. DAKE.

NASHVILLE, TENN., April, 1880.

THE NEXT "WORLD'S HOMŒOPATHIC CONVENTION."

LONDON, ENGLAND, January, 1880.

TO THE EDITORS OF THE "HAHNEMANNIAN MONTHLY."

DEAR COLLEAGUES: At the close of the World's Homœopathic Convention which met in Philadelphia in 1876, it was determined to hold a similar meeting every five years in some principal city of Europe or America; and a general wish was expressed that the seat of the next gathering might be London.

On this determination and desire being communicated to the Congress of British Homœopathic Practitioners, meeting in Bristol, in September, 1876, it was unanimously resolved that such a convention should be held in London in 1881, and that the Congress would undertake the arrangements necessary for the purpose. A committee, consisting of the undersigned, was thereupon appointed to draw up a plan of proceeding; and its report, which is herein inclosed, was accepted at the Congress of 1877, and the committee reappointed, with instructions to obtain adhesions and contributions.

The latter, viz., reports of progress and papers to be discussed at the meetings, we are soliciting from individual physicians practicing homœopathically throughout the world. But we now request your good offices towards interesting the readers of your journal in our proposed gathering, by bringing the subject before them, and also towards making it known to the homœopathists of your city in such way as you may think best.

The exact time and place of meeting, with the office-bearers, etc., will be finally decided at the Congress we shall hold in September, 1880; and information thereof will be duly forwarded to you, and published in all British homœopathic journals.

Hoping to hear from you ere long, and to find your services enlisted in the cause, we remain,

Very faithfully yours,

R. E. DUDGEON, *Chairman*, A. C. POPE,
W. BAYES, R. HUGHES, *Secretary*.
A. CLIFTON,

All communications to be addressed to the Secretary, Dr. Hughes, Brighton, England.

Report of the Committee appointed to make Arrangements for holding a World's Homœopathic Convention in London in 1881. Presented to and Adopted by the British Homœopathic Congress Meeting in Liverpool, September, 1877.

Your committee beg to report that they have had several meetings; and after much consideration, and in conference with the lamented President of the last Convention, Dr. Carroll Dunham, have agreed upon the following recommendations, which they present for the acceptance of the present Congress:

"*Scheme for the World's Homœopathic Convention,* 1881.

"1. That the Convention shall assemble in London at such time and during such number of days as may hereafter be determined.

"2. That this meeting take the place of the Annual British Homœopathic Congress, and that its officers be elected at the Congress of the preceding year; the Convention itself being at liberty to elect honorary Vice-Presidents from those foreign guests and others whom it desires to honor.

"3. That the expenses of the meeting be met by a subscription from the homœopathic practitioners of Great Britain; the approximate amount to be expected from each to be named as the time draws near.

"4. That the expenses of printing the *Transactions* be defrayed by a subscription from all who desire to possess a copy of the volume.

"5. That the Convention shall be open to all medical men qualified to practice in their own country.

"6. That all who attend shall present to the Secretary their names and addresses, and a statement of their qualifications; and, if unknown to the officers of the Convention, shall be introduced by some one known to them, or shall bring letters credential from some homœopathic society, or other recognized representative of the system.

"(*a*) That the members of the Convention, as above characterized, shall be at liberty to introduce visitors to the meeting at their discretion.

"7. That the committee be authorized to enter into communication with physicians at home and abroad to obtain—

"(*a*) A report from each country supplementary to those presented at the Convention of 1876, recounting everything of interest in connection with homœopathy which has occurred within its sphere since the last reports were drawn up.

"(*b*) Essays upon the various branches of homœopathic theory and practice, for discussion at the meetings and publication in the *Transactions;* the physicians to be applied to for the latter purpose being those named in the accompanying schedule.

"8. That all essays must be sent in by January 1st, 1881, and shall then be submitted to a committee of censors for approval as suitable for their purpose.

"9. That the approved essays shall be printed beforehand, and distributed to the members of the Convention, instead of being read at the meetings.

"10. That for discussion the essays shall be presented singly or in groups, according to their subject-matter, a brief analysis of each being given from the chair.

"11. That a member of the Convention (or two, where two classes of opinion exist on the subject, as in the question of the dose) be appointed some time before the meeting to open the debate, fifteen minutes being allowed for such purpose, and that then the essay, or group of essays, be at once opened for discussion, ten minutes being the time allotted to each speaker.

"12. That the order of the essays be determined by the importance and interest of their subject-matter, so that, should the time of the meeting expire before all are discussed, less loss will have been sustained.

"13. That the chairman shall have liberty, if he sees that an essay is being debated at such length as to threaten to exclude later subjects of importance, to close its discussion.

"14. That the authors of the essays debated, if present, shall have the right of saying the last word before the subject is dismissed.

"15. That, as at the first Convention, the subjects of the essays and discussions shall be—

"(*a*) The Institutes of Homœopathy.
"(*b*) Materia Medica.
"(*c*) Practical Medicine.
"(*d*) Surgical Therapeutics, including diseases of the Eye and Ear.
"(*e*) Gynæcology."

At a subsequent meeting of the committee, it was determined that the gathering shall be known as the "*International Homœopathic Convention.*"

QUILLAYA SAPONARIA.

BY E. A. FARRINGTON, M D.

(Read before the Hahnemann Club of Philadelphia.)

THE California physicians have, for some time past, used a new drug, called QUILLAYA SAPONARIA. It has gained quite a reputation throughout the West as a certain remedy in common colds and in influenza.

As a separate plant it has never, so far as I know, been proved. But its alkaloid, *Saponin*, has received a thorough examination by Dr. Hills, of New York.

The *Quillaya* is a genus of plants belonging to the order *Rosaceæ*. The bark of some of the species, notably of the QUILLAYA SAPONARIA, is used in South America, and quite generally, too, among the Spaniards, Mexicans, etc., in California, as a substitute for soap. Its saponaceous qualities are due to the Saponin, contained in the bark.

Dr. William Bœricke, who for eight years had charge of the San Francisco pharmacy, informs me that he has had frequent calls for the tincture of the *Quillaya*, and that several physicians have pronounced it an invaluable drug in the beginning of coryza and sore throat. He adds his personal experience also in its favor. It is claimed to cure when there are sneezing, stuffed feeling in the nose, soreness and rawness in the throat, aching all over the body, chilliness, etc.

Now, in the absence of proving of the individual plant itself, our next best thing is to examine into the produced symptoms of the *Saponin*.

Allen, vol. viii, tells us that Saponin is a "glucoside, the active principle of many plants belonging to the Caryophyllaceæ, Polygalaceæ, etc.; principally obtained from Saponaria officinalis, Gypsophila, Struthium, Polygala, Senega, and Quillaya."

From the symptoms collated in his *Encyclopedia*, I glean the following:

Frontal catarrhal headache; sneezing; cannot breathe through the right nostril; dull pain at the root of the nose, and at the temples; tongue yellow-white on the back, edges red and papillæ elevated; hard palate rough when touched with the tongue, the papillæ are raised. Tenacious mucus from the posterior nares; throat raw, scraped, sore, with feeling of constriction on swallowing. Tonsils swollen, bright red. Cough at every forced inspiration through the nose. Muscles ache, feel weak, as after great exertion; numbness; tingling, especially of fingers and soles of feet; chilly, feel faint;

feel as if covered with cold stockings; head hot, skin dry. Diarrhœa, painless but urgent, 4 P.M.

In the *New York State Transactions*, 1875, Dr. Hills records that *Saponin*, when locally applied to the heart, retards its action, like Digitalis. When applied to muscles, it paralyzes them. Given in appreciable doses to act, it caused dysphagia, rattling of mucus in the larynx, flow of saliva, loose cough, clay-colored but formed stools, or green and offensive; stupidity and inclination to keep quiet. Death is said to result from paralysis of respiratory centres, of cardiac nerves, and of the muscles.

It has been used accordingly for local anæsthesia, consistently with its recorded symptoms of formication, numbness, etc.

The depressing effects of the drug account for the general feeling of muscular soreness and want of energy, and remind us of *Gelsemium*, which, too, is indispensable in catarrhs, occurring in spring and summer, when the heat so depresses both the muscular and nervous systems. It would seem, then, that the QUILLAYA ought to relieve colds, which are produced by a damp, relaxing atmosphere, such as is common enough in our latitude, from May to mid June, and from mid August to far into October, or even November. It exhibits quite a contrast to ACONITE, NUX VOMICA, Belladonna, *Cepa*, etc., but seems to concord with Ferrum, GELSEMIUM, *Mercurius*, *Ipecac.*, *Bryonia*, *Carbo veg.*, etc.

Like *Nux vomica*, it is said to be adapted mainly to the initiament of a cold; but the Nux is curative when the cause of the cold is exposure to dry cold air, sitting or lying on cold stones, etc. Like Mercurius, there are rawness and soreness in nose and throat, and general muscular soreness; but *Mercury* suits late in catarrh, when the discharge is thick, yellow, or green; or, in the beginning, after exposure to wet, to damp evening air, to foggy weather, and when the discharge is watery, burning, and excoriating. There is, also, generally present fever and sweat, the latter exhausting rather than relieving the patient. Like *Gelsemium*, the SAPONIN (QUILLAYA), cures colds contracted in warm, relaxing weather. Both have muscular languor, desire for rest and quiet, general bruised feeling, even of the eyeballs, etc. The one, however, has more a stuffed sensation in the nose; the other, the *Gelsemium*, cures a fluent, excoriating coryza; and there is generally neuralgia of the face, and even of the head, with pains rising from the occiput to the forehead.

THE

HAHNEMANNIAN

MONTHLY.

A HOMŒOPATHIC JOURNAL OF

MEDICINE AND SURGERY.

Editors,

E. A. FARRINGTON, M.D. PEMBERTON DUDLEY, M.D.

Business Manager,

BUSHROD W. JAMES, M.D.

Vol. II. Philadelphia, Pa., May, 1880. No. 5.

☞ The Editors consider themselves responsible for the maintenance of the dignity and courtesy of the journal, but *not* for the opinions expressed by its contributors.

Editorial Department.

THE MAIN QUESTION.—There has always been a conviction in the minds of most honest physicians that the "distinctive lines" which divide the profession of medicine into antagonistic factions are a disgrace to our civilization and a hindrance to medical progress; and the desire to see these lines obliterated has led to a good deal of earnest thought and labor. Quite recently it has been suggested that we, as homœopathists, should abandon our distinctive name and disclaim an exclusively distinctive practice, in order thus to further the prospects of medical union. There can be no reasonable doubt of the honesty of those who make this suggestion, for some of them at least, have done and are now doing most important work for medical science in other directions.

It has always seemed to us that to abandon a principle in order to obtain peace, is to pay an enormous price for a very unmusical whistle, and that to surrender a conviction for the sake of union is to attach to union a value which it does not possess. In regard to the question before us, we had better, first of all, consider whether a union of all medical factions at present would not be more disgraceful and more obstructive to the progress of medical science than the present state of discord. Such a union could be but a name at best for nearly all the homœopathists of the world, and would in reality be merely a surrender to the behests of the American Medical Association.

The great parties to the present medical controversy are, not allopathy on one side and homœopathy on the other, but the American Medical Association, claiming to represent allopathy, is arrayed against all physicians of all schools in an endeavor to get the control of medical thought and medical practice. The question is not whether we shall believe and practice allopathy; not whether they shall believe and practice homœopathy; but whether any physician, homœopath or allopath, shall be allowed to form and hold his own opinions, and practice in accordance therewith. Disguise the matter as we may, make excuses for it as we will, the war which that Association is waging against the advancement of medical science consists in an effort to crush out all medical practice which its members, in caucus assembled, have declared or may hereafter declare to be out of accord with their own opinions.

Of course the allopathist will make answer just here, that the anathemas of the Association are directed, not against liberty of medical thought and action, but only against those "whose practice is based upon an exclusive dogma," to the rejection of the clinical experience of a past medical age; that all the Association wishes to secure is the exercise of that true eclecticism which proves all things in medicine, and holds fast that which is good; and that the homœopathist, because he refuses to do this, is to be persecuted, and, if possible, driven from the profession. This is the sophistry behind which the American Medical Association seeks to hide its infamy; as if any medical man, possessed of an ounce of brains, did not know that the exercise of a judicious eclecticism might be just as likely to result in the adoption of one general principle of practice, as in the selection of here a little and there a little from each and all systems, and the exclusive homœopath be thus as true an eclectic as the sanctified allopath, who takes whatever he wants from all systems, not forgetting to steal all he can lay his hands on from homœopathy itself.

That medical body, which claims the right to say that men shall not practice "upon an exclusive dogma," has an equal prerogative to prohibit any other particular form or method or principle of practice, which in their judgment or lack of judgment, seems to them unwise. Nobody denies that medical men have the right to associate themselves under any system of by-laws, and even to hold themselves aloof professionally from whoever they please, but it is a matter of history, that the A. M. A. has gone farther, and sought to make laws for other physicians as well as for its own members, and has done its best to drive out of the profession those who had the audacity to denounce them and contemn their medieval code. Can any physician—both thoughtful and honest—desire to unite with such a community of intolerant and arrogant spirits? Can such a union fail to involve medicine and its practitioners in deepest, darkest disgrace? It is all very pretty to talk about the lion and the lamb, "the young lion and the fatling," lying down together, but it is only a fool of a lamb that will lie down beside the lion without first securing proper guarantees that the lion is going to behave himself; and all past history shows that our allopathic lion is not a beast to be trusted. He hasn't yet begun to "eat straw like the ox," and until he does, the medical millennium has not arrived, and the lamb's only safety consists in eternal vigilance.

Our voice, then, is still for war—for a controversy defensive and aggressive, to be maintained with vigor and determination. And if to-day every member of the American Medical Association should become an avowed homœopathist, we should still keep the sword unsheathed until that Association should abandon and utterly repudiate all claim to the exercise of a censorship over the medical opinions and practice of the age.

WEDDINGS.—Whenever it lies within the power of the doctor, let him be prepared to administer wholesome advice concerning the management of weddings. There is no ceremony which should be more delightful to all interested than this wedding of two souls into one complete man. And yet, as it is ordinarily managed, many a bride has had her health ruined and not a few have lost their lives.

The lady is supposed to house herself for the conventional number of days, during which it is exceedingly vulgar to show herself on the street under any pretext. Her time is occupied with the minutiæ of her *trousseau* and with—thinking.

Pale and exhausted, she is but poorly prepared for the nervous ordeal of a more or less public ceremony, followed by that abomination, the reception. Then her bridal adornments are removed, and, arrayed in a more sombre suit, she is hurried away, to add to her exhaustion the fatigues of travel and sight-seeing. Is it to be wondered at that she falls an easy victim to disease?

We are not in favor of robbing weddings of their joyousness and festivity. But let the lady's preparations be less hurried. Let her give up the silly fashion which dooms her to the house and steals away her freshness and rosy hue. Neither rouge nor the excited hectic can take the place of the bloom of health. And above all, let her forego the trial of the reception, until she has sought recreation in her needed journey. It will be time enough on her return to receive the congratulations of friends—congratulations which can be truthfully and heartily extended, since they will greet the wife, refreshed and happy in her new state.

The gynæcologist will suffer sadly from such advice. But it will help to make healthy wives, healthy mothers, and consequently, more vigorous children. So in the long run, all doctors will lose, while the community will gain, both as to numbers and vigor.

Female Eunuchs.—Among the revolting perversions of religion, is that which requires both men and women to submit to the operation of castration. History records numerous instances of male eunuchs, but its pages are silent concerning the unsexing of women.

It is not very generally known that there exists in Russia a religious organization whose members hope to reach heaven by removing the possibility of venereal temptations. The process of emasculation is comparatively easy, and belongs to common surgical practice; but the removal of the ovaries is a more serious operation, and demands an expert. Until recently there was only one Russian surgeon who was fully qualified for this hazardous work. Educated in Paris for his nefarious occupation, he returned to his own country, and has since amassed an enormous fortune.

The Russian Government is not at all in sympathy with these fanatics, and is strenuously endeavoring to suppress the rite; but the task is a difficult one, because it is practiced among the noble and wealthy as well as among the commonalty.

So is added another offence to the disgusting chapter of sexual frauds. On the one side we may array illicit gratifications of the sexual passions, and on the other, mutilations of the body, under the absurd notion that removing the physical mea s is equivalent to removing the spiritual cause of sinful desires.

A Charge and its Refutation.—One of the most unfortunate circumstances connected with the recent controversies on the subject of triturations and potencies, is the personal feeling engendered between certain of the opposing parties. Partly as an apparent outgrowth of this feeling, charges affecting professional character have been preferred against certain members of our school. We have refused to publish these charges or to aid in their dissemination, so long as their truth or falsity remained in doubt.

We are now at perfect liberty to state, that one of these charges affected Dr. Samuel Potter, of Milwaukee—a member of the American Institute of Homœopathy and a contributor to this journal. The accusation, which was published in a medical journal, charged the doctor with an irregularity in his graduation. In reply to the charge, Dr. Potter submitted the documentary evidence of his studies and graduation to three ex-presidents of the American Institute,—Drs. Holcombe of New Orleans, Dake of Nashville, and Burgher of Pittsburg. These gentlemen, after examining the evidence, have written letters unanimously acquitting him of the charge.

A proposition.—We desire to call especial notice to the following letter from the veteran homœopathist of Baltimore. The writer's standing in, and services to the cause of homœopathy ought to secure him a careful hearing:

Messrs. Editors: I hope that the solid hour, promised to me at the last meeting of the American Institute of Homœopathy, held at Lake George, will be accorded at the next meeting, at Milwaukee. I hope to be present, and to give the results of my *investigations of forty-three years* into the curative power of the thirtieth attenuation of homœopathic remedies. I feel assured that I can convince the greatest skeptic upon this subject, if fair and honorable, and that too, without the aid of the microscope. Respectfully,

F. R. McManus.

Transactions of the Homœopathic Medical Society of the State of Pennsylvania. Tenth, Eleventh, Twelfth, Thirteenth, and Fourteenth Annual Sessions, 1874 to 1878, Vol. II.—We have the above long-looked for volume at last before us. It is handsomely gotten up in neat black cloth binding, and printed in Sherman & Co.'s best style. We had intended to print this month a careful review of this volume, but, owing to the pressure upon our columns, we are obliged, much to our regret, to defer it until our June issue.

☞ WE have received from a writer, who signs as "Boston," a communication, evidently intended for publication, but cannot print it because the writer's real name does not accompany the article. If "Boston" will send his or her name,—not for publication, but as a guarantee of good faith,—we will publish the article in our next number.

CORRECTION.—In the editorial on "The Proving of Drugs" in the April number, page 237, third line from bottom, the word "not" should be omitted.

Book Department.

CURABILITY OF CATARACT WITH MEDICINES. By James Compton Burnett, M.D., F.R.G.S., etc. London. Boericke & Tafel. New York.

Says the author, in his preface :

"My original intention was to write nothing on the subject until I could prove the curability of cataract by an extensive experience and a consequent array of facts likely to convince the ophthalmic surgeons themselves; but mindful of the fact that the pretension of being too complete too often results in sterility, I have decided to delay it no longer."

On p. 106 he says :

"It might be well perhaps to say that I lay no claim to any special knowledge of the diseases of the eye in general, or of those of the lens or its capsule in particular."

In a monograph of 208 pages he has, however, given his views concerning the restoration of the transparency of an opacified lens, with cases from his own practice, as well as a summary of those found in homœopathic and other literature. Upon this subject he is most certainly an optimist, and if we accept unquestioned the record which he presents to us the outlook for the cataractous patient is certainly a hopeful one. But it is to be greatly regretted that throughout the book is found *not one single case of undoubted cataract, cured by any method whatsoever.* Absolute tests of visual acuity are in no instance recorded, and improvement in sight vaguely expressed in the very untrustworthy testimony, as all oculists are aware, of the patients themselves. Differential diagnoses are not made with that care that science to-day demands, and we are constrained to say that many of the cases in which benefit followed the administration of the drug were lenticular scleroses.

In the first case mentioned the writer is not aware whether the cataract is capsular or lenticular, although the fact of its being a part of a chronic ophthalmia would render the former the more probable. No test was made at the beginning of medication, and no accurate record of the sight taken at its close; hence we are justified in accepting the patient's extravagant statement, that she saw "almost as well as ever," *cum grano salis.* These facts are of such vital importance that their absence seriously affects the worth of a record that might otherwise be valuable. Those of the homœopathic school who treat eye diseases extensively, are aware that much can be accomplished in a resolution of the products of intraocular inflammatory disease, and that this was really done in some of the "cataract" cases is, it seems, clearly shown.

Case XII, for instance, is taken from Raue. The following symptoms were found after an attack of intermittent fever:

"The eye had a *dead look, pupil enlarged and immovable; in the middle of the lens there was an opacity as if punctured by a needle; lids and conjunctiva reddened.*"

These are not evidences of cataract. It was in all probability a case of aquo-capsulitis.

In the probable cases of true cataract the lens was not examined by oblique illumination, and hence objective differences following treatment were not discovered. The subjective sensation of clearer sight may have been due to removal of undiscovered amblyopia or corneal opacities. We would not be hypercritical, because the power of our antipsorics is indeed wonderful, but no tissue in which absolute disintegration has occurred can ever be restored to its integrity. A siliculose or Morgagnian cataract can no more be restored to its original transparency than an atrophic globe can be transformed into a healthy eyeball. That incipient cataract may perhaps be cured, and further clouding of the lens prevented, by careful prescribing, we do not doubt, but that a nuclear sclerosis can be overcome by medication we do not believe.

In some respects the book is to be commended. It is clearly printed in good type on heavy cream-laid paper. The grouping of cases in convenient form will prove of value, even though the diagnosis in some of them may be questioned. As an original production, however, we fear that it will add but little to our knowledge of the subject.

BUFFALO, N. Y. F. P. L.

PHYSICIAN'S OBSTETRICAL REGISTER. By *Joseph M. Reeves, M.D.*, Philadelphia. 1880. Price, $2.00.

This book is designed to furnish a convenient form, by which physicians may keep a record of their obstetric practice, both for immediate use and for future reference. The record of each case occupies a single line, running across two opposite pages. On the first page are recorded matters of information, which can be obtained previous to the confinement, viz., names of parents, residence, occupation of father, mother's age, number of pregnancy, date of last confinement, character of delivery, date of last menses, confinement expected. On the opposite page this record is completed as follows: date of confinement, hour, length of labor, presentation, character of delivery, natural or operative, sex of child, child's name, color, page of remarks, charges. The "page of remarks" refers to the latter portion of the book, where convenient space is provided for recording any matters of interest connected with the case. Like all other good books, this one is provided with an alphabetical index.

There are many physicians who do not preserve a careful record of their obstetric cases, but there are probably none of this large number who do not sooner or later regret the omission. Such a record cannot fail to be of interest as a subject of reference, and its pages are liable to be drawn upon at any time for most valuable information by those most directly interested. We especially recommend that those, who are just commencing practice, should inclose $2 to Dr. Joseph M. Reeves, 842 North Sixth Street, Philadelphia, for a copy of his handy register. D.

OUR HOMES. By *Henry Hartshorne, A.M., M.D.*, Formerly Professor of Hygiene in the University of Pennsylvania, etc., Philadelphia. Presley Blakiston, 1012 Walnut Street. 1880.

We have here still another of the popular American Health Primers. Like its predecessors in the series, it contains little, if anything, to condemn, while its pages are replete with matters presented in a form adapted to the general reader. Small and compact as the book is, it supplies a vast amount of necessary information, relating to the building and management of dwelling-houses, with a view to the highest health of its inmates. The subject is judiciously arranged under the following heads, a short chapter being devoted to each of them: I. Situation; II. Construction; III. Light; IV. Warmth; V. Ventilation. VI. Water Supply; VII. Drainage; VIII. Disinfection; IX. Population; X. Workingmen's Homes. The chapter on Drainage is illustrated with numerous wood-cuts. The price of the work is fifty cents. D.

STAMMERING AND ITS RATIONAL TREATMENT, WITH REMARKS ON CANON KINGSLEY'S ELOCUTIONARY RULES. By *E. B. Shuldam, M.D.*, Trin. Coll., Dublin; M.A., Oxon. London. Homœopathic Publishing Company, 2 Finsbury Circus, E. C. 12mo. pp. 72.

The author attributes the prevalence of stammering partly to the indifference with which it is regarded by so many of those having in charge the training of children, and this indifference he ascribes to the widespread, but too often erroneous notion that the victims, if left to themselves, will "grow out of it." As a result of this neglect, the habit, upon which the volume treats, affects quite a large proportion of the inhabitants of all countries, some interesting statistics being given in illustration.

In the opening pages the directions given by Canon Kingsley for the cure of stammering are taken up and discussed, some of them approvingly, and some of them otherwise. It is very evident from these directions, that while

Kingsley may have been an expert elocutionist, he was not a physiologist, and some of his assertions and deductions, respecting the physiology of the organs of phonation and articulation, are rather amusing to the professional reader. Our author holds,—and all medical men will agree with him,—that the treatment of stammering involves the development of functional powers whose exercise cannot be controlled and directed by any one except an educated physician. At the same time he believes that in many cases the treatment must be chiefly elocutionary, and special principles are laid down for the management of individual cases. We could wish that the mention of the homœopathic remedies, found useful in these cases, had been accompanied by the special indications for the use of each of them. The work is well worthy of careful study on the part of any who may be interested in the causes and cure of stammering. D.

Gleanings.

Occlusion of the Duodenum.—Dr. Goodhart reports the case of a child, apparently healthy at birth, but which was soon attacked with vomiting of mucus. Death ensued in 126 hours. Autopsy revealed an occlusion of the duodenum without any communication whatever with the gut below. This malformation is rare, only seven or eight cases being on record. —*Lancet*, February 28th, 1880.

Uterine Phlebitis appears from fifth to twelfth day or later. Chill followed by complete apyrexia, but soon removed. Pain absent or slight, and deeply seated, at the level of the uterine cornua. Pulse strong, full, and dicrotic, of variable course. Temperature normal at certain hours of the day, showed a marked rise during accession of fever. Face sub-icteric; delirium and restlessness. Recovery rare.

Uterine Lymphangitis appears shortly after delivery. Single chill, moderate or absent, sometimes before chill. Pain limited by the border of the uterus. Continuous febrile state follows chill. Temperature ranges from 104° to 105.8° F. Face animated; eyes brilliant; cheeks red, later shriveiled; eyes sunken. Expression dull, when tympanitis, vomiting, and peritonitis supervene. The peritoneal symptoms now mask the former. Death often in seven or eight days.—*N. Y. Medical Journal*, April, 1880.

Formiate of soda, given in larger doses than 1.0 gram to the kilo of body weight, causes toxic symptoms. The approach of death is preceded by shallow inspirations, between which pauses of expiration occur, becoming shorter and shorter. Respiration ceases with an expiratory effort, and cardiac movements last some fifty seconds longer, becoming weaker and weaker in the systole.—*Philadelphia Medical Times*, April 10th, 1880.

Differentiation of three forms of puerperal diseases:

Septicæmia.—Slight or no chill; temperature 100° to 106° and 107°. Temperature falls rapidly before a fatal termination, and may rise again immediately after death. Significant absence of pain. Patient dull, heavy, even comatose; wandering, but never violent delirium; diarrhœa. Vomiting in severe cases; thirst; tongue dry. Sweat often profuse at first, but skin, dry and flabby, later.

PYÆMIA.—Repeated chills. Rapid rise in temperature, reaching its height at the end of the chill. Skin feels cold. Dry heat and then sweat. Face leaden or yellow, while in Septicæmia cheeks are dark scarlet. Rapid emaciation. Abscesses, purulent effusions into joints, etc. Chill, often slight, rarely repeated.

PUERPERAL FEVER.—Sudden development of abdominal pains, vague and uncertain as to seat, though often beginning in the hypogastrium. These pains are seldom absent. Abdominal walls soft, with not much distension, hence different from idiopathic peritonitis. Can lie on either side generally. Rapid gaseous distension of abdomen just before death. Temperature 102° to 106°. The oscillations in heat are increased when pyæmia is combined, and the temperature exceedingly high when septicæmia is also present. Great frequency of the pulse; a constant symptom, 110 to 160 per minute. Respirations 24 to 60. Tongue moist, white, and often indented by the teeth; dry and cracked only when patient keeps the mouth open. Delirium slight; generally she is tranquil during the day, though excited at night. Vomit dark, greenish, bilious. Hiccough, diarrhœa. Lochia may be increased or diminished, fetid or not. In fatal cases death often ensues on the fourth or fifth day. See Dr. Barker's *Puerperal Diseases.*

A LACERATION OF THE PENIS, which occurred during coitus, involved a complete severance of the urethra, with infiltration of urine and subsequent abscess, leaving a urinary fistula. The patient had gonorrhœa twenty years before, and had noticed that he was always longer than natural in urinating. Erections were in the shape of a bow, and the urethra was stretched like the string. The urethra, evidently, when the organ was erect, gave way. The penis was doubtless struck upon the right and violently crushed down upon the left, lacerating the right corpus cavernosum with its fibrous covering. Great difficulty was found in drawing off the urine; but it was finally accomplished with a No. 5 rat-tail gum catheter, which was allowed to remain in. The urethra was not only lacerated, but completely severed. A free opening was made, followed by the escape of pus and dark blood. A fistula was thus made, through which catheterization was managed, to the great advantage of the wounded tissues. Artificial healing of the fistula seemed to induce severe symptoms, so its closing was left to nature. The patient fully recovered.—*Philadelphia Medical Times*, April 10th, 1880.

BENZOATE OF SODA AND MAGNESIA.—Professor Klebs writes to the *Allg. Wiener Med. Zeit.*, No. 1, 1880, that tuberculous miliary eruptions can be made to proceed to self-limitation or retrogression under the use of Benzoates, especially Benzoate of magnesia. He employs the Benzoate of soda in inhalations, gram 1.0 a day, together with the internal administration of Benzoate of magnesia.—*Medical Current Record*, March 20th, 1880; see also HAHNEMANNIAN MONTHLY, volume i, p. 160. But in the London *Medical Times and Gazette*, several failures with this drug are recorded. Drs. Wenzel, Guttman, Fritsche, and Waldonburg, agree in their record of the inoperativeness of Benzoate inhalations. An editorial in the last issue of the *Medical Record* (March, 27th), refers to exaggerated and conflicting reports respecting this drug, and adds, that "it is hard to believe the salt has any special effect upon the disease." Klebs's original claim was that Benzoate of soda is the best known antimycotic. Inoculations with diphtheritic or tubercular matter were innocuous when followed by its administration. It is the same old story repeated. Born in theory, subjected to a checkered life of varied experience, and then buried in oblivion amid the disgust of a deluded profession.

USES OF THE PERINÆUM.—Dr. Gaillard Thomas regards the perinæum as useful in sustaining the anterior rectal wall and posterior vaginal wall. He described it as a wedge-shaped body, acting as a keystone in preventing a destruction of the equilibrium of the pelvic organs. In health the vagina, instead of constituting an open canal, is a collapsed tube, its anterior wall lying directly upon its posterior. Its curve is double; the first a decided bend from behind forwards, then a lesser one downwards and slightly backwards; its second, a slight curve from above downwards and backwards. Instead of being a flat surface, consisting of skin, areolar tissue, etc., filling the space between the anus and vulva, the perinæum was described as a triangular body, composed of strong layers of adipose and elastic tissue, etc.

At its upper portion the vagina is furnished with a depression, which receives and supports the cervix uteri.

During the discussion of Dr. Thomas's paper, objection was raised to the keystone action of the perinæum, and Dr. Thomas replied that he had submitted the view to two engineers, both of whom admitted that it was the keystone of an arch, upon which the lateral portions rested.—*Medical Record*, March 20th, 1880.

News and Comments.

CLAUDIUS GALENUS, the illustrious physician of ancient Pergamos, was wont to speak of his vocation and work as "a religious hymn in honor of the Creator."

THE WESTERN INSTITUTE OF HOMŒOPATHY will hold its annual meeting at Minneapolis, Minn., June 1st, 2d, and 3d, in joint session with the Minnesota State Society.

J. B. MCCLELLAND, M.D., has returned from his year's service at Ward's Island Hospital, and commenced practice with his brother, J. H. McClelland, M.D., of Pittsburg.

EDWARD S. SHARPLESS, M.D. (Hahn., Phila., 80), has been elected Resident Physician of the Children's Homœopathic Hospital of Philadelphia, located at N. E. cor. Eighth and Poplar streets.

ALONZO P. WILLIAMSON, M.D., late of the State Homœopathic Asylum for the Insane, at Middletown, N. Y., has been appointed Chief of Staff in charge of the Homœopathic Hospital at Ward's Island, New York.

PROFESSOR J. E. JAMES, M.D., of Philadelphia, will sail for Europe about May 12th, in quest of health and needed rest. We but echo the sentiment of a large number of physicians and laymen in wishing him a pleasant voyage, a complete restoration to health, and a safe return to his family, his friends, and his useful labors in the cause of Homœopathy.

ORIGIN OF YELLOW FEVER.—The opinion of the Philadelphia *Ledger* on the above subject may be gleaned from the following, which we clip from its editorial columns:

"Importation of yellow fever, it is hoped at New Orleans, will be stopped by quarantine below that city. So far, well; but what is being done about the indigenous article, the fatal seeds of which have been planted so profusely up the Mississippi,—at and around Memphis, for example."

CHICAGO HOMŒOPATHIC COLLEGE.—The Annual Commencement of the Chicago Homœopathic College was held, March 20th, in Hershey Music Hall, in presence of a large audience. The Annual Report was presented by the President, J. T. Mitchell, M.D., and shows the institution to be upon a sound financial footing with, and excellent prospects. Twenty candidates received the degree of the college, and the valedictory was delivered by Professor E. M. Hale, M.D.

CLEVELAND AND THE WOMEN.—We have received no information as to the commencement exercises of the Homœopathic Hospital College of Cleveland, nor of those of the Woman's Medical College of New York, though we have endeavored to obtain it for publication. There is a small slice of the universe lying outside of New York and Cleveland, and the inhabitants thereof would like to know, etc. The University of Michigan does not hold its commencement until June, at which time we expect to receive encouraging news from Ann Arbor.

HAHNEMANN HOSPITAL OF NEW YORK.—The position of Resident Physician of this hospital will be vacant July 1st. There will be a competitive examination for the position, early in June. The doctor will receive his board, lodging, washing, also thirty dollars per month. Applicants may address

JOHN H. THOMPSON, M.D.,
Secretary of Medical Board.

36 E. Thirtieth Street, New York.

SETTLEMENTS.—Members of the class of "80," Hahnemann College of Philadelphia, have located as follows. We shall announce others as we hear from them:

Alfred E. Baker, M.D., 623 N. Eighteenth Street, Phila.
W. H. Baker, M.D., 811 N. Sixteenth Street, Phila.
Charles H. Conover, M.D., 500 N. Eighteenth Street, Phila.
Eduard Fornias, M.D., 612 S. Tenth Street, Phila.
Edward M. Gramm, M.D., 1656 Vienna Street, Phila.
Lewis B. Griffith, M.D., 809 N. Tenth Street, Phila.
F. O. Gross, M.D., 1240 N. Fourth Street, Phila.
A. B. Kehrer, M.D., 1208 Pine Street, Phila.
James Kemble, M.D., 1804 Columbia Avenue, Phila.
Levi J. Knerr, M.D., 112 N. Twelfth Street, Phila.
John McDonald, M.D., 468 N. Sixth Street, Phila.
Edw. K. McGill, M.D., 1807 Girard Avenue, Phila.
Horace J. Shinkle, M.D., Manayunk, Phila.
Alfred P. Stoddart, M.D., 939 N. Twelfth Street, Phila.
William W. Van Baun, M.D., 1039 Spring Garden Street, Phila.
Willis H. Proctor, M.D., Binghamton, N. Y.

THE HAHNEMANN CLUB OF ST. LOUIS.—This body of homœopathic physicians, which was organized in July, 1873, now consists of the following members: Drs. T. G. Comstock, G. S. Walker, C. H. Goodman, Charles Vastine, Charles Gundelach, S. B. Parsons, H. S. Chase, W. A. Edmonds, William Collisson, and James A. Campbell. Drs. J. T. Temple and N. D. Tirrell, both now deceased, and Dr. A. S. Everett, who has since removed to Denver, Col., were formerly members of the club. The total membership is limited to twelve. The meetings are interesting and profitable and are well attended. The most perfect harmony has prevailed from the beginning. The club, it is said, has exerted a quiet but wholesome influence upon professional affairs in St. Louis, and helped to bring peace and prosperity out of chaos and trouble, so that homœopathy in that city has perhaps never enjoyed more cheering prospects than at present. At the last meeting of the Hahnemann Club of Philadelphia a communication was received conveying the hearty fraternal greetings of the Hahnemann Club of St. Louis and of its members. The communication elicited very earnest expressions of interest in the twin-sister organization, and the secretary was instructed to respond to it in suitable terms.

The Medical Charities of Philadelphia.—A meeting of the homœopathic physicians of Philadelphia has been held recently to consider a proposed plan for co-operation of the medical charities of the city with the ward associations of the Philadelphia Society for Organizing Charitable Relief and Repressing Mendicancy. The meeting was the result of a movement looking to this end, upon which the Homœopathic Medical Society some time ago took definite action by appointing a committee to draft a circular. In this circular the objects of the proposed union were stated to be "to protect the medical charities and the members of the medical profession from imposition on the part of applicants for out-door relief of hospitals or for dispensary relief, who have the ability, either wholly or in part, to pay for their treatment, and to avoid the lowering effect upon the self-respect and independence of our people induced through indiscriminate relief."

The committee were intrusted with the further duty of preparing a plan of co-operation. Dr. H. Noah Martin, chairman of this committee, after calling upon Dr. A. R. Thomas, Dean of the Hahnemann Medical College, to preside, stated the object of the meeting, and presented the plan agreed upon by the committee. It proposed to establish by the Medical Charities, a standard charge of, say ten cents per visit or for medicine, unless the case should be specially exempted after investigation, or the charter of the institution should prohibit any charge being made. It recommended,

1st. That all applications for relief should be made in the first instance at the office of the Medical Charities.

2d. That applicants with families in receipt of nine dollars a week or more, unmarried persons receiving six dollars or more, persons living out at service, are able to employ a physician, and should be refused treatment; and that applicants should be so advised through the cards of the Medical Charities, as well as by notices placed on the doors of the service rooms.

3d. That applicants who may be admitted to treatment shall be required to pay for their medicine, or to deposit ten cents at each visit in a box provided for the purpose, unless exempted through procurement of a certificate of the ward superintendent of the Society for Organizing Charity, on which the words "*unable to pay*" shall be noted. This condition should also be placed on the cards, and on the notices on the doors of the service rooms.

The plan was stated to have been introduced into other cities, where it was attended with salutary effects. Dr. Martin read a few extracts from the annual reports of a New York institution, where certain of the reforms proposed had been tried and found to accomplish great results.

Dr. J. K. Lee offered the following, which was adopted:

Resolved, That this meeting recognizes the need of a grand and uniform plan to protect medical charities and the members of the medical profession from imposition, as was proposed by the committee of the Homœopathic Medical Society, subject to such modifications as each individual institution may require.

Resolved, That a committee, consisting of one member from each ward and a representative of each local charity, if deemed desirable, be appointed to carry out the plan under consideration, and that it shall be called "The Committee on Co-operation of the Medical Charities with the Ward Associations of the Philadelphia Society for Organizing Charity."

The allopathic physicians of Philadelphia have taken similar action.

THE

HAHNEMANNIAN MONTHLY.

Vol. II, New Series } Philadelphia, June, 1880. No. 6.

Original Department.

NEURASTHENIA—PSORA.

BY AUG. KORNDŒRFER, M D, PHILADELPHIA, PA.

(Read before the Hahnemann Club of Philadelphia)

THREE-QUARTERS of a century have elapsed since Hahnemann gave to the world a few deep and comprehensive truths, clustered around that great central law of cure, for the discovery and promulgation of which, he was made the honored instrument.

Never before was the scientific world more thoroughly aroused, certainly never before did the medical world have to contend with such organized theories and such pointed and demonstrable facts. This weak thing of tiny pellet fame aroused the then dominant school of medicine to an opposition, which three-quarters of a century have not been sufficient to overcome, though quite sufficient to prove that truth is mighty.

Much of this opposition depends upon the lack of willingness, on the part of many, to accept truth when not arrayed in garb to their taste, and especially when she has not been introduced by some self-constituted aristocracy, recognized by them as authority in medicine. Much, however, also depends upon the want of fidelity—we might say want of loyalty—in the adherents of our school; while not a little has been owing to a lack of knowledge in regard to the teachings peculiar to our school. Since the law was given, many have attempted to apply it without even so much as reading a single line of the most masterly exposition of the same, as it fell from the pen of its great discoverer.

A careful perusal of his greatest works—the *Organon* and the *Chronic Diseases*—must lead to many valuable thoughts, while at the same time it will enable one to see, how as science advances, how as allopathy comes up higher into the light through which Hahnemann viewed nature, the truth shines so brilliantly, that some light makes itself manifest, even to unwilling minds.

Among the foundation principles to which Hahnemann called attention, and on which he laid great stress, may be mentioned that which asserts the importance of the mental symptoms over the mere physical, both as related to disease and to the selection of an appropriate remedy. In § 210 of the *Organon* we find the following: "The state of the mind and temper varies in all so-called diseases, and it ought to be considered as one of the principal symptoms which it is important to notice, in order that we may trace a faithful image of the disease." In § 211: "This extends so far that the moral state of the patient is often that which is most decisive in the choice of a remedy, for this is a symptom of most precise character, and one which can by no means escape the notice of a physician accustomed to make precise observations." In § 212 he again says: "To this principal feature in all diseases, namely, the changes in mind and disposition, the Creator of all healing means has given especial care, in that there is no powerful drug which does not, when taken into the healthy system, change in a marked manner both mind and disposition, and indeed no two substances act alike;" while in § 217 he says, "It is requisite to proceed with care in searching for the entire signs," "especially the principal and characteristic state of mind and disposition."

From these few passages we have adduced such undeniable evidence, as to the high position to which Hahnemann assigned the mental symptoms, that nothing further need be said to strengthen the assertion.

So new and revolutionary were these teachings, that they called forth but opposition and ridicule from the adversaries of the new system, while in the minds of at least some of its advocates, there existed a doubt as to the high degree of importance claimed for them by Hahnemann. Even to this day, comparatively little attention has been bestowed upon the nice distinctions of mental states as given in our provings; many of our school still failing to see any necessity for attention to such symptoms.

The time, however, is fast drawing nigh, yea, has even now arrived, when the physician, who would claim a true knowledge of nature in her diseased states, must show evidence of his knowledge and appreciation of the emotional disorders. The writings of some of the adherents of the old school of medicine must bring the blush to the cheeks of such of the new faith, who, from lukewarmness, ignorance, or fear of ridicule, have buried this one talent, instead of putting it to use. Recent allopathic writers, when treating of nervous diseases, make open avowal of views which certainly savor strongly of the teachings of Hahnemann in this particular direction. They now see that those who have heeded these pleadings for aid, pleadings made known in strongest language through the many and varied mental symptoms, have, in their efforts to assist nature thus enslaved, been most successful in breaking the bonds which disease had fastened upon her, and that, too, when she showed least power to free herself from the thrall.

For years, those who gave both time and attention to the study of the various forms of nervous disease were led to interpret such peculiar symptoms as but "odd fancies," "mere imaginings," "hallucinations," not worthy the notice of the learned, scientific physician! The much-neglected sufferers were called hypochondriacs; as such were regarded as unworthy of sympathy; looked upon as being, at least in part, fools. They were informed that nothing ailed them; that their symptoms were but the result of perverted imagination, and might readily be removed by a simple effort of the will. The poor hapless sufferers were urged to desist from such folly, *will* the symptoms away, and it would be gone. Who was the fool?

Yet, despite this learned advice, such patients but grew worse; the very will-power which they were directed to use, was wanting. They sought comfort and aid from their trusted advisers, and were sent empty, unprofited and comfortless away, soon to become a burden to themselves, while to their more sympathizing friends, they became objects of pity, yet shunned as though contaminating the very air in which they lived, by their gloomy forebodings and complaints. Happily the day of deliverance is dawning upon these outcasts, for such they but too often in effect become, avoided even by those who love them; pleasure palling in their presence.

The common school of medicine has at last opened its doors to the reception of the great truth, *i. e.*, that such nervous states are but expressions of disease, being a part thereof, and almost invariably connected with more or less annoying bodily complaints. Erb says: "Abundant experience has shown me that these cases are not rare, and are of great practical consequence;

for they cause much anxiety not only to the patient, but also to the physician." Again he says: "The chief contingent to this army of sufferers comes from neuropathic families." Beard remarks: "These disorders are transmissible." "They run in families more demonstrably than scrofula, cancer, or consumption. Indeed, one great cause of the rapid increase of these disorders, has been inheritance." And again, after detailing the various symptoms common to neurasthenia, he says: "The above detailed symptoms are not imaginary, but real; not trifling, but serious; although not usually or immediately dangerous. In strictness, *nothing in disease can be imaginary*. If I bring on pain by worrying, by dwelling upon myself, that pain is as real as though it were brought on by an objective influence."

Thus, clad in apparel so strange as scarcely to be recognized, we find Hahnemann's instructions, relative to the importance of the mental symptoms, embodied in the teachings of to-day, as found in the writings of the old-school specialists in nervous affections. Failing as they do to accept Hahnemann's theory of psora as being the foundation on which all chronic and hereditary non-syphilitic and non-sycotic diseases are based, they, nevertheless, are steadily advancing toward, and we hope for their ultimate arrival at, a knowledge of the whole truth,—a hope inspired by the fact that on carefully reviewing the various symptoms treated of under the title "Neurasthenia,"—a disease which but rarely presents marked objective phenomena—we are deeply impressed with the striking resemblance existing between the same and many of those which Hahnemann pronounced as dependent upon psora; such symptoms or conditions being, as per former quotation, transmissible even more demonstrably than scrofula, cancer, or consumption. Thinking it might prove interesting, I have appended a list of symptoms common to neurasthenia, all of which find their counterparts in the list given by Hahnemann as characteristic of the psoric miasm:

MIND AND DISPOSITION.—Gloomy. Melancholy mood. Hopelessness. Anxiety. Tearful mood; easy flow of tears. Irritable about trifles. Desire to be alone. Fear to be alone. Fear of man. Fears to go into crowded places. Fear of close or narrow places. Fear of contamination. Fear of disease. Fear of death. Fear of everything. Fear of being afraid. Fear of lightning. Inability to concentrate the intellect. Mind wanders in every direction.

SENSORIUM.—Vertigo.

HEAD.—Headache, especially sick headache. Pressure in the head; in the vertex; in the occiput. Tenderness of the scalp. Hair seems sore; even to touch the ends causes pain.

EYES.—Neurasthenic asthenopia. Muscæ volitantes. Pupils dilated or unequal. Congestion of the conjunctiva.

EARS.—Roaring in the ears. Subjective odors before the nose. Hay fever.

FACE.—Easy flushing of the face. Blushing.

MOUTH AND THROAT.—Tenderness of the gums and teeth. Neuralgic pains in the teeth. Easy decay of the teeth. Dysphagia. Mouth dry, or in some cases salivation.

GASTRIC SYMPTOMS.—Bitter or sour taste. Want of thirst. Desire for stimulants. Aggravation from coffee, tea, etc. Nervous dyspepsia; worse on empty stomach, better after eating. Flatulence, with annoying rumbling in the bowels.

URINE.—Urine often contains an excess of oxalates; in some cases of urates. Urine abnormally acid. Urine contains spermatozoa.

MALE GENITALS.—Involuntary emissions.

FEMALE GENITALS.—Irritable uterus. Irritable ovaries.

VOCAL ORGANS.—Speech stuttering or stammering. Voice faint, weak, want of clearness of tone, timid.

CHEST.—Oppression of breathing. Oppression in the region of the heart.

HEART AND PULSE.—Palpitation of the heart (irritable heart). Pulse tremulous, variable, easily excited.

BACK.—Tenderness of the spine, either general or localized in small spots. Pains in the back, changing place frequently, sometimes with heat and burning, at others with biting, penetrating sensations, or feeling as though ants were crawling just under the skin.

SUPERIOR EXTREMITIES.—Arms, hands, or only the ends of the fingers may either be numb, or excessively sensitive. Burning sensation in thumb and fingers, with pain running up the arm.

INFERIOR EXTREMITIES.—Cramps in the calves. Pains in the feet. Feet feel as if walking on velvet, rubber, or wool. Heat and burning in the feet. Painful spots on the feet. Shooting pains in the limbs. Heaviness of the loins and limbs. Limbs "go to sleep."

NERVES.—General aggravation from over-exertion. Flying neuralgia. Sudden jerking of single muscles. Tremors. Fidgety. Convulsive movements, especially when falling asleep. Faints easily. Sensation of utter prostration. Temporary paralysis.

SLEEP.—Insomnia. Cannot get sleep. Wakefulness worse after midnight. Gaping. Drowsiness. Dreams, troublesome, of snakes, monsters, etc.

TEMPERATURE AND WEATHER.—Great sensitiveness to change of weather; the so-called "barometers."

CHILL AND SWEAT.—Creeping chills up and down the spine. Coldness of single parts. Coldness of knees. Sweating of the hands, especially the palms. Sweating of feet.

TISSUES.—Dryness of the joints. Cracking of the joints on motion. Dryness of the mucous membrane.

SKIN.—Hyperæsthesia, local or general. Tenderness of parts, or of the whole body. Formication. Pungent feeling. Ticklishness. Itching without eruption. General dryness of the skin.

IDIOSYNCRASIES.—Marked idiosyncrasies to certain drugs, as to Opium or to narcotics in general.

All the foregoing symptoms are found, either in *Erb on Neurasthenia*, Ziemssen's *Cycl. of Prac. of Med.*, vol. xiii, or in Beard's monograph, more recently published; and though they by no means cover all the possible symptoms found in this widespread and multiform affection, they nevertheless give a comprehensive idea of its mode of manifestation.

In conclusion, allow me to present a few repertorial notes made while studying the treatment of this affection. No new remedies have been introduced, and many of the known symptoms are not even noticed; still it is interesting to find the antipsorics always in the foreground; in addition to which, a careful perusal will show some remedies to be of importance, that a more superficial study would have excluded from our consideration.

Finally, it may not be amiss to remark that, as far as possible, only such remedies have been included under each symptom as have undoubted authority:

Fear to go into a crowded place: Acon., Phosph. (fears he may be run over).

Fear in a narrow place: Argent. m, Valer. (in a room).

Fear of contamination (of disease): Ambra, Bell., Borax, Calc. os., Hyosc., Laches. (of cholera), Mercur., Natr. c., Nux vom., Rhus tox., Alum. (epilepsy), Arnic., Fluor. ac., Phos. (apoplexy), Ignat. (of gastric ulcer).

Fear (dread) of death: Acon., Alum., Anac., Arsen., Calc.

os., Cupr. m., Digit., Graph., Hepar, Ign., Laches., Mosch., Nux vom., Phos., Platin., Rhus tox., Sep., Stram.

Fear (dread) of thieves: Alum., Arsen., Aurum, Bell., Con., Ignat., Laches., Magn. c., Magn. m., Mercur., Natr. c., Natr. m., Phosph., Silic., Veratr., Zinc.

Fear of man: Acon., Anac., Aurum, Baryt. c., Bell., Cicut., Con., Cupr., Ignat., Hyosc., Lycop., Natr. c., Puls., Rhus tox., Selen., Sep., Stann.

Fears to be alone: *Arsen.*, Calc. os., Con., Dros., Kal. c., *Lycop.*, Ran. bulb., Sep., *Stram.*

Anxiousness: Acon., Æthus., Agaric., Alum., Ambra, Amm. c., Amm. m., Anac., Ant. cr., Argent. m., Argent. nit., Arnic., Arsen., Asa., Asar., Aurum, Baryt. c., Bell, Berb., Borax, Bryon., Calc. os., Cann. sat., Canth., Capsic., Carb. an., Castor., Caust., Cham., Cinch., Cic., Coccul., Coff., Coloc., Con., Crocus, Cupr. ac., Cupr. m., Digit., Drosera., Dulc., Ferr., Graph., Gratiola, Helleb., Hepar, Hyosc., Ignat., Ipec., Kal. c., Kal. chl., Laches., Lactic., Lauro., Ledum, Lycop., Magn. c., Magn. m., Menyan., Merc., Mosch., Mur. ac., Natr. c., Natr. m., Nitrum, Nitr. ac., Nux vom., Op., Petrol., Phosph., Plat., Plumb., Puls., Ran. scel., Rhus tox., Ruta, Sabad., Sabin., Sarsap., Secale, Sepia, Silic., Spigel., Spong., Squill, Staphis., Stram., Sulph., Sul. ac., Tabac., Thuja, Valer., Veratr., Zinc.

Blushing: Amyl nitrite, Coca,—Aur. (bashful).

Face flushes easily; Ambra, Amm. mur., Ferrum, Ignat., Lycop., Phosph., Nux vom., Sepia.

Anxious feeling about his disease: Acon., Amm. c., Arnic., Arsen., Asa., Calad., Canth., Cham., Dros., Kal. chl., Natr. m., Natr. ac., Phosph., Phos. ac., Valer.

Anxious feeling about his health: Alum., Amm. c., Calad., Calc. os., Coccul., Gratiol., Kal. c., Lach., Natr. c., Natr. m., Nitr. ac., Nux vom., Phosph., Phos. ac., Puls., Sepia, Sulph.

Anxious feeling around the heart: Ambra, Arsen., Aurum, Bell., Calc. os., Camph., Cann. sat., Caust., Cham., Coccul., Coff., Con., Croc., Cupr. m., Cycl., Digit., Euphorb., Helleb., Lycop., Menyan., Merc., Nux vom., Op., Platin., Phosph., Plumb., Puls., Rhus tox., Sec. c., Spong., Therid., Veratr., Viol. tr.

Trouble or anguish of conscience, as if he had done evil: Alum., Amm. c., Arsen., Carb. veg., Caust., Cina, Coccul., Coffea, Cyclam., Digit., Ferr., Graph., Ign., Magn. sul., Merc., Natr. m., Nitr. ac., Nux vom., Pulsat., Ruta, Silic., Stront., Sulph., Veratr., Zinc.

Apprehensive of evil; of misfortune: Aconit., Agaric.,

Alum., Amm. c., Anac., Arsen., Baryt. c., Calc. os., Carb. an., Carb. veg., Castor., Canst., Cicut., Clemat., Coccul., Coffea, Colch., Digit., Dros., Dulc., Graph., Helleb., Kal. hyd., Laches., Magn. c., Magn. sul., Menyan., Merc. Nux vom., Phosph., Rhus, Ruta, Sabin., Spong., Sulph., Tabac., Veratr.

Solicitude about domestic affairs: Baryt. c., Puls., Rhus, Sepia, Sulph.

Solicitude, want of: Citr. ac.

Desire to be alone: Acon., Alumina, Aurum, Baryt. c., Bell., Bufo, Calc. os., Cinch., Con., Cupr., Cyclam., Digit., Ferr., Graph., Hep., Hyosc., Ignat., Kal. c., Laches., Ledum, Lycop., Magn. m., Menyan., Natr. c., Nat. m., Nux vom., Phos., Rhus tox., Sepia, Stann.

Gloominess: Anac., Aurum, Bovis., Caust., Cham., Cinch., Con., Digit., Graph., Iod., Meny., Petrol., Plumb., Rhodod., Stann., Sulph., Sul. ac., Tabac., Tarax., Veratr., Zinc.

Sadness: Acon., Bell., Caust., Cham., Graph., Ignat., Lycop., Natr. m., Platin., Puls., Rhus tox.

Melancholy: Acon., Agn. cas., Alum., Anac., Arsen., Asar., Aurum, Bell., Cact. gr., Calc. os., Canst., Cinch., Coccul., Crocus, Cupr., Cyclam., Digit., Graph., Helleb., Hyosc., Ignat., Kal. c., Laches., Lycop., Natr. c., Natr. m., Nitr. ac., Nux mos., Nux vom., Phos., Phos. ac., Platin., Plumb., Puls., Rhus tox., Secale, Seneg., Sepia, Silic., Stram., Sulph., Sul. ac., Tabac., Veratr.

Hopelessness: Arnic., Arsen., Aurum, Bell., Calc. os., Caust., Coccul., Con., Graph., Hyosc., Ignat., Lach., Lycop., Natr. c., Puls., Rhus tox., Sulph.

Tearful mood: Acon., Amm. mur., Arsen., Aurum, Bell., Calc. os., Canst., Cham., Coff., Digit., Hepar, Ignat., Iod., Lycop., Natr. mur., Platin., Puls., Rhus tox., Sepia, Staphis., Sulph., Tabac., Veratr.

Irritable mood: Acon., Arsen., Asar., Aurum, Bell., Bryon., Cham., Coffea, Ferr., Ignat., Lycop., Natr. m., Nux vom., Phosph., Puls., Sepia, Stann., Sulph., Veratr.

Inability to think or incapacity for thought: Acon., Agaric., Alum., Ambra, Amm. c., Arsen., Coff., Digit., Helleb., Hyosc., Laches., Lauro., Lycop., Mezer., Natr. c., Natr. m., Nux vom., Oleand., Selen., Sepia, Stann., Verat.

Unfitness for bodily or mental work: Agn. cas., Alum., Amm. c., Aur., Borax, Cyclam., Lactuc., Mercur., Natr. c., Nat. mur., Nitr. ac., Nux vom., Oleand., Phos. ac., Sarsap., Selen., Sepia, Stann., Zinc., Zinc. ox.

Inability for connected thought: Zinc.

Paucity of ideas: Phos. ac., Rhus tox., Veratr.

Thinking seems to be done in the stomach: Acon. (This symptom I have observed in but one case, accompanied by marked depression of spirits. Acon.θ, 2 drops in 12 teaspoonfuls of water. Dose 1 teaspoonful every 2 hours removed the symptom in 48 hours, and the patient recovered. The accompanying nervous symptoms approached nearly to insanity.

Irritable heart: Acon., Actea Rac., Agaric., Argent. met., Argent. Nitric., Arsen., Asaf., Aurum, Bryon., Cactus, Calc. os., Cann. sat., Chamm., Cinch., Coccul., Digit., Ferr., Gelsem., Ignat., Kali Brom., Kali c., Laches., Lilium, Lycop., Mag. mur., Merc. sol., Mosch., Naja, Natr. m., Nux mosch., Nux vom., Phosph., Platin., Pulsat., Rhus tox., Sepia, Silic., Spig., Sulph., Zinc.

Sensitiveness of scalp: Æsc. hip., Agaric., Aloes, Ambra, Amm. c., Ant. cr., Ant. tart., Argent. met., Arsen., Arum tr., Baptis., Baryt. c., Bell., Borax, Bovis., Bryon., Calc. os., Calc. ph., Cann. ind., Carb. an., Carb. veg., Cinch., Coloc., Croton, Ferr., Gratiol., Hepar, Iod., Kreos., Lachnan., Laches., Ledum, Lycop., Magn. c., Mar. ver., Natr. m., Natr. sul., Nitr. ac., Nitrum, Nux mos., Nux vom., Paris, Petrol., Phosph., Psorin., Rhus tox., Sabin., Sarsap., Selen., Sepia, Silic., Spigel., Spong., Squill., Stann., Staph., Sulph., Tarax., Thuja, Veratr., Zinc.

Muscæ volitantes: Agar., Amm. m., Aurum, Bell., Calc. os., Cann. sat., Caust., Cinch., Coccul., Coffea, Con., Dig., Dulc., Hepar., Hyosc., Lactuca, Magn. c., Merc. viv., Natr. m., Nitr. ac., Op., Phosph., Plumb., Puls., Rhus tox., Ruta, Secale, Sepia, Silic., Spigel., Stram., Sulph., Tereb., Thuja, Zinc.

Amelioration of stomach symptoms after eating: Acon., Alum., Ambra, Anac., Baryt. c., Bovist., Cann. sat., Caust., Chelid., Cinch., Graph., Gratiol., Kal. c., Laches., Magn. c., Nitr. ac., Nux v., Petrol., Stront.

Involuntary emissions: Agaric., Alum., Arsen., Borax, Bovis., Calc. os., Cann. sat., Carb. an., Carb. veg., Caust., Cinch., Con., Digit., Diosc. v., Kal. brom., Kal. c., Lactuca, Ledum, Lycop., Merc. viv., Mezer., Natr. c., Natr. m., Nuphar. l., Nux vom., Petrol., Phosph., Phos. ac., Picric ac., Plant. m., Plumb., Puls., Ran. bulb., Rhodod., Sabad., Sarsap., Sepia, Silic., Staph., Therid., Thuja.

Irritable uterus: Aletris, Ars., Asaf., Aster. rub., Aurum, Bryon., Calc. os., Caust., Cham., Cinch., Coccul., Coffea, Con., Croc., Ferr., Graph., Helon., Hyosc., Ignat., Ipecac., Kal. c.,

Lilium., Magn. m., Natr. m., Nux vom., Op., Phosph., Phos. ac., Platin., Puls., Rhus tox., Sabin., Sec. corn., Sepia, Sulph., Tarent., Thuja, Zinc.

Irritable ovaries: Actea rac., Amm. mur., Arg. met., Arg., Nitric., Arsenic, Coloc., Con., Hamam., Kali brom., Kali c., Laches., Lilium, Naja, Platin., Sepia, Sulph., Thuja, Zinc, Zinc-val. (See also Irritable Uterus.)

Voice, feeble: Amm. caust., Ant. cr., Baryt. c., Bell., Cann. sat., Crotal., Hepar, Lycop., Tart. em.

Voice, trembling: Acon., Arsen., Canth., Ignat., Merc., Phosph.

Voice, weak: Amm. caust., Angust., Ant. crud., Canth., Carb. veg., Canst., Daph. ind., Gelsem., Hepar, Ignat., Laches., Lauroc., Lyc., Nux v., Opium, Paris, Phosph., Prunus, Puls., Spong., Stann.

Voice, timid: Agn. cas., Canth., Lauro.

Spinal irritation, intervertebral spaces feel sore: Actea Rac., Agaric., Cinch., Cinch-Sulph., Con., Ignat., Kali c., Natrum m., Nux vom., Phosph., Phos. ac., Pulsat., Sepia, Sulph., Zinc, Zinc phos.

Stitching pain in the spine: Angus., Arg. met., Aurum, Bell., Berber., China, Cina, Dulc., Gins., Helleb., Ignat., Menyan., Mephit., Merc. viv., Mosch., Phosph., Phos. ac., Ratan., Ruta, Stann., Sul. ac.

Stitching in the dorsal vertebræ: Cann. sat., Chelid., Gratiol., Ledum, Nitr. ac., Sabin., Verbasc.

Stitching in the lumbar vertebræ: Arg. met., Aurum, Bryon., Mezer., Phosph., Prunus, Thuja.

Cutting pain in the spinal column: Lobel. inf.

Cutting pain in the cervical vertebræ: Graph.

Cutting pain in the lumbar vertebræ: Digit.

Drawing pain in the spine: Bell., Daph. ind., Mosch., Ruta, Stram., Sulph., Zinc.

Pain as if in the spinal cord: Lactuca.

Pain in the spine: Acon., Aurum, Calc. os., Chinin., Coccul., Petrol., Ruta, Sabad., Silic.

Pain from touch: Aspar., Berb., Chinin., Ignat., Kal. c., Natr. m., Phosph., Rhus tox., Stram.

Pain in the lumbar vertebræ: Kreos., Nux mosch.

Aching in the dorsal vertebræ: Ailanth. gl.

Aching in the lumbar vertebræ: Jugl. c.

Bruised pain in the spinal column: Helleb., Ruta, Spigel.

Bruised pain to touch: Graph., Nux vom., Stront.

Bruised pain as if in the cord: Magn. m.

Bruised pain in the cervical vertebræ: Sabin.

Bruised pain in the sacrum: Coccul.

Sore pain in the cervical vertebræ: Digit., Sepia.

Soreness in the lower dorsal vertebræ, Chelid. m.

Cracking of the joints: Acon., Anac., Ant. cr., Camph., Caps., Cocc., Crocus, Ledum, Merc. viv., Nitr. ac., Nux vom., Petrol., Phosph., Rhus tox., Sabad., Sulph., Thuja.

Sleeplessness: Acon., Arsen., Bell., Borax, Bryon., Calc. os., Caust., Cham., Cinch., Cocc., Coff., Con., Cros., Graph., Hepar, Hyosc., Ignat., Kal. c., Laches., Merc. viv., Natr. c., Nitr. ac., Nux vom., Op., Phosph., Puls., Ran. bulb., Rhus tox., Selen., Sepia, Silic., Sulph., Thuja.

In addition to these, all the other remedies mentioned under after symptoms, have sleeplessness, but generally in less marked degree.

Sleeplessness, before midnight, especially: Arsen., Bell., Borax, Bryon., Calad., Calc. os., Carb. an., Carb. veg., Cinch., Graph., Hepar, Ignat., Kal. c., Laches., Ledum, Lycop., Marum, Merc. viv., Mur. ac., Phosph., Puls., Ran. bulb., Rhus tox., Selen., Sepia, Silic., Spigel., Sulph., Valer.

Sleeplessness after midnight: Arsen., Asaf., Aurum, Cann. sat., Capsic., Coff., Dulc., Hepar, Kal. c., Magn. c., Natr. c., Nux vom., Ran. scel., Rhodod., Sepia, Silic., Sul. ac.

Sleeplessness with drowsiness: Acon., Arsen., Bell., Bryon., Calc. os., Caust., Cham., Cinch., Con., Hepar, Kal. c., Merc. viv., Natr. c., Nux vom., Phosph., Phos. ac., Puls., Rhus tox., Sepia, Silic., Sulph.

Aggravation from changes of weather: Bryon., Mangan., Merc. viv., Nux mosch., Phosph., Rhodod., Rhus tox., Silic., Sulph.

Aggravation from windy or stormy weather: Bryon., Cham., Cinch., Laches., Mur. ac., Nux mosch., Nux vom., Puls., Rhodod., Rhus tox.

Aggravations from thunderstorm: Bryon., Caust., Laches., Natr. c., Natr. m., Nitr. ac., Petrol., Phosph., Rhodod., Silic., Elaps. (fear of rain).

Sensation of fatigue: Agaric., Alum., Ambra, Arnic., Bryon., Calc. os., Calc. phos., Camph., Cann. sat., Caust., Coccul., Con., Crocus, Hepar, Ipec., Magn. c., Merc. viv., Nux vom., Paris, Platin., Puls., Rheum, Rhodod., Rhus tox., Sulph., Tart. em., Veratr.

Weakness: Agaric., Anac., August., Arsen., Baryt. c., Bell., Bism., Bryon., Calc. os., Calc. phos., Cact. gr., Camph., Cann. sat., Canth., Canst., Cham., Cinch., Colch., Cupr. m.,

Digit., Ferr., Fluor. ac., Ignat., Iod., Kal. c., Lycop., Merc. viv., Natr. c., Nitrum, Nitr. ac., Nux mos., Nux vom., Oleand., Petrol., Phosph., Phos. ac., Plat., Puls., Rhodod., Rhus tox., Sec. corn., Sepia, Silic., Stann., Sulph., Sul. ac., Thuja, Veratr., Viol. od., Zinc.

Fainting: Acon., Arnic., Arsen., Bryon., Camph., Cann. sat., Cham., Cinch., Coccul., Coloc., Creos., Digit., Ferr., Hepar, Hyosc., Ipec., Laches., Mosch., Nux mos., Nux vom., Phosph., Sepia, Silic., Stram., Veratr., Viol. od.

Coldness along the spine: Baptis., Gelsem.

Chill on the knees: Cinch., Menyan., Puls.

Coldness of the knees: Agn. cast., Carb. veg., Puls.

Sweat of the palms: Acon., Amm. m., Anac., Calc. os., Cham., Con., Dulc., Fluor. ac., Ignat., Ledum, Merc. viv., Nux vom., Sulph.

Sweat of the feet: Angust., Baryt., Calc. os., Cann. sat., Canth., Carb. veg., Coccul., Coloc., Cupr. m., Fluor. ac., Graph., Iod., Kal. c., Ledum, Lycop., Magn. m., Natr. m., Phosph., Phos. ac., Puls., Sepia, Silic., Staph., Sulph., Thuja.

FLORIDA AS A CLIMATE CURE.

BY A. G. AUSTIN, M.D., WILLIAMSON, NEW YORK.

HAVING been induced, partly by friends and partly from a sense of duty, to set forth some of the many facts that have come under my observation during a sojourn of three and a half months in Florida, I deem it proper to give a geographical sketch of the country, which will enable the reader to judge more correctly as to the condition of things as they actually exist in that State.

Florida is heralded in many papers and periodicals and loud-toned voices, to be the great haven where invalids may find rest, comfort, a good climate, and final restoration from their diseases.

Jacksonville is located about twenty-five miles from the ocean on the St. John's River. This place is said to have fifteen thousand inhabitants, and lies above the river high enough to prevent overflowing. I have been told that there is no drainage of any account in the city and never has been; all the excrement of the city lies upon the surface of the ground, mouldering and infesting the atmosphere to such a degree, that upon rising in the mornings its odor is plainly perceptible, so that any one can smell it very plainly. The hot sun and perchance a sea-breeze may dissipate it, so that the air seems quite pure during the middle of the day. In the month of last December, I stayed in Jacksonville for a few days, during which time I learned of several cases of sickness of a malarious character. About the 20th of March I came through there again, and was told by people living there, that there was any amount of typhoid fever, and that many were dying from its effects. Some of the cases of sickness take on the intermittent, some the remittent, and some the true typhoid form. Most of these latter die, or else the constitutional health is left badly impaired.

The St. John's River is slow, rather shoal, and from two to three miles wide. Its waters are of a dark color (the color of lye), caused by the tannin from the palmetto roots. From Jacksonville I went up the river seventy-five miles to Pilatka, another place quite noted—on paper—for health and happiness. On my way up I found the river studded on both sides with low grass, peats, or swamps, that in many instances extend a considerable way inland and end in some low hole, dignified with the title of "lagoon," or lake. The river has low banks, with now and then a rise of two to ten feet, extending back from the river a short distance, and losing itself in a swamp, or what is called a "flat-wood." These "bluffs" are generally planted with orange groves. If great care be not exercised, the atmosphere will generate a mouldy vegetable growth on the surface of the trunks, and impart a sort of pallor to the tops of these trees, and they contract what Floridians call the "die back." The people all along this river are pale, lean, shrivelled, sallow, and hungry-looking, with sunken eyes and hollow cheeks.

Pilatka is called a very healthy place. It is built on one of these bluffs. One-fourth of a mile back, in any direction, will be found a low wet swamp, quite as low as the surface of the river, and hence undrainable. Indeed there is no drainage in Pilatka itself. All the excrement of the town is left on the surface to fester and rot, and help make up the health record. I found here several individuals who had come in search of health, among whom were two young men from New York city, who said that since their arrival in Florida they were bothered to get their breath, and that there seemed to be no stimulating properties in the atmosphere. These men were able to walk about the streets, yet I prognosed in the case of one of them, a fatal termination of his case within one week, if he remained in that climate,—a prediction which was speedily verified. His young companion soon left for home.

Another case I saw was affected in the same way, and he started further up the river to "find a place where he could breathe." Several other cases I met with were pale, weak, and just able to be out of doors a part of the time. They would answer invariably that they had the fever.

Not feeling very well satisfied with Pilatka, we took a steamer, about the middle of December, and ran up the St. John's twenty-five miles, and then struck out into the Ocklawaha,—a river much like the St. John's, only a little more so. It is bounded on both sides by swamps, lagoons, low wet pine-lands, prairies, etc. There are not on this river half a dozen huts—they call them dwellings—for a distance of two hundred miles. The swamps are cypress, covered with water, as are also the pine-lands, and useless for cultivation. All this country seems to be good for, is pasturage, and a residence for herons and alligators. Two hundred miles above the mouth of the Ocklawaha we found a few marks of civilization, on Lake Griffin, Lake Harris, and Lake Eustace, all lying near together in Orange County. Around these lakes are high pine-lands, just high enough to catch all the malaria that rises from the lakes, lagoons, and marshes, lying in close proximity thereto. I stopped on Lake Eustace for two weeks, and looked the country over closely. The inhabitants are all of the same cast and color, and ready to put off until to-morrow what ought to be done to-day. Quinine and bilious pills are the staple articles of commerce. Those families that can afford it, put Quinine on the table and take a dose of it all around in lieu of asking a blessing, and as a prelude to the hog and hominy. In the counties of Marion and Alachawa, the foundation is sandstone, and I have been informed by a man who owns property in Marion County, that it is very sickly in those counties, the prevailing malady being malarial fever, with some yellow fever in the summer season. He further stated that many families have left those counties in consequence of sickness. In Orange County the lands are principally pine-lands, the soil being dry and sandy, and the thermometer ranging through December and January, from 70° to 85° through the day, and running down at night to 45° or 50°, with a fog, four nights out of seven, so heavy, that it drips off the trees in the morning sufficiently to wet a person through in a little while. I saw several cases of phthisis, catarrh, angina, and general debility, while in that vicinity, and all except one went away no better than when they came. The remaining one had just arrived, and of course, did not know how it would affect him.

I got tired of this kind of weather and food, and went across the country thirty miles by wagon, and reached a point on the St. John's River, some two hundred and fifteen miles up, at a place called Sanford. Did not stop here long enough to learn the state of health around the country. I saw at Sanford several cases from the West, in search of health. Three of the party were getting worse every day, and one of them told me they should go home as soon as one of their party got well enough to start, as Florida was no place for them. Several others were creeping around in search of something they could not find,—health.

From Sanford we went up the river into Lake Jessup and travelled the country over in that vicinity for two weeks. This lake is skirted all around with a green vegetable growth, that on a foggy morning, would stink a dog out of a tan-yard. I found, back in the country, low pine and hummock lands, wet and swampy, and the Floridians call this a healthy country, except about eight months in the year, when they have a low grade of chills and fever. The celebrated Dr. Foster, of Clifton Springs, New York, notoriety, has an orange grove and a cottage two and a half miles back from the lake. He also owns other lands (as I am informed) which he would like to dispose of, and, in order to accomplish this end, is blowing aloud for this dilapidated hell-hole. There are several families located in that vicinity, all praising up the country, and three out of every four of them wanting to sell out and get away. They are all poor, that is, thin in flesh, sallow, and poorly fed. A robust, fleshy man you cannot find, unless he has recently came from the North or West. A rosy-cheeked girl is a thing heard of but not seen in that country.

I suppose that it takes a certain given amount of certain elements to make an atmosphere, no more and no less, in all countries. Well, suppose this atmosphere becomes pregnant with malaria from swamps, rivers, lagoons, and in most of the towns, all the effluvia from decayed vegetation, out-houses, cesspools, etc., and then add heat enough to make it 70° to 96° in the shade, and some days 115° in the sun, and falling at nights to 45° and 55°, with a moisture every three out of five nights that will wet a person through and through; then add a poor, feeble diet, and I will leave it for any intelligent physician to decide what to think of the prospects of a case of phthisis, catarrh, or any other form of exhausting disease, coming perhaps from a clear, pure, bracing atmosphere, and a bountiful table, to place itself under such sanitary (?) influences as those I have described.

THE HYGIENE OF MEDICAL EDUCATION.

BY A. C. REMBAUGH, M.D., PHILADELPHIA, PA.

(Read before the Philadelphia County Homœopathic Medical Society.)

BY the term education, is meant discipline of the intellect, establishment of principles, culture of the heart, and healthy development of our bodies. This embraces education in general. Our theme is the hygiene of *medical* education. It is unnecessary here to go further into definitions. When first thinking over this subject I intended to write *general* instead of medical, but found that there was enough to be said in a brief paper on medical education alone, and especially so as all general culture should be a copy of the education which we ought reasonably to expect in connection with the science and art of medicine.

But, according to my ideas, the doctors are only blind leaders of the blind, together falling into the same pit. The same cramming system, from first to last, in medical as in general culture. The question is, how much and how fast, not the cultivation of all the powers and senses practically.

Would it not be just as reasonable to attempt to make a shoemaker or a tailor by having him listen to a couple of courses of lectures in two years, or a three years' graded course, of five months each, and from six to eight lectures a day; as to follow the present mode of making doctors? I maintain that a doctor, with proper qualifications for his calling, cannot be made in this way (any more than Charlemagne could convert his subjects to Christianity by simply having them baptized, as he was foolish enough to try to do). This I say from personal experience. The school and the college are the places for laying a foundation, broad, deep and enduring; and, if it is not laid there, there will be one endless groping about and uncertainty, and a very unsatisfactory career. The college course in medicine should be extended to four years at least; the lecture term, to nine or ten months of each year, and the six to eight lectures a day of an hour each, either be reduced to one-half that number, or the lecture be shortened to one-half hour; the lectures to be alternated with practical manipulative instruction in all the various branches.

The lectures should, whenever possible, be made object lessons, and supplied with every obtainable means for illustrating to the eye as well as the ear. Each student might be supplied with a lump of clay to model the various bones and organs of the body as the lecturer proceeded. It would be a greater assistance to him than the expensive models now used. If physiological and many other lectures were illustrated by means of the projecting microscope there would be the keenest interest manifested, as the eye can take in at a glance, a story that might take an hour to tell or illustrate by drawings or the blackboard.

The past few years have shown great advancement in the use of ocular demonstrations in medical teaching, and with a great saving of mental strain to the student. Now add to this practical manipulations, and the advancement will be far more rapid.

Taking notes and memorizing them, after a day passed in the lecture-room, is a species of refined cruelty common to all institutions of learning; and, after the lecture-course is completed, a learned essay on some abstruse scientific subject is required from the student's already overtaxed body and brain. Then comes the dreaded examination, when every nerve is wrought up to its utmost tension, and a still more refined cruelty is added, by making this examination competitive for some little bauble or other. All competitive examinations are an abomination, a vice of this crowding and crowded age. Following all this, in too many instances we meet with cases of broken health, and even loss of life. We always hear of them after each commencement day, and class them among the heroes and martyrs of a glorious cause, instead of placing them where they belong, among the victims of voluntary manslaughter and suicide.

I might add something about the ventilation of our classrooms. The atmosphere, heavy with the fumes of tobacco, and the exhalations from exhausted bodies, are enough to overcome an occasional visitor, though the student becomes inured to them, our bodies can so accommodate themselves to impurities and impure surroundings, for a time at least, with immunity. The tobacco vice is one that physicians should be exempt from. I think the co-education of the sexes would modify this practice very much. All sex distinctions are a violation of the best laws of hygiene.

FOOD AND ITS PREPARATION.

BY J B. KNIFFIN, M D., PHILADELPHIA, PA.

(Read before the Philadelphia County Homœopathic Medical Society.)

A FOOD is a substance, which, when introduced into the body, supplies material which renews some structure or maintains some vital process. The preparation of food should, therefore, always have reference to its perfect assimilation to the powers of digestion.

The great law, "know thyself," is of no less value in the physical than in the moral being. As homœopathists we individualize, and each human being should endeavor to do this in his food. But the preparation of it is of the utmost importance. The habits of life of a people inhabiting a belt or zone are quite uniform, and will be found to conform to a general law remarkably well. Thus, in the hot regions, succulent food, as fruits and vegetables, with but a small portion of meat, is required. As we proceed toward the colder parts of the earth, this condition of things is changed, until we find man requiring an almost entire diet of fat from animals and fish, which would seem to furnish proof that it is by the combustion of this, with other non-nitrogenous food, that animal heat is produced.

In this climate, where so great a variety of food is in use, there should be the best possible education in the culinary art. And, as I desire this paper to have somewhat of a practical value, I shall speak of a few of our most common foods and give some rules for their preparation.

The nitrogenous elements found in muscular flesh and in albumen furnish, to a large extent, the material for building up the body, and supplying its waste tissues. Beef stands at the head of this list, and its preparation for the table should be by roasting or boiling, that the fibres may not be toughened by heat or coated by lard, which is often done in frying. I think that beef tea is a popular delusion, as it contains little else than the flavor with some of the salts, while much that is nutritious is left undissolved. Unless it is prepared by some process that will preserve its fibrin and albumen, it will fail of its purpose. There is an excellent article sold, known as "liquid beef," made by subjecting it to muriatic acid, then to pepsin, and lastly to pancreatin, which will readily be seen to be easily assimilated by a patient with feeble digestion. Mutton, being of a lighter, looser texture, is better suited to persons of sedentary habits, and those who are physically weak, and is always preferable to beef in dysenteric patients. Pork is the poor man's meat, for although it contains less nourishment than beef or mutton, the process of "curing" renders it very palatable, and the price brings it within his reach. It is, unfortunately, subject to disease, and being presented uncooked in the form of sausages, highly seasoned and dried, it may contain the cysticercus or trichina, rendering it an unsafe article of diet, unless well and thoroughly cooked.

Albumen, as found in eggs, is very nutritious, and is more easily digested when but slightly coagulated by heat, than when rendered hard by long boiling. The flesh of fowls is less nutritious than beef or mutton, but being rich in phosphates is suited to brain-workers, and the same may be said of fish.

Butter comes among the first on our list of non-nitrogenous foods, and the manufacture of this directly from the fat of animals has given rise to some discussion as to its real standing in the market. It is undoubtedly butter, with all its elements, but retains the tallow taste and odor. It is stated that there were 98,000,000 pounds sold last year. These fats have always been used as a substitute for butter, by those unable to procure that article, and even by others, and the manufacture of oleomargarine may yet prove to be a great public boon.

Passing now to the vegetable kingdom, we find them divided into the same two classes: nitrogenous and non-nitrogenous. This has given rise to the opinion that man could live without meat and suffer no loss, mental or physical. The late Professor Mussey advocated this view, and adopted it through a long life in the practice of surgery. In our climate the demand is irresistible for a variety from both sources. The attempt has often been made, in the treatment of diabetes, to cure the disease by restricting the patient to muscular flesh, but without success.

This class of aliments is largely represented by seeds, especially the cereals,—wheat, rye, oats, barley, etc., but the first is our great staff of life, because it contains in the greatest abundance the elements we need. The best flour is not the whitest; but bran bread for nourishment is a delusion, being so difficult of digestion that it acts as a foreign substance in the bowels, thereby increasing unduly the peristaltic motion.

Flour is adulterated largely by the use of rice, potatoes, starch, plaster of Paris, alum, etc., which cannot be said to improve it.

Oatmeal is becoming a very popular article of diet, and we

recommend it for school children especially. It should be thoroughly cooked, and the only way to accomplish this is by means of the farina kettle, the arrangement of which is well known. It should be placed over the fire at night, and cooked until morning. It is then very palatable and wholesome. The same mode of preparing rice may be adopted with advantage.

In reference to liquids used with our food, the less the better, slow and thorough mastication calling forth sufficient secretion from the salivary glands for all purposes. But the question is asked on every hand as to the advisability of using tea and coffee. The answer is obviously against their use. Experiments with tea and coffee, show the one to be an antidote to the other. Tea increases the action of the skin, lessens the force of the circulation, cools the body, and does not cause congestion of the mucous membranes; whilst coffee, by diminishing the action of the skin, lessens also the loss of heat of the body, but increases the heart's action and excites the mucous membranes. In one experiment, the subject, after taking an infusion of two ounces, was thrown to the floor unconscious in consequence of a large amount of fluid being suddenly abstracted from the blood and thrown into the intestines.

In closing this subject I will speak of alcohol, as it has been claimed lately that it is a true food. The experiments with it have not proven it. It is true that all the alcohol taken into the system was not accounted for in the excretions, but that which was collected was still unchanged, showing that the difficulty was in its collection.

Lager beer, now so largely used, has some claim to being a food, but the mischief of beer-drinking, lies in its giving rise to an appetite for the more stimulating alcoholic drinks, and as humanitarians, it is our duty to discourage its use.

The succulent fruits and vegetables perform an important work in preventing scorbutic diseases, which is difficult to explain, but is very evident to one deprived of them for any great length of time. Many cases of intermittent fever will yield to a few glasses of lemonade. Vinegar in excess should of course be avoided.

We have had recently under discussion, the use of condensed milk as a food for infants, and, being opposed to the use of it, I would present some observations made by Dr. Daly, of London. He says, children become fond of it from its extreme sweetness, and refuse other food more suitable for them when the coming teeth indicate it. He now gives, as a reason for not using it, that while children seem to thrive upon it and look fat and healthy, the flesh is not solid, the appearance is deceptive, and when disease attacks the child, it has not the power of resistance, requiring a resort to stimulants much sooner than is the case with children fed upon new milk. He has noticed that children fed on condensed milk are much more backward in walking. He attributes the trouble to the excess of sugar, which lessens its nutritive value, and induces a tendency to starvation of muscular tissues.

SANITARY PRECAUTIONS IN MEASLES.

BY CHARLES MOHR, M.D., PHILADELPHIA, PA.

(Read before the Philadelphia County Homœopathic Medical Society.)

SANITARY precautions in measles are rarely, if ever, observed. This statement applies to the profession as well as to the laity; and even our Board of Health, so far as I can learn, has taken no other cognizance of this highly contagious disease than to note, perhaps, that the number of deaths from measles during the last three months has been unprecedentedly large. Mr. George E. Chambers, Registrar of the Health Office, has kindly furnished me with tables, a reference to which shows that for the three months, beginning February 1st and ending May 1st, the deaths from measles exceeded those from scarlatina and small-pox combined. I append the figures, viz.:

Measles:	Adults, 3;	Minors, 84.	Total,	. . . . .	87
Scarlatina:	" 1;	" 55.	"	56	Combined total, . 84
Small-pox:	" 7;	" 21.	"	28	

What ratio the deaths bear to recovery is not ascertainable, as in measles no returns of non-fatal cases are required by the Philadelphia authorities. This much is certain, however, that the cases of measles during the last few months have been quite virulent; and this has been the case not only in this city, but in other places, notably so in Brooklyn. Measles is not, as it is commonly held to be, a trivial disease. True, some epidemics of measles, as well as of scarlatina and variola, are quite mild and the deaths few; but it must be borne in mind, that like the other eruptive diseases named, measles has at times proved very fatal.

In our own city there were 248 fatal cases in 1835, and 221 fatal cases in 1866; but if the mortality during the balance of the year 1880 should be proportionate to the deaths since January 1st, the number will be much in excess of the totals of the years above mentioned.

According to Woodward, out of 21,676 cases of measles in the American army, over 2.5 per cent. perished merely from the fever, without reckoning the numerous complications. The greatest fatality, however, has been observed in other countries. Thus, in 1749–50 there died on the river Amazon, according to D'Alves, 30,000 Indians, and a similar excessive mortality occurred in British North America.

At Madagascar, in 1806, 5000 cases died in one month. According to Seidl, in the district of Zolkiew, in 1840, almost 13 per cent. proved fatal. The mortality in many other places in various epidemics has reached fully 10 per cent.

In the Children's Hospital at Stockholm, of 131 cases, 36 per cent. died. At the Children's Hospital in Würzburg, in the epidemic of 1863, 10.5 per cent. died. In the Vienna Children's Hospital the deaths in 1864–1867 were 98 out of 372 cases. Watson writes that, at the London Foundling Hospital, 1 in 10 died in one year, and in another year 1 in 3. According to statistics extending over eleven years, of 1000 deaths in London, 27 are due to measles.

We thus see that the mortality in some epidemics has been large; and the experience of the past few months leads us to the conviction that it may prove larger in this country during the next few years than it has been in the past. I believe the mortality has been larger really than the records at the Health Office show. Even physicians participate in the common belief that measles is a mild disease; and when a death does occur in their practice it is returned as due to some one of the various complications, viz., meningitis, hydrocephalus, convulsions, congestion of the brain, congestion of the lungs, bronchitis, pneumonia, croup, diphtheria, or dysentery. True, any one of these complications may have been the immediate cause of death, but the remote cause was measles.

In this connection it may be well to remind you that, leaving out of the question such complications or sequelæ as catarrhal ophthalmia, otorrhœa, and lymphangitis in strumous patients, it is not uncommon for children, apparently recovered from measles, or convalescent, to be seized anew with difficult respiration, and after a longer or shorter duration of the new disturbance to even die; sometimes of cheesy pneumonia, with or without tubercles; sometimes from general miliary tuberculosis, or tubercular meningitis, the causes of which, as it appears, must be especially sought for in the cheesy degeneration of the swellings of the lymphatic glands occurring in the course of the disease (Thomas).

Among the many dangerous complications, pneumonia is the most frequent, and appears, like capillary bronchitis, especially in and just after the cruptive stage. The fact that it *often* develops *in* the eruptive stage, and that, with the exacerbation of the fever, the intensity of the eruption at first increases, may justify us in considering the pneumonia, in some epidemics at least, as a stage of measles, rather than a complication.

Croup sometimes supervenes and cuts off young patients. It tends to be of the asthenic type, and is not unfrequently preceded by diphtheritic inflammation of the fauces, which gradually passes down to the larynx (Aitken).

As will be seen further on, the physicians of Brooklyn have repeatedly seen measles followed by diphtheria, some of the cases proving fatal. Severe chronic intestinal diseases, such as entero-colitis, with wearisome diarrhœa, intestinal ulcers and stenoses, etc., may result from affections of the small and large intestines in measles. It is a very common experience that, after epidemics of measles, the children who have been affected are more prone to all sorts of attacks than at other times, and, among the severe acute diseases, croupous pneumonia has frequently made its appearance for a period of several months after the conclusion of the epidemic, especially in winter and spring (Thomas).

During the present epidemic in our own city, several cases have been observed among my homœopathic and allopathic friends, exhibiting grave typhoid conditions, and in one case heart-clot was the immediate cause of death.

The literature of the subject, so far as quoted, gives us sufficient grounds to class measles among the graver affections. If time permitted we might quote largely to show, (1) that it is one of the most virulently contagious of diseases, and that its contagiousness is fully developed at a very early stage of the disease (Bristow); (2) that persons contract the disease from the miasm adherent to the clothes of those who have recently visited rubeolous patients (Flint), or from clothes sent home in boxes from schools where the disease has raged, and that no person can remain in the same room, or even in the same house, with an infected person without hazard of taking the disease (Aitken); (3) that one attack does not render a person non-susceptible to subsequent attacks.

With this array of evidence before us, is it too much to ask that we use the same sanitary precautions in measles that we do in other contagious maladies? The physician of the present day should not content himself with curing disease; his mission is also to prevent it! It therefore behooves us to combat the following prevalent notions concerning measles:

1. That every child must have measles at some period of its life.

2. That the younger the child the milder the attack will be, and hence, the sooner one has it the better.

3. That one attack protects from a second.

4. That attempts to isolate patients are useless.

5. That disinfection of clothing, bedding, etc., is unnecessary, as the disease can only be conveyed by a sick person.

As before remarked, Brooklyn, N. Y., has suffered greatly with measles, and from an article prepared by J. H. Raymond, M.D., Sanitary Superintendent, I glean much useful information; and, in respect to the prevailing idea, that measles is a trivial disease, he pithily says: "From practical local observation and careful investigation of the subject, together with the experience of Brooklyn physicians obtained from their answers to a series of questions sent them by the Board of Health, ... we believe that the general impressions . . . . are entirely erroneous, and, if permitted to go uncontradicted, liable to do great harm and injury even to the degree of sacrificing human life."

It is interesting to note that since January 1st, 1880, in Brooklyn, of 1864 cases of measles reported to the Health Department of that city, 82 cases proved fatal, while during the same time the deaths from scarlet fever numbered only 65.

The questions submitted to the physicians of Brooklyn by the Health Department, and the answers received thereto, I herewith append. 155 responses were received and analyzed.

a. Is measles, in your opinion, highly contagious?

139 answer, Yes. 15 answer, No. 1 answers, Moderately.

b. Is it, in your opinion, more or less contagious than scarlet fever?

60 answer, More. 46 answer, Less. 45 answer, Equally.

c. Is it, in your opinion, conveyed by *fomites?*

88 answer, Yes. 36 answer, No. 20 are undecided.

d. Is measles, at the present time, in your practice unusually malignant?

14 answer, Yes. 124 answer, No. 12 answer, Severe.

e. How many cases have you had in which diphtheria has supervened upon measles?

54 cases are reported.

f. In how many instances, *under your own observation*, has measles attacked the same person more than once? or more than twice? and at what intervals?

210 second attacks are reported, and 7 third attacks. The intervals vary between two weeks and twenty-eight years, the usual interval being about three years.

g. Have these recurrences been severe, or have prior attacks apparently modified them?

36 answer, More severe. 130 answer, No modification. 30 answer, Attacks modified.

In view of the facts elicited by these queries, the Brooklyn Board of Health has included measles in the same category with scarlet fever and diphtheria, and requires the following action:

1. Reports to be made to the Health Office by physicians, of all cases coming under their care.

2. The exclusion of the sick and of others residing in the same house from the schools of the city, both public and private, until a permit for their return is obtained from the Board of Health.

3. These permits to be given when the patient is no longer in condition to spread the disease, and when the rooms, clothing, and other infected materials have been properly fumigated.

4. The fumigation prescribed by the Board of Health is by the burning, for five hours, of sulphur, one pound to each thousand cubic feet of space to be fumigated, the apartment being tightly closed.

5. Certificates of physicians that these requirements have been fulfilled will be sufficient evidence, and on their presentation to a sanitary inspector, or at the office of the Board of Health, the school permit will be at once issued.

Pending whatever action our own Board of Health may take, it seems to the writer that our duty is plain. Let us report every case to the health officer, and use the same sanitary precautions, as far as they apply, in measles, that we do in other forms of contagious disease.

THE JESUIT'S TEST.

BY C. F. NICHOLS, M.D., BOSTON, MASS.

In these times of testing, with the journals full of microscopy and spectroscopy, your contributor may be pardoned for presenting a reminiscence.

In 1873, there occurred a practical test, by members of a

body held to be as inquisitorial as microscopists. Curiously enough, at that time certain practical men, detective in spirit, zealous, trained to research, on turning attention to a medical method, held its ability to remove disease to be of sole importance. They seemed to think this the final aim, service, and test of physicians.

In 1873 your contributor became acquainted with Rev. S. B., a Jesuit missionary, well known throughout the West as a successful pioneer of the Romish Church, the founder of an important college of the Jesuits. Of noble birth in France, and an erudite scholar, the reverend Father had known Hahnemann as his mother's physician and his father's occasional guest, and was familiar with the theoretical teachings of homœopathy. He now, from time to time, during several months, discussed with much subtlety and patience the doctrines of the school, expressing at last his conviction that they alone offer logical promise of explicable cures,—an interesting conclusion to be reached by a trained mind in view of the alleged absurd inconsistencies of Hahnemann.

Finally the following experiments and tests were instituted: Two sisters, of similar temperament, employed as domestics in an establishment where the reverend Father acted as confessor, were attacked, shortly apart, by abdominal typhus. Placed in separate apartments, with like ventilation and diet, these patients were treated respectively by the regular attendant of the institution and myself. The comparative comfort and rapid recovery of the subject of homœopathic treatment was favorably compared with the progress of the patient medicated by the old school. Convincing no one, these cases created interest in the treatment by homœopathy, and its similar success in other acute diseases finally gained the approval of the interested parties. Dunham's two-hundredth potencies were invariably used.

Now was brought forward a young girl whose troubles seemed likely to persist unless actively prevented. A dirty, phthisical remnant of small-pox; she had the itch; knew how she had caught it; had given it to another girl. The doctors had called it itch, and had ordered ointment, when the reverend Father captured her for the crucial test. Her *acari* we saw with the glass, between the fingers and on both feet. Such a cure was insisted on as should confirm § 246's footnote,* for I

---

* See Organon, Wesselhœft's translation, p. 215.—Eds.

was reminded that the perfect similimum *could* so vivify the body as to render its tissues distasteful to parasitic life.

This girl presented an excellent picture for sulphur's action. The fingers itched worse when washed; bathing the habitual dirt increased her catarrh and asthma; she had craving hunger and constipation.

Her garments and bedclothing were frequently washed and boiled. She bathed oftener as the skin grew less sensitive. Having given Sulph.^{200} twice during two weeks without apparent effect, the 12th potency was substituted, four doses, twelve hours apart, in water, every week, lengthening the interval when nearly well. Four months after, her general health was good, and she had no eruption.

Worms, acari, and other parasites ought to disappear under antipsorics; but I had then and have since usually failed to cause their disappearance until mechanically shocked.

I may add, that the reverend Father, who had submitted his protégés to this treatment, much after the manner of travellers who first try a new fruit upon another creature before partaking themselves, was now a steadfast advocate and patient of homœopathy, together with a portion of his colleagues and the inmates of the establishments under their control.

Nevertheless "there is nothing there." There isn't the true ring of gold nor the true grit of charcoal *higher* than the "mystick seven." How testily this is exclaimed! and so the rough shell inclosing a pearl, and the cotyledons withering from the full-juiced stalk which has pushed them aside, "must" be found.

Yet it is now unquestioned in the learned world, that most modern discoveries are the result of sheer observation of strange facts, which often become patent in science long before their explanation has been accomplished.

"It need hardly be said," says Professor Jevons, in a recent number of *The Contemporary Review*, "that it is to carefully planned experiments in the physical sciences we owe almost all the progress of the human race in the last three centuries."

RETENTION OF URINE—DISCUSSION.

BY JOHN COOPER, M D, ALLEGHENY, PA.

(Read before the Homœopathic Medical Society of Allegheny County, Pa, May, 1880)

THIS important, and frequently painful morbid condition is met with both among males and females, but occurs more frequently among males. When met with among men, from the formation of the parts concerned, it is generally more difficult to relieve, and from the greater difficulty in giving relief, there is oftener great distress arising from the retention. In women, the shortness of the urethra makes them less liable to this affection, and, for the same reason, it is in them more readily relieved, and when it does occur, pain is, as a rule, longer in coming on, owing to the greater capacity of the bladder.

As a morbid state requiring the interposition of art, it is important that the means for its relief be most carefully considered.

The causes of retention may have their seat either in the ureters, the bladder, or the urethra. When the cause is located in the *ureters*, it is due to a plugging up, or a constriction. A renal calculus may have lodged in some part of its course, preventing the urine from flowing into its natural receptacle, the bladder. When the cause lies in the bladder, there is either a condition of atony, or the sphincter vesicæ is spasmodically contracted, or contracted in consequence of an inflammatory condition. When the cause can be traced to the urethra, there is either an enlarged or hypertrophied prostate, a stricture, an abscess closing up the canal, an obstruction from a stone or other foreign body, or a congestion of the whole or part of the urethra. Injuries to the lower portion of the spinal cord should also be mentioned as causing retention through the medium of paralysis. Let us examine into these various causes, and determine suitable treatment for each individual case.

It may readily be seen, that when but one of the ureters is plugged, only a partial retention can occur, and, moreover, that we shall have to treat the patient for calculus instead of retention, which will disappear upon the passage of the calculus into the bladder.

We come next to the *bladder* to seek for the cause of retention, and find atony of that organ a prominent one. The patient has perhaps journeyed a long distance by rail, and from want of will-power has been unable to evacuate the contents of the bladder while the cars were in motion. The bladder has been overdistended, and atony is the result. The desire to void the urine has now ceased entirely. No amount of straining or pressure upon the lower portion of the abdominal walls will start the flow, but will only aggravate the distress of mind and body under which the patient always labors. We have been called, then, to relieve the patient, and it must be done with the least possible delay, for, aside from the danger of rupture of the bladder, or of uræmic poisoning, the patient is already the victim of a condition, to fully recover from which may take months, or even years. Every moment saved, therefore, is precious. We would recommend, then, that a piece of ice be placed underneath the prepuce, and if this mild stimulator should fail to start the flow, then try a hot sitz-bath, at the same time pressing gently, but firmly, against the lower portion of the abdomen, in the region of the bladder. One or other of these simple means, will very often suffice to afford relief; but should they fail to have the desired effect, we must promptly resort to catheterization. We should caution the patient to be very prompt in voiding his urine whenever he has even the slightest desire to do so, until the bladder regains its normal tone. But for a long time he may be unable to relieve himself, except by the use of the catheter, applied either by his physician, or by himself after careful instruction in the use of the instrument.

Spasmodic contraction of the sphincter vesicæ, or contraction from congestion, are other causes of retention. When it is spasmodic, Camphora will generally afford relief; or Nux, particularly if the patient has previously been drinking hard. When the contraction is due to congestion or inflammation, we have such remedies as Acon., Bell., Canth., and Puls. Should we fail with remedies, we still have the catheter as a final and sure resort. In the spasmodic form we may reach the sphincter with the instrument, but fail to effect an entrance to the bladder at once. Not at all discouraged by this circumstance, gentle and continuous pressure will either overcome the resistance in many cases or, failing in that respect, will so far distend the sphincter as to allow the urine to flow slowly into the urethra, and thence into and through the catheter. Having accomplished this, we have gained time to allow our medicines to act.

In the congestive or inflammatory form, a much smaller catheter than the ordinary size will be generally required (although some authorities debar catheters altogether), and must be used with the utmost gentleness. It is better to take the risk of doing a little harm to the inflamed and swollen cervix, than to risk having the very grave condition of atony supervene in consequence of delay. If, as happens in some cases, an entrance cannot be effected, we must resort to aspiration, either *per rectum*, or, in case we are unable to reach the bladder by this route, as in the event of a very large prostate shutting us off from this far preferable course, the supra-pubic operation may be performed. Either of these methods can be resorted to with perfect safety and very little pain to the patient. The puncture made by the stylet will usually give no trouble, but will close the instant the canula is withdrawn.

Coming next to the *urethra* in our search for the cause of retention, we find that enlarged prostate holds a prominent place in the catalogue. If it is so much enlarged as almost or entirely to close the urethra at this point, it may be that the aspirator will afford the only means of relief. But catheterization, skilfully performed, will very often help us out of the dilemma. If the enlargement be but temporary, as from inflammation, the urine may be drawn by means of the aspirator, until, by the action of remedies, the inflammation is subdued, when the urine will flow, as before, through the natural channel. If the enlargement is a real hypertrophy, such as falls to the lot of many elderly men, we can hope for no relief from remedies, but must rely entirely on instruments. Of the catheters, there are two forms which promise the best chances of success from their use. They are the English, overcurved, and the French, nearly straight catheter, with an elbow half an inch from the point. With one or other of these it is generally possible to ride over the obstruction and enter the bladder, and, if the operation has to be repeated often, the patient may be taught to do it himself.

Stricture will frequently be found a cause of retention. It must be overcome by gradual dilatation. Still another cause, although of extreme rarity, is abscess in the walls of the urethra, stopping up the channel, and causing extreme pain. It may either be operated upon with the urethrotome or by bursting with the catheter or bougie.

Obstructions in the urethra from stones or other foreign bodies may be sufficient to stop the flow of urine. They may either be extracted by the urethral forceps or be removed by the operation of urethrotomy,

Injuries to the lower portion of the spinal cord, causing paralysis, will be followed by retention, which may last for an indefinite period or even be permanent. Our main dependence here is the catheter. Very little can be done with remedies.

The last form of retention I notice is that occurring in the newborn. If the urethra is perforate it will readily yield to a few doses of Acon. or Canth.

DISCUSSION.

Dr. Burgher: One important consideration in the use of

the catheter for the relief of retention due to atony of the bladder is, to withdraw only a portion of the urine at a time. The walls of the bladder will, by this means, sooner regain their tonicity and contractive power.

DR. J. H. MCCLELLAND: The paper brought out many important points in this affection. There is one symptom which is now considered to be an important diagnostic sign, and that is incontinence. Incontinence of urine in the majority of cases, is due to retention from an atonic state of the bladder, the result either of circumstances arising in the course of delayed evacuation of the bladder, so that it becomes overdistended, or from some affection of the cord, such as paralysis, or from an enlarged prostate. From this overdistension we have frequently an overflow of urine. Incontinence is this overflow. We should be particular in our inquiries in regard to the passing of the urine, as to quantity, regularity, frequency, etc. The attendant will often tell you that the patient is passing water frequently, and yet the bladder may contain a large quantity of water. This is true in fevers and prostrating diseases, where the mental faculties are clouded, and the patient makes no effort to evacuate the bladder.

One case which came to my knowledge was treated by a prominent practitioner for typhoid fever. There was an enlarged prostate, causing overdistension, and as a result, retention and incontinence. Attention was drawn to the frequent passing of water, but no careful examination was made. Another physician was called in consultation, who detected the difficulty, introduced a catheter, and drew off a large quantity of water. After a long sickness, the patient gradually recovered, but was compelled to use the catheter every day. I treated him finally, and he seemed to regain some power of the bladder under the use of Causticum. Catarrh of the bladder generally follows in these cases of long standing. Another I was called to see, in which fibroid tumor of the rectum had been diagnosed. The attendant said the urine was passed frequently, and that the catheter had been used without bringing away any discharge. I used the catheter, but could obtain no urine, although there was distension over the bladder. I requested the patient to stand up, but there was still no discharge for some time, then the water began to come away slowly, and by pressing on the tumor, about two quarts of urine was passed. There was no marked enlargement of the prostate, but from carelessness he had allowed the bladder to become gradually distended. We should distinguish carefully between the almost constant escape of urine, and those cases where there are distinctly marked intervals. When we find both incontinence and distension, the catheter should be used. Elongation of the prepuce in children is given as a cause of retention, and finally of incontinence.

Dr. McClelland here exhibited several steel spiral catheters, and called attention to their use, in comparison with other catheters.

Dr. Ferson: Would you suspect retention where there was constant dribbling, but no marked constitutional symptoms?

Dr. McClelland: In all these cases you will generally find some indications of distress, as for instance, slight fever and occasional pain.

Dr. Pitcairn called attention to retention following childbirth, as a condition to be guarded against.

Dr. Seip: In such cases Arsenicum is an important remedy.

Dr. McClelland: I used Stannum in one case.

Dr. Martin: Arsenicum is of value, also, in cases occurring in typhoid fever, or even in those in apparent health. In one case where a child was troubled with retention and pain in passing water, due to elongation of the prepuce, circumcision brought immediate and permanent relief. In cases requiring a steady use of the catheter, how often is it necessary to use it in twenty-four hours?

Dr. Burgher: I would say, once in from four to six hours. Where a physician cannot see the patient so often, relief can be obtained by leaving a flexible catheter in the bladder, and thus the patient be enabled to empty it at will, by simply removing a plug from the catheter.

Dr. Martin: I know that the books recommend that the urine should be drawn frequently. I knew, however, one case where the catheter was only used once in twenty-four hours, and the case did well.

Dr. Willard: I have found good results from the English catheter. I used it lately in a case, where the prostate was enlarged. In this case several physicians had failed to introduce a catheter. On making another attempt, the attending physician passed the English catheter very easily. He left it in the bladder, but on removing it, after some days, he could not replace it. A French gum catheter was then used successfully. This caused pain on being left in the bladder, and had to be removed. After this the English catheter could be freely used again.

Dr. Caruthers: In enlargement of the prostate the swelling is generally back of the gland, and in such cases I think the overcurved catheter would be the best. In one case reported, where the tumor was in the anterior portion of the gland, and had caused considerable trouble in attempting catheterization, it was not till a flexible catheter was used that the bladder could be entered. In enlarged prostate, the bladder is raised higher in the pelvis, and in such cases the long catheter here shown, would probably be of service. Retention from stricture, especially spasmodic, where there is inability to pass the catheter, often needs the aspirator to give relief. In these cases the stricture often disappears with the evacuation of the bladder by the aspirator, and thus the necessity for dilatation is avoided. In cases of extra-urethral abscess causing retention of urine, this should be opened before passing the catheter, otherwise rupture of the urethral walls may result.

DR. EDMUNDSON: In regard to the use of the aspirator in relieving stricture, I had one case where this was necessary, after a long attempt to relieve the patient by every other means. There was no trouble, whatever, in passing water the next morning when he awoke. In a second attack under another physician, the same means were used, and with like results.

DR. MARTIN: Anæsthesia will sometimes relieve, especially in children.

DR. EDMUNDSON: In the case mentioned, anæsthetics were freely used.

DR. MCCLELLAND: In the majority of cases, twice a day is sufficient for use of the catheter. In regard to leaving the catheter *in situ*, very careful discrimination must be made. Frequently the instrument becomes roughened or injured, and causes trouble in removing it. As a practical application of the catheter, where the patient can be seen but once a day, I introduce the catheter in the morning, and leave it in the bladder, telling the patient to empty the bladder once during the day, and in the evening, and then remove it. The next morning it is reintroduced.

DR. BURGHER: I do not advise the indiscriminate use of a retained catheter, but as being applicable to those cases arising from atony of the bladder, or causes producing similar results In such cases I would have no hesitation in allowing the catheter to remain in the bladder.

DR. WILLARD: In one severe case, in the beginning of my practice, where a severe inflammatory stricture had arisen from the use of nitrate of silver injections for gonorrhœa, the hot water sitz-bath, as hot as could be borne, together with opium in appreciable doses, gave relief. Both means had probably been efficacious in bringing about the desired result.

DR. HOFMANN: Has one case, where retention of urine frequently occurs, beginning always at 10 A.M., and lasting till 4 P.M. By taking Sarsaparilla[1], he obtains relief in a short time, but if the remedy is neglected, the trouble lasts as mentioned.

VOMITING OF PREGNANCY.

BY F. F. CASSEDAY, M D., STEVENS POINT, WIS.

I WAS much interested in Professor McClatchey's article in the May HAHNEMANNIAN on the above subject, but think he draws it a little too strong when he says he cannot conceive of a case where it would be necessary to procure abortion. I have recently treated a case, and now have it under my care, in which vomiting was persistent and continuous, and abortion was urgently indicated and performed.

I was called March 15th, 1880, to see Mrs. R—, a delicate blonde of 22 years. She complained of constant nausea, pain, and intense burning in the stomach, and the attendants informed me that she had been vomiting at short intervals for twenty-four hours. Very little nourishment had been given, as it was immediately ejected by the stomach. Suspecting pregnancy, I made an examination, and found the os soft and patulous, situated far back in the hollow of the sacrum, and well down on the floor of the pelvis. The fundus was thrown forward, and gave a sensation of pressure on the bladder. There had been no menstrual flow for three months. The pelvis was contracted, especially on the right side. Having settled my diagnosis, I prescribed Ipecac 3[x], gave directions for exhibiting small quantities of beef tea, and left. Called again the next morning, and found she was getting no better very fast. Vomiting had now become almost continuous, accompanied by painful retching and straining. The matter ejected was simply glairy mucus, together with the medicine and nourishment she had taken at short intervals. From this time until March 27th, the vomiting and violent straining continued with increasing severity in spite of the following remedies: Nux vom., Ars., Phos., Kreas., Carbol. acid, Apomorphia, Sepia, Ant. crudum, Nitrate bismuth, and Lycop. During this time the stomach had been intolerant of liquids of all kinds, and it was with difficulty that the most minute doses of medicine in trituration could be kept in the stomach or mouth long enough to be absorbed. Food was given during this time in liquid form per rectum, and consisted of beef tea and broths of various kinds. Having seen Hydrate of chloral recommended for this condition in the *Medical and Surgical Reporter*, I determined to try it as a last resort. I accordingly gave from 2 to 4 grains by the mouth every six hours, and 20 grains in solution per rectum, every evening. This controlled the vomiting and nausea completely, as long as she was under the influence of the drug, but they immediately returned on withdrawing it. She was kept under the drug continuously for four days, when it was gradually withdrawn. For two days after its discontinuance vomiting occurred but once. However, it soon returned with renewed intensity, accompanied with intense burning pain in stomach, œsophagus, and mouth, retching and violent general spasms. Her temperature and pulse, which previous to this time had been about normal, showed a marked elevation and acceleration. She also complained of chilly sensations at short intervals, cold feet and hands, and great faintness; "hardly had strength to breathe," as she expressed it. Stimulants, frictions, hot applications, and electricity improved her condition in this respect. From April 4th to 8th the following remedies were tried in vain: Puls., Oxalate of cerium, Acetate of morphia, and Sulphate of morphia. Counsel was called, and we decided to empty the uterus. Sound was accordingly introduced, hot water thrown against the os, and Ergotin given per rectum. No contractions were excited by this procedure, although the sound was introduced at intervals for ten days. During this time the following additional remedies were given: Acon. and Bryonia. Finally, on April 20th, the os was dilated by sponge tents and Atlee's dilator (this latter had been used previously), a mixture of Fl. ext. ergot and Gossypium was given by the mouth, expulsive contractions were excited, and the fœtus was discharged, followed by the placenta the next day. The uterus emptied itself of all the small clots and shreds of membrane on the third day, and the pains and vomiting ceased. There was a slight metritis developed on the sixth day, which was speedily controlled by hot fomentations and Aconite. She has gained strength and appetite steadily, and to-day (May 4th) she is in good condition. During her whole illness she was given ice freely, and liquid food, such as beef tea, chicken and mutton broth, Johnson's fluid beef, milk, cocoa, and Alkathrepta. Lime-water was used for a short time in the milk, but it was found to disagree, and was stopped.

I am just as firmly opposed to the production of abortion as my friend, Professor McClatchey, can possibly be, but I firmly believe it was absolutely necessary in this case, and especially so on account of the contracted pelvis. "But," I hear objectors say, "a few months more of gestation would probably have cured the vomiting, even if medicine did fail." Even so, my friends, provided her strength held out, and her system could stand the terrible strain. This kind of argument reminds me of the man, who was complaining over the fact that just as soon as he had taught his horse to live without eating, "the tarnal critter died."

Then, again, where vomiting does continue to full term, there is no certainty that emptying the uterus *then* will stop the vomiting. Cazeaux says that "cases of irrepressible vomiting are serious from the outset, inasmuch as, notwithstanding all modes of treatment employed, *abortion included*, it is impossible to know whether they will be certainly arrested." Of 118 cases collected by M. Guéniot, there were 72 recoveries and 46 deaths. Of the 72 recoveries, 41 occurred after abortion, either induced or spontaneous, and 31 recovered without abortion under very diversified treatment. Of the 46 deaths, 28 occurred *without abortion*, and 18 occurred *after* spontaneous or induced abortion. My conclusion, therefore, is, that induced abortion and premature delivery are valuable resources in intractable vomiting, and it is our duty to resort to them in cases where remedies fail and where the mother's life is in jeopardy. Finally, Cazeaux says: "When they reach the second period characterized by 1, almost incessant vomiting; 2, great debility; 3, continued fever; 4, and fetid breath (all of which my patient had); and when all medication has failed, it is right to advise abortion, leaving with the family the responsibility of deciding upon it as a last resort."

THE SANITARY CONDITION OF OUR HEALTH RESORTS.

BY B. F. BETTS, M.D., PHILADELPHIA, PA.

(Read before the Philadelphia County Homœopathic Medical Society.)

No one calls in question the fact, that climate is capable of exerting a powerful influence upon human health. This influence is the sum total of the influence exerted by the meteorological conditions, the condition of the soil, and the sanitary condition of the place. All of these influences should be taken into account before we decide whether the climate of a particular locality is capable of exerting a curative influence in a particular form of disease. *After* that, the experience of those who have personally tested the efficacy of the locality, should be considered.

This experience would be of very great value to the profession, if derived from a large number of persons, and accurate information in regard to the temperature, humidity, and sanitary condition of particular localities known as health resorts, would be of great service to the whole community.

When our municipal governments pay so much attention to the public parks and sanitary regulations of cities, it behooves the General Government to exercise a fostering care over our most valuable health resorts, so that the greatest amount of good may be accomplished by them, and their efficiency maintained for succeeding generations.

From a neglect of the proper sanitary regulations, some of our best health resorts are in danger of having soon to be abandoned. In view of these facts, I submit the following propositions:

1st. That the Bureau of Sanitary Science, Climatology, and Hygiene be requested to solicit from physicians (members of this society and others) their experience of the efficacy of the different health resorts for particular forms of disease, and incorporate such information in their next annual report to this society.

2d. That in view of the great advantage to be derived by the citizens of Philadelphia from the close proximity of our seaside resorts, and in view of the patronage our citizens give to these places, we urge the proper authorities to establish the very best sanitary regulations possible at these resorts, so as to insure for the future the same beneficial influences upon health, that a residence there now secures to us.

3d. That this society consider the propriety of petitioning the proper authorities at Washington to establish signal stations at health resorts wherever practicable, and that with the monthly meteorological reports from signal stations, there shall be rendered a statement of the mortality rate, disease tendency, etc., for the month, so that information required by physicians may be compiled by some central bureau, such as the National Board of Health, and distributed to such as make application for the same.

THE WARMING AND VENTILATION OF PUBLIC ASSEMBLY-ROOMS.

BY PEMBERTON DUDLEY, M.D., PHILADELPHIA, PA.

(Read before the Philadelphia County Homœopathic Medical Society.)

If the art of ventilation has seemed to be of slow growth, it has, perhaps, been as rapid as the advancement in our knowledge of the properties of the atmosphere would permit, except during the past few years. Its progress has, at any rate, been more or less steady, and has involved innumerable methods, from the crudest to the costliest; from Sir Christopher Wren's plan of cutting holes in the ceiling of the House of Commons—through some of which the warm air rushed out to irrecoverable waste, while through others the cold air from above, poured down upon the heads and shoulders of the British statesmen below,—on through various gradations to our own more costly and rather more efficient method, of mixing the warm air with the cold, the fresh with the foul, the clean with the dirty, and pumping out successive portions of the mixture through heated pipes.

It is certainly safe to assume, that if a knowledge of the atmosphere and its properties, and of man and his physiological necessities, can ever be sufficient to indicate a method of ventilating and warming apartments which shall be absolutely free from danger and discomfort, the time has already arrived, yea, it has been here for nearly half a century. We already know all about the local movements of the atmosphere and their causes, the changes occurring under the influence of heat and moisture, the causes and the quantity of its contamination in the presence of living beings, and the discomforts and perils consequent upon either a deficient or a vitiated supply of air to the lungs and the skin. It is possible that as regards the foundation principles, upon which we must learn to warm and ventilate our apartments, we never shall know much more than we know to-day. If, therefore, our present methods are imperfect and unreliable, it is because we have failed to apply the principles that underlie the subject, and which are sufficiently understood by the student of physical science.

In undertaking to decide upon the efficiency of present methods it is important first to know what constitutes perfect ventilation. In answer to this question it will be universally conceded that ventilation, to be considered perfect, must supply, in sufficient quantity, air of a proper *temperature* to secure perfect comfort, of a sufficient degree of *moisture* to maintain the health of the respiratory passages, yet not sufficient to prevent insensible perspiration, and of a *purity* equal to that of the external atmosphere for purposes of respiration, and that too without the necessity of opening doors and windows in cold weather. It may not be possible to come quite up to this standard, but I hope to show in the present paper, that we are falling very, very far short of it, while vast improvements in our methods are within easy reach.

The modern principle of ventilation includes the introduction of air, previously warmed, through grated openings, or "registers," located in or near the floor, and the removal of the vitiated air through similarly grated openings, or "ventilators," also placed in or near the floors, and communicating with a "shaft" or "upcast," so arranged as to be kept warm by the hot smoke and gases of the furnace chimney; the upward current or draft being aided, perhaps, by a "hood," "cowl," or some similar contrivance at the outlet above the roof. The relative position of the "inlet" and "outlet" is generally determined by the location of the chimney and the direction of the floor-joists; rarely indeed by the requirements of the room according to scientific indications. As a result of this plan (?), I can point you to a new schoolhouse in Philadelphia, provided "with all the modern improvements," in which the cold, foul air must pass *at right angles, directly through* the incoming current of warm, fresh air, in order to reach the outlet. Usually, however, the relative position of register and ventilator is much more reasonable than in the above instance. According to this method the idea is, that the warm, fresh air, upon entering the room, rises to the ceiling, distributes itself more or less evenly throughout the higher portion of the space, and gradually settles down to be used in respiration, and then to fall by its own increased gravity into the ventilators below. It would seem, however, that in some instances the air is supposed to rise at one side of the room, pass along the ceiling, then down the opposite wall, and along near the floor to the side of the room from which it entered, there to be received into the ventilating shaft, thus making a complete circuit of the apartment, and securing that wondrous desideratum of modern experts,—"a circulation of air,"—a phenomenon which may occur in a tornado, but never in an assembly-room.

Nearly all modern invention having reference to ventilation is designed to modify and improve this approved method; with what result we shall now proceed to show.

About five years ago the Board of Public Education authorized a sanitary inspection of the public school-rooms and buildings of Philadelphia. The writer was appointed to make this examination in the schools of the Fourteenth Ward, embracing some seventy school-rooms. In this ward, as also in the Second and Eighteenth, a large number of quantitative analyses of the air were made, for the purpose of testing the efficiency of the ventilating apparatus. Although in the three wards named we have some of the finest and most approved school buildings in the city, provided with the latest and best means and facilities for warming and ventilation, yet the investigation showed that in not one of the rooms so examined, could the air be maintained in even a tolerable condition of purity, notwithstanding the fact that the teachers were obliged in every case to supplement the action of the ventilators by opening windows, and thus involving the pupils and themselves in serious danger. From the reports of all the experts engaged in the inspection, it would seem that of the hundreds of modern school-rooms in our city, there is not even tolerably good ventilation in a single one of them. Thirty-eight modern rooms were subjected to the chemical examination above referred to, and the result showed that, although one or more windows were open in every case, yet there was an average of 14½ volumes of carbon dioxide ("carbonic acid," or CO_2) in 10,000 of air in all of them, *i. e.*, more than three times the normal quantity; while in some of them the quantity reached as high as 30 volumes or more. Had the windows been closed, and the whole work thrown upon the ventilating apparatus, the average according to present ideas, of course, would have been very much higher.

Surprising as these figures are, as exhibiting the inefficiency of our modern method of ventilation, our most interesting arithmetic is yet to come. It appeared that at the time these chemical estimates were made, each room contained an average of about forty scholars, their ages varying from six to perhaps sixteen years, or higher. Each scholar had an average of 187½ cubic feet of air space, and each room an average capacity of 7500 cubic feet. The inlet for warm air, exclusive of the grating, which partly covered it, averaged in section about 144 square inches, and was supplied by an ordinary furnace of large size. From some observations recently made, I am of opinion that such an apparatus, with the furnace kept just below a red heat on a moderately cold day, will furnish about 300 cubic feet of fresh warm air per minute; though this must, of course, be subject to great variation, depending much upon the freedom with which air is allowed to escape *from* the room, by ventilators or windows. These 300 feet of fresh air per minute will require at the shortest twenty-five minutes to fill the room, and a complete change of the air in the room, according to approximate calculations which I have made, will require from one and a half to two hours' time. Now, according to the observations of Andral and Gavarret, a person of twelve to sixteen years will exhale 915 cubic inches of carbon dioxide per hour, and a child of eight years 563 cubic inches. Let us then take 750 cubic inches as the average, and our forty pupils will exhale 30,000 cubic inches per hour, or 500 per minute. Reducing the 300 cubic feet of fresh air to inches, we have 518,400, or, to use round figures, just 500,000 cubic inches of air per minute. If with this we mix thoroughly our 500 cubic inches of carbonic acid, we shall have this gas constituting exactly 10 volumes in 10,000. Now add to these 10 volumes the 4 volumes which exist naturally in pure air, and it gives a total of 14 volumes in 10,000 of air. That is to say, if we place in a room, forty children, each about ten years old, and supply them with 5 feet of air per second, or 300 feet per minute, or 18,000 feet per hour, we may expect to find under the most unfavorable circumstances 14 volumes of carbonic acid in 10,000 volumes of air, and with our modern scientific method of ventilating rooms our experts actually do find 14½ volumes. In other words, our modern system is worth just a little less than no system at all.

But here the question will be asked, If under the conditions described it is possible to accumulate only about 14 volumes per 1000, how happens it that in some few instances the analyses showed the presence of 28 to 33 volumes? The explanation is, that in such cases, a large portion of the warm fresh air, almost immediately upon entering the room, has been allowed to escape at the top of an open window, without having first been mingled thoroughly and evenly with the foul air within. This, it will be seen, changes the conditions above given, just as completely as though a portion of the fresh air had been prevented from entering the room; and it is interesting as showing that when we open the windows of an assembly-room to obtain fresh air, we may be increasing the foulness of the atmosphere within, instead of diminishing it,—an apparent paradox that very few people have as yet learned to appreciate.

As a part of the investigation into the sanitary condition of our public schools, the committee of the Board of Education propounded to the teachers the question, "Does the ventilating apparatus give you enough fresh air, or do you have to open the windows?" This inquiry brought out from the 420 schools an emphatic, unanimous "No! we are obliged to open the windows even in cold and wet weather." It seems pretty conclusively shown, then, that of all the modern school-rooms of Philadelphia, provided with the best apparatus at present known, none of them are well ventilated; no! *not* ONE.

The reasons assigned by teachers for opening windows are, in a large proportion of the replies, first and chiefly, because of the foulness of the air, and, secondly, because the air is "too dry." This latter reason is probably not well founded, for it seems impossible to conceive of a crowded and illy ventilated room, in which the air would not be *over*charged with moisture from the lungs of the inmates. The real cause of the sensation of dryness is probably an unduly high temperature. If this be true, it only shows that the large quantities of CO_2, discovered by chemical analysis in the air of the rooms, is not to be attributed to any fault of the furnaces, or any deficiency in the consumption of fuel.

What is the remedy for this state of affairs? Is it possible, that for the balance of the lifetime of the human race, we shall have no better ventilation than such as we may hope to secure by some insignificant patching-up of the present methods? Does it not appear as if we should sooner or later be impelled to make *radical* changes in our plans, and to adopt principles entirely different from those in present use?

For a number of years past the writer has been impressed with a conviction that the warm, pure air, coming from registers placed in or near the floor, must of necessity be rapidly, and in a brief time completely, mingled with the cooler, fouler air, through which the column rises to the ceiling. This admixture is facilitated by a number of circumstances: 1st. The gratings of the register divide the ascending column into a large number of smaller columns, of various shapes and sizes, between which, the foulest, coldest air in the apartment makes its way to mingle freely and rapidly with the rising current. 2d. The natural effect of a current of any fluid, whether gas or liquid, is to draw a current toward itself from the surrounding liquid or gas in all directions; and particularly is this true, if the current increases its diameter as it flows, as is the case always with an ascending column of warm air. Here the lateral currents unite with and become a part of the ascending current, increasing its diameter, decreasing its velocity, and diminishing its temperature. 3d. The different temperatures of the various objects in the room—articles of furniture, window glass, wall surfaces, etc.—always excite local movements of the air in their immediate vicinity, thus aiding the intermingling process. 4th. The "diffusibility of gases," the property by which they are attracted by, and tend to mingle with each other, even when at perfect rest, also favors a complete admixture of the fresh air with the foul, the warmer with the cooler. If, now, we recall the fact already stated, that one and a half to two hours are required to completely change the air of one of our well-warmed school-rooms and replace it with fresh air from the heater, it will at once be understood how thorough and perfect this intermixing must inevitably be. If, however, any doubt on the subject should remain, it can easily be settled by the following very simple experiment. Let the general temperature of the room be first taken with a thermometer. We will suppose, for example, that it is 70° Fahr. Then note the temperature of the hot, fresh air at the moment it emerges from the register. Suppose it proves to be 170°, a very common figure. The difference between these two temperatures is just 100°. Now place the thermometer carefully in the very centre of the ascending current, and say four to eight feet above the register, when it will be found that the temperature has already fallen 50°, showing that the fresh, hot air has thus, in less than a second, perhaps, mingled with an equal volume of the cooler air which it encountered upon entering the apartment. I have made this experiment repeatedly, and I have here rather understated than overstated the results. In case the register is located in the side wall, instead of the floor, this degree of change will be affected by the time the air has reached a distance of *three* feet from the register.

We have thus shown that the fresh, warm air entering at the floor of a crowded assembly-room is pretty thoroughly mixed with fouler, colder air before it can be used in respiration at all, and that the foul air does not all remain near the floor, ready to be carried out by the ventilating apparatus, but that large portions of it are caught in the current of fresh air and whirled to the top of the room. The only place then, in which we shall find really pure air, is within a few inches of the register.

We have studiously kept all mere theories out of this discussion, and the facts we have presented make it almost unnecessary to say, that under the present system, perfect, or nearly perfect, ventilation is an absolute impossibility, and that even tolerably good ventilation can be obtained only by an enormous waste of fuel. The only way to secure excellence in the art of ventilating our churches, school-rooms, lecture halls, and hospital wards is by preventing, as far as possible, the warm air from mixing with the cold, the pure with the impure; for once they become so mingled, no art or contrivance can separate them again.

Practically, then, the warm air must be introduced in such a manner as to avoid swift currents. This may be accomplished in two ways. First, it may be introduced at a temperature only slightly raised above that of the room itself. This would prevent its rapid motion upwards, but it would fail to maintain a proper temperature of the apartment, and must therefore be rejected. The other method—and herein is the key to unlock this whole difficulty—consists in introducing the warm air through large and numerous openings, *not* at the bottom or sides, but *at the top of the room*, through the ceiling and cornice. If this current be directed downward, it will be speedily checked by the force of gravity, and the air will come nearly to a state of rest. There will, however, be a gentle movement of the whole mass of air downwards toward the floor, caused by the withdrawal of the cooler, fouler air through the ventilators below, and the constant influx of warmer air above. If the room be occupied by an audience, the respiratory "carbonic acid" will rise but a short distance above the "head line,"—four feet,—and will then fall towards the floor and flow off through the ventilators. I am of opinion that it would also be found practicable to introduce air at a considerably lower temperature than is done at present, and thus to increase the quantity of air without increasing the consumption of fuel, since under this method only the coldest air will be withdrawn through the ventilators, instead of a mixture of cold and warm air, as under the system in present use.

The method I have herein suggested, however, cannot be made available in its perfection, unless the warm air of the apartment is protected against the chilling effects of the window-glass, at least in very cold weather. The cooling effect of a window in freezing weather is precisely equal to that of a slab of ice of equal size. As a consequence, a rapid current of chilled air runs down along the window, and may be easily felt as a "draft" by a person sitting under it. The effect of a number of such windows, is to keep the air of the room in constant motion, a circumstance which would deprive our proposed method of much of its advantage. The remedy for this difficulty, consists simply in placing an additional sash a few inches inside the outer one, leaving an air-space between. This will be sufficient to secure the end in view, and will present the additional advantages of preventing waste of fuel and excluding noise.

In conclusion, there have been several objections offered against this method of warming and ventilating assembly-rooms, all of which have been very carefully considered, and it is gratifying to be able to say that no one of them appears to be well founded, or to involve the practical operation of our principle in any serious difficulty.

"OUR MATERIA MEDICA."

BY F R. MCMANUS, M.D, BALTIMORE, MD.

I READ, with great pleasure, an article upon "Our Materia Medica," in the May number of THE HAHNEMANNIAN, page 285, by E. B. Nash, M.D., of Cortland, N.Y. An extract reads thus:

"Several years ago I treated a child suffering from an obstinate attack of dysentery. The remedies which are usually successful, failed utterly. Counsel was summoned, but our combined efforts were equally unsuccessful. At one of my visits the mother chanced to be changing the child's diaper. I noticed that the anus was wide open. I could have inserted my little finger to the depth of two inches without touching the bloody mucus-lined walls. Neither Jahr's *Manual*, Snelling, Bell *On Diarrhœa*, nor Hering's *Condensed*, contain this important symptom. Finally I discovered this under Phosphorus, in Lippe's *Textbook*, 'Discharge of Mucus out of the Wide-open Anus.'" Dr. Nash cured his case with Phosphorus.

On reading Dr. Nash's article my mind was vividly called to what I had learned, forty-two years ago, in regard to that precise symptom and condition given in Phosphorus, recorded in the *first American* translation of the *first German* edition of Jahr's Manual, translated "by authority of the North American Academy of the Healing Art, Allentown, 1838." In the repertory of that volume, under the head of "Anus and Alvine Ejections," is found, "Openness, constant, of the anus." In the *Manual* Phosphorus has, "Escape of slime and blood from the anus, which *continually is open.*"

In Hempel's translation of Jahr, large edition, of 1848, ten years after the Allentown edition of Jahr, is found, as a symptom for Phosphorus, "Mucous discharge from the anus, which is constantly open."

Nux vomica has precisely the *reversed* condition of Phosphorus, the former having discharge of bloody mucus, with a sensation of *constriction*,—Phosphorus, a similar discharge, with *relaxation* and *openness*. It will amply pay any physician to look into Phosphorus in all cases of intractable dysentery, particularly when the seat of the disease is *confined to the rectum*, and *near to or involving the anus*. In cases, too, of a *reversed condition, inveterate constipation*, with disappointed calls, the trouble *being seated in the rectum*, the attention of every astute physician would be called to Phosphorus.

The importance of this subject will be my apology for asking for so much of your valuable space, and giving to it so much of my own valuable time.

A CASE OF PUERPERAL ECLAMPSIA.

BY CHANDLER WEAVER, M.D., FOX CHASE, PA.

Mrs. J. W., æt. 29, short and stout, of leucophlegmatic temperament, summoned me to see her, about 1 o'clock in the morning of March 28th, 1880. She had engaged the services of an allopathic physician for her expected confinement in two weeks, but he being sick, I was requested to take charge of the case.

She was very restless, sick at the stomach every time she moved, and very thirsty, yet water made her vomit. She attributed her illness to eating veal the day before, which had affected her in a similar manner upon previous occasions.

I prescribed Ars. 6th, which relieved her so that by 3 A.M. I left her quite calm and comfortable. I noticed considerable œdema, and learned that she had had three miscarriages,—the first one at the fifth month, the second at the sixth, and the last, which occurred thirteen months ago, was at the eighth month. She had never had a living child. When I called next morning, I found her quiet but unable to see, speech very thick, and she complained of dull frontal headache. I now made an examination of the uterus, which was attended with some difficulty, as she could not understand what it was for. The os uteri was partially dilated, flabby, and apparently uninfluenced by any uterine contractions. I could introduce the finger into the uterine cavity, but could detect no contractions.

Gave Gelsem.[1] in water every half hour, and informed her husband that if her sight did not return by noon I should want a consultation, and probably would have to deliver as soon as possible, in order to save the mother. At noon, before I returned to her, she had a convulsion, upon which I telegraphed to Philadelphia for Dr. B. F. Betts. After she came out of the second convulsion I found the os uteri in the same condition. Still continued the Gelsem. She had another convulsion, about 5 P.M., which lasted eight minutes. The interval between the convulsions had increased, but the last one was the most severe of any. It was followed by furious delirium, and force was required to keep her from throwing herself off the bed. Upon the arrival of Dr. Betts we etherized her, and drew off by the catheter a very small quantity of thick dark urine,—all that had collected since morning. This was unfortunately thrown away, but subsequently I examined her urine and found albumen present.

A third examination of the uterus was now made, and the cervix dilated so that the fingers could be introduced into the cavity of the uterus, yet no uterine contractions could be felt. After waiting for a time for labor to set in, it was thought best not to delay the delivery of the child any longer. The patient had lost two sisters in convulsions during parturition, and the character of the urinary secretion and the patient's condition made it probable that a similar termination might occur in her case. There was also a probability of saving the life of the child. The membranes having been ruptured the forceps were applied about 6 o'clock, and the child delivered alive at 7 o'clock. It was very weak, but got along nicely until the eighth day, when, from want of proper nourishment, and inattention on the part of a bigoted allopathic nurse, it died.

After the delivery, the Gelsem. was continued; the uterus contracted, the placenta was expelled, and but little hæmorrhage followed. The anæsthetic was discontinued and the Gelsem. administered until 10.30 P.M., when from the character of the delirium, pulse, and condition of the pupils, etc., I changed to Bell. in water every twenty minutes, until she became more quiet. Four strong persons were frequently required to control her. About 10 o'clock next morning she regained consciousness, but knew nothing of what had taken place since the night I first saw her. She had passed urine freely, and had no more convulsions. Her recovery was rapid under remedies specially indicated, without any complications.

She was able to sit up in bed on the eleventh day, and on the thirteenth day was about the room. The albumen has decreased to about 1 per cent., and is still decreasing under the influence of Ars. alb.

NUX MOSCHATA OR WHISKEY.

BY E. M. HOWARD, M.D., CAMDEN, N. J.

IN the May number of the HAHNEMANNIAN MONTHLY Dr. Josephine Van Deusen very sharply criticised my "Accidental Proving of Nux Moschata," published in the February number of the same journal.

It is apparent from the tenor of her criticism that she considers all the symptoms to have been produced by the whiskey, and would deny that the ounce of nutmeg, swallowed at the same time, could, or did, have any effect whatever; for, although she asks me to separate the whiskey symptoms from those produced by the nutmeg, she evidently does not think there are any to separate, as she states that "altogether it is quite apparent that the article of Dr. Howard is not properly titled."

In the first place it will be proper to mention, that the proving was an *accidental* one, and reported as such, and would not therefore be expected to be entirely free from elements of uncertainty. I took especial pains to recite all the surrounding circumstances, and have no doubt whatever but that the thoughtful readers of the HAHNEMANNIAN are fully able to judge for themselves, which of the symptoms were produced by the nutmeg, and do not, in this respect, need either my own or Dr. Van Deusen's assistance.

However, since a point of error has been raised, I will call Dr. Van Deusen's attention to the fact that the semi-unconsciousness from an overdose of whiskey does not usually last as long as it did in this case. Nor do "accidental" or any other drunkards "see double" for *two or three days* after the first effects of a debauch. If the doctor will take the trouble to again look carefully over the proving she will find a large number of the symptoms lasting a week (some for three weeks) or more; for instance: whirling sensation in head, throbbing in ovarian region, lascivious dreams, stammering, cramps in abdomen, etc. And, furthermore, if the doctor will compare the symptoms in this case with those given under Nux moschata in Allen's *Encyclopedia*, as I did before I offered them for publication, she will find a wonderful parallelism.

I, for one, am *very sorry* that Dr. Van Deusen should consider it her duty to thus discourage the careful publication of such cases of accidental poisoning; for although the same elements of uncertainty will be present in any symptoms occurring after a large dose of *any* tincture, it would have been a great misfortune if none of these cases had been reported in the past. And I must assert the necessity of reporting all cases that promise to give us the least insight into the action of drugs—whether to give us new symptoms, or confirm old ones. With this end in view, I have most carefully reported this proving of Nux moschata, to await the final winnowing which all our Materia Medica must undergo.

THE PHILADELPHIA COUNTY HOMŒOPATHIC MEDICAL SOCIETY.

REPORTED BY CHARLES MOHR, M.D., SECRETARY.

THE regular monthly meeting of the society was held on Thursday evening, May 13th, 1880, at the Hahnemann Medical College; the President, E. A. Farrington, M.D., in the chair. The minutes of the April (annual) meeting were read and approved.

The Censors reported favorably on the applications for membership of Drs. Ferris T. Price, Alfred E. Baker, H. H. Groth, and Charles F. Goodno, and these gentlemen were thereupon duly elected to membership. Applications were then made by Drs. F. Axt, W. K. Ingersoll, Edwin Simmer, Chandler Weaver, and J. Wandell. Referred.

By vote, the President was requested to appoint a delegate to represent the society at the meeting of the American Institute of Homœopathy at Milwaukee in June.

The report of the Bureau of Sanitary Science, Climatology, and Hygiene, was then presented by the chairman, Dr. Pemberton Dudley. The report embraces the following papers, which were read by their respective authors:

a. Food and its Preparation, by J. B. Kniffin, M.D.

b. The Hygiene of Medical Education, by A. C. Rembaugh, M.D.

c. The Sanitary Condition of our Health Resorts, by B. F. Betts, M.D.

d. Sanitary Precautions in Measles, by C. Mohr, M.D.

e. Warming and Ventilation of Public Assembly-rooms, by Pemberton Dudley, M.D.

The report was accepted, and a short discussion ensued.

Adjourned.

THE

HAHNEMANNIAN MONTHLY.

A HOMŒOPATHIC JOURNAL OF

MEDICINE AND SURGERY.

Editors,

E. A. Farrington, M.D. Pemberton Dudley, M.D.

Business Manager,

Bushrod W. James, M.D.

Vol. II. Philadelphia, Pa., June, 1880. No. 6.

☞ The Editors consider themselves responsible for the maintenance of the dignity and courtesy of the journal, but *not* for the opinions expressed by its contributors.

Editorial Department.

Is the Production of Abortion Ever Necessary?—Dr. McClatchey, in his article on "The Vomiting of Pregnancy" (see Hahnemannian Monthly, May, 1880), remarks: "It has been recommended that in the most severe cases, where apparently nothing is retained by the stomach, and there appears to be danger of death from starvation, an abortion may be procured. . . . . . I am not able, however, to conceive of a case where such procedure would be justifiable or necessary."

These sterling words have called forth considerable comment, and we are in receipt of two or three letters concerning the subject.

Dr. F. F. Casseday takes exception to the universality of Dr. McClatchey's views, and describes a case in point in an article which will be found upon another page of this number.

Dr. A. L. Monroe writes: "Dr. McClatchey's article, with its many valuable suggestions, brings to my mind a simple palliative, which has gained deserved popularity in our vicinity. Take an infusion of peppermint leaves, strong enough to produce its aromatic and pungent taste. Dissolve in this mixture sufficient common soda, to produce marked alkalinity. Give a swallow for each increase of the nausea. Having witnessed its exhibition in a number of cases, I recommend it with confidence for its power to render life endurable at a most trying time."

An exhaustive study of the question of "licensed fœticide" is contained in an address read before the College of Physicians and Surgeons of Michigan, and published in the *American Observer*, and is also issued in pamphlet form.

The negative answer to the question, is maintained with a force and spirit characteristic of the writer, Dr. N. F. Cooke, of Chicago, and is supported by the testimony of many respectable practitioners. "I have thus obtained," says Dr. Cooke, "an aggregate experience of over one thousand years of constant, active, obstetric practice, and the proportion results: As 20 is to 1000, so is the total number of 'justifiable' child-killings; or, in other words, one every fifty years! If now we deduct the cases of premature labor as not properly classifiable among direct fœticides, we have about 5 to 1000, or one in two hundred years of practice!"

Though strong language, this by no means over-estimates the subject under consideration, and should make the boldest man hesitate; ay, more, ponder long and seriously, and even then seek the concurrent advice of at least *three* of his fellow-physicians before he takes the life of one of these innocent, helpless "babes in the womb."

In the *Medical Tribune* for April, 1880, a writer concludes, from statistics carefully collated, that there are annually committed in the United States 150,000 abortions! Add to this the uncomputed number of miscarriages shortly after the first month, and for which women take pills without the doctor's advice, and the crime of abortion becomes as appalling in its magnitude as it is degrading in its effect on our national morality.

Let every physician, then, add his personal efforts, to the prevention and annihilation of this damnable crime. Let him use both pen and tongue to enlist the active co-operation of our national and State legislators; and, above all, let him beware how he concludes to induce abortion, deceiving himself with the excuse that it is necessary for the preservation of the mother's life.

Such cases may occur, although we agree with Dr. McClatchey, and many others equally sanguine, that we cannot conceive how such a case *can* occur. But it were better to obtain the concurrence of a dozen physicians than to err on the other side. Expense is an item so foreign to the subject that we bring it up but to reject it. What physician is there who would not volunteer his services or advice in so vital a matter as this?

We do not wish to criticise the motives of Dr. Casseday and his counsellor. The very fact that he offers his case for publication is evidence of honesty and purity of intent. But we have hitherto refused to publish such cases, lest they exert an unintended, but none the less serious, evil influence. And we insert Dr. C.'s article now because it affords an opportunity to express our earnest convictions on the subject.

In conclusion we urge upon the American Institute to consider this topic at its next meeting, and to report some feasible plan by which its members shall be governed. If we may be allowed to make a suggestion in advance, we propose that it be made obligatory upon every member of the Institute to refrain from the induction of the abortion of the unviable fœtus without the unanimous assent of at least *three* besides the physician in attendance.

The American Institute of Homœopathy.—The annual session of our national organization of homœopathic physicians will be held in Milwaukee, Wisconsin, commencing Tuesday, June 15th, and continuing four days. Judging from the preparations made by the various bureaus, the session promises to be one of the most interesting and valuable ever held. The meetings will open with an address by the President, T. P. Wilson, M.D., of Ann Arbor, and the Institute will almost immediately begin the work of receiving and discussing the reports of the bureaus, and the papers included therein. We already know, from the circular issued by the General Secretary, what the subjects of many of these papers will be. For instance, the Bureau of Sanitary Science, etc., will present a full set of papers on the subject of quarantine, international, national, state, and local; the disinfection and quarantine of mails, merchandise, etc. The Bureau of Materia Medica will discuss, in papers prepared by men of diverse shades of opinion, the vexed, and, alas! the vexing questions of the proof of drug presence and power, and of medicinal presence and efficacy in alternations above the sixth decimal. The Bureau of Clinical Medicine will give an exhaustive consideration of the history, causes, varieties, progress, pathology, contagiousness, prevention, and treatment of scarlatina. The Bureau of Pædology takes up the diseases of the infantile digestive organs in some ten papers. The remaining bureaus will, some of them at least, have reports equally valuable to present for discussion, and the various *specialties* connected with medicine give promise of being well represented.

Round-trip tickets, good for physicians attending the meeting, and their families, can be obtained *at excursion rates* (usually about two-thirds the regular fare) by applying to C. S. Halderman, 203 and 205 Washington Street, Boston; S. Carpenter, 526 Broadway, New York; J. N. Abby, 1348 Chestnut Street, Philadelphia; Edw. S. Young, Baltimore; Drs. Burgher and McClelland, Secretaries, Pittsburg. These tickets are good *to Chicago* and return. From Chicago to Milwaukee, members and their friends will pay full fare going, and one-fifth fare returning, on presentation of a certificate which will be furnished them by Dr. Olmstead previous to their leaving Milwaukee.

Messrs. J. F. Antisdel & Son, proprietors of the Newhall House, will entertain physicians and their friends at the reduced rate of $2.50 per day. The hotel is large, centrally located, convenient to the place of meeting, provided with an elevator and all the modern improvements, and elegantly furnished. Dr. C. C. Olmstead, of Milwaukee, chairman of the Local Committee of Arrangements, will give his personal attention to securing rooms in advance on application.

A banquet and hop in honor of the Institute will be given by the proprietors of the Newhall House on Thursday evening, June 17th. Special arrangements are also being made by the Local Committee, to promote the enjoyment of the lady friends of the physicians in attendance.

To those physicians who have formed the habit of attending these annual gatherings, we have not a word to say. *They* know all about it; and those of their number who can, by any sort of possibility, get to Milwaukee, will be there,—every man of them. But the HAHNEMANNIAN has on its subscription list a large number of *young* physicians, and we respectfully urge them, one and all, to do two things. First, write to the Secretary, Dr. J. C. Burgher, Pittsburg, Pa., for a blank application for membership, fill it out, get three members of the Institute to sign it (and, if possible, let one of them be a physician of the neighborhood in which you now reside), and return it to the Secretary, inclosing the admission fee ($5.00) and the first year's annual dues ($5.00). Secondly, attend the meeting at Milwaukee, if possible, and subsequent meetings, whenever practicable, and you will live longer, practice better, and die happier than if you shut yourself up in your shell, like a clam, caring nothing for the advancement of that grand profession, of which you form a part, but only for the little contracted circle of your own practice. "And don't you forget it."

A FUNNY ALLOPATH.—In the New York *Medical Record* of April 17th, there is an amusing editorial, entitled "Homœopathy in the Boston City Hospital." It seems that the homœopathic people of Boston propose now to take possession of what properly belongs to them,—a portion of the public hospital accommodations of that city. This leads the editor of the above-named journal to say, that "if a pure homœopathic practice could be introduced into the Boston City Hospital, and its results placed in comparison with those obtained by regular physicians, nothing more disastrous could happen to the so-called new school." True, there is not anything very mirth-provoking about that, until we learn, as we do further on, just what that word "disastrous" means. The editor goes on to say that "such an experiment is not new; that at Vienna and at Ann Arbor homœopathic education has been attempted side by side with instruction in scientific (?) medicine, and it has failed." Now we begin to see what that editor is driving at. Everybody knows about the "failure" they are making of it at Ann Arbor. The homœopathic faculty and all the homœopathic doctors round about are "tickled to death" over it. But those Boston people do not expect to be satisfied with one of your simple "failures." They propose to make a real first-class "disaster" out of it. Anything to beat Ann Arbor. Then the editor asserts (we do not know where he got his information) that homœopathy has been tried in various hospitals of Europe, and "has been given up as ineffective," and we learn what that means, a little farther on, in the statement that "the New York City Homœopathic Hospital has turned out to be a harmless institution." We do not just see why the editor should draw such a contrast between our practice and his own; still, we are glad to learn that in allopathic estimation a "harmless" hospital is considered "ineffective." The most amusing part of all that amusing editorial is seen in the remark that "homœopathy, in its pristine simplicity, is no longer practiced by intelligent men." We wish the same compliment could be paid to the opposing school, but even if it could be truthfully done, we fear that editor would not take it kindly. Advancement in medical science he seems to be afraid of. Perhaps he does not like the idea of being left all alone.

Our Journalistic Work.—We have not the least desire to parade before our readers the work which we, as editors, are doing for this journal. But we do feel like expressing a little honest pride in what OUR CONTRIBUTORS are doing for us. The present number completes the first half of the current volume; and we find, somewhat to our own surprise, on looking over these six numbers, that we have issued about SEVENTY-FIVE ORIGINAL ARTICLES; so that, leaving out of the account everything else contained in the journal as of no value, these articles have cost our readers just two cents a piece. We should dislike exceedingly to think that any *one* of our subscribers is dissatisfied with his bargain. As to the character and practical value of these contributions, our readers must judge for themselves. Here we desire to invite notice to the contributions contained in this number. Our opening article on "Neurasthenia and its Homœopathic Treatment," by Professor Korndœrfer, will prove, to more than one of our readers, of far more value than the whole cost of the journal for the year. And the same may be said of the article on "Retention of Urine," by Dr. John Cooper, of Allegheny, and the discussion on the same subject by the practical working members of the Allegheny County Society.

A Significant Straw.—In the *Physicians and Surgeons' Investigator*, of Buffalo, the editor, referring to matters homœopathic, speaks of our friend, Professor Wilson, of the *Medical Advance*, as "a leader in *that* school." The grammar that bothered our boyhood, taught us that "*this*" refers to an object holding a near position or relation, while "*that*" refers to an object *remote* in position or relation. Still we are not surprised at the above phraseology, as we observe from recent advertisements of the Buffalo College, of which the *Physicians and Surgeons' Investigator* is the organ, that that institution has dropped the word "homœopathic" from its title. The gentlemen connected with it, however, claim to be firm believers in the doctrine of *similia*. And why should they not be? The rankest allopaths "also believe and tremble," but that does not make them competent critics and teachers of Homœopathy.

CORRIGENDA.

In the May number, page 267, line 12 from bottom, "time" should be "twice." Page 268, line 16, "eructation" should be "evacuation."

Book Department.

PATHOGENETIC OUTLINES OF HOMŒOPATHIC DRUGS. By Dr. Carl Heinigke. Translated by Emil Tietze, M.D. Published by Boericke & Tafel. Philadelphia, 1880. Octavo, pp. 576.

Physicians nowadays, influenced by our hasty modes of living, demand books which shall afford them needed information condensed into the briefest possible space. Prescriptions must be hurriedly made, and so, hurriedly studied. The reception-room is full, and the frequent rings at the door threaten an overrun, which will sadly interfere with the prospective outdoor visits. The busy doctor, whose carriage is always needing new wheels, shakes his head emphatically, "No!" when an Allen's *Encyclopedia*, or a Hering's *Guiding Symptoms*, is offered him. Alas! what we gain in boldness we lose in thoroughness; what we gain for the emergency we lose for the slow, insidious, chronic case. And the effect on our Materia Medica, too, is serious and alarming. We are making but slow progress in the determination of positive drug-effects. The certain side of our remedies is not developing with that steady, healthful growth which characterized the labors of our predecessors.

In our hurry we can pause but to investigate the *general* features of drugs, neglecting *particulars* as useless refinements. The consequence is, our Materia Medica is shaping itself after the fashion of the minds of its moulders, and becoming daily more and more a collection of "glittering generalities." But still, even here, there are great differences. Some writers offer us the dry bones and shrivelled tissues, as void of life as a varnished skeleton. Others inflate the tissues with a windy supply of their own ideas, which, while they give them form, leave them scarcely recognizable as the children of Hahnemann and his plodding confrères.

But, concerning the work under review, we are happy to be able to say that its gifted writer has essayed more than some of the authors referred to. Each remedy is introduced with a brief account of its preparation, duration of action, and antidotes. Then follow the symptoms, arranged under the following headings: Generalities, Nervous, Circulatory, Respiratory, Digestive, Urinary, and Sexual Systems, and lastly, Employment Among the Sick.

Each of these headings displays a careful study, and the "outlines" are often precisely and tersely drawn. But we are of the number who believe that the integrity and perpetuity of our Materia Medica require more attention to the fine peculiarities of drugs. We are, as stated above, drifting into generalities, and this downward course is hurried rather than retarded, by clothing symptoms in a restricting garb of pathological terms. This is the only serious objection we have to Dr. Heinigke's book, and we know that here many will differ with us. But that we may be clearly understood as not underrating the doctor's labors, we will give an illustration of what we mean.

On pages 97 and 98 are given the symptoms of Cactus grand. Under the Mind we read: "Concealed, taciturn, sad, and melancholy mood." All this is true; but as the remedy is pre-eminently useful in cardiac diseases, why is the confirmed symptom, "Fear of death, ... believes his disease incurable," omitted? As the book only pretends to give outlines, it may be answered that all this is implied in "sad mood." Even if we grant this, the objection still obtains that such a rendering is too general for a practical book. Again, on page 98, it is written: "Sensation of constriction in the centre of the chest." This, too, is a genuine Cactus symptom, but is not distinctive enough. Why were not the more characteristic symptoms selected: Constriction like a cord tightly bound around the false ribs; constriction in heart as if an *iron band* prevented its normal movement? Constriction, indeed, expresses the pathological state; but needs the more definite iron-band sensation to distinguish it from Kali chlor., Cadm., etc.

Turning finally to Baptisia we find too general an outline of this remedy, which even the explanatory note, that the symptoms are taken mainly from "the observations of American physicians on the sick," will not wholly excuse. He has omitted the famous clinical indication of restless tossing, with confusion as to the patient's unity of person; restless tossing, wants to move from place to place; besotted appearance; tongue dry, and brown coated down the centre; muscles sore, compelling change of place; parts laid on feel sore; all necessary to a clear understanding, even in outline, of this valuable remedy.

Growing out of this same difficulty is another error, which has led physicians to the hap-hazard interchange of closely related drugs, regardless of their fine distinctions. Thus Iodine and Kali hydriod., Calc. carb. and Calc. phos., Natrum carb. and Natrum mur. are employed as though the combination did not materially affect the symptomatology. And Dr. Heinigke is inclined to this same mistake. Thus on page 101, under Calc. carb., he says: "No constant and well-marked differences of the other preparations of lime employed in practice, especially in the higher potencies, can be offered with regard to their action upon the healthy body." We must differ from the learned author here. We have pointed differences between the Calc. carb. and Calc. phos. which will generally, if not always, enable us to distinguish them in practice.

We are informed that the *Repertory*, which is referred to in the preface, will appear in the fall. And as it promises "to direct the attention to the comparison of the characteristic pathogenetic features of a definite category of drugs," we hope it will elaborate the chapters on "Employment Among the Sick," which are too limited and arbitrary.

E. A. F.

TRANSACTIONS OF THE HOMŒOPATHIC MEDICAL SOCIETY OF THE STATE OF PENNSYLVANIA: Tenth, Eleventh, Twelfth, Thirteenth, and Fourteenth Annual Sessions, 1874–1878, Vol. II. Philadelphia: Sherman & Co., Printers, 1880. 8vo., pp. 562.

This volume, so long waited for, may well make the members of the

Pennsylvania State Society feel proud. It is issued in handsome style, with close, yet plain, good type, on good paper. There is indeed, nothing mean about the whole get-up of the book, and its pages contain an amount of practical matter which, we venture to say, has rarely been seen in any similar work. Some of its shorter papers have, from time to time, appeared in the pages of this journal; but most of the more valuable and exhaustive articles have never before been published. Several of these articles are of such a character, as to make the work exceedingly valuable as a book for reference by the practitioner, while its value in this respect is greatly enhanced by the *repertorial* character of the index, by which any remedy mentioned in the work can easily be found and its application learned. This part of the work was done by our tireless and practical friend, Dr. Charles Mohr, of Philadelphia. The whole work reflects credit upon the Committee of Publication, and especially Dr. Joseph C. Guernsey, upon whom devolved the entire labor of superintending its issue.

In order to convey some idea of the work, imperfect and totally inadequate as it must be, we append the mere mention of some few of its papers; all of them being of the most practical character. First, we may state that the first sixty-eight pages contain the reported proceedings of the five annual sessions, from 1874 to 1878 inclusive. Then follow in order the constitution and by-laws, list of members, necrological reports, and the annual addresses.

In the Department of Materia Medica we find most important contributions: A Comparison of Calcarea and Silica, occupying twelve pages, by Dr. Farrington; a short essay on Pharmacy, by Dr. J. F. Cooper, of Allegheny; a Proving of Amorphous Phosphorus, by Drs. Gumpert and Kirk, arranged by Dr. H. N. Martin; a paper on the Progress of Homœopathy, by Dr. A. Lippe, and one on the Homœopathic Materia Medica, by the same writer. Next come some Verified Symptoms, by Dr. A. P. Bowie, followed by a complete Report of the very thorough and exhaustive Provings of Arseniate of Soda, by the Materia Medica Club of Allegheny County. This report covers forty-two pages, and is of such a character that no homœopathist can well afford to be without it. Next we have an interesting though brief essay on the Homœopathic Materia Medica as a Science, and its Application as an Art, by H. N. Guernsey, M.D.; a short paper on Acon. Nap., by Dr. Lippe. Then follow an exhaustive article of seventeen pages, by Dr. Farrington, on Antipsorics in the Dropsy of Infants, and a shorter one on Ferrum Iodatum, by the same author. These complete this first department.

In the Department of Clinical Medicine and Zymoses, the Allegheny County Medical Society has a paper on Sciatica, and an exhaustive treatise on Pneumonia and its Treatment. There are also two papers by our practical friend, Dr. Lilienthal, of New York, one on Dementia Paralytica, and the other a seven-page study of Diphtheria and Nephritis. Dr. W. J. Martin contributes an interesting article on Mercurius Cyanatus in Diphtheria, and Dr. T. L,

Bradford an exhaustive one on Croup, its Pathology, Diagnosis, and Treatment. There are several other papers in this department.

Under the head of Obstetrics and Gynæcology there are sixteen articles, among which we mention, an exhaustive essay of thirty-two pages on Puerperal Hæmorrhage, by the Allegheny County Medical Society, and other papers by Drs. H. N. Guernsey, J. H. Marsden, B. F. Betts, A. R. Thomas, and other of our representative writers.

In the Surgical Department, we have an Exposition on Hæmorrhoids, by the Allegheny County Society, and other papers of a practical type by Drs. McClelland, Macfarlan, Burgher, A. R. Thomas, C. M. Thomas, Betts, and Willard. There are also several valuable contributions on the subject of climatology.

Ophthalmology and Otology furnishes three papers: one on Our Imperfect Eyes, one on Retinitis Pigmentosa, both by Dr. W. H. Winslow, of Pittsburg, and one on the Abuses of Vision, by Dr. B. W. James.

To attempt the slightest critical notice of even the few papers we have mentioned would far outrun the limits of our space.

Of course it is understood that papers read before our societies do not, as a rule, profess to represent the well-settled convictions of the profession, as a whole, but rather of the individual writers. These papers help to *make* professional opinion. It is the province of the standard textbook to *reflect* that opinion. Hence, it will not do to criticise the former by the same standard that we apply to the latter. Such a criticism would simply bring out the varying opinions of the critic on matters which, after all, each reader properly expects to decide for himself. For the work before us, therefore, we have little but praise, and this we say, without undertaking either to indorse or to disapprove any of the opinions expressed in the papers. P. D.

Boston University Yearbook. Vol. VII, 1880.

This *Yearbook* is issued in the interest of the Boston University, an institution in which are taught art, agriculture, theology, law, medicine, and sciences in general.

It is the proud claim of this university, that it opens its doors for the benefit of all classes and both sexes. Its medical department, in particular, exhibits a matriculant list containing the names of quite a number of females. Among the theological students we notice the names of four or five ladies; one or two in the law department, and three or four among the post-graduates who attend the school of all sciences. The college of music, as might be expected, is well attended by females.

That which will especially interest the physician, is the excellent article by William F. Warren, LL.D., on "Hopeful Symptoms in Medical Education." The paper opens with a very ingenious description of "our American corpus medicorum" as sick. The cure of this troublesome invalid, Mr. W. thinks, can be brought about only by the laity, for doctors have widely and hopelessly disagreed. The treatment is preventive and hygienic. Any tendency to relapse is to be cured by the careful preliminary educational training of candidates for admission to medical colleges. Hygienic means are: lengthening of the time of collegiate study, grading of the curriculum, and the final examination by parties who have no pecuniary interest in the success of the candidates.

All this is sound doctrine, and we commend it to the profession.

We do not fully agree with Mr. Warren, however, in his hopeful prognosis concerning the obliteration of "the lines of party and sect." Allopathy is not trending towards homœopathy, even though some of its dignitaries may cry "anathema to old-time medicine." Many of all schools are shaking themselves loose from all restraint of law, and are sallying forth into the scientific world as free-thinkers, guided only by the results of experience. But lawlessness will never "render the catholicity of true science possible to the profession." E. A. F.

WOOD'S LIBRARY OF STANDARD MEDICAL AUTHORS FOR 1880.

Last year William Wood & Co., 27 Great Jones Street, New York, undertook the venturesome enterprise of the publication of one book every month, from some standard medical author, at the average nominal sum of $1 each to subscribers; the whole library at the end of the year thus costing but $12, for a set of the latest and best works of the kind then issued. This price was only one-third or one-fourth as much as the original works would have been sold at by retail booksellers, thus bringing into the hands of the practitioner the best medical thoughts of the day, and placing them within the means and reach of every practitioner.

Having fulfilled their promise faithfully during 1879, they are continuing in the good work this year, offering to subscribers twelve octavo volumes of from 250 to 400 pages each, and aggregating about 1000 more pages than the series for 1879; the price for the twelve volumes being $15. Already several valuable and standard works are out, and ready for the second year's shelf. This library for 1880 will consist in all of about four thousand pages of new and original medical writings from well-known authors and specialists. They are nicely bound in muslin, and issued in good style on fine paper, and although printed closely, the type is distinct and not objectionable. The following have already been received:

A TREATISE ON FOREIGN BODIES IN SURGICAL PRACTICE. In two volumes. By Alfred Poulet, M.D., Adjutant Surgeon-Major, Inspector of the School for Military Medicine at Val-de-Grace. Vol. I, pp. 271; Vol. II, pp. 320.

Every practitioner knows well the alarm of a patient or the relatives when a foreign body has accidentally become lodged in any of the passages or orifices of the body, and how urgently his services are importuned. Such an occasion is no moment for search over the scattered pages of a large standard work on surgery, to find out the best way to proceed in the case, to be rewarded only by a few meagre hints, and such perhaps as would naturally suggest themselves to his own ingenuity. In this work we have the whole subject treated fully from the experience of past generations, and condensed into a practical form for study and for every-day use, and those who are thrown upon their own surgical resources will not know how to do without it when they have once read the volumes; while for the medical student to acquaint himself with, it has no equal in that direction.

In treating upon the subject, Poulet has given in Part 1st, foreign bodies in general—their classification, nature, manner of introduction, fate, and treatment. In Part 2d, foreign bodies of the intestinal tract. Part 3d treats of those of the air-passages. Part 4th treats of those of the genito-urinary organs. Part 5th, of the ear. Part 6th, of the nasal fossæ. Part 7th, of the glandular canals.

Numerous illustrations and cuts of lodgments of and perforations by foreign bodies are given, and the various surgical instruments required, and now in general use, in this kind of surgical practice.

The chapter on the pharynx and œsophagus is particularly good, and four cuts of interesting pathological perforation-specimens from Dupuytren's Museum, and one from Langenbeck's *Arch.*, are shown. The treatise is a most valuable contribution, and we can highly recommend it to physicians and surgeons.

A Handbook of Physical Diagnosis, Comprising the Throat, Thorax, and Abdomen. By Dr. Paul Guttman, Privat Docent in Medicine, University of Berlin. Translated from the Third German Edition, by Alex. Napier, M.D , Fel. Fac. Phys. and Surg., Glasgow; with a colored plate and eighty-nine fine wood engravings. Pp. 344. 1880.

The frontispiece is a plate of the colors of urine (after Vogel) in nine tints: 1, pale yellow; 2, bright yellow; 3, yellow; 4, reddish-yellow; 5, yellowish-red; 6, red; 7, brownish-red; 8, reddish-brown; 9, brownish. black; all of which he explains in a section devoted to the subject in the latter part of the work, giving the conditions under which each color is to be found.

His method of examination of the organs of circulation is concise and to the point, but he devotes very little space to sphygmography; not nearly as much as the subject deserves in the light of recent researches, Waldenburg's "Pulsuhr" is described, by which the measurement with precision in definite figures, of the tension, fulness, and volume of the pulse is made, and not simply an estimate of the same as by ordinary sphygmographs. Marey's, Pond's, and Holden's instruments are all illustrated by cuts.

He seems to have almost overlooked laryngoscopy, but finally has devoted twenty pages to it in an appendix. This portion of the treatise is terse, yet describes all the essential phenomena requisite for an easy diagnosis.

B. W. J.

Gleanings.

Yellow Fever has lingered around Havana all winter.

Duboisin, according to Professor Ladenburg, is identical with Hyoseyamin, and Daturin with Atropin.—*New Remedies*, May, 1880.

VIOLA TRICOLOR, it is asserted, contains Salicylic acid, and this is one of the reasons why the plant may be preserved over winter.—*New Remedies*, May, 1880.

SMALL-POX AT NINGPO, CHINA, is always more prevalent in the spring of the year, owing to the custom of the people of having inoculation performed at that time.

SALICYLIC ACID IN INDOLENT ULCERS.—Salicylic acid, sprinkled on indolent or inflamed ulcers, is said to induce rapid healing.—*N. Y. Med. Journ.*, May, 1880.

CANDY EATERS should know that glucose, from which many confections are made, is being manufactured from old linen rags.—See *Chemist and Druggist*, April, 1880.

To detect the escape of gas, apply soap-suds to the suspected leaky joint in the pipe. The formation of bubbles will indicate the point of escape.—*The Sanitarian*, May, 1880.

MENTHOL is the name given to colorless crystals deposited from Oil of peppermint. It is powerfully antiseptic and promises to supersede Carbolic acid, etc.—*Chemist and Druggist*, 1880.

QUEBRACHO BLANCO.—Aspidosperma quebracho is the variety used in medicine. The wood of this white variety, as well as that of the red, is used in tanning.—*Chemist and Druggist*, April, 1880.

EPITHELIOMATA, says Atkinson, are of three forms: 1st, flat variety; 2d, papillomatous; 3d, infiltrating or deepseated. The rodent ulcer is regarded as epitheliomatous.—See *N. Y. Med. Journ.*, May, 1880.

RINGWORM OF THE SCALP is differentiated in cases where the hair grows over the diseased place, by the fact that some of the hairs break off short, presenting the appearance of black dots.—*N. Y. Med. Journ.*, May, 1880.

GENTIANA LUTEA should receive more attention. Its gastric and intestinal symptoms point to it as important in cases where either Nux vom., Puls., Ipec., Coloc., Merc., or Bry. may be selected, according to imperfect totality.

TRAINING YELLOW FEVER EXPERTS.—Surgeon J. J. Woodward, United States Navy, suggests that one or more experts on the subject of yellow fever, be trained at the expense of the General Government, to constantly prosecute inquiry thereupon.

CARE OF SURGICAL INSTRUMENTS.—Vasoline or Cosmoline is used by a sewing machine manufacturer to preserve polished metal or steel from rust. If effective, this will be a convenient way of protecting surgical instruments not in constant use.—See *New Remedies*, May, 1880.

DEATH-RATE OF NAPLES.—This Italian city has an annual death-rate of 54 per 1000 inhabitants, or about 24,000 deaths in a population of 461,571. Lung diseases cause about one-half the deaths. The sanitary condition of the town is probably worse than that of any other European city.

HIGH POTENCIES AND THE FOURTH STATE OF MATTER.—Dr. Buchman, of Alvensleben, looks upon the high potencies as radiated matter. In an interesting article, published in March last, he draws largely upon Cooke's brochure upon the fourth state of matter, which has been but recently translated into German.

CALC. PHOS. IN LARYNGEAL DIPHTHERITIS.—Dr. Cruwell, of Dantzig, thinks that Schussler's recommendation of Calc. phos. in laryngeal diphtheritis is based altogether upon theoretical grounds, his experience with it in practice resulting only in disappointment. Schussler's reply leads us to feel that Cruwell was right in his surmise.

MORTALITY REPORTS.—The National Board of Health receives weekly mortality reports covering a population of about eight and a half millions. About thirty large cities in this country offer reports, and during the first quarter of the current year the mean annual death-rate reached only 18.87 per 1000,—a lower rate than usual for the season of the year embraced.

NEPHRECTOMY was performed upon a man, aged 36, who had a diseased left kidney. The organ was removed by lumbar incision, under antiseptic precautions. The patient is doing well, and will probably recover, unless unexpected secondary hæmorrhage sets in when the pedicle separates.—*Lancet*, February 28th, 1880.

DANGERS IN USING SALICYLIC ACID.—In acute rheumatism, the heart is often affected as to its muscular tissue, myocarditis, when there are no signs of endo-or-pericarditis. The organ is then enfeebled and the use of a cardiac depressant, like Salicylic acid, may develop alarming, if not fatal, symptoms.—*Lancet*, February 28th, 1880.

LIGATURE OF THE FUNIS.—Dr. Budin considers, that where the gelatinous substance of the cord is abundant, the ordinary ligation may be insufficient to prevent hæmorrhage. He substitutes an elastic ligature. As its application is awkward, Tarnier has devised the plan of laying matches on each side of the cord, which are broken off and removed after the tying.—*N. Y. Medical Journal*, April, 1880.

News and Comments.

DR. HENRY N. GUERNSEY, after a sojourn of about a year in Europe, sailed from Liverpool May 19th. By the time this reaches our readers, we trust he will be safe at home again. His health, we are glad to know, has been fully restored.

SETTLEMENTS—CLASS OF 1880.—M. Eugene Douglass, M.D., Danville, Va.; T. Elwood Parker, M.D., Parkersville, Chester County, Pa.; William A. Wheeler, M.D., Phelps, N. Y., Harry W. Challenger, M.D., Rome, Ga.

A FEROCIOUS BULL AT LARGE.—*Caller.*—"Is the doctor in?" *Bridget.*—"No, surr! not now, surr! But, indade, he's been in twice since he wint out, surr." If any one captures the animal, please send him home to the office of our Business Manager.

INVITATION TO THE AMERICAN INSTITUTE.—The West Jersey Homœopathic Medical Society, at its annual meeting held May 19th, instructed its delegate to the American Institute of Homœopathy to invite that body to hold its session of 1881 at Cape May, N. J.

HOMŒOPATHIC HOSPITAL COLLEGE OF CLEVELAND.—The commencement exercises of this institution were held, we believe, in the latter part of February. Fifty candidates received the college degree, and the annual address was delivered by J. Crocker White, D.D.

LOCATIONS FOR HOMŒOPATHIC PHYSICIANS.—Dr. M. E. Douglass, who has recently settled in Danville, Va., writes that he is doing finely, and that "there are some fine openings in Virginia for homœopathic physicians." He will gladly render any assistance to those seeking a field of labor.

THE AMERICAN HOMŒOPATHIC OPHTHALMOLOGICAL AND OTOLOGICAL SOCIETY will hold its fourth annual meeting in the parlors of the Newhall House, Milwaukee, beginning June 15th, 1880. Papers are promised from leading specialists throughout the country. H. G. Houghton, Vice-President; F. Park Lewis, Secretary.

THE HOMŒOPATHIC MEDICAL SOCIETY OF WISCONSIN.—The sixteenth annual meeting of this body will occur at the Newhall House, Milwaukee, on Monday, June 14th, 1880, the day previous to the opening of the session of the American Institute of Homœopathy. The various bureaus will report during the day, and a meeting for general business will be held in the evening.

FAREWELL DINNER TO PROFESSOR J. E. JAMES.—On Monday evening, May 10th, the Hahnemann Club of Philadelphia tendered a complimentary dinner to Professor James, on the eve of his departure for Europe Among the invited guests were Hon. J. R. Reading, M.D., and Professor James's colleagues of the Hahnemann College Faculty. Short speeches were made by Dr. McClatchey, the President of the Club, also by Professors Gause, A. R. Thomas, and C. M. Thomas, Dr. J. R. Reading, and by several members of the Club. Dr. James sailed on the American line steamship Ohio, on Wednesday, May 12th.

R. J. MCCLATCHEY, M.D.—We are glad to know that the little daughter of our esteemed colleague and co-laborer, Professor McClatchey, has entirely recovered from her recent very severe illness. By the way, the doctor himself quite recently made a fortunate escape from severe injury, and possible loss of life. By the breaking of the front axle of his carriage, the horse, a spirited animal, became frightened, and ran, overturning the carriage, and dragging its occupants over the tender cobble-stones of the street. The doctor was fortunately able to check the animal, but not until the carriage had been badly wrecked, and himself badly bruised. He declares that for a week afterward he resembled in one respect Rip Van Winkle on awaking from his long nap, "every new motion discovering a new pain, for which Bryonia was not worth a cent."

THE LATEST FROM ENGLAND.—Just as we go to press, we receive three items of pleasant news.

ALFRED C. POPE, M.D., editor of the *Monthly Homœopathic Review*, was, on May 14th, elected to the Chair of Materia Medica, in the London School of Homœopathy, vice Richard Hughes, M.D., resigned.

E. W. BERRIDGE, M.D., has sailed for New York, and expects to be present at the session of the American Institute of Homœopathy, in Milwaukee.

PROF. J. E. JAMES announces, per cable, his safe arrival in England. He expects to return in September.

MARRIED.—CURRY—HINCHMAN.—On March 10th, 1880, by Rev. J. B. Gough Pidge, GEORGE H. CURRY, M.D., of Red Bank, N. J., to Miss MARY M., daughter of C. C. Hinchman, Esq., of Philadelphia.

WILLIAMS—DENNISTON.—At the residence of the bride's parents, April 29th, 1880, by Rev. G. Oram, E. C. WILLIAMS, M.D., of Lebanon, Pa., and Miss IDA M., daughter of E. A. Denniston, Esq., of St. Nicholas, Schuylkill County, Pa.

DECEASED.—MITCHELL.—Our readers will be pained to learn of the death, from pneumonia, of Mrs. FLORENCE L. MITCHELL, wife of J. Nicholas Mitchell, M.D., only daughter of Professor A. R. Thomas, M.D., and sister of Prof. C. M. Thomas, M.D., of Philadelphia. This sad event occurred on the morning of May 17th, after a few days' illness. Our colleagues, into whose homes and hearts this deep sorrow has so suddenly entered, will have the deepest sympathy of the whole profession in the loss of this most estimable wife, daughter, sister, and friend.

THE

HAHNEMANNIAN MONTHLY.

Vol. II., New Series } Philadelphia, July, 1880. No. 7.

Original Department.

THE AMERICAN INSTITUTE SESSION.

The thirty-third annual session of the American Institute of Homœopathy convened in Milwaukee, Wis., on Tuesday, June 15th, in the Court-house. The Institute was called to order at 9.45 A.M., and prayer was offered by Rt. Rev. Bishop Welles, of Wisconsin. Addresses of welcome were delivered by Hon. T. H. Brown, Mayor of Milwaukee, and Professor Danforth, on behalf of the Wisconsin Homœopathic Medical Society and the one hundred and seventy-five homœopathic physicians of the State.

The annual address was then delivered by Professor T. P. Wilson, M.D., of Ann Arbor, Michigan, President of the Institute. In his opening remarks he said that "since the organization of this society, one-third of a century ago, a generation of men has passed away, and we of to-day are but the lawful heirs of the noble men who founded this organization. Men die, but principles remain, and the truth lives on forever." He offered "words of cheer to the veterans who yet remain with us, who, in their distant homes, are looking with anxious eyes upon our proceedings, recalling, perhaps, those early days when they watched over the cradle of our cause, and rejoicing that over us all still floats the unsullied banner of Similia." The speaker mentioned two facts which hide from our eyes the real progress we are making: the cessation of hostilities that were formerly waged against us, and the fact that our work has become so widely distributed.

"The birth of homœopathy did not signal an epoch of medical reform merely. It was, and is in all respects, an epoch of revolution. A failure on the part of some to fully grasp this fact has resulted most disastrously to individuals and greatly hindered our cause. If men would only remember the sad fate of Lot's wife; if they would only recall the foolishness of the Israelites in their longings for the leeks and flesh-pots of Egypt, there would be in our ranks to-day less solicitude for the welfare of false and obsolete systems of practice, and a more jealous and zealous care for the honor and advancement of homœopathy. But in spite of this, we have been and still are advancing. And the ratio of advancement has been in direct proportion to the degree with which we as a school have adhered to the principles of homœopathy as taught by Samuel Hahnemann; and this, not because they were taught by Hahnemann, or were any better because he taught them, but because these principles are in themselves true, and therefore unalterable. . . .

"It must be conceded that Hahnemann thoroughly understood the problem with which he was dealing, so far as it related to the system of medical practice then in vogue. No man better than he understood the utter falsity of the theories and methods of his predecessors and contemporaries. This will be cheerfully acknowledged by all. It was not necessary that he should grasp, even after years of careful study and experiment, the whole scope of his discovery. I say it was not necessary, but if since his time there has risen a mind in the medical world possessing a deeper or truer insight into the arcana of therapeutics, he should be made to stand forth, that we may know him and crown him. And what, alas! if he whom we are seeking after should prove to be one of the modern gods of this bastard system taught by a Ringer, a Phillips, or a Bartholow! Hahnemann at least knew what he was striving to get away from, though he may have but dimly guessed whither his new path was leading him. It cannot be charged upon him that he was ever knowingly false to the principles of truth which were revealed to him. He made no compromise with error. No more did he apologize for ignorance. With the inspiration and fervor of genius, he adored that only which he saw to be true. You cannot conceive of such a mind as his framing an apologetic rule like this: 'The homœopathic law is coextensive with disease, but if any among us shall resort to any medical means other than those pointed out by the law *similia similibus*, the fault shall lie first of all at the door of our Materia Medica, on account of its incompleteness; or failing to make that excuse good, then it must be due to a want on the part of the physician of a sufficient knowledge of the remedies already possessed by our school.' In other words, and applied to other things, a man may not steal or commit murder according to the law, but if he does these things it must be because the authority of the government is weak, or the person so violating it is presumably ignorant of the law.

"To revive issues that are dead, to reassert what has been successfully denied, to declare that true which has been a thousand times proven to be false, to cling to those things which we have completely outgrown, to continue those practices which have become obsolete, to go back to the dead past instead of going forward to the living future, is not progress. Neither is it progress to go forward in a circle, while nothing can be worse than facing squarely about and attempting to retrace our steps. Dogs may return to their vomit, and sows to their wallowing in the mire, but the science of medicine, as developed and fostered in the homœopathic school of to-day, can never return to the chaos whence it came forth. . . . . . If we shall dare to compromise or surrender aught which is true, we will be recreant to duty and unworthy the trust confided to us. If, however, we shall strike the key-note of advancement, full, clear and loud, there will be many a fainting heart cheered, and along the whole line you may see the flashing of arms in serried ranks moving to fresh victory. . . . . .

"I beg now to call your attention to another most important fact. We have been advancing because the philosophy of our art is in consonance with the general advancement of science. During nearly a century of growth we have never been checked at a single point by any fresh discovery in the whole domain of science. I need not call your attention to the fact that empirical medicine has been, time and again, suddenly thrown back upon its haunches by the revelations of physiology, and of chemistry, and of microscopy, and of kindred subjects. I need not point out to you how, in spite of such revelations, the most absurd practices have been continued and taught by that same empirical school. On the other hand, the homœopathic school has found that not only its great central law of cure, but every corollary springing out of that law, has received the most cordial indorsement at the hand of kindred sciences. There can of course be no knowledge of a therapeutic law until we have come to a just comprehension of the true nature of disease. It has been most absurdly stated that Hahnemann rejected pathology. On the contrary we assert that he was the most profound pathologist of his age. What he did reject was the unscientific theories and the unmeaning jargon of those who assumed to teach pathology. What he especially rejected was the assumption that the tissue changes produced by disease was the disease itself, or was the thing to be treated by the intelligent physician. . . . . .

"The past year has been marked by an unusual amount of controversy. No one, I think, should call in question the right of either party to a full, fair, and candid expression of their views. Our only hope of present safety and future progress lies in continued agitation. But if I am to report upon the progress of homœopathy, it becomes my duty to say that we have been greatly hindered by controversies of a purely personal character, and it will be noticed that our literature has not been greatly enriched by contributions of this sort. A continuance of this is to be deprecated. There is such a wide field of future work before us, and it is so resplendent with the harvest of truth, that we cannot afford to exhaust our energies in any other direction, or upon any other cause. And I beg to call your attention to the fact that the general advancement of science is constantly widening our sphere of action. Who would have thought a few years ago what the microscope might do for us in the improvement of a certain class of triturations? Who would have guessed what a widespread interest might be created in these investigations? Molecular physics has received a new impetus from what has been already done in this direction by our Bureaus of Microscopy and Materia Medica; and it has also greatly enlarged our knowledge of both what is done and should be done by our pharmaceutists in their preparations of triturations. This department of pharmaceutical work may be said to have gone a long way forward within the past two or three years. It has been thought by some that the recent work of our microscopists has tended to cast a shade of doubt upon the validity of our so-called high attenuations. Nothing can be further from the truth. In the first place, the microscopic work alluded to, has but just begun, and has not assumed a finality upon any fundamental question. It the second place, it is not probable—I may, perhaps, say not possible—for any future revelations of the microscope to affect in any special degree the question of dynamics. The microscope deals with drug forms; it is left for another department to deal with drug forces. . . . . .

"I come now to speak of another cause of our progress, namely, the enlargement and perfection of our educational work. The homœopathic colleges of the United States are taking high rank among the best educational institutions in the country. It is not the fault of some of them that they do not take yet higher grounds. It is the fault of the profession which will not patronize, as it should, colleges that demand better scholarship. It is to be regretted that the Intercollegiate congress has met with so much to discourage its action. For the honor of our cause, let us hope that it will yet succeed in effecting a sodality among our colleges, and that together and in harmony they may carry on our educational work in accordance with the demands of the times."

Before concluding, the President also urged the necessity of prompt and decisive action to secure a due representation of the homœopathic profession in the medical department of the army and navy. He closed with an impressive tribute to the departed heroes of homœopathy: "I would lay a loving chaplet on the brow of all who are sleeping in yonder graveyards. I would exalt their virtues, and brighten the memory of their heroic deeds. I do not fear that they have perished, or that they will ever cease to be."

The regular business of the session was then taken up. The Secretary, Dr. J. C. Burgher, of Pittsburg, submitted the report of the chairman of the Publishing Committee, which showed the work to be in a backward condition. He asked to be relieved from duty on account of ill-health, and had at last been obliged to transfer his duties to Dr. Joseph C. Guernsey, of Philadelphia.

The Treasurer, Dr. E. M. Kellogg, of New York, submitted his report, which was referred to the Auditing Committee. It shows a cash balance on hand of $3664.15.

At this point in the proceedings, Dr. Berridge, of England, being present, was invited and took a seat on the platform.

The report of the Necrologist, Dr. Paine, of New York, was read and referred. There have been nineteen deaths reported to the Institute during the year.

The Bureau of Organization, Registration, and Statistics reported through its chairman, Dr. I. T. Talbot, of Boston, the following statistics: The most reliable register contains the addresses of 6000 homœopathic physicians in the United States, of whom 839 are active members of this Institute. The Western Academy has 150 members, and meets annually. There are 23 State societies, of which 17 are incorporated, with a total membership of 1859, of which 183 were added and 28 died last year. Of 89 local societies, 63 report to the bureau 1632 members.

The medical clubs are partly social and partly professional in their character. Six of these have 100 members.

Thirty-four homœopathic hospitals are established. Twenty-five of these report 1505 beds, occupied last year by 14,913 patients, 8455 cured, 2864 improved, 349 not improved, 355 (less than 2½ per cent.) died. The cost of 25 of these hospitals has been $1,189,175; debt $85,000; funds $41,206.

Of 29 dispensaries, 22 report 103,577 patients treated last year with 221,803 prescriptions at an average cost of 5½ cents per prescription in conducting the dispensary.

Eleven colleges, all in good standing, have had 1192 students and graduated 387 the past year. The alumni number 4822, and the instructors 159. The cost of establishing five of these colleges has been $230,000. Two special schools, ophthalmic and obstetric, have had 26 students, 18 graduates, and 182 alumni.

Sixteen journals are published in the United States; 4 quarterly, 10 monthly, 1 every two months, and 1 semi-monthly. These publish 22,250 copies, 700 pages, monthly, or 8400 yearly. One library association, one publishing society, and one homœopathic insurance company. All are in successful operation.

The Bureau of Anatomy and Physiology presented a paper by Dr. William E. Spaulding, of Massachusetts, on "The Sphincter Tertius," which was read, and afterwards discussed by Drs. Owens, J. H. McClelland and George A. Hall.

The Bureau of Psychological Medicine presented its report and papers as follows:

"Transitory Fury," by S. Lilienthal, M.D., of New York. As this paper had been already published, it was not referred for publication. Dr. H. H. Hoffmann, of Pittsburg, mentioned a case of the disorder referred to, occurring in the practice of Dr. C. P. Seip, of Pittsburg. The patient, from apparent health passed into a paroxysm of intense mental excitement, requiring force to restrain him. This lasted some hours. It was followed by heavy sleep, continuing 10 or 12 hours, and the patient then awoke to perfect health, and there has been no return of the disorder, and no recollection of the occurrence.

Dr. George F. Foote, of Stamford, Conn., read a paper on "The Causes and Prevention of Insanity, Inebriety, and the Opium Habit," taking the ground that the natural senses and instincts of the organism, if not impaired by abuse, will effectually prevent those forms of disease which are due to indulgence, and resist the invasion of many morbific matters and influences.

Dr. T. L. Brown, of Binghamton, N. Y., presented a paper, entitled "Morbid Vision." The author called attention to the fact that the condition of the brain and its relation to the quantity and quality of blood seem to control the phenomena of normal and morbid vision. The open air, well-ventilated rooms, strictly physiological food, exercise and sleep are conducive to correct vision. In the spiritual circle, held in a closed room, where bed-quilts and blankets are placed over windows and doors to keep out light and oxygen, and keep in carbon, the blood of each person in the room is carbonized, and the feeble-headed, small-chested medium, after hours of breathing the impure air, declares she sees her dead aunt or grandmother, in the darkness. An open door destroys the vision by purifying the air. The well-ventilated churches of this day have done away with the excitements of the revival, and they are now practically a failure, because the inmates are clear-headed in the pure air, and can think and act rationally. (The doctor was just for the moment somewhat disconcerted when a delegate suddenly interjected the question, "How about camp-meetings?"—a question which excited some laughter at the reader's expense.)

A paper on "Phimosis in its Relations to Insanity," was presented by S. H. Talcott, A.M., M.D., Medical Superintendent of the New York State Homœopathic Insane Asylum at Middletown, N. Y., embracing four interesting cases treated by surgical and homœopathic measures.

In the discussion which followed, Dr. Owens, of Cincinnati, said that there are hundreds of cases of phimosis without any attendant mental aberration. In Dr. Talcott's first case there was hereditary predisposition, and he thought this factor or masturbation or some other cause is frequently associated with the phimosis to produce the insanity. Dr. O. S. Woods, of Omaha, corroborated Dr. Owens. Dr. McClelland did not understand the paper of Dr. Talcott as implying that phimosis always results in insanity.

The Institute then took a recess until 8 P.M.

Evening Session.—The business opened with the reports of delegates from several State and county medical societies.

The Bureau of General Sanitary Science, Climatology, and Hygiene was then taken up, and Dr. B. W. James, of Philadelphia, acting chairman, called on Dr. D. H. Beckwith, of Cleveland, who read a paper on "Quarantine for Refugees Exposed to an Epidemic of any Kind by River, Railroad, or Wagonway." He gave a history of the spread of epidemic cholera throughout the principal cities of Ohio from a single case landed from a steamboat in Cincinnati, from which more than 6000 persons perished, and based an argument in favor of inland quarantine thereon. The greatest good to the greatest number was the correct rule, even if it did separate families and spread financial bankruptcy. The government should be empowered to compel States to establish quarantine, and stop railroad trains, steamboats, etc. Refugees from infected districts should be taken to hotel quarantines, kept for a suitable period, placed under the best possible sanitary regulations, and, upon leaving, be provided with new clothing; the infected garments being destroyed. He entered somewhat into the detail of the sanitary management of these hotel quarantine stations. The work of quarantining refugees should be under the control of the General Government, and its officials should be men learned in sanitary science.

Dr. Bushrod W. James read a synopsis of a paper on "The Cordon Sanitaire," by Dr. R. E. Caruthers, of Pittsburg; also one by Dr. M. S. Briry, of Bath, Maine, on "National Quarantine, Including that of the Seacoast." Dr. Briry spoke of the old Jewish quarantine against leprosy as consisting merely of isolation, and gave statistics of quarantine work. He mentioned instances of the transportation of the poison of cholera over thousands of miles in packed clothing, the unpacking of which was sufficient to originate an epidemic. He does not think this peculiar form of poison is transported very far by atmospheric currents.

The chairman then read a paper from Dr. L. A. Falligant, of Savannah, Georgia, on "Sanitation and Location of Quarantine Stations." Quarantine was not a cure for disease, but the means of preventing its spread, and its weight, therefore, fell upon the individual. The sick must be taken beyond the power of doing harm to the well. The site for a quarantine should be in a healthy place, so that the lives of the sick should not be endangered by their isolation. The generally prevailing winds also should be taken into consideration; a site should be selected, if possible, where the wind would neither blow miasma to the hospital, or the poisonous germs of the hospital to the dwelling-places of the healthy. In regard to distance, while it might be safe to locate a small-pox hospital one mile from human habitations, the yellow-fever hospital should be not less than five to ten miles off; this poison being peculiarly liable to be transported for long distances upon atmospheric currents.

Dr. B. W. James then read his own paper on "International Quarantine, Including the Seacoast." He spoke of the difference in the quarantine laws of different nations, which he deplored. The remedy, he thought, must come through the United States, whose coast line was so vast that a rigorous enforcement of wise sanitary and quarantine laws would attract the attention of the world, and make an example which would be followed. He gave a history of the endeavors of France to establish an international quarantine in Europe to prevent the spread of Asiatic cholera. He looked upon the International Sanitary Convention to be held in Washington as of vast importance, and hoped the golden rule would prevail in this congress of nations, but thought the example set by the United States would do more toward the establishment of a code of international quarantine laws.

The subject treated of by the bureau was then opened for discussion, and Dr. Dake, of Nashville, gave a history of the yellow fever scourge in Memphis. He argued that the disease was only spread by actual contact, and the germs were not conveyed in the air. In proof of this he cited the history of the yellow fever epidemic in New York, which had been confined to one part of the city by running a high board fence from river to river across the island. Dr. Bowen, of Fort Wayne, contended that infected clothes should not be destroyed by burning, as the disease was spread in the heat and smoke. Dr. Verdi, of Washington, said the clothes should be baked in ovens, the intense heat destroying the germs of the disease without destroying the clothing, which was an item with poor patients. Dr. Taylor, of Indiana, criticised the idea that the government should supersede the State authorities in the matter of quarantine. Dr. Verdi, of Washington, spoke against the doctrine of State rights bearing on this question, because the interest was an open one. He spoke of the shot-gun quarantine as revolution. It was impossible to stop any epidemic without a single and leading authority to direct operations. He defended the National Board of Health against the charge of interfering with local health authorities, and showed that, on the contrary, that board had during the last year given $150,000 to enable these local boards to carry out their own regulations. Dr. J. Pettet, of Ohio, spoke in favor of the use of superheated steam to disinfect clothing, as a dry heat to destroy the germs of disease would char and consequently destroy them. Dr J. E. Smith, of Cleveland, had been through two yellow fever epidemics, and contended that fear of the disease was a potent agent for its spread. The problem to be settled was, How to prevent the disease?

Dr. Bushrod W. James, of Philadelphia, offered the following resolutions, which were adopted:

Resolved, That the President appoint two delegates to represent this Institute in the next meeting of the American Public Health Association.

Resolved, That this Institute appoint delegates to present the views of this national body to the International Convention called by the United States Government; and if delegates are admitted to its proceedings from medical and other scientific bodies in this country, then our own delegates to be supplied with credentials to present to that body, and the delegates thereupon ask admittance to take part in the proceedings of the International Conference appointed to be held at Washington.

The Institute then adjourned until 9.30 o'clock the next morning.

SECOND DAY—*Morning Session.*—The Secretary read the statistical reports from the various medical colleges, showing all these institutions to be in a flourishing condition.

The Special Committee, consisting of Drs. H. C. Allen, J. P. Dake and J. C. Burgher, appointed yesterday to consider the report of the chairman of the Committee of Publication, made a report concerning the delay in the publication of the *Transactions of the World's Homœopathic Convention,* and of the session of 1879. They recommend that the work be committéd to the hands of the ex-Provisional Secretary, Dr. Joseph C. Guernsey, of Philadelphia, with instructions to bring them out as soon as possible. The recommendation was adopted.

The rules of order were then suspended, and Dr. E. W. Berridge, of London, England, read an address to the Institute on the subject "How Can We Best Advance Homœopathy?" In introducing his subject, he said:

"It cannot be denied that homœopathy has not advanced, and is not advancing as rapidly as we could desire, nor as rapidly as we once had just and reasonable grounds for expecting it to advance. In the United States, where it has taken firmest root, and where its spreading branches most widely overshadow the land with healing in their leaves, the old school is yet triumphant in point of numbers. In Great Britain we have but 275 avowed homœopathic physicians, and this number includes not a few who have not the slightest claims to this honorable title; and while there are many colleges and universities empowered by the state to grant degrees in medicine, we have not one legally recognized school of homœopathy. On the Continent matters are in the same unsatisfactory condition. More than forty years have elapsed since Hahnemann penned the fifth edition of his *Organon;* more than eighty since he first announced the law of Similia, and yet how little fruit has his life-work borne in comparison with what should have been. Why is this? To what causes are we to attribute the fact that the profession and the public have not more universally accepted homœopathy?

"There are those nominally amongst us who have a stereotyped answer to this question. Hahnemann, they say, was too dogmatic, too uncompromising, too visionary; and as a panacea for all the unbelief which now pervades the allopathic mind, they recommend that we should give up what they call our 'sectarian attitude,' that we should drop and disavow the name of homœopathy; that we should repudiate as untenable that which they term the extravagances of Hahnemann, such as his doctrine of chronic disease, etc., and finally that we should claim for Similia Similibus Curantur, not the position of a universal law, but only that of a very good and useful rule of practice to which there may be many exceptions. Do not let us be mistaken in this matter. If we wish the old school to amalgamate with our own, it will never be effected by compromise. Truth has no occasion to descend from her lofty eminence and ask permission to be heard. . . . . .

"Such has been the effect of our wavering upon the minds of our allopathic brethren; what effect has it had on ourselves? Ever since that fatal error was committed by one whose memory we nevertheless hold in honor, of proclaiming 'absolute liberty in medical opinion and action,' a change for the worse has taken place in our own ranks. Ever since that time the name of Carroll Dunham has been held to sanction every kind of empiricism. Forgetting that he himself in his teaching and practice was a true Hahnemannian, men have eagerly caught at his well-intentioned, though mistaken, perhaps misunderstood, words, and ever banded themselves together to overthrow those that remained true to the teachings of the master. I need not recount the various phases of the struggle, they are all well known to you; suffice it to say that the crisis is past, and convalescence has commenced. There are indications both here and in my own country of a desire to return to a purer faith and a truer practice. How can we best accomplish that great work? How are we to advance homœopathy, and render it the sole and universally received science and art of therapeutics. . . . . . The great error of the present race of homœopathists is their neglect to study the *Organon* of Hahnemann, and it is to this great work, the very Bible of homœopathy, that I especially desire to call your attention. I do this with the more earnestness because I find there are so many who have never even read it, much less studied it. 'The *Organon*,' they say, 'is full of Hahnemann's theories.' Leave out the theories then; Hahnemann merely gave them for what they were worth, as the best explanation he could give of certain facts. His theories were based upon his facts, not his facts upon theories. . . . . .

"Was there only one utterance that I could make during this visit to your mighty continent, it would be 'Study the *Organon* of Hahnemann.' It is not as a blind bigot, or a fanatical enthusiast, or a mere hero-worshipper, that I urge these matters upon your attention. I am as ready as any man to worship a hero, but his right to the title must be first demonstrated to me. Since I first discovered how I was misled in early days by teachers, and taught to believe implicitly much that reason and maturer judgment have compelled me to reject as fallacious, I have become skeptical in all things, and require absolute proof before I accept a statement as absolutely true. And my absolute and unwavering acceptance of the truth of the practical teachings of Hahnemann is based upon experience. It is now eighteen years since I first commenced the study of homœopathy; I have compared it with allopathy and with eclecticism. I have tested it in the most severe acute diseases threatening life, in the most chronic and inveterate diseases which had baffled all other treatment, and in incurable cases when only euthanasia was possible, and I have never once found Hahnemann's teaching to be wrong. Nay, more, though Hahnemann's faithful followers have made many discoveries in the same field in which he labored, so vast was his insight, and so profound his genius, that there is scarcely a single therapeutic discovery of modern times, of which you will not find at least the germ in his writings.

"Hahnemann's system is the true, the only science of therapeutics, and if my words will persuade any of you who may have departed from his standard, to adopt a purer practice and a truer faith, I shall feel that my visit to you has not been in vain."

Dr. Smith, of Chicago, moved that Dr. Berridge be requested

to give his article to the Secretary for publication, which was carried.

A motion to reconsider was made on account of objections being made to its being incorporated in the proceedings.

The matter was finally laid on the table.

The Report and Papers of the Bureau of Materia Medica, Pharmacy, and Provings were then presented by the chairman, Dr. J. P. Dake, of Nashville, Tennessee, who introduced the subject with some observations on the development of the Materia Medica, the issue of certain new publications, and the work on which the bureau had been engaged during the year. The general subject of the papers was "The Limit of Drug Attenuation and Medicinal Power in Homœopathic Posology." They were arranged under two heads, the first of which, viz., "The Proofs of Drug Presence and Power in Attenuations above the Sixth Decimal," being considered in the following papers:

(a.) "As Furnished by the Tests of Chemistry," by W. L. Breyfogle, M.D.

(b.) "As Furnished by the Spectroscope," by Conrad Wesselhœft, M.D.

(c.) "As Furnished by the Microscope," by J. Edwards Smith, M.D.

(d.) "As Furnished by Analogy from the Field of Impalpahle Morbific Agencies," by J. P. Dake, M.D.

(e.) "As Furnished by the Tests of Physiology," by Lewis Sherman, M.D.

The portion of the subject included under the second head, "The Proofs of Medicinal Presence and Efficacy in Attenuations above the Sixth Decimal," was presented in the following papers:

(f.) "As Furnished by Clinical Experience in the Use of Attenuations Ranging from the 15th to the 30th Decimal," by A. C. Cowperthwaite, M.D.

(g.) "As Furnished by Clinical Experience in the Use of Attenuations above the 30th Decimal," by C. H. Lawton, M.D.

Dr. Breyfogle's paper gave the results of carefully conducted chemical experiments with the 3d, 6th, 12th and 30th decimals of Arsenicum, Nux vom., Sulphur, etc. Perceptible results were obtained from Ars. 3d and 6th; but Sulphur 3d and upwards gave no results. Experiments were also made upon human subjects with material doses of the carefully selected homœopathic drug, for the purpose of ascertaining the largest dose which might be administered without danger of medicinal aggravation, the results showing that quite large quantities of Ipecac., in the vomiting of pregnancy, could be given with no other than a curative effect, and the same negative results were obtained with other drugs.

Dr. Wesselhœft's paper gave the degree of delicacy observable with spectroscopic tests, showing that by the best authorities the minimum quantity detected has been of Sodium, the 1-18,000,000th of a grain; Lithium, 1-6,000,000th; Strontium, 1-1,000,000th; Calcium, 1-1,000,000th. Cæsium and Rubidium have each been detected in the proportion of one grain to five tons of water. The author of the paper then quoted from his paper of last year the statement that modern research indicates the limit of the divisibility of matter to be reached at about the 11th centesimal, and cited the recent experiments of Crookes on the fourth state of matter, as confirming these indications. The paper concludes with an account of some spectroscopic experiments made by the writer himself with Sodium, in which the 1-100,000,000th of a grain gave ocular evidence of its presence.

Dr. J. E. Smith had entitled his paper, "Remarks and Suggestions Concerning the Study of Homœopathic Triturations." In presenting his subject he asked the privilege of correcting an almost universal misapprehension in regard to himself. "*I do* NOT *believe*," said he, "*that the microscope will enable us to discover the ultimate divisibility of matter*," and expressed himself further as being very anxious that his views in this particular should be no longer misunderstood and misrepresented.

He first gave a description of the apparatus and facilities at his command in pursuing his investigations and securing the most exact microscopic measurements of particles of triturated Aurum—the metal experimented with. He summed up in general terms the results of the microscopic researches recently made with homœopathic triturations of gold, as follows:

1st. A certain so-called trituration, sold for Aurum 3^x, contained no gold at all. 2d. Mr. Witte's triturations of Aurum fol. has been demonstrated to be almost equal in fineness of particles to the average triturations from the precipitate. 3d. Four-hour decimal triturations are not very far superior to the two-hour. 4th. Triturations of Aurum met. up to the 6^x from various makers vary considerably, no two being identical in the fineness of the contained particles. 5th. The popular idea that particles of gold are ten times smaller in the 2d than in the 1st, and ten times smaller in the 3d than in the

2d, is very far from being correct. 6th. In all the triturations of gold from the 1st to the 6th decimal examined by me, fully 33 per cent. of the metal escapes subdivision under the pestle, *i. e.*, does not become subdivided to anything like the extent formerly accepted. 7th. It is quite possible with careful manipulations to display particles of metallic gold under the microscope, which; in point of minuteness, challenges our most difficult test-objects.

The concluding portion of the paper described an improved method of preparing triturations of gold, this method having been devised after repeated experimentations by Dr. Smith and Mr. Witte. It consisted in recovering the gold from "amethystine fluid," and triturating. On adding water and alcohol to the trituration the same purple fluid is produced, which, after standing for a period of ten days or more, deposits a sediment, which consists chiefly of impurities from the milk-sugar used in making the triturations. This fluid under the microscope exhibits no suspended particles of gold, but evaporation on a glass slide imparts an appearance like that of "watered silk." Under this new method of triturating gold the 3d and 6th yielded particles having a dimension of 1-95,000th to 1-115,000th of an inch. We understood Dr. Smith to express the view that the metal contained in the amethystine fluid is not in solution, but in suspension, the particles being so minute as to be invisible even under his highest powers.

Dr. Lewis Sherman's paper referred to a comparison of Dunham's provings of Sepia^{200}, made in 1875, with the provings of milk-sugar, made by Dr. Wesselhœft, two years later; the object being to show that the great bulk of the symptoms was due to other than drug agencies, fear being probably one of them. This form of pathogenetic test, the writer argued, is unreliable for the reason above given. In the Milwaukee Test of 1879, most of the experimenters declined any attempt to designate the medicated vial, thus exhibiting a lack of confidence which the proposers of the test did not anticipate. Some of the experimenters had said that even the low attenuations would fail under a similar test. Accordingly Dr. Allen undertook to test the 30^{x}, and he (Sherman) undertook to test those still lower. Dr. Allen subsequently withdrew from the work. The tests made by Dr. Sherman and his co-laborers were guarded against unfairness and error as carefully as was possible, and the results, together with those of the "Milwaukee Test" proper, are in brief as follows:

3x,	9 blanks.	Tests, 5.	Correct selections, 4.	Incorrect, 1.
5x,	9 "	" 3.	" " 3.	" 0.
6x,	9 "	" 7.	" " 6.	" 1.
7x,	9 "	" 2.	" " 1.	" 1.
8x,	9 "	" 2.	" " 1.	" 1.
9x,	9 "	" 2.	" " 1.	" 1.
10x,	9 "	" 2.	" " 0.	" 2.
30x,	9 "	" 7.	" " 0.	" 7.
30x,	1 "	" 1.	" " 1.	" 0.

Dr. Dake's paper came next in order. It presented a host of facts in connection with various morbific agencies: malaria, miasms, electricity, etc., all going to prove that abnormal effects are producible by agencies not recognizable by the senses, or by the most delicate processes of the laboratory.

Dr. Cowperthwaite then introduced the "high potency" side of the question in an able and careful paper. He began with the proposition, that as man cannot live by bread alone, he must sooner or later acknowledge his physical relation to the unknown as well as to the known. When Hahnemann had repeatedly seen Acon.^{30} cause sweat in fever, he very properly adjudged that in Acon., medicinal power did not cease below the thirtieth potency. And Hahnemann's observations fully confirmed this opinion as to a considerable number of other drugs. The doctor then cited the comparative experiments made in hospitals with the 30th, 6th, and 15th decimals, continued for a long period, the disease selected for investigation being pneumonia. The observations showed that as regarded the processes of infiltration, resolution, exudation, and the total duration of the disease, the results were by far the most favorable to the 30th, or highest, and the least favorable to the 6th, or lowest. He also reminded the Institute of the historical fact that the early homœopathists of America had only the 30th potencies with which to demonstrate the truth of similia, there being no other potencies in the market. Had those 30ths been destitute of medicinal virtue, homœopathy would to-day be a matter of history. He argued that when clinical evidences are carefully and properly observed, they are useful in the same proportion as are the observations of the chemist and the microscopist. The paper closed with a number of carefully observed cases recorded by well-known practitioners, in which the 30th potency developed rapid and permanent cures, and added, "If men believe not these facts, neither would they be persuaded though one arose from the dead."

Dr. C. H. Lawton in his paper alluded to a natural obstacle

to the acceptance of high potencies. Facts must harmonize with known laws, else their convincing influence is limited. When men will not, or do not, experiment for themselves, we must present reason and logic by which to convince them. Observation gives evidence that medicinal power and efficacy extend beyond the supposed limit of the divisibility of matter, though we may not understand it. The writer argued that without potentization there can be no medicinal efficacy. He offered some interesting facts in support of his views respecting the value of potencies above the 30th, among which was a case of perityphlitis, treated by Dr. Pearson, of Washington, D. C., with Hepar sulph.^{m} (Tafel), and followed by recovery.

Adjourned till 7 P.M.

Evening Session.—Discussion was had upon the general subjects embraced in the report of the Bureau of Materia Medica, etc. Dr. Lilienthal explained that Dr. T. F. Allen, of New York, had declined to take part in the test of high potencies, because he was unwilling to have them prepared in Milwaukee. Dr. Lippe said such a test had been made in Vienna thirty years ago by Dr. Wadsworth, and resulted in overcoming the skepticism of that gentleman. Physicians decline to spend time in a repetition of that experiment simply because there is no need of it. Dr. A. E. Small did not see what chemistry, microscopy, or spectroscopy has to do with high potencies. He thought nature furnished abundant analogies of the action of infinitesimals, and illustrated his point by the germination of the seed and growth of the tree. Once, after having been enjoined never to give a certain patient Pulsatilla, he had secretly administered a dose of the 800th Jenichen, and had, the next day, been called to account for it. Dr. McManus had a patient in whom the presence of the common shrub, *Talicanthus*, produced syncope. Dr. Owens thought the bureau had gone entirely out of its own province for a subject, and he was disappointed at having heard nothing which in his estimation could promote our knowledge of the Materia Medica. Dr. McClelland defended the bureau; it had selected a subject connected with "Materia Medica, Pharmacy, and Provings," and adhered strictly to it. Some of the testimony offered was of a negative character it is true, still such testimony is of great value. The report shows that certain attenuations failed to show the presence of medicinal qualities, but this is not proof positive that such qualities do not exist therein.

He said that patients troubled with malignant typhoid fever were, through the enthusiasm of the reporters, represented as having been cured by a single dose of medicine in one day. These reports were palpably false and weakened men's faith in homœopathy and in homœopathists.

Dr. Wells, of Brooklyn, gave his experience in the treatment and remarkable cure of a case which had come under his own observation. Dr. Brown, of Binghamton, N. Y., complimented the papers presented by the bureau. He contended that medicines were matter and we were matter, and by watching the contact of the matters we could discover certain changes that formed data for future action. Dr. Pearson, referring to the papers, said they were a great improvement on those presented last year. Dr. Dake corrected a mistake of Dr. Lilienthal, and said that Dr. Allen's refusal to participate in the potency test could not have arisen from the cause stated, as the potencies were to have been prepared in New York and not in Milwaukee.

Dr. H. M. Smith, for Dr. J. J. Mitchell, chairman of the Committee on a Homœopathic Dispensatory, submitted a report.

Dr. Talbot, of Boston, said year after year we have a report on the subject of a dispensatory in an incompleted state. Twelve years of incubation was sufficient, and he moved the subject be indefinitely postponed. After some discussion the motion was adopted.

The Bureau of Clinical Medicine, having for its subject Scarlatina, was then taken up, and the chairman, Dr. C. Pearson, of Washington, read a paper on "Its History, Etiology, and Varieties." Dr. Lilienthal, one on the "Diagnosis, Pathology, and Course of Scarlatina." Dr. T. F. Pomroy, one on the "Contagious Nature of, Liability to, and Exemption from Scarlatina."

Adjourned till 9 o'clock to-morrow morning.

THIRD DAY—*Morning Session.*—On motion of Dr. D. S. Smith, of Chicago, the Institute voted to take from the table for reconsideration the address of Dr. Berridge, of London, delivered yesterday.

Dr. Talbot, of Boston, addressed the Institute in reference to a certain passage contained in the address of Dr. Berridge, characterizing it as a great wrong alike to this body, to the physicians of America, and to the memory of one who is held in reverence by every true friend of true Homœopathy. He read the passage referred to, as follows:

"Ever since that fatal error was committed, by one whose memory we nevertheless hold in honor, of proclaiming 'absolute liberty in medical opinion and action,' a change for the worse has taken place in our own ranks. Ever since that time the name of Carroll Dunham has been held to sanction every kind of empiricism. Forgetting that he himself in his teaching and practice was a true Hahnemannian, men have eagerly caught at his well-intentioned, though mistaken, perhaps misunderstood, words, and ever banded themselves together to overthrow those that remained true to the teachings of the master."

Can such words as those go out from the American Institute as its sentiment? When at Chicago, as those who were present well remember, there were some ready and endeavoring to break this Institute to pieces, and were proclaiming that there were only a few homœopaths, and all the rest were mongrels, then it was that Dr. Carroll Dunham uttered his ringing words proclaiming "liberty of medical opinion and action," which stand upon our record like letters of gold, and have done more to advance homœopathy—true homœopathy—than those of any other man that have ever been spoken. And when we find that from the platform of this Institute, an aspersion has been cast upon his name, we cannot let such words go upon our records without a solemn and indignant protest.

Dr. Wesselhœft, of Boston, said: "I desire to say what I had no opportunity of saying yesterday. A young physician from abroad was by courtesy admitted to a seat on the platform, and proceeded to lecture the Institute on its ignorance of homœopathy, and its neglect to read *The Organon.* This was not in good taste, and I object to the incorporation of that lecture in our transactions. Such accusations were successfully stamped out by the Institute years ago. Dr. Berridge was ill-informed and ill-advised. That is my apology for him."

Dr. Ludlam, of Chicago, thought that the remarks of Dr. Wesselhœft acquired additional force from the fact that Dr. Berridge does not come to us as the acknowledged representative of any foreign society. When he (Dr. L.) attended the sessions of the British homœopathic societies, Dr. Berridge was not present. He comes to us and speaks to us as a private physician only.

Dr. J. P. Dake, Nashville, Tenn., said that in America the progress of our cause has been steadily and not slowly onward, that whatever hindrances have come in our way have not arisen from any spirit of excessive liberality on our part. Probably the greatest obstacle, so far as our course has occasioned any, has been an extreme construction placed upon the teachings of the master and an excessive indulgence, on the part of some of our leaders, in measures obnoxious to the learning and the experience of the medical world. Dr. Berridge is mistaken in the supposition that the moderation and liberality advocated in this body by the loved and lamented Dunham has been the cause of any weakness or delay in our onward course. No man in all America did more, in the same number of years, to further the interests of homœopathy than Carroll Dunham. Although not given to hero-worship in this country, we do not fail to appreciate and defend the good name of those who, having wrought most nobly and successfully in life, now rest peacefully from all earthly labor.

As to the study of Hahnemann's writings, I venture to say that our practitioners are as familiar with them as any medical men in the world. While esteeming the words of the master as explanatory of the new system of therapeutics, in the day of its birth and the years of its youth, we do not regard all his sayings as infallible, nor his tenets as everlasting. Under the fostering influences of freedom, and persuaded that, in matters of science, there can be no limits to progress, we are ever looking for fresh facts and new principles to guide our way in the field of practice. We revere Hahnemann; we take his teachings for what they are worth; but we do not accept from him all the opinions held in his day as priceless treasures. As for the old school of medicine in this country we have no compromise with it. While there is much common ground for allopaths and homœopaths to occupy and cultivate together, we stand upon our own field, a peculiar people, when we come to the application of medicines for the cure of disease, acknowledging the law *similia* as supreme and final. We differ, sometimes, among ourselves as to the extent of the field covered by that law, and as to the preparation and uses of remedies under its guidance; but we forsake not the banner, years ago planted upon these shores, under which we have been gathered from the devious ways of old physic, and under which, our successors shall ultimately possess all this goodly land.

Dr. Ober moved that the paper be laid upon the table, and the discussion thereon expunged from the minutes. The motion was adopted.

The consideration of the Bureau of Clinical Medicine was then taken up where it was left by the adjournment on Wednesday evening, the subject being Scarlatina. Dr. J. P. Mills, of Chicago, read a paper on "Dissimilarity to Diphtheria and other Cutaneous Diseases." Dr. O. P. Baer, of Richmond, Ind., also presented an article on "Belladonna and other Prophylactics."

Dr. Lippe, of Philadelphia, then read a paper on "The Treatment of the Varieties and Symptoms of Scarlatina," and Dr. P. P. Wells, of Brooklyn, presented an interesting essay on "Specific Prescribing in Scarlatina."

Professor Ludlam, of Chicago, offered a resolution that hereafter the annual meetings of the Institute shall consist of one general morning session daily, and that the afternoons be given to bureaus for sectional meetings. The resolution was adopted.

Dr. Talbot, of Boston, offered a resolution indorsing the proposition of the homœopathic physicians of Great Britain for an international congress in London in July, 1881, which was adopted, and providing for the appointment of a committee to further that object. Adopted; the committee consisting of Drs. I. T. Talbot, E. M. Kellogg, and B. W. James.

The Bureau of Microscopy and Histology presented a paper by Dr. Wesselhœft on the "Relations of the Microscope to Materia Medica and Potencies," and one by Dr. J. E. Smith on "Modern Microscopes."

The Committee on Time and Place of Next Meeting reported that invitations had been received from Cape May, Long Branch, Manhattan Beach, Newport, Saratoga and New York city. It was voted to refer the whole matter to the Executive Committee, with instructions to hold the next meeting in or near New York city.

The election of officers to serve for the ensuing year was then held with the following result: President, J. W. Dowling, M.D., New York; Vice-President, William L. Breyfogle, M.D., Louisville, Ky.; General Secretary, J. G. Burgher, M.D., Pittsburg, Pa.; Provisional Secretary, J. H. McClelland, M.D., Pittsburg, Pa.; Treasurer, E. M. Kellogg, M.D., New York; Censors, F. R. McManus, M.D., Baltimore, Chairman, R. B. Rush, M.D., C. T. Canfield, M.D., William H. Leonard, M.D., P. G. Valentine, M.D.

The Bureau of Obstetrics presented its report through Dr. G. B. Peck, of Rhode Island. It embraced important papers, as follows:

"The Forceps and the Principles of their Use," by R. M. Foster, M.D.

"Extra-uterine Fœtation," by C. Ormes, M.D.

"Placenta Prævia," by Geo. B. Peck, M.D.

Dr. Foster's paper encourages the use of the forceps, and argues that just in proportion as their use increases, the mortality of mothers and children during labor diminishes. No instrument at all equals it in the saving of human life. He gave a history of its "development," and exhibited various modifications in illustration of his subject.

Pending the consideration of this subject the Institute adjourned until 3 o'clock.

Afternoon Session.—The consideration of the report of the Bureau of Obstetrics was resumed, and Dr. Peck's paper was read. It is based upon reports received from about 120 homœopathic physicians of this country, and the facts presented and conclusions drawn are exceedingly interesting and valuable. We are happy to be able to announce that some of these cases will appear in forthcoming numbers of the HAHNEMANNIAN.

Dr. Ormes's paper was also important, detailing an interesting case. After its reading, discussion was had on the various papers.

Under a suspension of the order of business, Dr. J. H. McClelland exhibited Vance's crinoline jacket for spinal curvature, and called attention to the advantages it possessed over the Sayre jacket, particularly because of its being removable at will for the purpose of securing rest and cleanliness.

The Bureau of Gynæcology reported through its acting chairman, Dr. Biggar of Cleveland, the following papers:

"Uterine Fibroma," a case with operation, by C. Ormes, M.D.

"How do Medicines Act on the Generative Organs of Women?" by E. M. Hale, M.D.

"Influence of Homœopathic Treatment on the Development of Ovarian Cysts," by B. F. Betts, M.D.

"Cæsarian Section," by S. S. Lungren, M.D.

"The Use of Intra-uterine Stem Pessaries," by Mrs. E. C. Cook, M.D.

Adjourned until Friday morning.

FOURTH DAY—*Morning Session.*—The Bureau of Pædology, Dr. William H. Jenney, chairman, reported the following papers:

"Acute Gastritis; Its Causes, Diagnosis, and Anatomical Characteristics," by W. H. Jenney, M.D.

"Prevention and Treatment," by W. Edmunds, M.D.

"Thrush," by T. C. Duncan, M.D.

"Prevention and Treatment of Stomatitis," by A. M. Cushing, M.D.

"Dietetic Rules in Digestive Diseases," by Mary A. B. Woods, M.D.

Dr. H. C. Allen offered a resolution, which the Institute adopted, providing for an inquiry into the preliminary qualifications required of students by the various medical colleges.

At 11 o'clock, in accordance with a previous arrangement, Dr. F. R. McManus, of Baltimore, delivered an address in which he gave his early experience with the thirtieth potencies. He detailed his first attempts to acquire such a knowledge of the homœopathic healing art as might enable him to put its principles to a practical test. For a whole hour the venerable doctor held the closest attention of his critical audience, while his humorous description of his cases and of the results of his treatment elicited applause and laughter from both high and low dilutionists. Amongst the many cases treated experimentally was a gonorrhœal orchitis, for which Arnica^{30} was prescribed, and *the patient* (a cooper) *was ordered to continue at work*, lest the beneficial influence of rest should modify the action of the remedy. In spite of this precaution (?) the patient, three days afterward, reported himself well. A case of pain in the knee-joint, which the doctor had treated allopathically for years, yielded promptly to Puls.^{30}. A case of intermittent neuralgia of six weeks' standing disappeared permanently in 24 hours,—scared off with a single dose of Spig.^{30}. A number of other similar cases were reported. The whole address was calculated to add materially to the force of the papers presented by Drs. Cowperthwaite and Lawton in advocacy of the thirtieth potencies. His closing remarks are well worth transcribing: "The greatest enemy homœopathic physicians have, is to be found in themselves. That man is a fool, who, in using vaccine virus as a prophylactic, inserts it into a child's arm every morning and evening for five days. One dose, well selected, and allowed to have its full effect, is better than indecision and needless repetition."

The Bureau of Ophthalmology and Otology reported papers on "Diseases of the Lids," by F. Park Lewis, M.D.; "Tumors of the Lids and Diseases of the Lachrymal Glands," by J. H. Buffum, M.D.; "Stricture of the Lachrymal Passages," by D. G. Maguire, M.D.

The Bureau of Surgery presented papers on "Staphylorraphy," by I. T. Talbot, M.D.; "Injuries of the Abdomen," by Professor Hartshorne; "Hernia," by J. H. McClelland, M.D.; "Radical Cure of Hernia," by C. M. Thomas, M.D.; "Sphincterismus," by George A. Hall, M.D.; "Prolapse and

Foreign Growths of the Rectum," by E. C. Franklin, M.D.; "Acute Peritonitis; Its Relation to the Diagnosis and Surgical Treatment of the Abdominal Viscera," by John C. Minor, M.D.; "Acute Intussusception," by N. Schneider, M.D.

Some general business of minor importance was transacted, appointments of committees announced, and then at 12 o'clock, the thirty-third session of the American Institute of Homœopathy was declared adjourned. It was estimated that about 250 physicians were in attendance, and forty new members were received.

CALCAREOUS INFILTRATIONS.

BY A. R. THOMAS, M D, PHILADELPHIA, PA.

(Read before the Philadelphia County Homœopathic Medical Society.)

Among the changes of structure which the tissues of the body are capable of undergoing, are prominently those known as degenerations.

Degenerations are characterized by certain transformations of the elements of a structure, which may originate either in the tissue itself, or may be the result of deposits from without; the change in either case impairing the vitality and function, first of the tissue, and second of the organ of which it forms a part. The causes leading to these conditions are undoubtedly various, and many times difficult to determine. Among the more evident may be enumerated: disturbances in the circulation, from either arterial, capillary, or venous obstructions; insufficient nutritive supply; excessive or prolonged waste, as in diabetes, albuminuria, hæmorrhage, etc.; diminished or increased functional activity; inflammation; the action of various substances when taken into the system, as Iodine, Mercury, Bromine, Lead, etc.; and finally, nervous influence. Many of these causes may act first to induce simple atrophy, this being accompanied or followed by degeneration.

It is usual to divide degeneration into, first, metamorphoses, and second, infiltrations. In the former there is a conversion of the albuminoid elements of the tissues into new materials, this being followed by such destruction of histological elements as to ultimately remove all trace of original structure, and to arrest all functional power. Fatty, mucous, and colloid degenerations are instances of such metamorphoses.

Infiltrations differ from *metamorphoses* inasmuch as the new material which is found in the tissues is not derived from a change of any of their elements, but is deposited from the blood. This condition is rarely followed by destructive changes in the elements of the tissues, and hence they are less disturbed functionally. The infiltrations include frothy, amyloid, calcareous, and pigmentary.

CALCAREOUS INFILTRATION.—While calcareous infiltration may be of less importance, pathologically, than many other forms of degeneration, yet the subject is one of interest and deserving of careful consideration. Having little to do with acute diseases it will be found to have important relations to many chronic affections.

A calcified tissue or organ presents certain characters, rendering it readily and unmistakably recognized. It is hard, rigid, rough to the touch, and grating under the knife. The deposits may occur in pilules or spiculæ, or exist in small granular pustules, or in rounded masses.

The chemical elements entering into the composition of these deposits are found to consist mainly of the salts of lime and magnesia, the phosphates and carbonates of these materials being the forms more generally found.

In looking for an explanation of this pathological condition we are to remember that both of the substances are freely soluble in one of the constantly present elements of the blood, namely, carbonic acid, as well also, to a limited degree, as in lactic and certain fatty acids, and physiologists tell us that they are always present in certain proportions wherever these acids are found. It is not difficult to conceive that under certain conditions there may be an excess of these salts of lime and magnesia held in solution, and that while the blood circulates slowly through the capillary vessels, the retarded flow facilitates the great tendency for diffusion of the carbonic acid, which escaping leaves the insoluble salts behind. Particle by particle being thus deposited, the complete calcareous change thus finally results. In some instances calcification may be looked upon as a variety of *metastasis*. In extensive caries of bone, where the resorption of earthy salts is more rapid than the elimination by the kidneys, there may be a deposit of the same, most frequently in the pyramids of the kidneys, more rarely in the lungs, in the mucous membranes of the stomach, and still more rarely in the mucous membranes of the intestines and of the sphenoidal and ethmoidal cells, in the dura mater and liver and walls of bloodvessels.

Nearly every tissue and organ of the body is susceptible of this pathological change. We find it occurring in cartilage, in muscle, both voluntary and involuntary, in the walls of bloodvessels—arteries, veins, and capillaries, in the several membranes, tendons, ligaments, connective tissues, etc. Among organs affected may be mentioned the brain, kidneys, valves of the heart, the placenta, and various glandular bodies. Morbid growth, also, and deposits of various kinds are liable to this change. Thus adhesions resulting from inflammatory actions, false membranes, hypertrophies, tumors of various kinds, and tubercular deposits are particularly liable to become calcified.

When involving normal tissues, the result of calcification is to gradually impair, and finally totally destroy their function, and thus lead to other complications and derangements. When taking place in abnormal growths, as in fibroma, enchondroma, struma, tubercles, cancers, etc., the process may be looked upon as a conservative one, frequently tending to arrest the original pathological development, and directly prolonging life.

Gouty deposits differ from ordinary calcareous deposits, 1st, in their chemical composition, these being made up mainly of the urate of soda; and 2d, in their being less diffused through the body, selecting first the articular cartilages, with that of the external ear, tendons, and ligaments of the joints, and very rarely the bloodvessels, skin, and kidneys.

RESPIRATORY ORGANS.—Calcification may appear in different portions of the respiratory apparatus. Of the larynx, the thyroid and cricoid cartilages are more frequently and more extensively involved. The same condition may develop in the cartilaginous rings of the trachea, or within the bronchial tubes, to their smaller ramifications. This condition is generally found in old persons who have suffered from severe and chronic catarrhs, the relation of the calcification to the catarrh in these cases, however, being that of an effect rather than a cause; the prolonged inflammatory action giving one of the conditions known to favor the formation of these deposits.

An interesting example of calcareous degeneration is found in the so-called lung-stones, *calculi pulmonales*, occasionally discharged from the lungs by expectoration. These bodies are small, rounded, and smooth, varying in size from half a pea to that of a pin's head, or smaller, as seen by the example presented. There is no question but that these bodies are calcified tubercles. They are not only occasionally expectorated during life, but are found post-mortem. The case from which this sample has been obtained is the only one that has come under my own personal observation. The patient is a lady of about 60 years, thin and feeble, and for many years subject to bad catarrhs, with harassing cough. For the past two years she has occasionally expectorated these bodies, a few only of which have been saved. The physical signs upon examination of the lungs, as well as the general appearance of the patient, indicated tuberculosis.

Calcification of tubercle is generally a favorable result in pulmonary tuberculosis. Those tubercles near the bronchial surfaces may be discharged into these passages and expectorated, while others may become encysted and remain comparatively harmless.

A remarkable specimen of interstitial deposit in the parenchyma of the lungs was obtained at a post-mortem examination made a few months ago for Dr. C. B. Knerr, of this city. Upon opening the chest, some pint and a half of serum was found in the right pleural cavity, and, as the hand was carried around the lung, at about the middle of the lower lobe a hard mass, half the size of the fist, was felt in the lung substance. Upon removal, this mass was found to be composed of numerous calcareous bodies, varying in size and shape, the larger being irregular, and quite a half-inch in its longest diameter. These bodies appeared to be formed in the connective tissue uniting the bronchial tubes and bloodvessels. There were no evidences of inflammation either in the lung substance or in the pleura covering that portion of the lungs. In none of the works on morbid anatomy can I find mention made of such extensive deposits.

The brain is not exempt from this pathological condition, the walls of the larger arteries being more frequently affected. Small calcareous deposits are occasionally found in the brain substance and in the dura mater, but it is more frequently in morbid growths of the brain that this condition of calcification is found. Tubercle, cancer, and the results of certain cysts may undergo this change. There are no symptoms by means of which these conditions may be detected during life.

LESIONS OF THE CIRCULATORY APPARATUS PRODUCED BY CALCAREOUS INFILTRATIONS.

BY W. B. TRITES, M D., MANAYUNK, PA.

(Read before the Philadelphia County Homœopathic Medical Society.)

It will be unnecessary for me to dwell on the general subject of calcification, so clearly has it been presented to you in the able paper of my honored colleague, Professor A. R. Thomas. Therefore, without further introduction, let us proceed to examine the lesions which this species of degeneration occasions in the circulatory apparatus.

The heart, arteries, and veins are favorite seats for the development of calcareous degeneration, their internal coat or lining membrane being the portion most apt to be involved. The muscular walls of the heart are not nearly so apt to become calcified, though Heschel reports a case occurring in a patient suffering with Bright's disease, and Luken another in which a calcified mass 3 cm. long and 2 wide had been developed idiopathically in the heart substance. Such formations result usually from the calcification of fibrous or connective tissue growths, which have penetrated the heart tissue and then become the subject of this degeneration; or, as Routh has pointed out, it may result from the contents of an abscess of the walls becoming encapsulated, and finally calcified.

But the serous lining of the heart, the endocardium and valves are very frequently invaded by calcareous infiltration. Indeed, so common is this, that it may be taken as one of the signs of advancing age. But the deposit of lime salts in these localities is not peculiar to old age. It may occur at an early period of life, while diseases of the kidney seem to be especially liable to produce it. Intemperate habits, overwork, and what has lately been rendered more than probable, the slavish use of tobacco, each tend to produce atheroma, and atheroma is usually but the forerunner of calcareous degeneration.

Calcification may occur in any part of the endocardium, but it is more commonly found in the left ventricle than in the other cavities, and in the aortic and mitral valves much more frequently than in the valves of the right side of the heart.

In 79 cases of valvular disease reported by Dr. Barclay in the *Medical and Chirurgical Transactions* for 1848, 12 showed marked calcareous deposits, 8 in the mitral valve and 4 in the aortic, and of these 12 cases 7 of them suffered from some form of kidney disease.

Chronic endocarditis, the primal cause of the development of this species of degeneration, is characterized by the production of cartilage-like, opaque, or translucent thickenings. Such lesions are especially seen in the fibrous zones surrounding the orifices, the chordæ tendinæ, and upon the ventricular surface of the aortic valves, and the auricular surface of the auriculo-ventricular valves.

These cartilage-like thickenings of the endocardium become

the seat of fatty degeneration, or of atheroma, and in these new formations a precipitation of calcareous matter takes place, resulting in the formation of bone-like plates, or of scattered scales of calcified tissue.

Owing to the situation of the coronary arteries, being imbedded in the endocardium, they are especially liable to undergo this process, hence it is not an uncommon thing to find them converted into calcareous tubes, or even entirely obliterated by the deposit of mineral matter. The pericardium, undergoing the same processes of chronic inflammation and the production of cornea-like tissue upon its surfaces, is often the seat of calcification. Some of these have been very extensive; Bauer relating a case in which the whole sac became converted into a hard calcareous capsule, enveloping the heart. The arteries are more prone to this pathological condition than any other portion of the circulatory apparatus. In them, as in the other instances of which we have spoken, calcareous degeneration is generally the result of a chronic inflammation of the internal coat. I say generally this is the case, but not always, for another form of calcification is met with in arteries of medium and small size, a form not attended with or consecutive to fatty degeneration, but apparently due to a calcareous transformation of the muscular cells of the middle coat, converting them into calcareous spindle-shaped bodies.* This species of calcification has no necessary connection with inflammation of the artery, and occurs most commonly in arteries of the lower extremity, and next in those of the arm and head. But, as before stated, a chronic endarteritis is the more common cause of the lesion. In endarteritis, as in inflammation of other serous membranes, there are produced scattered elevations of the internal coat, resembling in some instances, cartilage; in others, where the consistence is less, they look like mucoid or gelatinous growths. These elevations hold within themselves cells containing fatty granules. After the inflammation subsides this fatty metamorphosis continues until the patch loses its translucent appearance, becoming yellow ard opaque. The fatty degeneration continuing, the groups of granules which first had the form of cells are fused together, and there results a characteristic atheromatous focus. This atheromatous focus is situated, as Virchow has proved, in the thickened internal coat, and not between the internal and middle coats, as has been suggested. As long as the patch remains

* Virchow's Cellular Pathology, p. 407.

intact it is covered by the thickened endothelial layer of the internal coat. If we cut through this covering we find the contents composed of an opaque pulp resembling the contents of a sebaceous tumor, and consisting of cholesterin crystals, fatty molecules, and degenerated remnants of tissue. This constitutes atheroma, and is more or less constantly associated with calcareous degeneration. Calcareous molecules are deposited in the tissues intervening between these fatty degenerating cells, and the result may be the formation of either calcareous lumps, or more frequently of thin, more or less transparent plates, which are curved in conformity to the curve of the vessels in whose walls the lesion may take place. The calcareous plates thus formed at first are not exposed, but covered by a thin membranous lamellæ composed of the internal layer of the internal coat. The rush of blood along the vessel, however, soon strips this off and leaves the plates denuded.

Calcareous deposits are in some cases scattered irregularly along the walls of the arteries; in other instances these formations are so numerous and large as to convert the vessel in which they occur into a rigid bone-like cylinder. Rindfleisch supposes that the pathological deposition of calcareous salts, which in the blood are rendered soluble by the presence of carbonic acid gas, takes place at the periphery of cell districts, and is due to the difficulty of reabsorbing the nutrient matters which have found their way hither.

This difficulty favors the separation of the more absorbable from the less absorbable constituents, and thus the dissolved carbonic acid is removed, while the calcareous salts, which its presence had rendered soluble, are deposited in the tissue.

The aorta at its arch is more liable to the formation of such deposits than any other artery, though none enjoy entire immunity. It occurs least frequently, perhaps, in the pulmonary.

Küttner has described a case in which all the arteries were calcified, and more so the further they were situated from the heart. It occurred in a patient suffering from scrofulous caries of the dorsal and lumbar vertebræ, and had besides a purulent nephritis.

Calcareous infiltration is seldom seen in the capillaries, although sometimes it occurs, especially in those of the dura mater in the condition called psammomata by Virchow. The coats of the veins are less subject to degeneration than the arterial coats. Fatty degeneration is somewhat rare, but calcification is more common. By it, plates or rings are formed which are imbedded in the walls of the vessels. Especially are they apt to occur in dilated veins of the lower extremity.

These calcareous plates are developed in the fibrous portion of the middle coat. At first they consist of granules deposited in the fascicula of the connective tissue; the granules soon unite to form transparent plates which envelop the vein to a greater or less degree. The veins of the lower extremity are especially liable to such formations. Occasionally we meet with cases in which the whole venous system becomes infiltrated with mineral matter. Such a case is reported in the *American Journal of Homœopathic Materia Medica* for December, 1871, by Dr. Kitchen, of this city, and is one of the most remarkable recorded. At the autopsy the omentum could be lifted up in one stiff, hard mass, the veins being enlarged and calcified. The mesenteric veins were in the same condition. The liver grated under the knife, and was studded with calcified nodules, evidently the veins. The kidneys were in the same condition, the large venous trunks had patches of calcareous deposits here and there, while the veins of the lower extremities were transformed into perfect calcareous tubes.

This is a very remarkable case, and sad to say, the specimens of it which were procured were unfortunately lost by the pathologist into whose hands they were placed for examination.

GAS IN THE PERITONEAL CAVITY--A CLINICAL CASE.

BY W. B. TRITES, M D., MANAYUNK, PA.

(Read before the Philadelphia County Homœopathic Medical Society.)

THE presence of gas in the peritoneal cavity is looked upon as one of the most certain signs of intestinal perforation, but the following case will show that it may exist even when the walls of the intestines are unimpaired.

Mrs. A., a patient of mine, died on November 7th after a tedious illness, during which she had suffered excessively from dyspnœa and a sensation of tightness and pressure in the chest. She had had a troublesome cough, and was greatly emaciated. During the last week of her life she expectorated a quantity of bloody mucus, which seemed to relieve her. A large area of the chest was dull on percussion. Owing to this category of ills, I had half made up my mind that a growth existed within the mediastinum and was the cause of the symptoms.

But finally the patient died, and Dr. A. R. Thomas, who had

seen her with me, kindly came out and conducted the autopsy, which was made about fifteen hours after death.

On uncovering the body we found it greatly emaciated; the abdomen was quite tympanitic. An old-school physician who had been called in the emergency stated that this tympanitis had developed about twenty-four hours prior to her death, and had been attended with great dyspnœa.

In dissecting back the abdominal walls, a slip of the knife opened the peritoneal cavity, when, to our surprise, a quantity of odorless gas escaped, and led us to think that the bowels had in some way been ruptured. A careful examination of them, however, failed to reveal any such condition, the walls of both the stomach and intestines being found intact. The other abdominal viscera were found normal, with the exception of the liver, which was slightly congested.

Turning our attention to the thoracic viscera, we found the greater part of both lungs hepatized, and the fluid in the pleural cavity a little more than normal. On opening the heart the cause of all this mischief was revealed in a stenosis of the mitral valve. So narrowed was the opening that my little finger passed through it only with difficulty, although it should have admitted the tips of my three fingers with ease. The obstruction to the circulation caused by this contracted opening, had produced the pulmonary congestion, and this had caused the excessive and long-continued suffering of my patient. The cause of death had been determined, but the presence of the gas in the peritoneal cavity still remained unexplained. Dr. Thomas, in his extensive experience, had never met with such a case, and the books, so far as I know, record nothing like it.

The case remained unique until the December number of the London *Lancet* containing the proceedings of the London Clinical Society, reached us. In these proceedings I find a case of gas in the peritoneal cavity reported by Mr. G. Brown, which occurred in a patient of his suffering from enteric fever complicated with double pneumonia. In this case the abdominal parietes were punctured with a fine trocar during life, and the gas allowed to escape. It reaccumulated, and death resulting it was found at the autopsy to be in the peritoneal cavity. The intestines and the stomach showed no sign of perforation; the lungs were found to be greatly diseased, large portions of them solidified. Mr. Brown advanced the following theories as to the probable source of the gas, and as his case is so like mine I shall give you his views:

1st. He thinks the gas might have passed by diffusion through the intestinal walls, or,

2d. It might have been derived directly from the blood by exosmosis of carbonic acid gas through the delicate walls of the peritoneal capillaries, and this, he thinks, is the more probable, from the fact that for several days prior to death the blood of the patient had been highly charged with that gas in consequence of imperfect aeration in the lungs.

I merely record the case as a pathological curiosity, and give you Mr. Brown's views, not as settling the matter, but merely as an ingenious, and I must say plausible, effort to account for the presence of gas in the peritoneal cavity.

PERFORATION OF THE INTESTINE FROM A BLOW ON THE ABDOMEN.

BY J. M. REEVES, M.D., PHILADELPHIA, PA.

(Read before the Philadelphia County Homœopathic Medical Society.)

I DESIRE to call your attention to a case which is thoroughly unique in its character, and which will be of interest to you, I have no doubt. It occurred in the private practice of Dr. E. W. Meisenholder, of York, this State.

An auctioneer, 65 years of age, a short, chunky man, who had been brought home from a sale to which, in the enjoyment of his ordinary health, he had gone in the morning of the same day. He attempted to move the box of a large Conestoga wagon, and in doing so he placed his foot on the wheel and slipped, and threw his whole weight on the edge of the box. He struck himself with great violence in the abdomen on or near the upright piece used to keep the box in place and more secure.

He immediately complained of intense pain in the region of the abdomen, but managed to read the conditions of the sale. He was carried to the house, where such means as were at command were used to give him ease, but without avail. He was finally taken to his home, and on the doctor's arrival he was suffering with symptoms of shock, and extreme anxiety depicted on his face. Cold clammy skin, and pulse 130 and 140 beats per minute, sharp and wiry. He complained of severe pain over the whole of the abdomen. The doctor was satisfied of the fact that there was some grave injury. On seeing him in the evening found no improvement except less pain. In the morning he was worse, except so far as pain was concerned.

It was ascertained on this visit that he had been suffering with a right inguinal hernia in times past, and for which he had been wearing a truss. Thinking the symptoms might be due to a strangulated hernia, the doctor examined the right inguinal region. There seemed to be some enlargement of the hernial sac and integumentary thickening, yet the doctor was not satisfied of any strangulation.

After due deliberation a consulting physician was called in, and he felt somewhat like operating, thinking there might be a hernia, and giving the patient the benefit of the doubt; but his low condition and generally failing powers induced them not to operate. In thirty-three hours after the injury the patient died, never having rallied from the shock.

The family granted a *post mortem*, which was made forty hours after death, No abnormal appearance was found on the abdomen. However, a well-marked livid discoloration was apparent upon and underneath the parietal layer of the peritoneum. The small intestines were covered with a profuse quantity of semi-organized lymph, everywhere abundant. The bowel contained in the hernial sac passed readily out of it, and presented no trace of strangulation, but partook of the other characteristics present. Corresponding to the livid spot on the abdominal wall, a complete perforation of the intestine was found,—a perfect solution of continuity,—the size of a split pea, which would readily permit the passage of the intestinal contents into the cavity of the peritoneum. That this perforation was produced at the time of the accident by a powerful vulnerating force admits of no doubt, and it accounts readily and satisfactorily for all the symptoms present. Several ounces of serum, loaded with lymph, were found in the abdominal and pelvic cavities. The peritoneal inflammation seemed to start as a focus from the point of perforation, being there most marked, and nature had made prompt efforts at repair. This case shows with what extreme rapidity peritoneal inflammation manifests itself, and is interesting from its rarity.

RECENT OBSERVATIONS IN ANATOMY AND PHYSIOLOGY.

BY J. M. REEVES, M.D., PHILADELPHIA, PA.

(Read before the Philadelphia County Homœopathic Medical Society.)

HAVING been called upon by our worthy chairman to prepare a report on Anatomy and Physiology, I would desire to say in making up this paper, that it must be apparent to us all that there can be but little new information gathered from journals or other sources on these important subjects, and as we are supposed to be posted in fundamental principles, it is unnecessary to report on textbook matter; hence, we can see the difficulty in making a paper of interest. However, I have abstracted from such journals as were at my command the following:

ANATOMICAL ANOMALY.—Dr. Blackwood, of Philadelphia (in *Medical Times*, October 26th, 1879), found a case of double vagina and cervix uteri in a virgin. Each vagina was moderately capacious, and presented no abnormal features. The cervix on the right side presented at an angle of about 10 degrees, bending towards the right; the left probably 20 degrees, pointing towards the left. Each cervix was normal in size and character; both canals patulous to the sound, but only so far as the os internun, beyond which passage was impossible with any justifiable force. The uterus was single, with double cervix; body of uterus was of usual size. The sound passed to the fundus at the depth of 2½ inches through the right cervical canal, after it had been dilated; and 2¾ inches through the left, the extra distance being attributable to the length of the cervix. The uterus was found divided into two cavities by a complete septum. It was found that the pain which accompanied menstruation was referred to the left side, and was intensified at every second menstrual period. On examination the flow was found to come only from the right side. At the appearance of the menses at the next period the flow was from the left cervix alone, and the discharge less than from the right side, showing that the discharge came from either side alternately.

LOCALIZATION OF THE FUNCTIONS OF THE CEREBRUM.—M. Jaccond relates two cases which in his opinion tell against the view that there are two separate centres in the cerebrum. The first is that of a man æt. 42, suffering with suppurative meningitis. The right hemisphere was very hyperæmic, but presented no adhesions of the meninges, but the pia mater of the left hemisphere was infiltrated with pus, especially in the regions of the central convolutions and central sulcus. The pia mater was adherent over two-thirds of these convolutions. During the last two days of life the patient suffered with convulsions of the left side of the body, but there was no hemiplegia. He sees in this case an example of unilateral convulsions in consequence of a stimulating lesion of the motor region of the same side. The second case was a woman æt. 83, who survived two days after an attack of apoplexy. During this period she suffered from hemiplegia of the right side, with anæsthesia. Speech was not disturbed, and death the result of advanced phthisis pulmonalis. The left hemisphere was intact; the right presented an extensive flattened hemorrhage between the dura mater and pia mater, covering the upper border of the hemisphere, so that the central sulcus was about its middle. No other lesion was visible. He refers the hemiplegia in this case to compression of the upper parts of the central convolutions, but mentions also its occurrence on the same side.—*Lancet*, January 3d, 1880.

DEFECT OF THE CEREBELLUM.—Dr. Fraser, in Glasgow *Med. Journal*, March, 1880, describes the case of a brother and sister in whom a defect of the cerebellum was present. The brother walked like a drunken man, reeling very much, body inclined forward, head thrown back, mouth open, and eyes turned up, seemingly in constant danger of falling on his face, though he seldom fell, and could walk a considerable distance. Later on he grew worse, and often fell. Could walk but short distances, and would stand for hours leaning against a door-post, his body stooping forward and swaying, his head thrown back with a constant nodding motion, as if too heavy for his neck. His general health good, and no mental unsoundness. For first year or two of life was healthy, after that began to reel and stagger slightly, and gradually grew worse.

The sister presented similar symptoms. There was a family history of tendency to diseases of the nervous system. At the death of the brother from phthisis, a post mortem revealed nothing remarkable in the brain and cord except a very small cerebellum. The weight, when separated by cutting through the peduncles, was 1260 grains (2 ℥ 5 ʒ). The changes were: 1. The cortical gray substance of the cerebellum was little more than half its normal thickness, and there were gaps at the surface, probably caused by the collections of fluid in the soft membranes. 2. The white substance presented little apparent reduction, and, in proportion to the gray substance, appeared of undue thickness. 3. The cells of Purkinje in the cortex were greatly shrunken and contorted, their processes being indefinite and altered in direction.

INFLUENCE OF SWEATING ON THE POWER OF THE GAS-

TRIC JUICE, AND ON THE ACIDITY OF THE GASTRIC JUICE AND URINE.—M. Sassicki writes a paper containing his results in the investigation of the influence of sweating on the power of the gastric juice, and acidity of the latter and the urine. The object of his research was to ascertain whether gastric juice and sweating stand in the same relationship to each other as gastric juice and urine, *i. e.*, whether the acidity of the two remaining fluids decreases if one of the three is either eliminated or neutralized. He takes his idea from the fact that individuals who perspire much, suffer from dyspepsia. He comes to the following conclusions: 1. Sweating decreases the power of the gastric juice. 2. Acidity of the gastric juice is decreased. 3. Both the absolute and relative acidity of the urine is diminished. 4. The stronger the perspiration the more the digestive power and acidity of the gastric juice are lessened, as well as the acidity of the urine.—London *Med. Record*, December 15th, 1879.

ABSORPTIVE QUALITY OF GRANULATING WOUNDS.—There are few at the present day who are willing to believe that granulations are good absorbing surfaces; for it has generally been supposed that as soon as granulation is established there is no danger of absorption of poisonous matter, and when blood-poisoning did take place before this period it was supposed to have received the poison prior to the completion of granulation, and yet there are several facts which demonstrate that some substances at least may be introduced into the circulation in this way. Bonnet, in 1852, confirmed this by the absorption of Strychnine by granulating wounds. Also with Iodine, especially if applied in the form of an ointment.

A Dr. Hock published a paper in a German journal of surgery in which he desired to know the absorptive power of granulating wounds at different periods, and whether the form of administering affects the result. A large piece of skin was removed from the back of a dog, and a suitable dressing was applied. When granulation was complete, the wound was tested. Two classes of substances were tried, such as could be found in the urine, as the Ferrocyanide of potassium, Salicylic acid, and Sulph-indigotate of soda, and such as showed their presence by the production of constitutional effects, as Pilocarpin and Apomorphia. Applied in a solution to a sore four days old, treated with water-dressings, the Ferrocyanide appeared in from 17 to 20 minutes, while the same substance applied to a freshly cut surface appeared in 15 minutes. Used as an ointment it was absorbed more rapidly; still more so when the salt was sprinkled over the wound in the form of a powder. A like result when Pilocarpin was used, the ointment and powder producing constitutional effects more quickly than when applied in same quantity to a freshly cut surface of the same size. Apomorphia was absorbed from wounds thus treated only during the 12 hours immediately after infection. As the wounds became older it was found that though the first traces of absorption of the Ferrocyanide could still be detected about the same period as in those of four days old, yet no marked precipitate could be obtained in the urine till some days later. Chloride of zinc in 8 per cent. solution at once arrested absorption by granulation. Sloughs caused by the application of stray Carbolic acid absorbed with extreme readiness. Glycerin also aided absorption. Granulated wounds, treated antiseptically, absorbed in larger amounts and more rapidly than freshly cut surfaces. And such substances as Apomorphine, which could not be taken up by wounds treated with water-dressings, produced their physiological effect with great rapidity in this instance even after the removal of their dressings. About two days elapsed before the granulations assumed the character of those treated with water-dressings.—*British Med. Journal,* January 3d, 1880.

ANTHRAX.

BY A. C. REMBAUGH, M D., PHILADELPHIA, PA.

(Read before the Philadelphia County Homœopathic Medical Society.)

OPINIONS on the subject of anthrax differ, and especially in regard to its origin, as they do regarding all other subjects observed by scientists. The popular idea may differ from the scientific and be held just as firmly. It may be considered hereditary, a father and son having died from the effects of this disease, appearing on the same part of the body, as each arrived at about sixty years of age. Another case was attributed to gluttony, the victim having been a confirmed epicure. Another case was attributed to poverty of the blood, the patient having been a poor working-girl, confined by night and day in limited apartments, very poorly ventilated. Another case occurred in a gentleman, a perfect model in all his habits and mode of life; and still another case—a carbuncle—appeared on the wrist of a young man, who dressed and looked after the last-mentioned case.

There seems to be no more satisfactory solution to the question than the bacterian theory, as advocated by Ziemssen in his *Cyclopædia*, viz.:

"The results of microscopic examinations are of the greatest importance. Davaine, with Raimbert, was the first who demonstrated bacteria in them. Davaine found the bacteria, after two or three days' development of the carbuncle, imbedded chiefly in the centre of the pustule, in the Malpighian layer, beneath the cuticle layer of the epidermis. On the third day of development the bacteria constituted the exclusive and essential element of the tumor."

So far as a judgment can be formed from the small number of cases thus far known, anthrax in man seems to be distinguished from that of the domestic animals in the respect that the bacteria are much less often so regularly distributed through the blood of man. The human organism affords far less favorable conditions for the increase and reproduction of bacteria than does that of the herbivorous animals.

Anthrax bacteria are found in the cellular tissue of the intestines, in the blood and chyle vessels, in a great number in the swollen hæmorrhagic, infiltrated mesenteric glands; also in the liver and spleen.

Anthrax is common in manufactories and establishments where animal products are worked up, especially hair, wool, bristles, and hides.

Intestinal anthrax is much more rare. It is difficult to make a diagnosis from the symptoms and appearances alone. A simultaneous appearance of carbuncular or œdematous affections of the skin naturally goes far to assist the diagnosis. The microscope alone can give a final and satisfactory diagnosis, in showing the presence of filamentous bacteria. Inoculation of animals can be resorted to, such as rabbits, guinea pigs, etc.

While anthrax carbuncle preferably occupies a portion of the body habitually uncovered, simple carbuncle generally chooses the skin of the back and neck.

Lengyel and Rorangi, out of one hundred and forty-two cases of anthrax carbuncle, lost only thirteen; Niçolai, out of two hundred and nine cases, lost only eleven.

Davaine has found (estimated) in a single drop of blood eight to ten millions of these fine, rodlike bodies, seemingly of vegetable origin, and claims to have produced anthrax by the millionth dilution of such a drop. He also produced anthrax by the inoculation of dried anthrax blood twenty-two months old.

Einke relates the following case as very well illustrating the violence and tenacity of the poison. The skin of an ox (from whose flesh two persons got carbuncle) which died of anthrax in the fall of 1852, was soaked in the following spring in the water of a pond, and then made up by a saddler into harness. The saddler got carbuncle. From a flock of sheep which were washed in the pond four weeks later, twenty perished in a few days of anthrax, and both the horses (for whom the new harness was made), after they had worn it for four days, died of the disease in twenty-four hours.

In 1864 there died in Russia of the Siberian boil plague seventy-two thousand horses. Virchow reports as perishing from anthrax more than fifty-six thousand horses, cows, and sheep, and five hundred and twenty-eight men, from 1867 to 1870, in Government Novgorod.

Anthrax in man has almost entirely yielded to the domain of surgery, works on this subject containing all obtainable information relating to it. But this pest should have the same claims upon the physician as upon the surgeon. Its spontaneous origin in man is decidedly denied. Its transportation over long distances has also been distinctly recognized. It can be proven to have entered Europe from Siberia and South America.

Anthrax pustules chiefly occupy uncovered portions of the body (84 per cent.). Man is more like the carnivorous and omnivorous animals, which take the disease with greater difficulty than herbivora. Men are more liable (59 per cent.) than women (41 per cent.), and there is increased liability in those from ten to fifty years of age.

Huisinger describes a case where a woman, after eating some liver taken from a diseased animal, died in twelve hours without the formation of any carbuncle.

I cannot, of course, agree with Mr. Ziemssen in his treatment, "a thorough destruction of the local affection;" "extirpation with the knife, followed by cauterization;" "excision;" "deep crucial incisions;" "fuming nitric acid;" "caustic potash;" "carbolic acid."

Bæhr's hints on the treatment of anthrax are excellent. He says: "Here, too, as in the case of boils, we urgently advise against the artificial opening of the carbuncle, more especially if it is premature. An early access of atmospheric air favors the development of gangrene; pus is but too readily taken up by the cut-vessels, and the inflammation is allowed to spread."

Professor Helmuth relates a case in his work on surgery, of M. Paget's, of St. Bartholomew's, where the more a carbuncle was cut the more it spread, and only ceased to spread when the cutting ceased. Cold water compresses, with dilute Calendula, covered with oiled silk, proves a very effectual application. Helmuth, Bæhr, and other homœopathic writers, give indications in full for the necessary homœopathic medication.

REMARKS ON SEVERAL SUMMER REMEDIES INFREQUENTLY USED.

BY E. A. FARRINGTON, M.D., PHILADELPHIA, PA.

THE season has come which is so unrelentingly severe on the very young, the old, and the weak. Concerning the first class it behooves us to study well, remedies particularly adapted to their ailments, which are provoked or aggravated by heat. Prominent among such affections are bowel complaints.

Well-tried remedies, such as Aconite, Bryonia, Sulphur, Ipecac, Arsenic, Carbo veg., Podophyl., Verat. alb., etc., should be uppermost in our armamentarium, for they will be most frequently needed; but there are several newly added drugs which must not be forgotten in the limited number of cases calling for them. We subjoin a few.

Œnothera biennis,—the evening primrose, common in fields and waste places, is an invaluable remedy in exhausting, watery diarrhœa. It does not act, as has been suggested, as an astringent, by its tannic acid, but is a genuine homœopathic remedy, producing and curing diarrhœa. The evacuations are without effort, and are accompanied by nervous exhaustion, and even with incipient hydrocephaloid.

Gnaphalium causes a watery, offensive, morning diarrhœa, which repeats itself often during the day. The provers were children, and well have they portrayed a very common group of cholera infantum symptoms. They had rumbling in the bowels, colicky pains, and were, at the same time, cross and irritable. The urine was scanty, and the appetite and taste were lost. A writer in the *Homœopath* used this drug very successfully last summer, and Dr. Hale refers to it in his *Therapeutics*.

Geranium maculatum is also a successful baby's remedy. Dr. Hale devotes eight pages to Geranium and other astringents, dividing their action according to his rule of primary and secondary symptoms, and deducing thence two propositions for use in practice. The provings, brief though they are, help us in the choice of the drug: constant desire to go to stool, with inability for some time to pass any fecal matter; then the bowels move without pain or effort. Mouth dry, tip of tongue burning. Allopaths use it as an astringent.

Paullinia sorbilis has been suggested for diarrhœa which is green and profuse, but odorless.

Opuntia comes to us recommended by so careful an observer,—Dr. Burdick—that although we have not used it, we do not hesitate to present it anew. Nausea from stomach to bowels; feels as if the bowels were settled down into the lower abdomen. Confirmed in adults. In infants we may perhaps look to this drug when the lower part of the abdomen is the seat of disease, as this seems to be its characteristic seat of attack.

Nuphar luteum causes a yellow diarrhœa, worse in the morning, either with colic or painless. It has been employed for diarrhœa during typhoid, and indeed seems to cause nervous weakness. Whether it will be of service for infants remains to be seen. We should look to it when Gamboge, Chelidon., etc., fail, and when exhaustion is a prominent attendant.

Kali bromatum has been several times given successfully in cholera infantum when there were great prostration, cool surface, and symptoms of hydrocephaloid. Compare Cinchona (incipient hydrocephaloid, following prolonged or oft-repeated diarrhœic discharges), Calc. phos., Carbo veg., Verat. alb., Camph., etc.

Among dietetic adjuvants, Koumiss and Lactopeptin are comparatively new.

THE CURE OF CATARACT BY MEDICINES.

BY R. J. M'CLATCHEY, M.D., PHILADELPHIA, PA.

Apropos to Dr. Lewis's review of Dr. Burnett's book on curing cataract by medication, in the May number of the Hahnemannian Monthly, I noticed, in reading the *Revue Homœopathique Belge*, that Dr. H. Bernard gives some bits of experience of his own while reviewing Dr. Burnett's book in that journal. He says that he *benefited* a lenticular cataract of the left eye, in a person eighty years old, where the sight was gone, with Cannabis tincture, the sight returning in six months. He also treated a lady, seventy years old, having the arthritic diathesis, with Spigelia, and with marked benefit. He also refers to a case occurring in a young girl, in consequence of disappointment, which he relieved with the Hypophosphate of soda; and in a number of instances he has helped similar cases of cataract with Cannabis tincture and Natrum mur. 1ˣ, in alternation. As a piece of personal observation I may remark that Dr. Bushrod W. James, of Philadelphia, has brought about a great change within a few months, in a case of cataract occurring in a patient, and, indeed, a relative of mine, so that the lady, from groping about with much difficulty and uncertainty, is now able to go anywhere, and last night danced with great ease and enjoyment. The medicines used thus far in this case have been: Chimaphila umb. 6th, for four months, thrice daily, and Graph. 3ˣ trit., a powder every morning, noon and night, during the past three weeks.

AN EPIDEMIC OF CROUP.

BY M. B. TULLER, M.D., MILLVILLE, N. J.

(Read before the West Jersey Homœopathic Medical Society, May 19th, 1880.)

DURING the months of October, November, December and parts of January and February, membranous croup was alarmingly prevalent in Millville. Under allopathic treatment the deaths amounted to some forty or fifty children, despite the "scientific treatment." So rapid was its course that a fatal result often followed in from twenty-four to thirty-six hours' illness.

The epidemic assumed three distinct forms. Some, as is commonly the case, were taken suddenly in the night. Others suffered for several days from hoarseness and running from the nose. When the nose became very dry, the voice would fail entirely, and the little patient would quickly succumb, unless promptly treated with the similimum. My cases of these two varieties numbered thirty-five, and, by dint of hard study and the faithful application of homœopathic principles, I succeeded in saving them all.

The third variety differed essentially from any form of croup I have ever met with or read of. Indeed it is a question whether it was croup or not. The children would be sick a week or more with an apparent nasal catarrh, sore throat, and cough, but with little if any hoarseness; otherwise they seemed well. In one case the child's mother thought that there was some slight feverishness. At the end of a week these patients would be seized with a severe loud wheezing, without either sawing respiration or barking cough, the voice remaining clear until death. The cough was dry and somewhat wheezing, and followed by a slight greenish sputum. The allopaths returned these cases as croupous pneumonia. It certainly was not laryngeal croup. Was it tracheal or bronchial? After a careful study I have concluded that it was not tracheal, since this form is not so fearfully fatal as were our cases.

Was it bronchial catarrh or bronchial croup? Both have many symptoms in common; but only the former has the long-lasting catarrhal symptoms; so we decide in favor of bronchial catarrh.

Homœopaths used Acon., Hepar, Lach., Spong., Bell., Phosph., and Kali c. I subjoin one case. In the latter part of February I was summoned to a case which had been sick ten days without treatment. This neglect arose from the ignorance of the parents, who were not aware of the character of their child's illness. I found the voice gone, cough worse on lying down, face red, becoming engorged with blood with every coughing spell; the pupils were dilated, and there was drowsiness attended with restlessness and full pulse. Bellad.^{200}, every half hour.

At 8 P.M. found her sinking rapidly, her extremities cold to the hips. So certain was I that she had the right remedy to cure if the case was curable, that I gave Sac. lac. every five minutes, and awaited the result. Gradually the breathing became easier and the body warm, until finally she began to expectorate large pieces of membrane; when satisfied that the child was better, I went home. Next day, improvement.

Monday, still improving. Tuesday, not so well. Gave Bellad. 40^{m}. Wednesday, very much worse; had coughed all night; worse after 12 P.M., the face becoming red with every coughing spell, pupils dilated, with the same restlessness and with thirst. Consulting Lippe's *Key to the Materia Medica* I found under "Cough with red face," Kali carb. Some time ago, it will be remembered, I stated that when the face presented the appearance of Bellad., but the remaining symptoms did not agree, I selected Kali c. The aggravations after midnight in the present case also suggested this drug. I gave the 200th potency, which was followed by prompt relief and recovery.

In treating croup I observe the following rules: 1st. Select carefully the indicated remedy. 2d. Keep the patient in a dry room, of a temperature not varying much from 70°F. 3d. Do not allow the child to sleep longer than an hour at a time, especially after it has begun to expectorate.

ON NICOTIN POISONING.

TRANSLATED BY S. LILIENTHAL, M D., NEW YORK.

NICOTINUM and its effects was the subject of discussion at the meeting of the Medical Society of Prague, February 13th, 1880.

Professor Zaufal spoke of the symptoms which smoking produces on the organ of hearing: subjectively, sensations of hearing, vertigo, catarrhal affections of the tube and tympanic cavity by direct transmission from the chronic nasal and pharyngeal catarrh. Snuffing is injurious, not only on account of constant irritation of the mucous membrane, but it is also well known that some of the snuff may be carried into the tympanic cavity, and thus become a mechanical irritation. People of hard hearing should neither smoke nor snuff.

Dr. Bulowa, as physician to a tobacco manufactory, where five hundred girls made cigars, frequently observed even severe cases of anæmia, with such symptoms as muscular debility, especially of the lower extremities; dragging, oscillating gait. Sometimes there was the muscular asthenia without anæmia; spasms, especially of the muscles of the forearm, clearly brought about by the intoxication, and not by over-exertion of the muscles, as lacemakers, who abound in this neighborhood, exercise to a far greater degree these muscles, and never suffer from spasms of the forearm; facial spasms, dilatation of pupils; in one case, general spasms. All of which disappear by leaving the manufactory and attending to other duties, but return with their return to cigar-making.

Dr. Petrina relates the case of a man who from adolescence smoked the strongest cigars, and suffered by-and-by from chronic Nicotin poisoning, evincing itself by emaciation, neuralgia, oppression, præcordial anguish, trembling, total insomnia, frequency of pulse and respiration. Only total abstinence for some time produced a transient relief; as soon as he smoked again his state grew worse, and he died with all the symptoms of general anæmia. The abduction proved a high-graded anæmia of the brain and spinal cord, corresponding to the physiological experiments with this poison, which causes a spasm of the peripheral bloodvessels. A second similar case recovered under hydropathic treatment.

Dr. Popper remarks that Zenker was the first to describe a peculiar pulmonary disease, tabacosis pulmonum, where the lungs show brown spots, which are accumulations of tobacco dust.

Dr. Lazansky found in syphilitic smokers, plaques in pharynx, larynx and choanæ, which he never yet discovered in syphilitic women.

The amblyopia from tobacco has been often observed, but still deserves to be mentioned.—*Med. Central. Zeitung,* No. 33, 1880.

THE PHILADELPHIA COUNTY HOMŒOPATHIC MEDICAL SOCIETY.

REPORTED BY CHARLES MOHR, M.D., SECRETARY.

THE regular meeting of the society was held on the evening of June 10th, 1880, at the Hahnemann Medical College. The President, Dr. E. A. Farrington, occupied the chair, and beside him, by special invitation, sat Dr. E. W. Berridge, of London, England.

The Secretary, after making a few appropriate remarks, nominated Drs. Constantine Hering and James Kitchen as honorary members. They were unanimously elected.

The Bureau of Anatomy, Physiology, and Pathology, Dr. A. R. Thomas, chairman, presented several papers. (See articles in this number.)

By request of the chairman of the bureau, Dr. W. C. Goodno presented a diseased liver, with sections under microscopes. He said:

The patient was a lady, about 50 years of age, who for about one year past had been in miserable health, but not until one month since did she experience serious symptoms, when her digestion became impaired, her strength failed, and jaundice supervened. These symptoms steadily progressed until her death, which occurred six days ago. Upon post-mortem examination, I found upon one nipple a shallow ulcer, which had been examined by Professor Gross a month or two ago, and diagnosticated as epithelioma. A section of the nipple is upon the table, and will be found to corroborate the diagnosis. The liver, as will be observed, weighs 8¼ lbs., owing to cancerous growth of the usual encephaloid variety. Its entire surface was quite uniformly covered with depressed grayish circular spots, looking like cicatrices, and about ½ inch in breadth, with the exception of two, which measured about four inches. The lungs contained disseminated nodules, averaging about the size of a small pea, and presenting the same microscopical appearances as those in the liver. The fact of interest in connection with this case is the existence of a very fine reticulum among the epithelial elements, discernible only by the use of a high power and careful preparation, which fact is contrary to the generally received opinion. I have seen one similar specimen in the possession of a pathologist of this city. Since the post-mortem, I have learned from the husband that the patient had complained of uterine symptoms, and an examination some six months previous to her death revealed the existence of a fibroid polypus; also that soon after the examination she noticed a hardness upon one side of the vagina, which gradually increased until the canal was quite closed. In answer to a question by Dr. Morgan, Dr. Goodno stated that there was no obstruction of the large bile-ducts.

After acceptance of the report of the bureau, the following discussion ensued:

DR. H. N. GUERNSEY: I should have been better pleased if some recognition of homœopathy had been made in the papers. Some morbid influence is set to work on the vital forces, and step by step disease is produced. At the commencement of such a condition, we should at once take into consideration all the symptoms, according to Hahnemann's method. All abnormal formations are developments from diseased vital force, and by collecting the symptoms and conditions we have assumed to be at the back of them, we find a remedy which shall control that vital force in its abnormal demonstrations. I have treated many cases of anthrax, hundreds of them, and only one proved fatal, and that within three hours after my first visit. That case had been treated with cold-water dressings. If I had seen it early it would have been relieved without applications, without anything but the correct homœopathic remedy. In prescribing, remember that the mind itself often gives the clue to the needed remedy. One case commenced on the nape of the neck, and spread so that it had taken off the scalp. Maggots crawled all through the putrid mass. I did not swerve one particle from the teachings of my master, SAMUEL HAHNEMANN. The remedy was found, and the patient, though nearly fifty years of age, made a fine recovery. The treatment had the effect of renewing his age, so that he became a vigorous man. It gave me pain to hear all these papers so beautifully describing the subjects, without a syllable in regard to their genuine origin. I am sorry to come back home and make these horrible remarks to-night, but I may not have another opportunity. How did these calcareous formations you describe begin? No well person ever had them. Let it be taught that all such developments come from a disturbed condition of the vital forces.

What are we here for except to learn how to cure the sick, as Hahnemann says?

DR. J. C. MORGAN: I am glad to hear Dr. Guernsey sound the note of homœopathy. At the same time I have no doubt that our friends went no further because they feared infringing on the Bureau of Clinical Medicine. I think Dr. Guernsey is right in asking that physiology and anatomy be connected with the etiology instituted by Hahnemann. Dr. Trites alluded to what Virchow has called psammoma or sand tumors. These are malignant growths which have undergone calcareous degeneration. Now in treating a sarcoma, if Dr. Guernsey would endeavor to convert it into a psammoma, he would do the best that can be done.

Respecting anthrax, it is well to bear in mind that English surgical works identify it with carbuncle, while the German authors confine it to gangrene of the spleen, malignant pustule, and speak of mycosis intestinalis as the same condition of the intestines. I think homœopathy bears an important relation to bacterial poisoning. The formation of bacteria is a symptom of incipient dissolution. If this be true, we should prevent our patients getting into such a condition.

DR. A. KORNDŒRFER: Dr. Guernsey has evidently fully regained his health, and we are so well pleased that we can stand a little scolding. Shortly after he left Philadelphia we changed our plans and instituted the bureau system. Now the members of the bureau reporting to-night on anatomy, physiology, etc., have nothing to do with practice. There is not a member here who does not agree with Dr. Guernsey as regards the dynamic origin of disease, and I may be allowed to set him right, as he has wholly misjudged us.

In regard to carbuncle, *Anthracinum* is a remedy which is too often overlooked. Where *Arsenicum* symptoms are apparently present, with burning and severe pain, frequently of a throbbing character, nervous feelings, marked burning in the parts, much aching, dull, dusky appearance of the surrounding parts, excessive sensitiveness of the parts affected, great prostration, and yet lacking in the peculiar *Arsenicum* restlessness, periodicity, and thirst, *Anthracinum*, given in the 2^c or higher, acts promptly and cures. In the earlier stages, symptoms agreeing, it will avert the disease. In one bad case it afforded marked relief, but the patient died after the slough had been removed, leaving a clean, open wound, the patient dying from exhaustion. The carbuncle was nine inches long by seven inches wide, involving the occipital and posterior cervical regions down to the spinous process of the second dorsal vertebra. It extended laterally from ear to ear. It had burrowed under the angle of the jaw on one side. All remedies were employed with the greatest care, but the case progressed from bad to worse. *Anthracinum* seemed to check the process but for a season. The patient improved, especially in his mental state, and I hoped for a recovery, but he sank very rapidly. The causes of calcification of arteries, I think, are neglected in the earlier stages, owing to the fact of its being impossible to discover any physical symptoms which would lead us to suspect them, many of them going on without marked constitutional symptoms until these changes have taken place. Dr. Friese, of Harrisburg, whom I lately attended, had suffered for years from trifling symptoms, never suspecting any marked heart disease. He attended to his professional duties, and was always active until within the last few years. On making the post-mortem, however, I found the mitral valves in a state of ossification. Remedies, though carefuly chosen, give only temporary relief. If we treat a case in the early stages no doubt it may be cured. When Hahnemann differentiated so nicely according to the symptoms, and according to the pathological formations on the skin, between purple rash and scarlet rash, he was teaching us how to treat disease. First, we must collect symptoms from the patients; secondly, we must obtain indications by physical exploration. It is this complete history, this totality, that is required in order to bring homœopathy up to the standpoint of a science. Now, if we give the indicated remedy and failure results, and post-mortem examination reveals a certain pathological condition, we have gained a fact. Such facts confirmed frequently will teach us in certain conditions to exclude certain remedies, which fail, despite the apparent similarity.

DR. H. N. GUERNSEY: Why bring up all these disordered conditions, and speak of the cause according to this great man and that great man, and never say a word about Samuel Hahnemann?

DR. A. KORNDŒRFER: We all know that what Hahnemann taught was true. These are the actual causes. The true fundamental cause for the maintenance of disease lies in the dynamic change. But the immediate, superficial cause is one which we can grasp only by carefully studying each individual case. It is just for studying these immediate causes that this meeting is held. If we merely reiterate the theories laid down by Hahnemann, we convene for the admiration of Samuel

Hahnemann. We want to get at the immediate causes, knowing full well the other.

At this point the President asked if any member had been able to add any medicines to those already known in the treatment of malignant pustule, namely, Bufo, Lachesis, etc.

DR. H. N. MARTIN: I cured two cases of malignant pustule with *Ant. cr.* 2c. This drug has intense burning pains, with localized inflammation. I was led to it particularly on account of a case of dry gangrene which it cured. Something was said about sarcoma. In the fall of 1876 I had a case of cancer of the breast in a lady, forty-four years of age. This was removed by Dr. J. H. McClelland. The tumor weighed 5 lb. 6 oz. The wound healed nicely. I gave the patient, as an experiment, Carbolic acid 2x dilution, gttæ x in 12 teaspoonfuls of water, a dessertspoonful to be taken every two hours. She has taken the drug every two hours for four years. The cancer has not returned, and she has no drug symptoms!

DR. E. W. BERRIDGE: I fully agree with my friend Dr. Guernsey in regard to applying the rules of homœopathy. We must first take up the symptoms of the case in order to find the right remedy. On this point I am quite satisfied. In my country some physicians try to carry all the Materia Medica in their heads. When we think of the ten volumes of Allen's *Encyclopedia* we know how impossible such a task is. I am always in the habit of carrying my repertory with me for reference, although I do not always use it. I never found any patient who objected to my using it excepting one old lady. She did not like it. She dismissed me in consequence. She died two days later! (Laughter.) Now in regard to pathology. All collateral branches of course ought to be developed. Whether pathology would enable us to treat the patient any more intelligently I very much doubt. Taking, for instance, calcareous degeneration, in what provings do we find that? We might find it in cases of chronic poisoning in animals. Now there are but few medicines which have been pushed to the extent of producing pathological changes. We have a case, and the totality of the symptoms corresponds to one remedy, the pathological condition corresponds to another; are we to take the totality of the symptoms or the pathological condition?

My experience has been that if we get the totality of the symptoms and prescribe the indicated remedy one of two things will happen. If the patient is curable he will be cured; if he is not curable then he will be benefited. Now the cases of which Dr. Korndœrfer spoke, in which the similimum had been prescribed without any benefit, should be published. Then the profession could work up those cases to see if the similimum had been given.

Dr. Korndœrfer (rising to explain): I said that when a remedy was given and failure was the result and a given pathological condition was discovered post-mortem, then we would have one fact positive gained, that a remedy with its symptoms so similar as to lead to its selection with a pathological state existing, and that remedy having failed despite the apparent similarity of symptoms, then it should be placed among the questionable remedies, when in a future case we find a similar pathological condition existing. Thus we are able to exclude remedies. I have not referred to original provings.

Dr. J. C. Morgan: Syphilis, which is one of the Hahnemannian miasms, is a prominent cause of calcareous degenerations, hence anti-syphilitic remedies are to be thought of in that connection. Dr. Hering has informed me that Hahnemann himself wrote: "Whenever pathology becomes a science it must be taught in our colleges." The letter containing this sentence was stolen, but Dr. Hering attests the fact.

Dr. C. Mohr: Dr. Guernsey, in finding so much fault with the work of this evening, forgets that some months before his departure for Europe he gave me the hint which has led to the adoption of the bureau plan of work. I am sure, however, that he is laboring under a misconception. Had he been present at our meetings during the past six months he would have found them very pleasant. After the bureaus reported, a discussion of papers ensued, carried on temperately, and no matter how abstruse the subject may have been, enough was found to give rise to a good talk and a "pressing home" of some of the principles of homœopathy. For one, I am glad the bureau made the report just as presented. The papers recall many experiences that might be spoken of with profit from a homœopathic standpoint. For instance, this pathological specimen before me, presented by Dr. Goodno, reminds me of a most interesting case, that but for such a reminder might never have been recalled. In May, 1877, I was called to treat a lady aged 52 years, who had been suffering for 3 years with terrible burning pains deeply seated in the hepatic region. A careful examination revealed an enlarged, nodulated liver. The emaciation was progressive, and the patient presented all the appearances of a cancer cachexia. Dr. Korndœrfer and others examined the case, and it was pronounced carcinoma. At this time her daughter was under the treatment of Dr. Betts for carcinomatous degeneration of the cervix uteri. The physical symptoms already described were associated with others, such as swollen, tender abdomen. The subjective symptoms, sharp pains, with burning in *sudden paroxysms*, the distended abdomen, made worse from pressure and jars, led me to give *Belladonna*, which, during a year, was given as needed, in potencies rising from the 3, to the 40^m. After the last prescription a rapid improvement set in. I was astonished last fall to see the lady, with every vestige of an enlarged liver gone, and looking absolutely *well*. A few months since I was called to see her for retention of urine. After catheterization and *Bellad.* she improved, and has been able to attend to her household duties until to-day, when she called on me, complaining again, this time of bearing down in vulva, burning pains in uterus, associated with an offensive leucorrhœal discharge. Suspecting cancer, from subjective symptoms and former history, I requested Dr. Betts to make an examination for corroboration. What he found, Dr. Betts can tell this meeting, as I have not yet heard his report myself.

Dr. Betts: I examined the case of which Dr. Mohr speaks to-day, and I found the cervix undergoing cancerous degeneration. I believe that the ostium vaginæ is also affected in the same way. One of the ovaries is undergoing cystic degeneration. The daughter of this lady was sent to me for epithelioma of the cervix, which was relieved by the galvano-cautery. The patient was very comfortable for three or four years under homœopathic treatment. It however returned and was again removed as far as possible, and after the operation she came near losing her life, but homœopathy again rescued her. We were considering the advantages and disadvantages of the study of pathology. I do not believe that pathology will aid in our ability to treat disease. Hahnemann starts out by saying that it is the physician's only duty to cure the sick as readily, as speedily, and as permanently as possible. I do not think we have emphasized the *permanently* sufficiently. Homœopathy claims to cure a disease permanently if it cures it at all. Frequently, from pathological knowledge, we can trace diseases back to embryonic tissue. Now if we will trace thence the disease clear up to its final development, we find it then presenting several stages, in some of which, at least, we can cure.

In order to determine whether the removal of symptoms

means permanent cure, and, still more, in order to determine if our patrons are less liable to develop structural diseases than those under allopathic charge, we must faithfully tabulate the pathological histories of our families and compare results. This work will demand a thorough knowledge of pathology, as well as a most intimate acquaintance with our method of cure.

HOMŒOPATHIC MEDICAL SOCIETY OF PENNSYLVANIA.

THIS society will hold its next session in September, in Easton, a town beautiful for situation, renowned for the culture and social refinement of its inhabitants, and within easy reach of the Delaware Water Gap, where the physician can pleasantly enjoy a brief respite from his toils, and return with renewed vigor to the scene of his active duties. To enable this organization to act with efficiency and fulfil its purpose, the name of every homœopathic practitioner in the State should be enrolled on the list of its membership. If we reasonably expect to enjoy the patronage of the State, and share in the management of its charities, we must create a public sentiment that will give cogency to our appeals and command respect for our rights. More than this, each physician is the depositary of some fact derived from experience that would add to the wealth of the profession and promote the interests of humanity. And in giving we also receive, and thus confer a twofold benefit. The rust of disuse will be worn off by the friction of new thought, the cobwebs that have been woven around our torpid natures will be brushed away, and we will feel the inspiration of a new life and rise to a fuller appreciation of our duties and privileges. In the name of the society I would especially invite our young men to give us their support and co-operation. We need your enthusiasm and strength to enable us to carry forward the work in which we are engaged for the advancement and triumph of our cause.

The older men, from the infirmities of years and the inexorable demands of old mortality, will soon be forced to retire from the contest, and upon you will fall their mantles and their responsibilities. Here you will receive the necessary training and experience to enable you to accept the leadership, to bear our banner in the van of progress, and vindicate the law of similitude and its just claim to recognition as a boon to suffering humanity.

J. K. LEE,
President.

THE

HAHNEMANNIAN MONTHLY.

A HOMŒOPATHIC JOURNAL OF

MEDICINE AND SURGERY.

Editors,

E. A. FARRINGTON, M.D. PEMBERTON DUDLEY, M.D.

Business Manager,

BUSHROD W. JAMES, M.D.

Vol. II. Philadelphia, Pa., July, 1880. No. 7.

☞ The Editors consider themselves responsible for the maintenance of the dignity and courtesy of the journal, but *not* for the opinions expressed by its contributors.

Editorial Department.

OOPHORECTOMY.—A few months ago we referred to the digusting castration of women, as required by a certain Russian body of religious fanatics. And now, in the light of recent surgical practice, we are persuaded that the operation of oophorectomy, as a radical means for the cure of reflex nervous ailments, is becoming alarmingly frequent.

Surgical skill is so rapidly mastering the dangers of the knife that the dignity of medicine is fast fading away.

At the late meeting of the American Medical Association, held in New York, the unsexing of women was discussed without the slightest opposition. The only question raised was concerning the best and safest method to be pursued.

Alas, for the fate of this wonderful structure, man! Disease converts its happiest motions into painful throes; the therapeutist, through defective method, looks on helpless, and finally the cruel knife robs it of its parts, and leaves it ill-shaped and comparatively useless.

How tenaciously woman holds on to her functions is shown by the fact that the smallest fragment of the ovarian stroma left, keeps up the menstrual stimulus, and defeats the main object of oophorectomy.

Reason and common-sense are outraged by modern medicine, and the body cries out against its destroyers.

We are forcibly reminded of the urgent appeal of Dr. Dunham to institute thorough provings upon females. Will not the profession—the homœopathic profession—bestir itself, and add to our collection of symptoms peculiar to women?

The surgical operation should be the last resort, not the early expedient, to mark the physician's ignorance of medicine.

WHAT WAS DONE AT MILWAUKEE?—This question has doubtless been asked scores of times since the close of the Institute session, and any one who was present at the meeting knows how utterly impossible it would be to convey an adequate idea of all the good things served up at that intellectual feast. We have tried, in our report of the proceedings (see page 385) not only to present the chief items of general business transacted, but also and more especially to give our readers some idea of the scope of many of the papers presented, together with the drift of the scientific discussions, believing that such a report would be of far more interest than mere minutes of the meetings. As will be seen, the exceedingly condensed report we have made occupies a large space in the present number, and crowds some other valuable matters over into the August number; an arrangement with which we think our subscribers will be fully satisfied.

The opinion, expressed very freely, was that the session had been in all respects a success. We heard from several of the older members present the intimation that the papers presented, as a rule would compare very favorably with those of previous sessions. It was noticeable that even in the papers bearing upon controverted points, and upon subjects on which the writers were known to entertain very profound convictions, there was always exhibited that conservatism and moderation of tone, without which controversial discussion loses so much of its convincing force and effect. Furthermore it was observed that in the essays based upon research, more or less original in character, there was evident an entire absence of any desire to twist and contort the facts to suit preconceived notions. In the discussions too, while members expressed themselves very freely, there was, with but few exceptions, a due deference to opposing views. To crown all, there was an earnest and untiring devotion to the business of the session, which elicited comment from the entire newspaper press of the city. These remarks apply not only to the general meetings of the Institute, but to the sectional meetings as well. If there was any attempt to trespass upon the right of free expression or free opinion, it was made outside of the Institute, and not under its sanction or recognition.

Annual Address of the President of the American Institute.—Dr. Wilson's Annual Address before the American Institute is full of interest and instruction. It is really refreshing in these days of homœopathic degeneration to see the president of a large body of physicians stanchly upholding the true principles of our art. Especially gratifying is his defence of Hahnemann's great discovery, the potentization of drugs. "It is the inherent force of the drug we use and not the drug form. Hahnemann clearly taught these things more than three-quarters of a century ago, but even in the homœopathic school they are not understood. . . . It is an error to suppose that 'high dilutions' or greatly attenuated preparations have been affected by the discoveries of the microscope. . . . Drug forms and drug forces are separate departments of investigation."

We fully agree with the doctor in his conclusions, except so far as he seems to separate force from matter. We are prepared to deny utterly that attenuations legitimately end with the 11th or 12th of Hahnemann, microscopic investigations to the contrary notwithstanding. The limit of potentization has not yet been reached, if, indeed, it ever can be. But we are not prepared to admit that potentization transfers the force of the drug thus treated to the potentizing medium.

We believe that all force is spiritual, but its manifestation in this world demands the intervention of some form of matter.

The fallacy which deceives the microscopist is the assumption that the molecules which they observe, are the ultimata of the substance examined. There are forms of matter too subtle for any known magnifying glass, and yet they are as real as the most tangible objects; and, in a sense, they are more effective; for they present their forces less incumbered, and so more active, more potent. Every substance is animated by a motion of its parts, varying with the individual object. Thus this motion is of one kind in gold, of another in silver, and of still another in zinc, and so on. That this power is limited by so-called molecules, is a bold assertion. Every object, animal, vegetable, or mineral is enveloped in an emanating effluvium of its own matter. Who can deny that medicinal power may have to do with such emanations? And yet the microscope avails nought here. It is matter in a form not yet explained by physics. We do not see, then, that any one is justified in severing force and matter, and so we differ from Dr. Wilson in this regard, but agree with him in his enunciation of truths which are far above the crude investigations of those who would subvert them. F.

NOTES.—Very odd, sometimes, are the calls we receive from anxious patients. We have several times been requested to "call and see" so and so "*before we go out*," meaning, of course, before we go our rounds. The other day we were amused by an importunate servant who persistently forced a note upon us, though several in the office had a prior claim. The note read: "Dear Doctor, please send me some striking-out medicine, etc." After closely questioning the messenger, we found that a child had premonitory symptoms of measles, and the anxious mother, impressed with the danger of the rash striking *in*, desired some medicine to make it strike *out!* "What's the meaning of this pain through my stomach to my back, doctor?" "Gastralgia," was our brief reply. "Oh! well, I told mother I thought there was a great deal of gas in my stomach!" The patient has just left, so we are sure that we are reporting her correctly.

EXTRA MEDICAL RECORD.—We are indebted to the editor and publishers of the *New York Medical Record* for their kindness in sending us daily their extra issue, containing full reports of the proceedings of the American Medical Association, during its recent session in New York.

DR. SIMS ON LICENSED FŒTICIDE.—We call attention to the remarks of Dr. Sims on "Vomiting of Pregnancy," which we have included under the head of "Gleanings." It is pleasant to meet with such high confirmation of our position as maintained in the editorial pages of last month.

WE invite special attention to the article of Dr. J. K. Lee, President of the Pennsylvania State Society. The *necessity* for a large attendance at the next meeting is something imperative. We Philadelphians, in particular, ought to do far better in this respect than heretofore. There is room for improvement, however, in all parts of the State.

Book Department.

THE VENEREAL DISEASES, INCLUDING STRICTURE OF THE MALE URETHRA. By E. L. Keyes, M.D., Professor of Dermatology and Adjunct Professor of Surgery in the Bellevue Hospital Medical College; one of the Surgeons of Bellevue Hospital; Consulting Surgeon to the Charity Hospital, etc. William Wood & Co., New York, 1880. 8vo., pp. 348.

The author has aimed at giving as clear a description as possible of the various venereal disorders and the best remedies he considers useful in their treatment, leaving out theoretical points and conflicting opinions of various writers upon the subject.

We are glad to find him an advocate of diminished doses, and that he does not favor the heroic "weighing down" of the sufferer with enormous quantities of Mercury; and in general he deems it better to wait until secondary symptoms in syphilis show themselves before beginning its use, if it has to be used at all. He believes in a prolonged treatment (three or five years) in secondary cases, and administers Mercury in such developments. He believes in the *cure* of syphilis.

The book treats first of chancroid, in part second of syphilis and its various phases, and in the third part of gonorrhœa and its complications. In urethral stricture he differs from the general writers of the day, and does not favor promiscuous cutting in such cases, and complains that those who constantly incise do not give any prominence to the cases which have not been relieved thereby, and urges careful study of each case.

There are numerous cuts throughout the book. The chapter on syphilis of the skin and the part on syphilis affecting the lymphatics are particularly well illustrated in this manner. The work forms a most valuable addition to the literature of the subject. B. W. J.

A TREATISE ON THERAPEUTICS. Translated by D. T. Lincoln, M.D. From the French of A. Trousseau, Professor of Therapeutics in the Faculty of Medicine of Paris, Physician to the Hôtel Dieu, etc.; and H. Pidoux, Member of Academy of Medicine, Honorary Physician to the Hospitals, etc. Ninth edition, revised and enlarged with the assistance of Constantine Paul, Professeur Agrégé in Faculty of Medicine of Paris, Physician to the Hôspital Saint Antoine, Sécrétaire-General of the Société de Therapeutique. Vol. I. Wm. Wood & Co., 27 Great Jones St., New York. Octavo, pp. 302.

This work is another of the series of Wood's Library of Medical Authors for 1880. It contains four large chapters of therapeutic agents arranged in the usual manner of the old-school classification under the following heads: 1. Reconstituents—iron; tonic treatment in general. 2. Astringents. 3. Alteratives. 4. Irritants.

Written for the school of practice that does not believe in the "proving" of drugs upon healthy individuals, and obtaining in this way the entire drug symptomatology of the remedies as well as their general action, either as irritants, alteratives, or other such properties, the book is no doubt in that direction well adapted to its mission. But such works ought to fill a much wider field of usefulness, even in the homœopathic school, than they do. For instance, when the authors attempt to reply to the question, "How should iron be given in chlorosis, in what dose and how long?" they insist upon their minutiæ, and theoretically explain why it should be so particularly administered; and, after asserting that chlorosis is a very serious disease, into which many patients are prone to relapse during the remainder of their lives, they state: "It is a fact which is observed as one grows older in practice, that iron, after relieving the worst symptoms, sometimes becomes all at once impotent." Now the physician who practices upon the principle "*Similia similibus curantur*" has quite a handful of remedies adapted to the symptoms of the different cases of chlorosis, and he uses them, successfully too, in the removal of all the symptoms, not merely the most violent. Trousseau and Pidoux see but one remedy for chlorosis, and that is iron. If that fails they are "out at sea, without compass or rudder;" it is iron or nothing, and if iron does not cure, or disagrees with a given case, the patient is pronounced incurable.

The much-abused homœopath takes these incurables of his medical brother, selects from a score of remedies having many symptoms similar to those observed in chlorosis, and in some manner mysterious to the "regular" practitioner the symptoms fade away as dew before the morning sun. When that is fully accomplished there is not enough pathology left in the case to hang a spider's web upon.

Under alteratives, the authors give a section to substitutes for cod-liver oil, in which they accord with other writers that whale, or fish oil, poppy-seed oil, lightly fried bacon, and butter, are just as efficacious in scrofulous and rachitic cases. While at the head of a large hospital for children Trousseau compared the effects of butter and cod-liver oil upon some of the inmates. He gave two to five ounces of butter per diem to some rachitic children, and they improved quite as rapidly as those who were fed on cod-liver oil. This quite disposes of the claims to *peculiar* medicinal virtues on the part of cod-liver oil. The habit he sometimes practiced of adding cod-liver oil to the butter he was feeding to the children merely to make the parents believe he was giving the oil, and not a simple pleasant agent, butter, was certainly a matter of very bad taste, and quite reprehensible.

The use of irritants for issues and for vesication and counter-irritation we cannot in any way agree with from our standpoint of medical education.

The book is neatly bound in cloth, and is printed in the customary fine style of Wood & Co.'s publications in general.

B. W. J.

HANDBOOK OF DISEASES OF THE SKIN. By J. R. Kippax, M.D. Published by Duncan Brothers. Chicago, 1880.

In these days of massive books it is refreshing to read a brochure which condenses the pith of a large work into a small compass.

We do not wish to discourage exhaustive treatises on any branch of science direct or collateral to medicine. But we do approve of practical little books, disrobed of all theories and extended accounts of investigations, and presenting the unmistakable outlines of the subject under consideration. Such an essay is Dr. Kippax's *Handbook of Skin Diseases.*

To these advantages to the busy practitioner and the student are added in this little book excellent type and paper, and plenty of interspace to prevent the wearying of the eyes. And now let us examine into the quality of the subject-matter.

After a brief account of the anatomy and pathology of the skin, the author defines terms used in dermatology. Next he treats of etiology. Here we must object. Hahnemann's *Chronic Diseases* and *Organon* are neglected, and the wonderful etiological teachings therein propounded are silently passed by. We hope Dr. K., in his next edition, will give his readers the benefit of Hahnemann's years of experience in skin diseases,—an experience which is as superior to that of modern writers as truth is to falsity.

The classification of skin diseases is concise and very useful. This is a difficult task well performed.

Part II contains the description and treatment of skin affections arranged in alphabetical order. The definitions are printed in small caps, which brings them prominently before the eye, and helps in their comprehension.

Part III comprises a chart of characteristics, with diagnostic, therapeutic, dietetic, and hygienic hints.

The remaining three parts include a glossary, metric tables, and bibliography of works consulted by the author.

In regard to the treatment, the work is quite complete for a handbook. Under anthrax are collected indications for 14 remedies; under eczema, for 52, etc.

We note two serious objections to Dr. Kippax's management of skin diseases. One objection, which has already been referred to in considering etiology, applies here also. In the treatment of itch, for example, our author utterly ignores Hahnemann's explicit directions, and calmly dismisses the matter in these words: "A high potency of *Sulphur* given internally has the reputation of curing scabies. But perhaps the best and most prompt results will be had from well-directed local treatment, . . . as the removal depends upon the death of the insect." These are bold words, which would sweep away the vast experience of a decade of Hahnemann's best years!

The remaining objection to this otherwise excellent work grows out of the first. He who subscribes to the precepts of the founder of our school needs no resort to ointments, tar-soaps, and other so-called adjuvants. He recognizes the skin as a part of the man, and so dependent upon the man for its diseased states. Local cuticular symptoms are but one item in his study, and his remedy is selected accordingly. Allopathic researches have added immensely to our store of facts; but how can works, written in open defiance of the true law of cure, guide us in therapeutics? Will they not, unless we are thoroughly indoctrinated in the truth and firm supporters thereof, rather tend to wean us away into their own insidious teachings? Have they not done so in the work before us? E. A. F.

On Pyrexin or Pyrogen as a Therapeutic Agent. By John Drysdale, M.D. Published by Balliere, Tindall & Cox. London, 1880. A pamphlet of 16 pages.

Perhaps no remedial agents have been so severely criticised both within and without our ranks as those derived from the products of disease. Despite the clinical proofs of their value, Psorinum, Variolinum, Syphilinum, etc., are discarded by many, and denounced as nasty filthy inventions. Sepsin or Pyrexin, however, prepared according to Dr. Drysdale's formula, may not seem quite so offensive as those enumerated above. And this fact derives additional support from the doctor's own description of the properties of Pyrexin. He regards it as probably of the nature of peptones, and finds that mice poisoned by its subcutaneous injection are not so infected as to admit of a spread of the affection by inoculating healthy mice with their blood. He believes that, by a careful preparation of the fluid from exposed decomposing meat, he has obtained "a simple non-reproducible chemical poison," like Atropin, Serpent venom, etc. He recommends that it be employed in fevers of a typhoid type.

The four positive symptoms which he gives were obtained from mice. The animals became dull, languid, ceased to eat; then restless, with dim, sunken eyes, bleeding from the anus; stupor, lasting until death.

The dose proposed is from one to five minims, administered subcutaneously. While it is not denied that it may act given internally, the other method is preferred, "as we do not know how far the stomach or the mucous membrane may not impair its activity, as they certainly do with snake-poison. This also can only be determined by experiment, and it may turn out to be effective in the much more convenient way of administration by the mouth."

Since, however, Lachesis and other snake-poisons are wonderfully effective in the potencies, we are not prepared to accept Dr. Drysdale's method of using the Pyrexin. And, that so promising a substance may find its proper position in our Materia Medica, we urge a careful proving of it.

What led Dr. D. to his interesting experiments was a remark of Dr. Burdon Sanderson: "Let me draw your attention to the remarkable fact that no therapeutical agent . . . . is known which possesses the property of producing fever. The only liquids which have this endowment are liquids which either contain bacteria or have a marked proneness to their production." We agree with Dr. D. in denying this sweeping assertion, while at the same time we approve his efforts to test the value of Sepsin in certain typhoid types, with which it has, of course, a striking similarity. But protoplasmic theories will not aid us one whit. What we must have is a thorough proving which will place us above theories.

The pamphlet is short and so full of interest as to demand the time and attention of all who are interested in medical progress. E. A. F.

Gleanings.

PISCIDIA ERYTHURIA (Jamaica dogwood), used to stupefy fish, is now employed as a hypnotic.—*Therapeutic Gazette.*

GENERAL PARESIS finds a thoroughly indicated remedy in Alcohol, in small, but appreciable doses. Amelioration follows, but not cure.—*Hom. Times*, May, 1880.

TOBACCO USING may, it is again asserted, be cured by substituting the "pineapple," a fungus growing upon pine-trees. Dr. Millard never knew it to fail.—*Med. and Surg. Reporter.*

CARICA PAPAYA acts on flesh like pepsin. It contains a ferment which converts blood-fibrin into peptone. It can dissolve gluten, albumen, and flesh at 102°. It also dissolves croupous membranes.—*Therapeutic Gazette*, March, 1880.

TAYUYA again. Additional reports tend to confirm the value of this drug in scrofula and syphilis. See *Therapeutic Gazette*, March, 1880. According to Stillé and Maisch, p. 304, this root is said to come from a species of Bryonia.—EDS.

ASPILIA LATIFOLIA, belonging to the compositæ, is used in Africa as a hæmostatic. The natives prefer it to any treatment introduced by Europeans. It is employed internally and topically.—*Phar. Jour. and Trans.*
This plant should receive an early and careful proving.—EDS.

ROBINIA bark, chewed, caused sleep, stupor, dilated pupils, staggering, spasmodic muscular movements, drawing of the knees to the chest, burning in throat and stomach. A very young child had pallor, pulselessness, livid lips, sunken eyes, and complete prostration and insensibility for three hours.—*Pacific Medical Journal*, April, 1880.

REMEDIES FOR DORSA OF HANDS.—**Pix liquida*, cracks, bleeding; intolerable itching at night. Bovista, moist tetter; also after use of tar ointments. **Natrum carb.*, skin dry, chapped. **Rhus tox.*, rhagades. Sambucus, blueness. *Calc. ostr.*, *Petroleum*, *Sulphur*, rhagades from working in water; the last two especially worse in winter.—EDS.

A CAUSE OF INFANTILE COLIC and sleepless nights is a too frequent nursing of the babe, by which it takes continually a fresh mammary secretion over-rich in casein. This the child digests imperfectly, with consequent pain and curdled stools.—See *Management of Children*, by Annie M. Hale, M.D Published by Presley Blakiston, Philadelphia.

TO EVACUATE SMALL CALCULI.—Make the patient lie on the belly; then the calculi will fall to the anterior part of the bladder. The patient is then allowed to rise slowly on all fours. He micturates in this position, and the calculi, which have not yet had time to return into the cul-de-sac behind the prostate, are carried away in the stream of urine.—See *Medical Times*, April 24th, 1880.

BROMIDE OF ETHYL, of growing popularity, finds something of a check in the following: "With my fingers on his pulse, I perceived a sudden cessation; his face was cyanotic, with both venal and arterial turgescence; respiratory movements were imperceptible, the eyes turned upward and immovable, jaws locked, and the entire body somewhat stiffened."—*Phil. Med. Times*, May 22d, 1880.

PAINS IN THE CHEST-WALLS.—*Calc. ostr., soreness, worse from touch. *Sepia, the same, but pressure relieves. *Senega is somewhat similar to the lime, because needed often in fat persons. It cures soreness, worse when moving the arms. *Anisum stellatum (Jeanes) cures a pain at the junction of right third rib with its cartilage. *Pix affects the left cartilage. *Ranunc. bulbosus will often relieve soreness and stitches in the chest-walls from taking cold.—EDS.

FIBROIDS OF THE UTERUS have been successfully treated with dry earth. Dr. Hewson, of Philadelphia, has used it for twelve years. He makes a paste of the ordinary brick clay and encircles the abdomen of the patient with it, covering it with batting and securing it with a many-tailed bandage. He reports fifty successful cases. Potters' clay does not work so well as the fine yellow clay employed in making the best Philadelphia bricks.—*Med. Record, Extra,* June 4th, 1880.

CALCIUM SULPHIDE is very valuable in skin lesions attended with suppuration. In *acne* of the pustular form, in hordeolum and boils, it is useful; it not only relieves the symptoms, but prevents further crops of boils. —*Med. Rec. Extra,* June 4th, 1880. We fully agree with the learned author of these remarks, as will every homœopath, since Calc. sulph. is virtually our Hepar, with which we have successfully battled suppurations for years past. *Que palmam meruit ferat.*—EDS.

LOCOMOTOR ATAXIA is indubitably incurable, though it may be moderated, and the fatal day postponed. Patients should escape the extreme heat of summer, and should avoid cold, as it is an exciting cause. Sea-air and sea-bathing are generally undesirable. Exercise must be regulated by the individual case, some requiring rest, others moderate exercise. Great care should be taken to prevent decomposition of urine retained in the weakened bladder. Tobacco is injurious.—Dr. Weir Mitchell, *Phila. Med. Times,* May 22d, 1880.

DIALYZED IRON is a comparatively new antidote for arsenical poisoning. According to Stillé and Maisch a spoonful of salt should be administered at the same time to insure the conversion of the iron into a ferric-hydrate. Otherwise it will fail. It must also be remembered that iron cannot reach such of the poison as has been absorbed into the system. Dynamic antidotes should be used for such symptoms, especially Cinchona, Verat. album, Ipecac., and, if chronic skin symptoms follow, Graphites.

VOMITING OF PREGNANCY has been frequently cured by Copeman's method of forcing the finger into the os and carrying it along until the first joint enters the cervix. The internal os must not be opened in the least. Only one case is reported as having resulted in abortion.

With the light before us now, let us hope that we shall hear no more of deaths from pregnancy-vomiting, nor even of miscarriages induced to save the lives of mothers.—J. Marion Sims, M.D., *Arch. of Med.,* June, 1880.

FOOD FOR BABIES.—Boil a teaspoonful of powdered barley and a gill of water with a little salt for fifteen minutes; strain and mix with half as much boiled milk and a lump of white sugar. See *Management of Children,* p. 49. We insert this item, not as entirely new, but as a composition likely to be needed in the coming months. Although starch is not readily managed by infants under three or four months, yet a modicum of farinaceous food with the milk aids the digestion by separating the caseous particles of the latter.—EDS.

ABORTION.—Here are some more telling words from that indefatigable opponent of the abortionists, Dr. W. Goodell: "Now, gentlemen," having sent the woman out of the room, "I am free to say I don't believe those miscarriages were honest. This crime of abortion is so shockingly prevalent in this country that I cannot believe her. When I am called to a case of pelvic peritonitis, not after natural labor, I generally think it is due to criminal abortion or to preventive measures, as astringents after coitus. The latter is a more frequent cause than the former."—*Phila. Med. Times*, May 22d, 1880.

GOUT, in the form of "suppressed gout," is becoming quite common in middle life. Palpitation, vertigo, angina pectoris, dyspepsia, etc., are all relieved, if the disease develops itself and attacks its wonted place, the big toe. Excess in animal diet is as likely to produce gout, as abuse of alcohol. Fish diet retards its development. An intermittent pulse is regarded as a sign of the disease.—*Lancet*, February 28th, 1880.

To develop "suppressed gout," we remind our readers of the following: Natrum phos., Lithium c., Colchicum, Antim. crud., Lycopod. Concerning the first, a prover had pains at the heart, when pains in great toe were better. The second has cardiac symptoms with gouty pains in the joints. The last two are excellent in "gout of the stomach."—EDS.

DILATING THE CERVICAL CANAL, to modify or remove the vomiting of pregnancy, is a comparatively new suggestion. This procedure is by no means scientific, and its necessity throws opprobrium on the efficacy of medicines. Yet, rather than resort to the almost criminal induction of premature labor, physicians should accept any expedient which offers the best chance for both mother and child.

Schröder seems to have a dread of tents in the dilatation of the cervix uteri. So many serious consequences have followed their use that he prefers a bilateral cervical incision even as far as the vaginal junction. Fritsch objects to tents because they tend to induce sepsis (see *N. Y. Medical Journal*, April, 1880). Homœopathicians have less concern than old-school physicians, because their medicines so readily control the possible after-effects.

CALOTROPIS GIGANTEA seems to have gained some deserved reputation in the treatment of leprosy, lupus, etc. Flückiger and Hanbury state that the plant was known in India prior to the Christian era.

It is said to have removed double chin, flaccidity of the muscles, and thickness of the neck in middle life.

A writer in the *Homœopathic World* (April, 1880); reports a cure of lupus with this drug. Cartilage of the nose gone; dark-brown crusts on cheeks, each side of the nose; thick crusts on the upper lip, which is internally thickened; skin surrounding the crusts shining and inflamed. The medicine seems to create a discharge of matter, resulting in an increase of appetite and improvement in the health. This drug should receive a thorough proving, as from the tendency of its symptoms it is no doubt an antipsoric.

PLANTS IN THE SICK-ROOM cannot materially affect the amount of carbonic acid and oxygen in the air, for absorption and exhalation are carried on very slowly. It has been determined that soft-leaved plants, as the geranium, lantana, etc., give forth $1\frac{1}{2}$ ounce by weight of watery vapor from each square foot of leaf-surface during 12 diurnal clear hours. At this rate the Washington elm at Cambridge, with its 200,000 square feet of leaf-surface, would give off $7\frac{3}{4}$ tons of water in 12 hours. An indoor plant will transpire more than half as much as one in the open air. As many of our rooms are warmed by dry air, a number of thrifty plants may prove quite beneficial by supplying needed moisture. Especially are consumptives benefited by the moist atmosphere which plants produce; and a profusion of foliage plants in the room will greatly assist in the prolongation of their lives. In the selection of plants avoid those of strong scent, and choose those rich in leaves.—*Philadelphia Medical Times*, May 8th, 1880.

News and Comments.

A FOURTH YEAR IN THE MEDICAL SCHOOL OF HARVARD UNIVERSITY.—The medical faculty of Harvard College have adopted the following plan of study:

First Year.—Anatomy, Physiology, and General Chemistry; and an examination upon these at the end of the year.

Second Year.—Topographical and Practical Anatomy, Pathological Anatomy, Medical Chemistry and Materia Medica; and an examination upon these at the close of the year, General Anatomy excepted.

Third Year.—At the end of the third year there will be an examination in Therapeutics, Theory and Practice, Obstetrics and Surgery.

Fourth Year.—Clinical Medicine, Clinical and Operative Surgery, Clinical and Operative Obstetrics, Ophthalmology, Otology, Dermatology, Syphilis, Mental and Nervous Diseases, Laryngology, Hygiene, Legal Medicine, Diseases of Women and Diseases of Children, but the main studies of the third and fourth years will be more or less continuous.

The instruction in the special branches, in which an examination is now for the first time instituted, is intended to be more clinical and individual in character than that heretofore given.

The degree of Doctor of Medicine will be given to candidates who have passed a satisfactory examination in all the studies of the four years' course. The new plan of instruction goes into operation at the beginning of the next academic year.—*Harvard Register*, April, 1880.

All medical men and women are agreed in the opinion that a lengthened term of medical study is fast becoming an absolute necessity in view of the rapid extension of medical knowledge and the thoroughness now required in the various specialties. Yet it does not follow that medical graduates are learned and skilled in medicine in proportion to the length of their pupilage. It will, doubtless, be found that American graduates, after a three or four years' course of college and hospital study, are little, if any, less successful in practice than their European cousins, who spend half a dozen years within the college walls.

As to the course adopted by Harvard, we shall not be suprised if a radical change should soon be found necessary, especially in the arrangements for the study of the fundamental branches—Anatomy, Physiology, Chemistry, and Materia Medica.

A NEW LECTURESHIP IN THE PHILADELPHIA COLLEGE.—A new lectureship on Histology and Morbid Anatomy has been created in the above-named institution, and Dr. William C. Goodno, formerly Demonstrator of Surgery, has been elected to fill the position. Heretofore, Normal Histology has been taught by the Professor of Physiology, and Morbid Anatomy by the Professor of Clinical Medicine. The new arrangement will give the last-mentioned Professor additional time for teaching Physical Diagnosis, and as the Professor of Physiology will now take the department of Sanitary Science, it will to that extent relieve the chair of Gynæcology, and allow an additional hour each week for practical instruction in this most important branch. Dr. Goodno is one of the best practical microscopists in Philadelphia, thoroughly conversant with the subject he is called upon to teach, and withal is unusually pleasing and lucid as a lecturer. Every feature of the new arrangement promises new advantages to the students.

THE HOMŒOPATHIC HOSPITAL OF PHILADELPHIA.—The annual report of this institution, just issued, shows that, notwithstanding the inadequate facilities and other serious disadvantages under which the board of managers are carrying on their work, there have been a larger number of patients treated in the hospital than ever before in one year. The statistical portion of the report presents the following figures:

Patients in hospital, May 1st, 1879, ...	18	
Admitted during the year, ...	408—	426
Discharged cured, ...	385	
Discharged improved, ...	17	
Died, ...	5	
In house, May 1st, 1880: Males, 8; females, 11; total,	19—	426
Surgical cases, 342; medical cases, 84; total, . .		426
Besides these there were treated in the office by the physicians and surgeons connected with the hospital, 360 cases; making the total number of patients for the year, ...		786

The causes of death are given as follows: Fracture, 1; ovariotomy, 1; hæmorrhage, 1; phthisis, 1; pyæmia, 1; total, 5.

In the dispensary connected with the hospital the following shows the number of patients treated:

Medical, 5158; surgical, 381; total, ...			5539
Outdoor visits, ...	1385		
Prescriptions, ...	9753		
Patients cured, ...		2764	
" failed to report, ...		2593	
" died, ...		25	
" still under treatment, ...		157	
Total, ...			5539

There were also treated in addition to those above mentioned:

Eye cases, ...	480	
Ear cases, ...	158	
Gynæcological cases, ...	202	
Confinement cases, ...	82	
Total cases in the dispensary, ...		6461

The board of managers in their report speak very forcibly of the extreme necessity for increased hospital accommodations, and in a location better adapted to the needs of hospital work; and they express the hope that, with the hearty aid of the friends of homœopathy in Philadelphia, this most desirable object may perhaps be secured at a very early day.

SETTLEMENTS—CLASS OF 1880.—S. W. Hurd, M.D., Akron, N. Y.; L. Willard Reading, M.D., Hatboro, Montgomery County, Pa.; H. P. Challenger, M.D., is at Atlanta, Ga., and *not* at Rome, as we wrongly stated last month.

DECEASED.—GUERNSEY.—On Wednesday, June 23d, FLORENCE GERTRUDE, infant daughter of Dr. Joseph C. and G. T. Guernsey.

DR. JACOB SCHMIDT, of Baltimore, Md., died March 23d, 1880. He was an efficient member of the Maryland Homœopathic State Medical Society, having held the office of treasurer therein from the time of its organization until his health failed him. For a period of twenty-five years he was not absent from his post of duty for a single day. The society above named have adopted resolutions of respect to his memory.

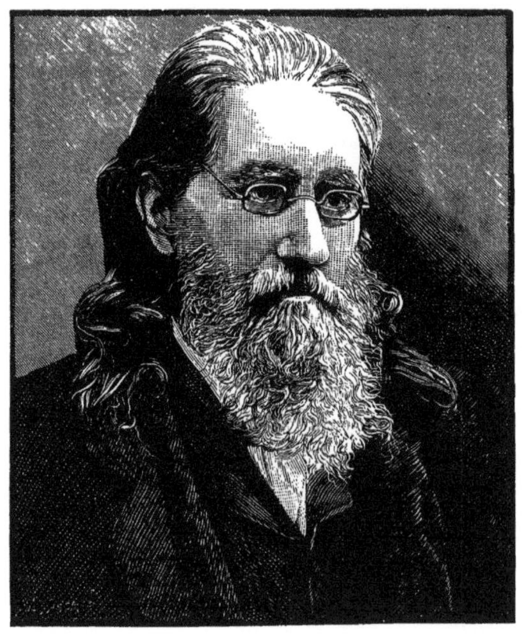

CONSTANTINE HERING, M.D.

Born January 1st, 1800. Died July 23d, 1880.

THE

HAHNEMANNIAN MONTHLY.

Vol. II., New Series } Philadelphia, August, 1880. No. 8.

Original Department.

STUDIES IN MATERIA MEDICA—LACHESIS.

BY E. A. FARRINGTON, M.D., PHILADELPHIA, PA.

ANIMAL KINGDOM.

It is our purpose in the following series to consider the most important symptoms of the Materia Medica. If, therefore, unconfirmed symptoms are exceptionally mentioned, they are so designated that their value may not be overrated.

The plan adopted is easily understood. Drugs are to be treated according to their place in natural history, beginning with those derived from the animal kingdom. Each order or class is to receive a separate examination, its resemblances and differences noted, and the individual members compared with related remedies. Thus is preserved a uniform progression from generals to particulars.

If the student comprehends the general qualities of a drug, he is prepared to apply its particulars. Given, for instance, a special symptom: sleepy, but cannot sleep, Bellad., Apis, etc.; if the general properties of these two remedies are known, the choice is easy.

Still, it must be remembered that it is only by the multiplication of particulars that the general character can be distinctively drawn, just as a strange object becomes more and more familiar and separable from its similars as we recognize more the relation of its parts to the whole. And here we may call attention to a serious error, which has damaged homœopathy.

Recognizing that the totality is to be employed rather than single symptoms, some teachers have neglected the latter, and

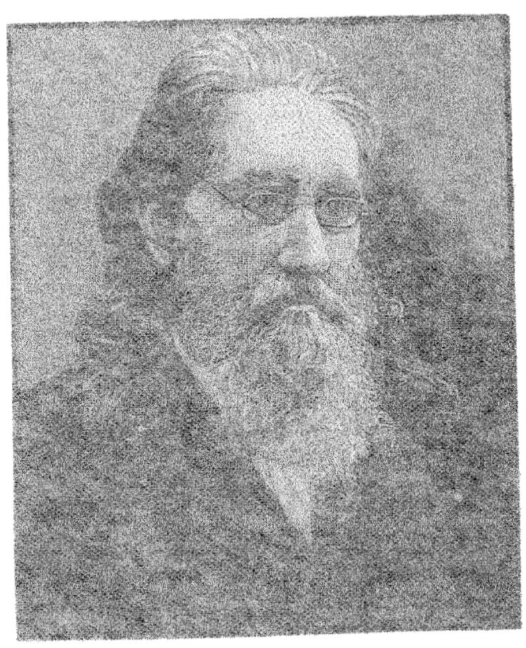

CONSTANTINE HERING, M.D.

Born January 1st, 1800. Died July 23d, 1880.

THE

HAHNEMANNIAN MONTHLY.

Vol. II., New Series. } Philadelphia, August, 1880. No. 8.

Original Department.

STUDIES IN MATERIA MEDICA—LACHESIS.

BY E. A. FARRINGTON, M.D., PHILADELPHIA, PA.

ANIMAL KINGDOM.

IT is our purpose in the following series to consider the most important symptoms of the Materia Medica. If, therefore, unconfirmed symptoms are exceptionably mentioned, they are so designated that their value may not be overrated.

The plan adopted is easily understood. Drugs are to be treated according to their place in natural history, beginning with those derived from the animal kingdom. Each order or class is to receive a separate examination, its resemblances and differences noted, and the individual members compared with related remedies. Thus is preserved a uniform progression from generals to particulars.

If the student comprehends the general qualities of a drug, he is prepared to apply its particulars. Given, for instance, a special symptom : sleepy, but cannot sleep, Bellad., Apis, etc.; if the general properties of these two remedies are known, the choice is easy.

Still, it must be remembered that it is only by the multiplication of particulars that the general character can be distinctively drawn, just as a strange object becomes more and more familiar and separable from its similars as we recognize more the relation of its parts to the whole. And here we may call attention to a serious error, which has damaged homœopathy.

Recognizing that the totality is to be employed rather than single symptoms, some teachers have neglected the latter, and have published descriptions of drugs, hewn out after the fashion of their own synthetic thought. This error arises from a misunderstanding of the procedures of the so-called symptomists. Few, if any, prescribe for one symptom; for, although such a single indication may lead them to a drug, their knowledge of the drug as a whole immediately comes into consciousness, and they intuitively fit the fact into its proper place. Now, because this understanding of the whole was acquired by a long and patient attention to details,—to characteristics,—they really have a more accurate mental picture than most of their accusers. A correct generalization of a drug, then, can only be made after a full and complete analysis of its particulars. The mental impress formed by a reconstruction of these particulars is the true general. Always afterwards in prescribing, when a single characteristic presents itself, it is to be measured by its relation to the whole. This is the true value of HAHNEMANN'S "totality."

In general, medicines derived from the animal kingdom act energetically and rapidly. They vary in intensity from the fatal snakebite to corals, sponges, etc., which are more or less modified by their mineral constituents.

OPHIDIANS.

The OPHIDIANS are characterized by their paralyzing action upon the nerves. They directly weaken the brain and heart-action. Then follow decomposition of the blood, changes in the muscular tissue, and local death from gangrene. At first there is developed a condition of anxiety, mental excitability, and oversensitiveness of the brain, with hallucinations, anxious fear, etc. Afterwards arises nervous depression, varying from such a debility as is observed in severe or protracted disease and advancing age, to mental confusion, stupor, low delirium, and paralysis. *Constrictions* are noticed, as in the throat, larynx and sphincters in general. *Hæmorrhages,* blood usually dark, decomposed, oozing from any orifice of the body. *Face* sickly, pale, anxious; earthy, gray or yellow-red; bloated, dark red or bluish. *Special senses* altered; dim vision; ocular illusions; noises in the ears, with hardness of hearing; irritability; excitableness of brain and spinal nerves, accounting for the mental restlessness and bodily sensitiveness. This latter is most marked in LACHESIS, in which it is present even during unconsciousness. Predominant even with the pains are torpidity, numbness, twitchings, formication. *Inflammations and fevers* of a low, destructive type, etc., as gangrene, malignant ulcerations, diphtheritic deposits, typhoid, pyæmia, etc. With all there are tendency to faint, muscular prostration, trembling, as in drunkards, in nervous fevers, etc., irregular circulation, some parts being hot, dark-red, others cool, clammy, livid, or bluish; flushes of heat; apoplectic congestions, with great prostration or paralysis. Livid swellings. Ulcers which are purplish, offensive, with inefficient granulations and thin, ichorous discharges.

Periodicity: symptoms return the same time each year.

LACHESIS has been most frequently used, and consequently more fully confirmed clinically. It may be distinguished from the others with a degree of certainty; but the latter need further proving and testing.

MENTAL SYMPTOMS.—Loquacity, with a constant shifting from subject to subject; vivid imagination; jealousy; frightful images; proud; sadness and anxiety, worse on awaking.

Mental activity; he sits up late at night at mental work.

Memory weak; makes mistakes in writing and reading; has to stop to think how to spell.

Loss of consciousness, with cold feet; cold, clammy sweat.

Muttering delirium; tendency of lower jaw to drop; eyes sunken; tongue protruded with difficulty; it trembles and catches behind the teeth; tongue dry, red, or cracked; stupor, with anxious expression; debauched look.

CROTALUS is almost identical in its action on the brain and in its effects on the sensorium and vital forces. Both may meet in the treatment of scarlatina, yellow fever, erysipelas, especially with meningitis, diphtheria, typhoid, etc. Clinical experience with CROTALUS has been chiefly in yellow fever, erysipelas, and diphtheria. Both have mental excitability, ecstasy. LACHESIS only seems to have the *peculiar* loquacity, though simple garrulity may belong to both. In the epistaxis of diphtheria, thin, persistent, dark red, the rattlesnake has acted best, other things being equal. In erysipelas CROTALUS affects the right, LACHESIS the left side, with dark-red puffiness, delirium, stupor, and suspicious coolness of the extremities. Yellow skin is most marked under CROTALUS.

NAJA TRIP. also excites the mind, and conversely causes depression and forgetfulness. Like the LACHESIS there is a state of moral persuasion. In the former this is expressed as a consciousness of some duty to be performed, but attended with an unaccountable inclination *not* to do it. In the LACHESIS it is described as a feeling as if the patient was under the control of some superhuman power. NAJA develops sadness, which is characteristically connected with an intense frontal headache, fluttering of the heart, and spinal pains—a group more marked than in LACHESIS. And, besides, the latter remedy causes pains down to the root of the nose, or over the *left* eye.

Related Remedies.—In Loquacity compare STRAMON., *Hyosc.*, *Bellad.*, Lachnanthes, Mephitis, Actea rac., Paris q. The first is distinguished by the red face and other signs of sensorial excitement. The second exhibits hasty talking, and, moreover, is accompanied with symptoms of cerebral irritation. The relation of BELLAD. and LACHES. is often one of degree. Both are suited to meningitis from erysipelas, to scarlatina, apoplexy, etc.; but the former represents the initial stages of these diseases or states in which, even though there be stupor, still there are evidences of irritation and not wholly of depression. Thus, the patient often starts from his heavy sleep, cries out, grinds the teeth, awakens frightened, etc. His pulse is usually strong and the surface congestions are bright red, or from intensity, deep red, livid. If there is an eruption, as in scarlatina, it is red, even if sparse, and vitality is not so low that the extremities are cool, the rash bluish, and the cellular tissue infiltrated and threatening an unhealthy suppuration, as in the snake-poison. Often, however, after the use of BELLAD. we find evidences of cerebral exhaustion, or blood-poisoning, or impending paralysis, when LACHESIS may be required. The patient still cries out in sleep or awakens frightened, the tongue still shows elevated papillæ, the head is hot, and the face is red; but the pulse is quicker and more feeble, the feet are cool, surface heat is irregularly distributed; the mind is more befogged and drowsiness is stealthily creeping on; the inflamed part, or the pseudo-membrane, or the eruption, as the case may be, is becoming more purplish,—these indicate the change.

In Mephitis the loquacity is as if one were drunk. Under *Actea* the symptom is found associated with menstrual suppression, with puerperal mania, or as a part of delirium tremens. In the former cases the absence of the snake-debility is a sufficient distinction. But as LACHES. is especially useful in the latter affection, the choice may not be so easy. *Actea* cures wild imaginings of rats, etc., sleeplessness, wild, crazed feeling about the head, incessant talking with continual change of subject, must move about. LACHES. has more marked trembling of the hands, diarrhœa, and great exhaustion, with the loquacity and hallucinations.

Paris q. causes a garrulity which is much like that caused by tea, a sort of vivacity, with love of prattling. See also Rhus, Hyosc., Lycopod.

In Delirium compare HYOSC., LYCOPOD., *Rhus tox.*, *Bellad.* (see above), *Opium*, *Apis*, Baptisia, Muriatic acid, Arnica.

The first two resemble LACHES. in severe cases where the vital powers are waning, and paralysis of the brain seems imminent, as shown in stupor, dropping of the lower jaw, involuntary stool and urine, etc. These three, together with *Opium*, *Arnica*, MURIATIC ACID, *Apis*, RHUS, and LYCOPODIUM, have trembling or paralysis of the tongue. *Opium* has, in distinction, dark brown-red face, cheeks flap in breathing, more stertor; body hot and sweaty. *Arnica* pictures apathy, stupid expression, suggillations; even in stupor, restless as if bed was too hot and hard, and seems momentarily relieved when position is changed. *Muriatic acid* displays a sunken face, tongue smooth, as if deprived of papillæ, or brown, shrunken, and hard; slides down in bed from muscular weakness.

Apis has not so markedly dropping of the lower jaw; but resembles LACHESIS in muttering delirium, trembling tongue, etc. The bee-poison, however, causes a nervousness, restless from an irritable fidgety condition, sleepy but cannot sleep; shrill outcries; later, muttering delirium, happy, strange expression; tongue trembles, but is studded, especially around the edges, with blisters; in typhoid, particularly, abdomen swollen and extremely sensitive; hands and forearms cold; involuntary thin stools. This sensitiveness is a bruised feeling, differing from the hyperæsthesia of LACHESIS; and this fact may be elicited from the patient while he is unconscious, for in the *Apis* he resists pressure as well as touch, while in LACHESIS slight touch is more annoying than more firm pressure or friction.

LYCOPOD. is a drug which induces depression of function, from a slight *ennui* to complete stupor. This quality often demands the fern, and happily frequently yields to it. If we examine Hahnemann's masterly provings we shall see numerous illustrations of this property. Thus, talks rationally on exalted subjects, but is confused when conversing on everyday things. Prostration and paralysis of the arms, he must let them fall; but while at work they are strong. Thus we see, that by an exertion of the will, functional activity is somewhat aroused. Now carry this effect farther, and we see the patient becoming drowsy; he is worse from 4 to 8 P.M. [which is the time of *minimum* tension of electricity of air]; he is worse after sleep, or arouses cross, frightened, and very irritable; his muscles refuse their support, his face looks sunken, lower jaw drops, breathing becomes rattling, eyes filled with mucus; rumbling in the bowels and constipation—all picturing just such a giving out of the vital forces as may suddenly or insidiously follow some poison, as that of scarlatina, or diphtheria, or typhus. And experience teaches that LYCOPOD. acts well after LACHESIS.

HYOSCYAMUS bears strong symptomatic resemblances to LACHES., but it does not act so profoundly. It causes, at first, perverted sensorial action, strange hallucinations; he grows suspicious and fears being poisoned; he talks in a rambling manner, jumping in a meaningless way from subject to subject; he seems more *agitated* than violent; he talks with imaginary persons. Now such illusions are not foreign to the snake-poisons, but the HYOSC. has, as very characteristic, the following group: suddenly sits up in bed, looks inquiringly around, and then lies down; talks of his business; answers correctly, but immediately becomes delirious again; scolds, raves; stares, pupils dilated; starts in terror and tries to escape. Lascivious, throws off the clothes, and uncovers the genitals. Muscular twitchings in single groups; plays with his fingers. Now, this picture may change, for underneath all these maniacal manifestations is a systemic weakness, which existed from the beginning. The patient is weak, ataxic, his muscles fail him, and he may fall into a typhoid state. Then he grows stupid, lies with eyes closed, distorted features, dropped jaw, twitchings of muscles, tongue trembles, black sordes on the teeth; tympany, stool and urine involuntary; respiration stertorous, with suffocation and rattling; pulse weak, irregular, etc. If, now, the case grows worse, with cracked *bleeding* lips, horribly offensive stools, cold extremities, Hyosc. will be of no further service, while LACHESIS may yet save. If not, compare ARSENIC, *Baptisia*, Muriatic Acid.

RHUS TOX. in one phase of its action may simulate LACHESIS; that is, when drowsiness supervenes, delirium with muttering, dry, cracked tongue, sordes, involuntary stool; and in affections like scarlatina and diphtheria: eruption scant and livid, epistaxis, drowsiness, cellulitis, swelling and suppuration of the (left) parotid, ichorous coryza. In degree the snake-poison is undoubtedly lower than the RHUS, and so, other things being equal, is indicated later. RHUS has its well-known restlessness; loquacity is not prominent, the patient remaining silent, or answering abruptly as if nettled and too weak to waste words; later his answers grow more and more incoherent. The tongue has a red triangular tip, while in LACHESIS the point is often cracked and bleeding. The stools are watery, often greenish-brown and flocculent, and are passed involuntarily at night; but they are never so offensive as those of LACHESIS. RHUS is an erethistic remedy, and must be very similar to existing symptoms, if it is to be continued after torpidity sets in without the erethism. [In such a case compare with it Phos. acid, Carbo veg., Lachesis.] Its cellular infiltration usually partakes of the erysipelatous inflammation; thus, if about the neck, as in scarlatina, the surface looks red,—a sort of dusky red. The patient is also very drowsy, and at the same time restless; worse after 12 P.M. The left parotid swells and threatens to suppurate, and the uvula is dark red and œdematous. Under LACHESIS the engorged throat presents a dark-bluish cast; patient arouses from sleep as if smothering; the least touch upon the throat induces suffocating spells; sleep always aggravates, while in RHUS this is not so uniformly so. The latter has much restless tossing in sleep; nosebleed or some other symptom becomes aggravated or appears about 3 A.M., arousing the patient; after awhile he falls asleep, and upon again awaking feels heavy and sore, as if he had not slept; these sensations pass away after he has stirred about his bed. In LACHESIS the torpor is supposed to be farther advanced, the adynamia more marked, the swollen throat is hard and dark, and the fever is low, with cool extremities and weak pulse. In threatening suppuration the snake-poison is preferable when the swelling softens here and there, presenting ash-colored or livid points, which "break" very tardily or degenerate into sloughing, as if vitality was wholly inadequate for the work imposed.

In Jealousy, compare *Apis*, HYOSCY. In Pride, compare *Lycop.* (imperious, commanding), Hyosc., Stramon., Veratrum alb. In Ecstasy, compare Crotalus, Tarantula, Cuprum, *Opium*, Anacard., the latter having: soul feels as if freed from the body; *Antim. crud.*

Anxiety and apprehensiveness are symptoms of many animal poisons, especially of the ophidians. In the latter, exciting reading may be a cause. It is also præcordial in LACHES., Crotalus, and *Naja*. In *Elaps* it is developed as a fear of rain. In LACHESIS it is attended with sensitiveness of the brain; it returns when riding in the open air. We may likewise note an anxiety when mixing with the world, seeing many people, suggesting LACHESIS in uterine affections. Dreads going to bed from fear of apoplexy. *Naja* brings about a depression of spirits, during which any little imaginary trouble brings about mental agony. Elaps has a fear of being alone, lest rowdies break in; apprehensive of some fatal disease, with faint feeling in the pit of the stomach. Compare LACHES.

Compare ARSENIC, *Lycopod.*, Hydrophobinum, the latter having strongly marked apprehensiveness, *Actea rac.;* which, like Lachesis, is indicated in the distressing forebodings of women; ACONITE, which is anxious in crowded streets; *Phosph.*, which fears being run over; LYCOPOD, etc.

Weak Memory is a natural result of a poison which so powerfully depresses the mind. After the intellectual excitement, which is especially noticed in LACHESIS and *Naja*, the mind grows confused, speech and writing are performed imperfectly and incorrectly. This is common to all ophidians. As a part of a typhoid condition we have already sufficiently dwelt upon this mental state; but it may be profitable to further compare the snake-poisons in defective memory as a symptom of senility, idiocy, apoplexy, etc. LACHESIS, as quite thoroughly known, may be useful in the impaired memory of drunkards; also after partial recovery from an apoplectic stroke with paralysis of the left side; or, again, the stroke may have been preceded by absence of mind, vertigo. As exciting causes, violent or protracted emotional disturbances and intemperance have been noted. Overstudy, entailing severe taxation of the mind, may also lead to loss of memory, and, *cæteris paribus*, LACHESIS be needed.

Related Remedies.—In Apoplexy, compare *Nux vom.* Arnica; here there will be also left-sided paralysis, but it is rather suited to stout persons, and suggillations are also present; patient remains indifferent for weeks. The *Nux* precedes LACHES. for inebriates. Opium, Apis. From overstudy, NUX VOM., SULPH., Picric acid, *Phosph.*, Coccul., Sepia, Anac., LYCOP., CALC. OSTR. For mistakes in spelling, compare Nux v., Fluor., LYCOP., SULPH.

Lasciviousness, amativeness, is a part of the ophidian excitation. The provings of Elaps do not mention it; but it is present in the remaining members of the group under consideration. Indeed it is related that some of the Lachesis provers were thus urged into hasty marriage. The latter drug is useful for epilepsy from onanism. Emissions at first relieve, leaving the mind clearer and more active; later they weaken, and are followed by profuse, exhausting sweats. Lasciviousness attends the feeling as if the patient (female) was in the hands of some stronger power. *Naja* has palpitation, spinal pains, and mental gloom from sexual irregularities.

Compare PLATINA, nymphomania, epilepsy from onanism; Bufo, onanism, spasms; HYOSC., PHOSPH., both for lasciviousness; *Picric acid*, headache, excessive erections; Agnus castus, excesses cause impotence, but lascivious thoughts remain; Zinc, Conium, Tarent., Origanum, etc.

All the ophidians cause vertigo, congestion to the head, frontal pains, mental confusion, and general weakness. Fainting from cardiac weakness.

LACHESIS.—Vertigo: after rising, on awaking, mornings, with feeling as if he would have a fit; worse on closing the eyes; on awaking occiput feels heavy, with sick, weak feeling and dizziness; the joints feel as if sprained; with pale face and fainting; with staggering to the left; in forehead, with misty vision.

Headaches generally worse on the left side; caused by heat of the sun, menstrual irregularities, climacteric disturbances, abuse of alcohol, rheumatism, catarrh, etc.; throbbing in head from the least movement; whizzing; congestion, with bright-red nose-bleed.

Forehead: bursting, throbbing, undulating pain in the forehead, worse after sleep and on stooping, with vertigo, nausea, weak mind and weak, numb limbs; sore aching above the eyes, extending to the root of the nose; sore pain in left frontal protuberance, worse early in the morning; frontal headache faint on rising.

Temples and sides: pulsating headache, usually in left temple and over the eyes, with mental confusion, before the development of a coryza; pains from right side of head to neck; muscles tense; rheumatic headache.

Vertex: burning, as at climaxis; boring.

CROTALUS is provokingly similar in character. Clinically, LACHESIS has cured more headaches on the left side; CROTALUS, on the right. Both have congestive headaches with abdominal ailments, CROTALUS having relieved when constipation seemed to be the cause; LACHESIS, with hæmorrhoids. Although both have attendant bilious vomit, it seems strongest in the rattlesnake-poison.

In ELAPS the vertigo is accompanied with inclination to fall forwards, rather than to the left. The headaches increase and decrease gradually—a useful symptom, if confirmed.

NAJA simulates the LACHESIS very closely, with headache on waking, fluttering at the heart, and melancholy. But, if the provings are correct, the former has relief from alcohol; the depression of spirits is very marked, and there are more spinal pains. NAJA also has weight and pressure on the vertex, with cold feet and flushes in the face.

Related Remedies.—In Vertigo, Fainting, etc., compare *Theridion.* Here, too, the dizziness is worse with eyes closed; but a distinctive feature is that vertigo, pains, and nausea are intensely aggravated by noise. Both have sun pains. *Arsenic, Hydrocyanic acid,* Digitalis, Veratrum alb., Camph., in vertigo and fainting from cardiac weakness.

Ill-effects of heat of sun, compare Glonoin., Bellad., Camph., Natrum carb., Therid. (See above.) The first two, with bloated red face, paralytic weakness (Glon.), unconsciousness, etc., resemble LACHESIS; but the latter displays the effects of heat upon one already exhausted. All the ophidians are intolerant of warm, relaxing weather, and so we find many ailments returning in spring and summer. In the LACHESIS case the patient may be an inebriate, or one prostrated by mental fatigue. The sun's heat makes him languid, dizzy, faint, or, if congestions ensue, the face is dark red, and looks at the same time sunken, cadaverous; extremities cold. Here Camphor may be demanded if vitality is ebbing away, the fainting spells grow worse, and the body is icy cold and bathed in cold sweat. Both LACHES. and Natrum carb. are useful when hot weather fatigues, in which case compare, also, Selen. and Natrum mur.

In intense pains, as in meningitis, remember the relation between LACHES. and Bellad. (See above.) Compare here, also, Baptisia, Rhus tox.

In catarrhal and rheumatic headaches compare MERCURIUS, Cinchona, *Pulsat.*, Bryonia, Gelsem., etc. Undeveloped or suppressed coryza, especially in the debilitated, is serious, because so distressing. Pains over the eyes, languor, and mental confusion combine to make the sufferer miserable. LACHES. often relieves, as do also Cinchona, when the head is worse from the least draft of air; Bry. and Puls., when the checked catarrh is thick yellow and green respectively; Gelsem., when motility is lessened, patient drowsy, with neuralgic pains from occiput to forehead and face. Apropos of nerve pains, PULSAT. relieves when they go into face and teeth; LACHES., as well into neck.

(To be continued.)

LARYNGISMUS STRIDULUS.

BY F. M. HALE, M.D., CHICAGO, ILL.

(Presented to the Indiana Institute of Homœopathy, May, 1880.)

LARYNGISMUS STRIDULUS has been described under the various names of asthma of Millar, thymic asthma, child-crowing, spasm of the glottis, false croup, etc. Many physicians of extensive practice have never seen a case. The writer has seen but three in thirty years, though practicing largely among children. In Guernsey's *Obstetrics* may be found an exhaustive description of its etiology and symptoms.

The case which I purpose narrating was so intense and prolonged and the relief so brilliant that I have been led to examine all our authorities in relation to its therapeutics. I will not take up the time of the Institute in describing the various opinions as to its pathology, but will merely state, as my opinion, that while a proportion of the cases may be due to mechanical pressure on certain nerves, a large majority must be due to simple paresis of the vagus and its branches. The therapeutics, as given in our textbooks, seem to me singularly inadequate to cope with this distressing malady.

A genuine case of the disease is very rarely met with, though cases bearing a resemblance to it are quite common. It may be simulated by spasmodic croup, catarrhal croup, catarrhal laryngitis in nervous children, etc. In these cases the remedies commonly recommended often remove the symptoms. Guernsey recommends Ars., Bell., Gelsemium, Ipecac., Lachesis, Laurocerasus, Moschus, Phosphorus, Sambucus, and Stramonium. Of these Sambucus and Phosphorus are suitable only for catarrhal cases. The others may be useful for transient cases due to acute attacks supervening on catarrhal affections. In the three cases under my care the above were tried faithfully without apparent benefit.

Lilienthal, in his *Therapeutics*, mentions, besides the above. Aconite, Cuprum, Iodine, Chlorine, Nux, Mephitis, and Bromine. Of these the most valuable are *Cuprum*, with which I cured one of my cases, and *Bromine*, with which, in the form of Bromide of potassa, I cured another. Iodine is also recommended by Baehr, who recommends, in addition, Ignatia, Veratrum alb., and Plumbum; but he gives no proof that the last are useful. With Iodine 6th he claims to have cured five cases.

Farrington (HAHNEMANNIAN MONTHLY, May, 1880), in

a paper originally read before the Hahnemann Club of Philadelphia, gives an excellent and condensed history of this malady. His therapeutics is quite extensive, giving all mentioned above, and, in addition, recommending a host of other remedies, some of which are new, namely, Lobelia, Phytolacca, Physostigma, Strychnia, and Naja. His paper is the best which has been written on the subject up to this time. It is suggestive that he mentions Bromide of camphor, and this lead me to narrate the last and most remarkable case I have seen.

The little patient was a weakly, poorly nourished child, ten months of age, which had been fed on cow's milk, cream, an other artificial foods. It had but one tooth, an upper in cisor, with the eruption of which, at eight months, dentitio was arrested.

The attacks of spasms of the glottis developed shortly afte this period. At first they were not severe. The child was then being treated by an allopathist, but without benefit, but rathe with a steady increase of the disease. Another allopath wa called in, who treated the child for two weeks. At the end o this time the symptoms became so severe that the physicia informed the parents that "effusion of water on the brain had occurred, which would soon bring a fatal termination.

At this juncture the case came into my hands, and a ver unpromising one it was. The child was greatly emaciated haggard, and semi-comatose. The skin was cold and clammy the eyes dull, and the pupils contracted. The spasms, fo nearly two weeks, had recurred every fifteen or twenty minutes It had been drugged with Quinine, Cod-liver oil, Iron, and Bromide of soda, which were probably the cause of many o its symptoms, including the extreme prostration. The bowel were constipated, and digestion so impaired that nearly every thing taken was vomited.

For two days I tried Cuprum and Veratrum, which, how ever, did not lessen the intensity or frequency of the spasms.

At this time an eminent allopathic neurologist was sent fo by the father, and kindly met me in consultation. I had pre viously advised a wet-nurse, but, as the child would not tak the breast, it was fed with the nurse's milk after it was artifi cially drawn. The consulting physician confirmed my diag nosis, and advised that the patient be kept in a dark room with only one calm attendant, and that the neck be comfort ably swathed in dry cotton, remarking that it should be treate like a case of Strychnine poisoning. He so strongly urge injections of Chloral that the parents insisted that they shoulc be given. After the first enema of ten grains the child slept four hours, but awoke worse than ever. The enemata were repeated for forty-eight hours as often as it awakened; but even in this artificial sleep the spasms occurred just as frequently, and the patient was evidently fast sinking. I refused to allow them to be continued any longer, and, after letting their effects pass off and giving Nux^{30} as an antidote, I tried for several days Lachesis, Arsenicum, Sambucus, Iodine, and Gelsemium. It occurred to me one evening to resort to the Monobromide of camphor. I gave the 1^{x}, a powder containing about the $\frac{1}{15}$th or $\frac{1}{20}$th of a grain, every hour.

The next morning the nurse informed me that the child had slept several hours, and that the spasms had not averaged more than three or four an hour. The remedy was continued as before. The attacks were now reduced to two an hour, and the general appearance of the patient greatly improved. The extremities were warmer, the skin felt better, the eyes were brighter, and the child seemed to be more quiet. The medicine was continued every two hours with such steady and real improvement that at the expiration of four days, after commencing the Camphor bromide, the spasms ceased, and did not return.

At the time of this writing there has been no appearance of spasms, and the little girl is rapidly improving in every respect.

I will add that owing to the swollen and tender state of the gums I scarified them very freely every two or three days, but I do not think this had much to do with the cure, for it had been practiced by my predecessors and by myself for a week before the improvement set in.

The child is now being fed with one-half fresh cow's milk and one-half water, sweetened with sugar of milk, which agrees with it perfectly.

I shall be gratified if the result of my experience in this case will be of service to others in combating this frightful and often dangerous disorder.

P.S.—Since writing the above, one month ago, my little patient enjoyed apparently good health up to the night of May 25th. On that night the child was restless, and next morning a small ball of hardened wax dropped from each ear. The following night she was again restless, with frequent sudden screams, and the next day the ear discharged a brown, thick, excoriating matter. Notwithstanding the use of Ars. iod. and Sulph.[30], the discharge steadily increased until June 2d, when it suddenly ceased, and a livid, pustular eruption showed itself on the head, face, hands, and feet; the child became stupid, and evinced the signs of pressure on the brain, followed by the convulsions usual in that condition. On the 5th of June it died. No local application had been used in the ear except warm water and glycerin. *No laryngeal spasm occurred during its last illness.* The question arises whether the cause of the laryngismus stridulus was located in the brain, or whether it was in the inner ear, and was identical with the ear trouble which succeeded. No post-mortem was allowed, but it is not improbable that both troubles had a similar origin, although the latter condition may have been independent of the former.

COMPARATIVE CHARACTERISTICS OF NEW REMEDIES.

BY J. E. WINANS, M.D., N. J.

(Read before the West Jersey Homœopathic Medical Society.)

THE following annotations embrace clinical verifications in cases in which the single remedy has been employed. Many of them, though apparently insignificant, may become of great moment in instances where the leading indications for our best-known remedies are wanting.

To distinguish between similar drugs is an essential study which will ever demand the attention of the careful prescriber. Every comparison made helps to lighten the burden.

The sequence of remedies is another important subject which has not received deserved attention. Investigations in this direction demand the use of one drug at a time, and the most careful consideration of symptoms as they develop. Especially must we be particular to record symptoms in the order of their occurrence, and note such as disappear under the action of the administered drug. The remaining symptoms suggest the next remedy, which, if it often follow the preceding, should be recorded as worthy of remembrance in such relationship.

As liberal men let us interrogate nature as to facts without regard to any preconceived theories and without prejudice. If we are sure of our choice, if we have selected the similimum according to the strictest rules of our art, let us not hesitate to try potencies of all degrees up to 1000th and higher. If we allow prejudice to prevent our ever stepping beyond a certain mental limitation in the scale of attenuations, we will remain strangers to some of the most beautiful illustrations of the superiority of our law of cure.

The most notable exception to the rule of the single remedy is in the treatment of remittent fever, in which affection the selected drug must be alternated with material doses of Quinia, and then, if continued after the suspension of the latter, when the fever is under control, will prove vastly superior to Quinia alone. Intermittent fever, like the former, presents many difficulties in the selection of the appropriate remedy, but here Quinia should not be given as in the remittent fever. When the well-chosen remedy fails, give a dose of Sulphur anywhere from the 30th to the 1,000,000th as an intermittent, resuming the old remedy upon the accession of the next aggravation. This, together with hygienic, dietary, and similar adjuncts, will help us through the most obstinate cases.*

With this preparatory statement we take up in brief review a few new remedies and their clinical application:

ACTEA RACEMOSA, or CIMICIFUGA, is especially suitable for nervous females, tall, dark complexioned, and subject to rheumatic and uterine troubles, resembling in this latter respect Caulophyllum and Sepia; and in neuralgias and rheumatism Bellad. and Rhus, which are complementary. Its action on the male organism is more analogous to that of Bryonia. In alcoholism and delirium tremens Cimic. is indicated when the patient has a frightened look and changes rapidly from subject to subject. Like Lach., Rhus, and Thuja it affects especially the left side; like Bell. the upper dorsal spines; and like Bell., Bry., and Rhus the lumbar muscles. Characteristic indications are: Sleeplessness; intermittent neuralgia; pains in eyeballs and under left mamma; sensitiveness to draughts of air (China); sinking at epigastrium; palpitation, especially after full meal or overexertion; left-sided prosopalgia (Coloc., M. biniod., Mezer., and Spig.). Tongue clean, but pointed as in

---

* We are at a loss to understand why Dr. Winans, who seems so expert in symptomatology, should resort to alternation in the treatment of remittent fever, especially as he discountenances such a course in a kindred disease. We hope that Bönninghausen's Intermittent Fever (translated by Dr. Korndœrfer), and the able little work of Dr. H. C. Allen, will induce all homœopaths to remain true to the principles of Hahnemann, and not be deluded by alternations "with Quinia in material doses."—EDS.

Rhus; frequent ejaculatory sighs; short, dry cough; leucorrhœa (*post* menstrual). Rhus or Sepia follows well.

ÆSCULUS HIPPOCAS. has, as a leading symptom, a severe aching about the sacrum and hips when bending over at washing in persons subject to hæmorrhoids. In other respects better suited to constitutions like those produced by Bry. or Podophyll. Best results from ψ or 1^x.

AMBROSIA ARTEMISIÆFOLIA (rag-weed), will probably prove a valuable addition to the therapeutics of "hay fever," viz.: Aralia rac., Arsen., Alb. and Iod., Aurum m., Gelsem., Grindelia, and Sticta p. The effects of the pollen, when brought in contact with the Schneiderian membrane, coincide so wonderfully with the earlier symptoms of this curious affection as to suggest to our minds an interesting question for solution in its etiology, viz., whether this pest to the farmer may not also be responsible for the production of the so-called "hay asthma?" At all events this circumstance furnishes an incentive for further investigation, with the desire of ascertaining its cause and most successful mode of treatment.

BAPTISIA TINCTORIA, like Verat. viride, which it resembles in some respects, will, doubtless, be better appreciated as its true range of usefulness becomes more unfolded. At present its widespread empirical use in typhoid conditions has prevented that individualization so requisite to true success in this, as in all other forms of disease. In the early stages of typhoid fever Gelsem. and Verat. viride, among the new remedies, and Bell., Bry., Arnica, and Rhus of the old, seem to compete with it. It seems to be especially applicable to diseases of a septic nature or origin, in which fetor and great prostration are prominent features. Hence its reported success in diphtheria and diphtheritic croup. In this marked prostration its analogies are notably Arsen., Gelsem., and Rhus t. In the appearance of the tongue, and in the "sore, bruised feeling," it resembles Arnica. We turn to the mental symptoms for a distinction. The Arnica patient says "there is nothing the matter" with him, or else "he forgets the world while speaking." The Baptisia patient either "falls asleep in the midst of a sentence" or "he cannot sleep because his head feels as though it was scattered about." This latter symptom, first given us by that indefatigable worker, Dr. J. B. Bell, has led to its successful administration in intermittents, thus showing the superiority of this mode of treatment over any petty theories. In some leading symptoms it also somewhat resembles Cimicifuga.

BERBERIS VULGARIS is a remedy which promises to be prominent in the treatment of Bright's disease, especially in those addicted to the use of spirituous liquors. Indications are: Albuminous urine, with great distress in region of kidneys; worse on stooping, especially after use of gin. Suits persons who are irritable, dyspeptic, of a Carbo veg. constitution, after this remedy has relieved the gastric irritability caused by a debauch. It also seems to affect the liver and portal circulation to a marked degree, insomuch that it is spoken highly of in jaundice and anal fistula. Here it certainly deserves to be more thoroughly tested. Its rheumatic symptoms resemble those of Puls.

Boracic acid, lately in the *Investigator*, is referred to as "a valuable remedy in pruritus,"—no special variety being referred to; hence empirically used. We certainly have need of some additional mode of treatment for this distressing and troublesome affection. The remedies generally used are Dolichos, Rumex, Rhus, and Sulph.; for pruritus vulvæ, Ambra, Calad. s., Plat., Sepia, and Zinc., and of the new remedies, Collinsonia, Ham. v., and Helonias. Dr. Lilienthal, in his *Therapeutics*, italicizes M. protiod. for simple itching.

Caulophyllum suits tall, slender females (Phos.) who are of a dark complexion and are inclined to rheumatism (Cimicif.). Its peculiar affinity for the uterus is well known. No less remarkable is its relation to rheumatic affections of the wrist and finger-joints, especially of the right hand (Viola odor.). The swelling of the finger-joints is pale; pains worse every other evening and on attempting to close the hands. Also recommended for stomatitis and leucorrhœa when occurring in women with "moth patches" upon face and forehead. As in Kali bich., rheumatism and gastric symptoms alternate, so here rheumatism may alternate with asthmatic attacks, where Kali c. and Phosph. may also be required.

Eucalyptus globulus, given empirically, cures obstinate cases of ague, in which relapses are frequent. A teaspoonful of the fluid extract to a cup of milk, two or three times a day. In the *Homœopath* of August, Eucalyptus is cited as a remedy likely to prove of use in acute coryza. Mention is made therein of the benefits resulting to two foreign observers from chewing the dried leaves. Here, too, is a troublesome affection for most of us to treat, expecting a complete cure. Allium cepa, Bellad., Bry., Euphras., Kali b. and iod., Merc., Nux v., Puls., Rhus, and Spigelia have been most serviceable among the old remedies; of the new, Aralia r., Gelsem., the Deutiodide of merc. and potash, and Sticta pulm. have severally been recommended.

GELSEMIUM in its general effects resembles Acon., Bell., Puls., and Verat. v. In throat affections it seems to be complementary to Lachesis, which it follows well. Like Bell., it is most often called for in diseases of women and children. For nervous females it quite resembles Cimicif., and may be needed, even more often than it. Most Gelsem. patients have as characteristic, drowsiness, vertigo, and great muscular prostration. No remedy, not even Bry. or Cocculus, has vertigo more marked. Its headaches are usually attended with irregularities of vision—either dimness or diplopia—and heaviness of the eyelids. In this latter respect it resembles Caust., Rhus, Sepia and Verat. alb. For sudden loss of sight in acute diseases it has an analogue in Stram.; for diarrhœas induced by depressing emotions, in Podoph.; for slowness of pulse, in Chinin. s., Digit., Kalmia, Opium, Stram., and Verat. vir. On the muscular system it causes either a loss of voluntary motion or spasmodic movements in a lateral direction, as in eyeballs and lower jaw. Legs give way on bending the knee (Calc. c. and Lycop.). In fever characterized by cold hands and feet and thirstlessness (Apis m. and Pulsat.). In diphtheritic conditions, throat symptoms begin on right side passing to left (Lycop. and Podoph.).

HAMAMELIS VIRGINICA has especial relation to the nervous system. Its range extends from simple venous congestions and varicosities to passive hæmorrhages. Its analogues among the older drugs are Aloes, Arnica, Carbo v., China, Puls., and the mineral acids; among the new, Acalypha ind., Æsculus h., Collinsonia, Erigeron, and perhaps Podoph. and Trillium. It seems to exert a special influence over congestions of the pelvis and generative organs. Its empirical uses are manifold and require no repetition here. In epistaxis analogous remedies are Arnica, Carbo v., Phosph., and Trillium. In hæmoptysis, Acalypha, Cinchona, and Millef. In orchitis it is valuable, resembling Pulsat. For females it has been recommended in pruritus, vaginitis, vaginismus, dysmenorrhœa and leucorrhœa. It is said to especially affect blondes, with brown hair and leucophlegmatic temperament, who sleep late in the morning, are depressed in mind, irritable and languid after awaking, and who, at each menstrual period, pass into a state resembling stupor. For hæmorrhoidal troubles it is a leading remedy. Compare Æsculus, Aloes, Collinsonia, Mur. ac., Nux v., and Podoph.

JATROPHA CURCAS is a plant which should be more widely

known and employed in choleraic diseases. Indications for its use are: Profuse evacuations, coming out with a gush (Croton tig. and Gratiola), and attended with much gurgling in abdomen; violent thirst, cold perspiration, cramps in legs (especially right), or indifference to pain and vomiting of albuminous substances. Attacks brought on from eating watermelons.

KAVA KAVA, PIPER METHYSTICUM, will doubtless prove a valuable addition to our Materia Medica when its range of usefulness has once been fully ascertained. It is a bush found in several of the Pacific Islands, of which the Sandwich (?) group is said to furnish the best specimens. The natives make an intoxicating beverage from the roots. Its free and continued use is said to develop skin symptoms similar to lepra and elephantiasis. Every now and then we see some new mention of its clinical employment in the various journals of our school. In the *Investigator* of January 15th Dr. Wolff reports excellent results from its use upon his own person in chronic cystitis, with fetid urine of a dirty color, with a crystalline sediment on bottom and sides of the vessel (Apis), but, especially, depositing a stringy gelatinous mass, very adherent. The above cleared up under K. kava, but the urine became sour, greenish in appearance, with variegated pellicle floating upon the surface, and a deposit of very fine sand, which may be mingled with the above gelatinous mass. Later the urine became frothy, and so remained for a protracted period. Under the continued use of the θ, strangury resulted, followed still later by thick, lumpy mucous discharges, obstructing the passage of the urine. On stopping the remedy these symptoms gradually disappeared, the pellicle alone being present some ten days later. Upon a return of the old symptoms a month or two later, Brachyglottis seemed to follow well. In the report of a case of metritis, some two years ago, by Dr. Hiller, which had been previously under allopathic treatment for six weeks, the patient complained of "a sharp pain from right ovary through to back, with tenderness of abdomen to touch and cold extremities." Patient of a dark complexion and constipated habit. Pains were aggravated and rendered unbearable after Cham. θ, but were promptly relieved by K. kava θ in water. (From the above, this drug may be an addition to the antidotes of Cham.) In this year's June *Homœopath* Dr. H. also reports its successful employment in the case of "a lady suffering from nervousness and tremulous weakness as a sequel of pneumonia. She was fearful; short-breathed on ascending; loss of appetite and impaired digestion; complained of pain under right shoulder-blade and through right chest, directly down right side and hip, with extreme weakness in loins." She received ten drops of fluid extract four times a day. Improvement commenced immediately, and at the end of eight weeks the number of drops was reduced to four; was apparently perfectly well at the end of ten or twelve days. In the same number of the *Investigator* as that in which Dr. Wolff's article occurs, Dr. Skinner, of Liverpool, contributes some valuable verifications of the mental symptoms of K. kava. These are: "Sleeplessness and restlessness, compelling change of position (Ars. and Rhus.); toothache or earache." The pains were "agonizing (Acon.), with tossing, twisting, and writhing, and were temporarily relieved by the attention being diverted." (Baryta c. has a similar toothache.) Good results from both θ and 500th attenuation. From Dr. Hiller's observations it seems to affect the right side especially.

LAC CANINUM in the 100,000th potency is reported to have cured a case of long standing. "Heavy pain in the eyeballs, accompanied with outward pressure." This remedy, introduced, we believe, by Dr. Swan, has achieved for itself a wonderful reputation in the more malignant forms of diphtheria. For this it is deserving of the very highest encomiums, instead of the heartless indifference to which it has been subjected by many from no other cause than the mere fact of its origin. Dr. C. Lippe, of New York, gives the following indications for its use in various forms of ulceration other than diphtheritic: "Ulcers in any part of the body, of a shining, glistening appearance. In diphtheria the ulcerations and swelling of the glands shift from one side to the other and back again (Kali bich.). It may be accompanied also by an excoriating nasal discharge, similar to that of Arum t."

From what we can glean, the left side is more frequently the chief seat of the affection (like Bellad.? Gelsem., Kali bich., and Lach.). It has been found most efficacious in attenuations ranging from the 200th to the 100,000th.

MELILOTUS, were its reported symptoms clinically verified, would prove an efficient remedy for certain distressing nenralgic headaches, congestive in character, lasting several days, and finally relieved after a profuse nosebleed. (Antimon. c. is somewhat similar. Alumina, Carbo a., Coffea, and Dulc. have also epistaxis with headache.) The remedies most used in this annoyingly frequent trouble and neuralgic headache are: Acon., Ars., Bell., Bry., Cimic., Gels., Ignat., Kalmia, Lach., Nux v., Paullinia, Phosph., Puls., Sang. canadensis, Silic., Spig., Sulph., Verat. alb. and viride, and perhaps Rhus tox.

PHYTOLACCA.—The special affinity of this remedy for the female breast is well known. Its complete sphere of clinical application, like that of numerous other drugs, is yet to be learned. From its empirical use—or rather abuse—much that would otherwise have become of great clinical value has been lost to the profession. The pains are mostly of a shooting character (Acon.); its throat and urinary symptoms show its applicability for diphtheritic angina, where its characteristic symptoms are also present. These are: "Rawness in the throat, with corrosive pain on swallowing, as from a red-hot ball. Swallowing frequently attended with severe pain at root of tongue. Pain on swallowing hot liquids or solid food." We remember to have cured a severe case of tonsillitis with Phytol. 1^x in which the latter two symptoms were prominent. Left tonsil most affected. (Lycop. has a desire for cold drinks in Angina.)

In diphtheria the membrane is usually dark; urine dark red and albuminous, leaving a mahogany stain in the vessel; fever, with severe pains in head, back, and limbs. Its influence upon the liver is shown by pain in right hypochondrium and constipation. The eruption on skin and rheumatic pains suggest its use in syphilis.

PODOPHYLLUM is a grand remedy, whose beauties will never be fully revealed to those who employ only the lower dilutions. In chronic hepatitis it rivals Nitric acid when given in the 500th and upwards, and in acute cases is used, perhaps, next to Bry. and Merc. in frequency, about as often as Bellad. (?) or Chelidonium. Calc. c. and Gelsem. are probably its nearest analogues. Similar to Calc. c. in its nse in lymphatic children, with softness of skin and flabbiness of muscle, especially during dentition. Similar to Gels. and Lycop. in sore throat, passing from right "to left;" in "diarrhœa induced by exciting emotions," especially news of distressing character; diarrhœa worse in morning and after eating, generally breakfast. (In diarrhœa of teething children when Podoph. proves insufficient, Sulph. ac. follows well.)

In hepatitis, Podoph. is indicated when, with tongue showing imprint of teeth (Merc.), there is distension (painless to pressure) of right hypochondrium, with a "desire to frequently rub or stroke the same;" appearance of "liver spots" upon arms and face (forehead especially); anorexia; great belching;

stools preceded by griping pains in region of umbilicus; or, later, in hypogastric region from presence of hæmorrhoids.

In meningitis, with "rolling of the head" (Bellad.) and grinding of the teeth, it has done good service. Is likewise claimed to have cured pneumonia, and even to have checked hæmorrhages from various parts.

These are but a few of its many uses.

RUMEX CRISPUS is indicated in patients who experience a dulness in the head after waking; itching in the ears; heat and pricking in face; fluent coryza with sneezing and discharge of mucus from posterior nares. (Ipecac., dry coryza, with sneezing; Squills, sneezing, with cough; Bellad., cough ending in sneezing.)

It has also a morning diarrhœa (Aloes, Nuphar, Podoph., and Sulph.); also a cough from tickling in throat-pit, worse from cold air, from pressure on throat, and from lying on left side; soreness in larynx and behind sternum; pain in left lung and coldness of hands. There is "much tough mucus in larynx, with ineffectual hawking;" hoarseness, with altered voice, changing frequently (Arum t.). Indicated in children with a "hoarse, barking cough at night or early in A.M. on waking." Turning over in bed causes palpitation (Spig. ?). A symptom peculiar to Rumex, so far as known, is a prickling itching of the skin (lower extremities especially) upon exposure to cold air, as while undressing; relieved somewhat by warmth, more so upon the appearance of perspiration, with which the attack usually ends. Noticed more in those of a Bry. or Lycop. constitution, and may be accompanied by a fine red pimply rash. The left side is mainly affected. Characteristic of Rumex patients is the desire to "cover themselves up warmly," as instanced by those suffering from cough, who "cover their heads with the bedclothes," in order to render the air warmer to their sensitive skins.

VERATRUM VIRIDE.—We predict a future for this remedy second only to Acon. and Bellad. Analogues are: Bapt., Gels., Hydrate of chloral, Physostigma, Tabacum, Verat. alb., and the "Bromides." In its action upon the vaso-motor and cerebro-spinal systems its closest resemblance is to Acon. and Bellad. Though occupying a position midway between them, it can never, from its very nature, supplant either of the above useful polychrests. It causes, and therefore cures, active cerebral and cerebro-spinal congestions; hence must ever remain a useful remedy for convulsive diseases, especially cerebro-spinal meningitis and eclampsia, resembling more or less closely

Bell., Cicuta, Gels., and Stram. Upon the base of the brain and origin of the pneumogastric, its action is such as to markedly reduce both the frequency of the pulse (Digit., Gels., Kalmia, and Opium) and respiration. It seems to be useful in headaches proceeding from the nape of the neck, and where the cerebral congestion is such as to induce mania. In meningitis we may also find vomiting, or face pale and cold, with slow pulse.

The sensation of "tongue as if scalded," reminds us of Coloc., Magn. mur., and Rhus ven.; the "red streak in the middle" of that organ, of Arg. n. and Phos. ac. Baptisia, Kali b., and Phos. have each a yellow streak; Arnica, a deep chocolate-brown, but not furred, streak down the centre; while Leptandra has a tongue which is black down the middle.

For its employment (*0* or 1^x) in the earlier stages of typhoid, with "stabbing pains in right iliac region," we are indebted to a friend and former classmate. In metritis and puerperal fever it is also claimed to have done excellent service. It has been recommended by some in the first stage of pneumonia, but we are inclined to adhere to Acon., Bell., and Bry.; all but the former giving better results when used in the 1000th attennation than when lower.

Should a case present the characteristic tongue with "red streak in the middle and yellow edges," Verat. v. might prove the similimum for the entire case. Is said to especially suit full-blooded, plethoric individuals.

Yethia helenoides is highly recommended (by those who have used it) in late numbers of the *Investigator*. In the October number of 1877 we find the following symptoms recorded: "Dryness of fauces, with constant hemming in order to clear throat; dryness of epiglottis, with a burning sensation." These symptoms, together with reported cures of pharyngitis based upon them as characteristics, mark for it an important place among remedies in the treatment of this affection. In the above it resembles Bell., Canst., and the Iodides of merc. Additional symptoms are a marked slowness of pulse; cold sweat over entire body, coming and going in flashes; prover felt "very weak, nervous, apprehensive that some dire calamity was about to occur;"—a useful mental symptom.

PUERPERAL CONVULSIONS.

BY ROSS V. PITCAIRN, M D., ALLEGHENY, PA.

(Read before the Allegheny County Homœopathic Medical Society, June 11th, 1880.)

THE violence of the expulsive efforts in many labors, exhibiting the agitation and agonies which the sufferer bears, would suggest that this state must often border on that of the convulsive affections, and convince us that convulsions cannot be of very rare occurrence.

The convulsions occurring during the gestative and parturient states are classed as puerperal. They are subdivided, however, according to their forms and symptoms, into three varieties: hysterical, apoplectic, and epileptiform.

Hysterical convulsions are confined to the early stages of pregnancy, and they do not differ from the usual manifestations of hysteria. This period of gestation is seldom visited by the other varieties, although epilepsy may make its first appearance during the early stages of pregnancy, as at any other period of life, among those predisposed to it by inheritance or from other influences.

The apoplectic variety is precisely similar to apoplectic convulsions occurring under other circumstances. The paroxysms appear principally during parturition. A slight spasm soon followed by a comatose condition, with the general apoplectic symptoms, make up the distinguishing features of this variety.

Eclampsia, or puerperal convulsions proper, present during the spasm all the characteristics of epilepsy, and from this resemblance are spoken of as epileptiform. They should not, however, be confounded with true epilepsy, since with the exception of the symptoms during the convulsion, there is no other similarity. The term *eclampsia* was applied to this variety to indicate its position as a distinct affection.

The "aura epileptica" is seldom, if ever, felt preceding the puerperal convulsion, and epileptic convulsions are entirely suspended during parturition, to again resume their usual frequency when this condition is past.

All researches have failed to find a clear and satisfactory cause for this latter form of convulsions. An essential feature necessary in their development seems to be a peculiar irritability, sometimes induced by gestation.

This condition, however, does not always ensue, or, at least, not to the same degree during every gestation period, else when the same proximate causes are brought to bear upon the patient, convulsions would be the result. It can only be said in regard to the etiology that, following this impressible or sensitive nervous condition, any source of irritation acting primarily or secondarily on the sentient nerve centres may be sufficient to excite convulsions.

Puerperal convulsions are most frequent in primipara. Varions reasons are given for this fact, such as firmness of the bdominal walls and rigidity of the womb; also the anxiety, which is naturally more common and more intense during a first gestation period. It is claimed by some that those of small stature present greater liability to this disease, but this view is not supported by sufficient evidence. The reasons assigned for its occurrence among this class are the same as those given for its greater frequency in primipara. Women of a naturally irritable nervous temperament seem more susceptible to the causes producing these attacks. Those who have been subject to spasmodic and convulsive attacks, not epileptic, on previous occasions, would probably be more likely to become the subjects of this disorder. It often happens where such a case occurs, that it is accompanied by others in the same locality, and, as a consequence, atmospheric influences have been held to be exciting causes, but without any special evidence on which to base such a theory.

The retention of urea in the blood, inferred from the presence of albumen in the urine, and caused by a morbid action of the kidneys, has received much attention in relation to eclampsia. Although in the majority of cases the attack is preceded by some œdema and albuminuria, still the kidneys cannot be said to have any direct action in the production of the convulsions; the numerous cases of albuminuria during gestation not followed by convulsions, and of convulsions not preceded by œdema or albuminuria, together with modern pathological investigations, all tending to confirm the view that the convulsive disorder is not, as a rule, dependent upon renal difficulty.

Marsden refers to a work, *On the Nerves of the Uterus*, by J. Frankenhauser, of Jena, in which the author claims to have demonstrated an intimate connection between the nerves of the uterus and the renal ganglia. From this discovery he is led to believe that the condition of the kidneys is sympathetic with the irritation of the uterus. "He infers that the sudden occurrence of convulsion following all external sources of irritation (as the pressure of the fœtal head on the cervix, digital examinations, etc.) and emotional causes, would tend to show that the nervous system, and not the vascular, is the starting-point of the disease, and thinks the pathological changes of the kidneys, as observed in women dying from convulsions, are too slight and of too short duration to indicate a long-continued congestion; and in confirmation of this view is the evidence of convulsions where no albuminuria existed."

In a late number of the *North American Journal of Homœopathy* appears a partial translation of an article by Professor Spiegelberg, of Prussia, who claims that cases of convulsion of this form without albuminuria are acute epileptic attacks, and that true eclampsia depends upon uræmic poisoning. Another theory advanced in regard to their pathology (and which appears in Playfair's work) is an anæmic condition of the brain. This anæmia is accounted for primarily from the hydræmic condition of the blood naturally attendant on the pregnant state, and when albuminuria is present it would increase this fluidity; hence the association of the urinary and convulsive affections.

As the heart is normally hypertrophied during pregnancy, any slight cause tending to produce a hyperæmic condition of the brain (when this state of the blood exists) might result in an extravasation of the blood into the nervous structure, causing subsequent compression of the minute vessels, and consequently anæmia.

It is thought by some, however, that the preponderance and great impressibility of the nervous system during pregnancy is the main factor in the production of puerperal convulsions, just as slight irritations in children, owing to this state of the nervous system, give rise to a similar class of affections.

Convulsions of the greatest severity may appear suddenly, without any previous indication of their approach; generally, however, as in other grave affections, they are preceded by precursory symptoms, such as headache, giddiness, noises in the ears, injection of the conjunctiva, dimness of sight, confusion of the mind, rambling incoherent mutterings, and sometimes nausea and vomiting.

The termination of the convulsions varies in different patients. A few cases continue in the comatose condition, into which they commonly subside in the intervals of the convulsions, and this condition gradually extends to a state similar to that of apoplexy, and ends in death. Some remain in a condition of semi-consciousness and exhaustion for a length of time, and gradually recover. In other cases the patient becomes maniacal, and continues so for a long period, but ultimately recovers.

The degree of danger from these attacks, considered in relation to the time of their occurrence, is said to be greater when they appear during labor and continue afterwards than those appearing after delivery, and the most favorable are those occurring during the progress of gestation.

Convulsions coming on after delivery generally appear about four hours after the birth of the child. The mischief is attributed to some injury occurring during labor, though its location cannot be specified.

TREATMENT.—The early recognition of the symptoms preceding the convulsions will prove of much importance, by enabling the proper precautions to be taken to lessen their severity, and possibly to avert the attack. The remedies most likely to be prominently indicated are: Bell., Cimicif., Gelsem., Cuprum met., Nux v., Cicuta vir., Apis, Mel., Opium, Stram., Hyosc.

When the paroxysm is present, restraint should be made on the movements of the body to prevent injury, and some article placed in the mouth to prevent laceration of the tongue. Notice should be taken of the bowels and bladder if not already attended to. A measure recommended by Playfair—compression of the carotids to prevent congestion—may not be unworthy of trial on the approach of a paroxysm. A valuable adjuvant in the treatment is Chloroform inhalations, given either continuously or at intervals, as may be deemed best.

Hydrate of chloral may be administered if, on account of the cyanotic condition of the patient, chloroform should not be admissible. When it cannot be given by the mouth it may be administered by enema.

In ante-partum convulsions this treatment, by relaxing the muscular tissues, will prepare the way for such further expedients as may be necessary. If the mitigation thus secured is not considered sufficient, and the os is dilated or dilatable, the membranes should be ruptured, and delivery expedited by the forceps. When it is apparent that artificial measures will be necessary to terminate the labor, for the purpose of controlling the convulsions, and securing the patient against danger, it should be performed at such time as may prove most beneficial also to the child. Forcible dilatation is contraindicated, unless the convulsions rapidly increase or the patient's strength rapidly diminishes. All needless irritation of the cervix by examinations should be avoided, and the patient should not be examined, or interfered with, unless fully anæsthetized.

DISCUSSION.

Dr. Hofmann: The hypotheses in this disease are well stated in the paper, but none of them are as yet thoroughly proven. I have had only three or four cases in thirty-four years' practice. One occurred during, and another after, pregnancy. A third case was in the seventh month of pregnancy, and died under the care of another practitioner soon after the delivery of the fœtus.

Dr. Martin: Have had but one case, and that occurred a few days ago. She was a primipara,—a stout, healthy woman; had never had any form of convulsions. On the morning of June 7th she first began to complain of slight headache with nausea. Slight delirium followed. In the afternoon she had a convulsive attack, and I was called. Gave Hyoscy.^{30}. The spasms continued, but at longer intervals. The os was slightly dilated, and at 3 P.M. the membranes were ruptured. With the assistance of Dr. Z. T. Miller forceps were applied, and she was delivered; the child was living but nearly asphyxiated. She had several convulsions while under the Chloroform, and also after its use was suspended. At no time did she return to consciousness during the day. The convulsions continued through the night, but at longer intervals. The Hyoscy. was the only remedy given. On the 8th she had no more convulsions, but there was some muscular twitching and jerking of the limbs. To-day (11th) she is rational, except that she has some imaginary visions. The first return to consciousness was accompanied with desire to pass water. The urine was not tested. No dropsy was present, nor was there any untoward symptom till the day of delivery.

Dr. Winslow: I had two cases of puerperal convulsions during my early practice. The first might be denominated epileptiform, the attacks occurring during gestation. There was œdema of the limbs and slight convulsive attacks during the seventh month of pregnancy. From an examination of the urine, I diagnosed congestion of the kidney, and feared Bright's disease. Gave Bromide of potash (being still in old-school therapeutics), but the disease was not arrested. She would have an attack about once a week, and always at night. Gave a farinaceous and fruit diet, and forbade the use of meat, continuing the Bromide at intervals. These attacks would come on without any apparent reason, and would be severe enough to cause her to injure her tongue during the paroxysm; in the morning she would have a feeling of exhaustion. Labor came on in the afternoon, and the child was born before I reached the house. Perfect restoration to health followed.

The second case was a young lady of good muscular development, in labor with her first child. She had not suffered from any marked symptoms during pregnancy. except melancholy from fear of trouble occurring during labor, some sluggishness of the bowels, headache, and a bilious condition, due probably to want of exercise. At the onset of labor I found that the pelvis was small but not deformed, the muscles of the perinæum tense and strong. Labor was tedious for eighteen hours. The head came down into the lower strait and stopped. The child was in the first position, but the head was large and firmly fixed in the pelvis, so that it could not be moved in any direction. I tried several times to apply the forceps, but could not deliver. While I was watching her, twitching of the eyelids began and the face became of a bluish color. Fearing trouble I sent for consultation, but before the consulting physician arrived she had a convulsion, during which I administered Chloroform. Some stupor followed the convulsion. The forceps was again tried, and failed. The convulsions continued and the face was pallid. Craniotomy was advised and performed. The child was delivered, but only with great difficulty, after partial crushing of the thorax. Convulsions continued for two hours after delivery. A sort of stupor followed this, although she seemed quiet and was breathing easy. Milk-punch was given. As I was about to leave her I noticed a sudden prostration; I administered Ammonia, but she died in fifteen minutes. I would not use Chloroform so freely in another case. The well-known depressing action of this agent upon the heart, combined with the shock of delivery, were sufficient to produce paralysis of that organ. We see this same result follow capital operations, where after ceasing the administration of the anæsthetic a profound shock will be experienced. I think we should be careful not to produce too deep a state of anæsthesia.

Dr. Shannon: Have had two cases. The first case died; the second recovered. I was called to the first case about 11 P.M. She was suffering from pain in the abdomen; the os was not dilated. Was called again at 6 A.M., and found my patient lying on the floor in a convulsion. She never returned to consciousness. The os was but slightly dilated at this time. Dr. J. F. Cooper delivered her with difficulty, but she died immediately afterwards. The second case occurred about two weeks ago. Labor was hastened by a blow on the abdomen. Saw her late in the evening, but could not reach the os. She complained of pains about the stomach similar to the first case. Had been feeling badly all day; pulse about 90; had vomited some. While sitting by her, she suddenly turned her head, looked upwards, and passed into a convulsion. Put her under the influence of Chloroform and delivered. It was a case of foot presentation, and the child was still-born. After delivery she fell into a quiet sleep, which lasted four hours. She did not return fully to consciousness during the next day. On the third day she had nosebleed and transient hallucinations. About three days after delivery she had severe pain in the epigastric region, with sleeplessness. Gave Argentum nit. with apparent relief.

Dr. Burgher: We may distinguish the three divisions of this trouble by the fact that the first is of a nervous character, easily controlled; the second class is due to uræmic poisoning to a greater or less degree, but still controllable by proper medication; the third class is, I believe, always fatal because due to cerebral lesion. I attended one lady in her fourth or fifth confinement, who had an attack of convulsions twelve hours after delivery, coming on without any apparent cause. The first convulsion lasted about fifteen minutes; the second one, which occurred after my arrival, lasted about the same length of time. I gave Hyoscy. as soon as possible. She has never had another convulsion, although she has passed through two confinements since then. I believe the cause was, to some degree, of uræmic origin.

Dr. J. B. McClelland: Will Dr. Winslow explain how an operation for the removal of the fœtus operates to produce shock upon the mother similar to that resulting from a capital operation?

Dr. Winslow: As soon as the child was delivered shock was manifested immediately, as evidenced by the sudden paleness. When a uterus is thus suddenly emptied there is a removal of obstruction to free circulation, the blood rushes to the extremities, the brain becomes anæmic, and syncope is the result; the heart depressed by Chloroform, and lacking the stimulus of blood supply, is not able to restore the disturbed circulation.

Dr. J. F. Cooper: Have had several cases of puerperal convulsions, some of which occurred before and others after delivery. Every practitioner should have full knowledge of the influences which tend to bring about this condition if he wishes to be successful in its treatment. We have, as has been stated, three kinds of spasms to which pregnant women are liable. In the early part of gestation we have slight spasms due to hysterical causes. These are amenable to treatment without emptying the womb. Many cases of this kind pass to term and are delivered without trouble. Another class among these are subjects of epilepsy or produced by epileptic causes. Finally we have eclampsia proper. The causes producing this disease are not regarded alike by every practitioner. Although it has been denied, still I believe there are few cases of severity which are not accompanied by albuminuria. Where eclampsia proper occurs near the end of pregnancy it is scarcely possible to control it and have the woman go to term. The womb must be emptied; this seems to be a necessity. If this cannot be done by medicinal means, other artificial means must be used. In my first case the patient had been in convulsions for a long time when first seen. The prognosis of death from shock was given. Forced delivery was the only thing which promised any success. The os was dilated a little over an inch. The patient was in the seventh month of pregnancy, and the convulsive attack was the result of fright. Could not reach the fœtus with the hand, so the blunt hook was passed up and caught in the popliteal space. The child was easily brought down and delivered in half an hour. The mother survived only a few minutes. She was in convulsions when the forceps was applied.

APHASIA AND ITS TREATMENT.

SYNONYMS: APHEMIA—ALALIA—LALOPLEGIA—PARALALIE.

BY S. H. QUINT, M.D., OF CAMDEN, N. J.

(Read before the West Jersey Homœopathic Medical Society, at its Annual Meeting in Camden, May 19th, 1880.)

"By aphasia is understood a condition produced by an affection of the brain, by which the idea of language, or of its expression, is impaired" (Hammond). Hamilton defines the same affection "as a partial or complete loss of speech, which does not depend upon any vocal or lingual impairment of function, but upon disease of the speech-centre, whereby the origination of forms of expression is suspended or deranged to a greater or less degree, or a kindred loss of writing or gesticulating power. The disease is generally conceded to be seated in the third frontal convolution, and is characterized by the disruption of the connection between the formation of ideas and their expression by the lingual apparatus."

This definition does not include those cases in which the individuals are able to speak, but will not, as among the insane; nor does it embrace those who cannot speak from paralysis of the tongue, or other muscles of articulation, or from any defects in the vocal apparatus. The distinction between aphonia and aphasia must also be made; for in the first the idea of speech is undisturbed and articulation is not interfered with, while in the aphasic, the stammering and incoherent speech is especially prominent.

There are many peculiarities connected with this form of disease, but I cannot undertake to consider these in detail. Suffice it to say, that it is a protean affection, involving in many curious ways the power of reading, reading aloud, speaking, writing, gesticulating, etc. General mental activity, in a majority of cases, is normal; but words are forgotten, or, if remembered, cannot be pronounced. In other cases words are substituted for those intended; while in still others there is a combination of incongruous syllables. Some patients, when the word is pronounced for them, can repeat it, but soon forget it again. Still further, a patient may transpose the letters of a word, as "gum" for "mug," or may use a word having some association with the correct one, as "cow" for "milk," etc.

When the disease especially affects the ability to write, it is termed agraphia. When the patient can write but cannot speak, it is termed aphemia. Most patients understand perfectly what is said to them. Some can even read to themselves, or express themselves by signs and gestures, but are always more or less unintelligible.

There seems to be little doubt as to the seat of this disease; the collected cases of various writers tending to show that it is located in the left anterior part of the brain, and that the third frontal convolution is the one most frequently involved.

According to Hammond, "Giving a full consideration to the facts and arguments presented, there is reason to believe, first, that the organ of language is situated in both hemispheres, and in that part which is nourished by the middle cerebral artery. Secondly, that while the more frequent occurrence of right hemiplegia, in connection with aphasia, is in a great measure the result of the anatomical arrangement of the arteries which favor embolism on that side, there is strong evidence to show that the left side of the brain is more intimately connected with the faculty of speech than the right.

"This disease depends not upon a defect of the apparatus for the receipt of impressions, nor upon the apparatus for the communication, but upon a loss of function in what has been called the 'central organ of articulate speech;' and both the inability to remember words and connect them with ideas, and the inability to *compel the organ* of articulation to form words, depend upon some change at this point. This loss of power to express ideas is symptomatized by aphasia, agraphia, or other defects in the communicating faculty. If there be amnesia, the central disturbance (whatever it is) is the same, and the variation of lost means for expression depends upon the manner of separation of organs from mental control. There seems to be little doubt as to the seat of this centre, and as to the circumstances under which it is impaired."

When we divide the faculty of speech into the two following categories, viz., 1st, the faculty of creating words as representatives of our ideas, and of recollecting them—internal speech, and, 2d, the power of co-ordinating the movements necessary for the articulation of the words—external speech, we have a classification which forms the basis of the division of aphasia into two varieties, the amnesic and the ataxic.

By the ataxic form we mean that the speech disturbance is accompanied by other cerebral or nervous lesions, and manifested especially by symptoms of hemiplegia. The amnesic form is characterized by the speech disturbance only. In the one the individual is deprived of speech because he cannot co-ordinate the muscles used in articulation; in the other because he has lost the memory of words.

Hammond claims that this point had not hitherto been noted, and says: "The phenomena indicate, I think, very clearly, the seat of the lesion and the physiology of the parts involved. The gray matter of the lobes presides over the ideas of language, and hence over the memory of words. When it only is involved, there is no hemiplegia, and there is no difficulty of articulation. The trouble is altogether as regards the memory of words." If, on the other hand, the "corpus striatum,—which contains the white or fibrous tissue coming from the anterior column of the spinal cord, and is besides connected with the hemisphere,—or any other part of the motor tract is involved, we have the accompaniment of paralysis on the opposite side." In the cases in which the power of co-ordinating the muscles of speech is lost, we have, without exception, hemiplegia or the ataxic form, indicating the motor tract as the seat of the lesion.

Aphasia is most frequently complicated with hemiplegia, and almost always of the right side, thus showing the cerebral lesion to be in the left hemisphere. It may be dependent upon any form of brain disease which produces disorganization of, or pressure upon, the third frontal convolution, or parts immediately adjacent. Among the common diseases leading to this, we find cerebral hæmorrhage, thrombosis or embolism, tumors or sclerosis, as well as certain forms of meningitis. Age has but little influence, excepting so far as it determines cerebral hæmorrhage, embolism, or the other diseases just mentioned, although but few examples in young persons and children have been reported.

Aphasia of a temporary character may depend upon functional conditions, such as cerebral congestion, indigestion, or as the result of fright or other emotional forms of excitement; or it may be connected with epilepsy or hysteria.

In diagnosing aphasia we must be careful to make the distinction between it and other difficulties of speech, and to avoid being misled by defects in articulation dependent upon incoordination or paralysis of the tongue, or by certain mental irregularities, or, in some cases, by congenital mutism. There may be transitory aphasia; but, as a rule, organic disease of the speech-centre is of a permanent character.

Speech defects which are of a local character are symptomatized by the patient's inability to speak, although he may fully convince us of his ability to form words and to appreciate their meaning; and, moreover, unless there be paralysis, can write his words. This is not the case in aphasia. In lighter forms of tongue paralysis there is no trouble about the selection of words, but a clumsiness in pronunciation, which, with other muscular weaknesses, points to paralysis. This is also met with in the general paralysis of the insane, but here it is combined with other mental impairment, as well as with muscular trembling.

Hysterical aphasia is characterized by the tendency to employ words irrelevant to the subject, or obscure and profane expressions; and, strictly speaking, should not be classed as aphasia.

In the early speech disturbances of left hemiplegia, or organic brain disease, the patient's attempts to articulate will result in clumsy mispronunciations; while in aphasia his articulation, be it ever so limited, will be rarely imperfect. He also generally evinces great impatience, embarrassment, and mortification, arising evidently from a full knowledge of his failing.

In looking for the causes of this trouble we should not forget that heart disease, parasites, and other extraneous disease may be the cause of a thrombosis or embolism, which may lead to aphasia. In some instances it will be found in connection with diabetes or albuminuria.

The prognosis, when due to the lighter causes, as fright, hysteria, or cerebral congestion, or to a gouty diathesis, is exceedingly good. When combined with paralysis it is always significant of deep trouble, and may last during the remainder of the patient's life. If there is softening or previous acute cerebral disease, or if there is evidence of arterial degeneration or valvular deposits, the case assumes a hopeless aspect. If due to traumatism, surgical aid may occasionally bring relief.

Treatment.—Lilienthal's *Homœopathic Therapeutics* gives the following: Aphasia, a symptom frequently observed before and after apoplexy: Calc., Canst., Con., Natr., Nux v., Oleander, Op., Plumb., Zinc. None of these remedies, however, were used in a recent case which came under my observation and treatment.

When this case was presented to me at the asylum, the patient had already been pronounced incurable by some of the leading old-school physicians; and this opinion had been acquiesced in by one of our leading Philadelphia homœopaths. They had, as I was informed by those who brought him to me, pronounced the case to be softening of the brain; but it afterwards proved to be the ataxic form of aphasia.

The patient on his arrival was quite excited and perfectly unintelligible. He was weak, emaciated, and his appetite poor. His efforts at conversation consisted of a perfect jargon, and his whole case seemed at first to be hopeless.

I tabulated the remedies of all the main points presented, and thus formed the following repertory, adopting mainly the classifications of Jahr and Bœnninghausen:

1. **Forgetfulness** (Amnesia).—1. Anac., Bell., Hyos., Lyc., Veratr. 2. Alum., Bry., Con., Cyclam., Graph., Guaiac., Hell., Laur., Nat. m., Nux v., Oleand., Petr., Rhus t., Selen., Spig., Stram., Sulph., Viol. od. 3. Acon., Ars., Bar., Bov., Calc., Carb. v., Colch., Creas., Croc., Ignat., Lach., Op., Puls., Sabin., Sepia, Staph., Verbas., Zinc.

2. **Hemiplegia.**—1. Alum., Anac., Cocc., Kali, Lach., Phos. ac., Sarsap., Sulph. ac. 2. Agar., Arg. n., Bar., Bell., Calc., Caust., Chin., Colch., Cyclam., Dulc., Guai., Hyos., Mezer., Mur. ac., Nat. m., Oleand., Phos., Plumb., Rhus t., Sabin., Spig., Staph., Stram., Stront., Zinc.

3. **Memory,** deficient for correct writing, Lach.

— — for letters while reading, Lyc.

— — for proper names, 1. Sulph. ·2· Anac., Croc., Guaiac., Oleand., Puls., Rhus.

— — for what was read, Guaiac., Hell., Phos. ac., Staph.

— — for what was just spoken or what one intended to say, 1. Bar. 2. Arn., Carb. an., Colch., Hell., Verat., Hep., Magnes., Merc , Mez., Rhod., Sulph.

— — for names of things, Lyc., Rhus t.

— — for things thought of, 1. Nat. m. 2. Cocc., Colch., Hyos., Staph.

— — for words, Bar., Lyc.

— — for words, or an inability to find suitable words, 1. Cham., Thuya. 2. Nux v. 3. Anac., Capsic., Phos. ac. 4. Con., Crotal., Kal., Lyc., Puls.

Memory, weakness of, 1. Bell., Hyos., Verat. 2. Anac., Con., Lyc., Nat. m., Petr., Stram. 3. Bry., Graph., Puls., Selen., Sil.

4. **Speaking**, mistakes in, 1. Amm. c., Calc., Cham., Chin., Graph., H ., Nat. m., Nux v. 2. Caust., Con., Kal., Mang., Merc., Sepia, Sil.

5. **Speech**, broken, Tabac.

— embarrassed, 1. Bell., Calc. c., Cann., Mez. 2. Amm. c., Anac., Aur., Caust., Cic., Con., Dulc., Euphr., Galv., Graph., Hep., Nat. m., Nux v., Op., Ruta, Secale, Stann.

— confused, Bry., Calc., Canst., Lach., Lyc., Sec.

— confused on certain words, Lach.

6. **Writing**, mistakes in, 1. Lach. 2. Amm., Cham., Chin., Graph., Hep., Nat. m., Nux v. 3. Bovis., Cann., Crotal., Natr., Puls., Rhod., Sepia.

7. **Sleep**, morbid propensity to, principally Acon., Ant., Bar. c., Calc., Caust., Crocus, Lach., Laur., Led., Mosch., Nux v., Op., Plumb., Puls., Secale, Sulph.; also Am., Bell., Bry., Camph., Carb. v., Chin., Fer., Lyc., Merc., Natr., Nat. m., Nux v., Phos., Phos. ac., Rhus, Spig., Sil., Staph., Stram., Verat., Zinc.

Sleep, morbid, in daytime especially, Podoph.

8. **Somnolency**, during the day, Bell., Calc., c., Carb. v., Chin., Con., Graph., Hep., Kal., Lach., Merc., Nat. m., Nux v., Phos. ac., Podoph., Sulph., Bar. c., Raphan.

9. **Paralysis**, following apoplexy, Arn., Bar. c., Bell., Nux v., Stann., Zinc; also Anac., Con., Lach., Laur., Stram.

— of tongue, Caust., Graph., Lach., Strych., Dulc., Euphr.

— of tongue following apoplexy, Bell., Hyos., Op., Stram.

10. **Apoplexy**, Arn., Bar. c., Bell., Cocc., Lach., Nux v.,

Op., Puls.; also Acon., Antim., Coff., Con., Dig., Hyos., Ipec., Merc., Nux m., Tart. em.

A careful study of the above showed that Anacardium was the remedy, and it was administered accordingly. He immediately began to improve, more in the general health at first than in any special symptom. At the end of a month or six weeks, its action appearing to be exhausted, I gave Lycopodium, beginning with the *θ*, and gradually going up, until finally, after the 200th was reached, he was discharged cured.

I have briefly compiled the symptomatology for the mental conditions only, with a few of the most important concomitants, which I will now give, beginning with the two remedies used in the case alluded to, and afterwards taking up the others alphabetically:

Anacard.—Great weakness of memory; memory quite useless, particularly for single names; trembling from every motion; motions awkward; want of words in speaking; confusion of ideas. Accompanied with impaired digestion, sleepiness after a meal, lassitude, and prostration; also paralysis.

Lycopod.—Great weakness of memory; errors in speaking words and syllables; confounds letters and forgets their names; chooses wrong words for every-day things; inability to think, with difficulty in finding the right expression and suitable words. Lassitude and emaciation; great dryness of the skin; difficult digestion (this symptom disappeared, however, after taking the Anacard.)

Calcar. c.—Frequent inability to recollect; easily commits errors and misapplies words in speaking. Emaciation; dry skin; cerebral congestion.

Caustic.—Distraction and inattention; slow march of ideas; pronounces words wrong, and confounds syllables with letters.

Conium.—Inability to express himself correctly in speaking; frequent errors in speaking; stupidity and difficulty of comprehending what has just been read.

Natr. carb.—Readily commits errors in writing; weakness of thought.

Natr. mur.—Thoughts wandering; easily commits mistakes in speaking and writing; inability to think.

Nux mosch.—Fits of complete thoughtlessness and distraction, with jumbling together of different alphabets in writing; omission of letters and syllables; want of power of comprehension while reading. Frequent sleepiness; cool dry skin.

Nux vom.—Distraction and difficulty in collecting his senses; easily commits errors in speaking and writing, with omission of words and syllables; inability to think, with confusion of ideas, forgetfulness; deficiency of words; uses unsuitable expressions, and errs in regard to measure and weight. Paralysis; inclination to lie down; sleepiness during the day; head congested, face dark red.

Oleander.—Obtuseness of intellect; difficult comprehension of what is read, with confusion of thought; weakness of memory.

Opium.—Misconception; wavering conceptions; weakness and complete loss of memory; weakness of intellect, and apathetic indifference to joy and suffering. Muscular flaccidity; red face, sparkling eyes; sleep comatose, and with snoring; paralysis; cerebral congestion.

Plumbum.—Equally as important in paralysis of mind and intellect as in physical paralysis; absence of mind. Paralysis; pale, miserable, cachectic appearance; dryness and falling off of the hair of the head; emaciation; sleepiness in the day time.

Zincum.—Slumbering condition of the mind; great forgetfulness and weakness of memory; difficult comprehension and association of ideas, with inability to exertion. Great sleepiness in the daytime; lassitude and depression; frequent vertigo and headache; indolence.

NATRUM MURIATICUM AND SEPIA.

BY DR. KUNKEL, OF KEIL.

(Translated by S. Lilienthal, M.D., New York.)

ARTICULAR rheumatism belongs to the affections which are not only a *crux medicorum* for allopathy, whose therapeutics are in such a desolate state that the ice-bag is considered one of their remedies, but even many physicians of our own school acknowledge the fruitlessness of their treatment in this affection. I intend to lead your attention to two remedies which were of essential service to me in such states: Natrum mur. and Sepia.

An articular rheumatism is in most cases the expression of a constitutional affection. We must differentiate two groups of symptoms: those of the *status presens* and the *antecedentia.* The former hardly ever give us sure indications for the selection of the remedy.

Both remedies develop profuse sweat, which under Sepia takes place especially during the morning hours. In Sepia the perspiration is often of a foul odor, or, as some say, to be compared to the odor of elder flowers. In Natrum mur. all symptoms, and thus also the perspiration, are more conspicuous during the forenoon.

Characteristic for Natrum mur. is the intermittent and irregular pulse with increased heart's action, too often based on a malarial dyscrasia, or even a pericarditis rheumatica. Natrum mur. in alternation with Spigelia acted repeatedly well with me in such cases. Natrum mur. gives us thirst with the fever, whereas Sepia has thirstlessness, notwithstanding the profuse perspiration. In Natrum mur. the pains are fixed, whereas we find them migrating under Sepia (Puls., Bell., Arn., Sulph., etc.). The tormenting sleeplessness, so often accompanying articular rheumatism, belongs rather more to Natrum mur. than to Sepia.

Natrum mur. is not an antipsoric in its strictest sense. It is rather the remedy for malarial dyscrasia. Sepia belongs to psora, and is related to Sulphur, Calcarea, and Lycopodium. Natrum mur. is a chief remedy in those cases of chlorosis based on a malarial dyscrasia. Such patients show most frequently the cardiac symptoms,—extraordinary mobility of the vascular system, dyspnœa, splenetic stitches, articular pains (especially in the knees), thirst, get easily tired, lachrymose humor,—all of which improve towards evening. Anæmia may not be necessarily present.

Whereas Natrum mur. has aggravation by motion, Sepia feels worse when quiet. All elements are sometimes silent during forced motion, supposing that the strength allows it. Only at the beginning of motion, worse,—stiffness, increased pains when rising after sitting, passing off by moving about. After motion, aggravation of all the symptoms.

Both remedies are of great service in headache. That of Natrum mur. is mostly seated in the forehead, appears in certain types during the forenoon and decreases in the afternoon or evening. Such periodically appearing headaches are often very severe Headaches, corresponding to Sepia, appear mostly in the morning when waking up, pass off in an hour or an hour and a half after walking about, or (more rarely) increase in intensity till evening. Nausea and vomiting with the headache.

Both remedies are necessary in affections of the eyes. The ophthalmia of Natrum mur. is frequently taken for a scrofulous one. The accompanying symptoms, sometimes also the typical character with exacerbation in the forenoon, may serve as effectual guides. The eye affections corresponding to Sepia have mostly a neuralgic character with exacerbation early in the morning.

Bloatedness of the face belongs to both; Natrum mur. of the upper lip, Sepia of the under lip. Color in Natrum mur., pale; in Sepia, pale or yellow, which also shows the hot flashes so characteristic of climaxis.

The gastric symptoms, subjective as well as objective, are similar in both. Disgust to fat and bread, momentary amelioration after eating, but the pains get more severe after ½ to 1½ hours (Lach). Natrum mur. has more relation to the spleen; Sepia to the liver. In relation to the sexual organs, we would remark, just as in psoric individuals, a thorough cure of gonorrhœa is hardly possible without the corresponding antipsorics, so Natrum mur. will find its place in the gonorrhœa of malarious persons. In chronic syphilis Sepia often shows great curative power, especially in cases which leave it doubtful whether we have to deal with syphilis or hydrargyrosis, always supposing that the symptoms correspond.

In skin affections both remedies are of great importance. A manifestation exclusively characteristic of Natrum mur. is large maculæ, like erythematous, somewhat bluish, over the whole chest, especially after becoming heated from preceding walking. Psoriasis, non-syphilitic, especially on the side of the joints, yields to Natrum mur. Sepia suits better in chloasma. We often recognize immediately the Sepia patient by his dirty, larger or smaller spots (sometimes the whole forehead is of a dirty yellowish-brown color) on forehead, around the mouth, or from the yellow or red saddle over the nose down to the cheeks.

Natrum mur. has aggravation during a thunderstorm (the patient becomes sleepy), from manual labor, especially knitting. Sepia: fog, murky atmosphere, sitting position, especially bent over, as in writing or manual work.

Experience taught me that the higher potencies act far more satisfactorily on these *apparently* acute affections. One cannot understand why physicians using the 10th or 12th potency show such a horror at the 200th. During the last month of March I cured three cases of articular rheumatism, *two with Sepia* 200th *in five days,*—young men of eighteen and twenty years, whose *status presens* and *anamnesis* clearly pointed to Sepia. The third case was a *perfectly healthy* young woman, whose affection arose under the influence of the genius epidemicus, and who was cured in a still shorter time with Mercur. 3d.—*A. N. L.*, 15, 1880.

FRAGMENTARY PROVING OF ERYTHROXYLON COCA.

BY DR. GRUBENMANN, OF ST. GALLEN, SWITZERLAND.

(Translated by S. Lilienthal, M D.)

OCTOBER 25th, 1879, I took at 8 A.M. one drop of the tincture. After eight hours, sensation of fulness in stomach, of tension in the head, excessive development of gas in the stomach, meteorismus, eructations without relief; after twelve hours, symptoms of gastric catarrh, perfect inappetency, watery eructations, nausea, dulness of head, mental depression, sexual nisus increased. After taking the first, second, third, fourth, fifth dilution, similar primary action, but in a less degree than after the mother tincture.

November 6th, 5 P.M., 5 drops of the sixth centesimal dilution; felt well the whole evening; woke up in the morning with great heat in the head, pain in vertex and occiput, boiling (*watlend*, which can also mean undulating), pulsating; the pain afterwards concentrating itself on the left side of the skull and occiput, where the trapezius muscle is inserted. No appetite; copious eructations without relief. No appetite for dinner (2 P.M.); the whole afternoon dulness of head; thirstlessness. After 4.30 P.M. large quantities of air were expelled from the stomach by eructations; without smell and without relief up to 7.30 P.M. The whole day sexual irritation, with discharge of a clear, thick, prostatic juice; sensitiveness of the perineal region even when sitting; also of the anus, where there is a sensation of burning tension. Pulse somewhat accelerated, but not much; stools only after thirty-six hours, usually every twenty-four hours. The symptoms gave the picture of a slightly febrile, gastric-dyspeptic state, with meteorismus of the stomach.

November 8th I felt well again with exception of the still severe ructus; flatus moderate.

December 5th took a few drops of the fifteenth centesimal dilution. In the evening nothing abnormal; the next morning a soft stool with slight tenesmus. In the afternoon again a stool, yellow and thin. Head somewhat tense, and about 5 P.M. sensation of fulness and gurgling in stomach and abdomen; tension and cutting in both hypochondria and back. After 5.30 P.M. tremendous discharge of air by eructation without great relief, so that I wondered what could have contained all that air without producing greater tension.

December 7th, passed still a great deal of wind without

diminution of the tension in gastric and hypochondriac region. No stool that day; one on the 8th. I felt afraid to take more of Coca[15], as my digestive organs are none the strongest. Coca[30] always gave great relief.—*A. H. Z., No.* 17, 1880.

In a paper read by Dr. Searle before the Medico-Chirurgical Society he showed that, like coffee, tea, tobacco, and alcohol, Erythroxylon Coca is used as a nutritive and stimulating beverage, taken the whole year round with less injury to the system than the others mentioned, and still what good remedies do we find in Caffein, Thein, Nicotia, and Tobacco when strictly indicated. Allen gives us a pretty fair pathogenesis, but still it needs working out, especially since Searle considers it nearly a specific for his "new disease." S. L.

THE HOMŒOPATHIC OPHTHALMOLOGICAL AND OTOLOGICAL SOCIETY.

THE fourth annual session of this society, which has become so well known of late, was held at Milwaukee during the first days of the session of the American Institute. The attendance from the East was not large, but the energy and earnestness of the Western men present rendered the meeting a decided success. The sessions were held in the parlors of the Newhall House. Papers were read by leading oculists throughout the country. The society during the past year has met with an irreparable loss in the sad death of its president, Dr. W. H. Woodyatt. In the absence of Vice-President Haughton Dr. Phillips was called to the chair, and, as Dr. Lewis was not present, Dr. Beebe acted as secretary. Dr. Haughton's address, which was read by the secretary, was a tribute to the memory of the lamented president of the society. Repeating the words spoken at the funeral, Dr. Haughton said: "Of our brother, who presented to us ever such a grand manhood, with its frank, open, earnest face towards truth, its fidelity to duty, its love of righteousness, what shall we say? Entering upon the other life in this faith I have been rehearsing, imagination may not follow nor attempt to picture the augmentation of delight with which he will enter into its realization. The story of a life is never told, and I shall not attempt it in the discharge of this grateful duty. Too many things are hidden, too many ministries are performed in the 'silent chamber' for us to trace the processes by which a man is made what he is. Well-balanced and strong, in society honored, in his practice trusted and beloved, instant in service, faithful at all times, it is a blessed thing to know of such a character that it has its roots in a deep central faith, planted early and growing like the rest of him, by cautious inquiry, but with a clear, earnest, and rational look into the revealed realities of the unseen world, and the righteous will of God."

Among the papers presented at this meeting were many containing original and valuable thoughts. Dr. W. H. Winslow treated his subject, "Conical Cornea," in a very thorough and scientific manner. In the case cited the result was certainly very remarkable. The beneficial effects of treatment, when we consider the hitherto unsatisfactory results that have been obtained, are especially gratifying. The Doctor also points out the value of combination glasses to meet the corneal astigmatism.

Eserine is evidently just now being very thoroughly investigated by homœopathic oculists. Dr. James A. Campbell, in opposition to Sanderberg's views, believes it to be a potent agent in acute glaucoma,—and certainly the effects in the case reported could not be happier. Even should the disease recur, as Sanderberg fears, the remedy is far to be preferred to its alternative, iridectomy.

Dr. George S. Norton offered a short but extremely interesting paper on "Amblyopia Nicotina." A perfect cure followed the use of Nux vom. 1^x.

Dr. J. H. Buffum presented a conscientious study of that formidable but fortunately rare disease, "Diphtheritic Conjunctivitis." The remedies employed were Bell. and Rhus; and when corneal ulceration occurred, Aqua chlor. and Eserine locally. The result was very gratifying. The Doctor also made some remarks on the use of the cotton drum-head, which we were not able to obtain, but which will appear in the *Transactions*. The papers by Dr. Alfred Wanstall exhibited a wide familiarity with ophthalmic literature. They will be read with general interest, and the specialist will find them most valuable.

Dr. Bushrod W. James gave a verbal description of recent improvements in the ophthalmoscope.

A very peculiar "Case of Symblepharon," by Dr. D. J. McGuire, will repay perusal.

Dr. J. F. Edgar gave three cases of "Atresia Canaliculi," with remedies adjunct to surgical treatment.

Dr. C. H. Vilas described a congenital coloboma of the iris and choroid. The defect was binocular and similarly situated.

Dr. E. W. Beebe presented a study of exophthalmic goitre.

Among the papers of general interest to the profession was one by Dr. Charles Deady, a "Proving of the Duboisia Myoporoides," as suggested by the society a year ago. A most accurate record was made of the physical changes, so far as they could be observed. The record of the effect of the drug on the ocular fundus and on the larynx is more complete than that of any remedy we possess.

Dr. F. Parke Lewis's paper embodies some aural clinical notes. The effects of Bryonia in acute otitis exb. and media is pointed out, and the sphere of action defined. The effects of Calcic sulphide (Hepar sulph. calc.) are considered more marked in subacute and chronic aural catarrh, when the drug is exhibited in low trituration, than those of any other remedy employed.

The *Transactions of the Society*, embracing the papers in full, will very soon be published, and as the number of copies will be limited, those desiring to receive them may secure them by writing at once to the secretary, F. Parke Lewis, 230 Pearl Street, Buffalo.

DR. BERRIDGE AND THE AMERICAN INSTITUTE.

DR. T. P. WILSON'S REPORT REVIEWED.

In the July issue of the *Medical Advance* appeared some editorial comments upon the address of Dr. Berridge and the treatment given him by the members of the Institute, which I desire briefly to notice.

The statements made as to what occurred at Milwaukee, and the comments upon them, are so far from correct and so unjust, not alone to "certain gentlemen," but to the entire Institute, that I shall be obliged to deal in plain contradictions and plain reflections.

Dr. Wilson says: "A distinguished foreigner, an English physician, was invited to read a paper. He obtained permission to do so only by a bare two-thirds vote, quite a number of the members boldly standing up to be counted against this courteous act. Why? Because they knew beforehand the opinions of the gentleman to whom the invitation was extended, and they did not propose to give him a chance to express his opinion. This is the liberty they boast of."

In regard to Dr. Berridge's being "invited to read a paper" I have no knowledge, but presume he was so invited by Dr.

Wilson, or Dr. Lippe, or some other member of the Institute, in his individual capacity.

Upon motion of Dr. B. W. James, a gentleman having as little use for Dr. Berridge's peculiar opinions as any man in America, our brother from England was invited to a seat upon the platform beside the President, every member of the Institute present voting in favor of the extension of the courtesy.

Business went on through the first day, and nothing was said about an address from our foreign guest.

On the morning of the second day, when the report of my bureau was in order, and I had arisen to read my introductory, I was suprised by a resolution, offered by one of my good friends from St. Louis, inviting Dr. Berridge to deliver an address *at the close of the first part of our bureau report.*

As soon as I had recovered from my surprise at such an extraordinary and annoying intrusion upon the order of our bureau papers, I arose and protested in as mild and courteous a manner as I could, asking the Institute to allow our papers to come in as arranged and not thus break in upon them in the middle. I distinctly stated that I was anxious to hear Dr. Berridge, but at a more fitting time, and without this unreasonable interference with our prescribed work. The papers from my bureau had been carefully arranged, so that one would follow another closely, like blocks of prepared marble in the walls of a rising structure, and I could not think of having such a *hiatus*, however agreeable in itself, brought in to disturb the connected consideration of what we were offering. Other members, realizing the injustice contemplated, spoke against the resolution, and it was defeated. It being then moved to have the address come before the report of our bureau, *no opposition was made*, and the motion was carried.

I do not hesitate to say that had the motion been made the day before, or at any time, to have Dr. Berridge address the Institute, *without coming in the middle of an important bureau report*, no opposition would have been met with.

The members of the American Institute are not wanting in courtesy, nor in a proper appreciation of "freedom of medical opinion;" but they have some regard for what is due to a bureau of earnest workers and to an important subject under consideration.

I cannot pass on without mentioning that I asked my friend from St. Louis how he came to offer such a resolution, contemplating such an interference with my bureau, and was told by him that the resolution was not his own, that he had been asked to present it by Dr. Wilson. Perhaps the latter may, after all, find himself responsible for the alleged discourtesy to the "distinguished foreigner."

Again Dr. Wilson says: "The paper was read and received, and the following day it was withdrawn because it did not happen to suit the notions of certain gentlemen. Fortunately for them their ill-considered remarks were stricken out of the proceedings, and it may be a question who was most sat down upon, the assailers or the assailed. No wonder, after what they had said, they hastened to have all record of it expunged from the proceedings. It was a clear case of self-protection."

True, the paper was read and hastily referred to the Publishing Committee; but shortly, when the old associates of Carroll Dunham, men who were familiar with Hahnemann's *Organon* before Dr. Berridge was born, began to think of the reflections cast upon their old friend, and, indeed, upon the Institute itself, they arose to object to the publication of the address in the *Transactions*, and a motion was made to reconsider the vote of reference.

After considerable debate the motion to reconsider was laid upon the table.

So things rested till the next morning, when the *Daily Sentinel* appeared with the full text of Dr. Berridge's address.

I have been in the Institute a great many years, and have seen its members much agitated by one affair and another; but I have never witnessed so profound and universal a determination to resent an indignity, to defend one of its honored and lamented dead and its own good character, as was evinced when the Institute assembled that morning, especially when our veteran pioneer, Dr. David S. Smith, moved to take the subject of the final disposition of the address off the table for present consideration.

Dr. Talbot opened the discussion with words well considered, plain, and to the point. He will never need to qualify one expression, nor to change a single sentiment. Dr. Conrad Wesselhœft said just what a sober, earnest, well-informed member, feeling the gravity of the occasion and the injustice attempted, should say.

Dr. Ludlam's inquiry as to the status of Dr. Berridge, whether he was with us and speaking as a delegate from the British Homœopathic Congress, or any other foreign society, or whether he was here and speaking simply as an individual, was exceedingly appropriate, and developed the fact that he had come in no official capacity, and had no claims beyond those of an individual.

My own remarks were deliberate, and such as I should make again on a like occasion. I have no changes to make.

We all objected to this language: "Ever since that fatal error was committed by one, whose memory we nevertheless hold in honor, of proclaiming 'absolute liberty in medical opinion and action,' a change for the worse has taken place in our ranks. Ever since that time the name of Carroll Dunham has been held to sanction every kind of empiricism." We not only objected to this statement, as to our certain knowledge *untrue*, but we objected to its being uttered in our faces, in the American Institute, and especially by a stranger honored by our courtesy, and having no claims upon our forbearance beyond those of any other respectable physician from abroad.

I am sure when the older brethren of Dr. Berridge in England read his address, they will agree with us that he overstepped the limits of propriety and well deserved the castigation received.

Imagine the "*three gentlemen*" referred to by Dr. Wilson (as having been the "recipients of special favors from the homœopathic medical profession in England") in attendance upon a meeting of the British Congress and honored with a seat upon the platform. Does any one suppose they would, upon being asked to speak, proceed to misrepresent the position and influence of the honored and lamented Dr. Quin, or to lecture those present upon the special need of their giving more study and heed to Hahnemann's *Organon?*

As one of the "three" referred to I say we would be very far from thus abusing the courtesy extended, even did we believe Dr. Quin had taken a wrong stand or uttered a wrong sentiment, years ago, when president of the Congress, or were we persuaded that our English brethren were quite neglectful of the teachings of Hahnemann.

I must correct Dr. Wilson's report where he says the address was "withdrawn because it did not happen to suit the notions of certain gentlemen."

After a free discussion, in which neither Dr. Wilson, nor Dr. Lippe, nor any other sympathizer with Dr. Berridge opened his mouth to say a word in his defence, it was decided, no one voting to the contrary, *that the address and all discussion relating to it be left out of the printed transactions of the Institute.*

The address was not "*withdrawn*," but REJECTED—not to suit the notions of a few members, but upon the deliberate judgment of the American Institute of Homœopathy in one of its very largest meetings. And when the address was "laid upon the table" there was no need of a report of the discussion that had taken place in regard to its character and tendencies.

But, as already intimated, all the blame seemingly attached to the overt act of Dr. Berridge does not lie at his door. We are told "he was invited to read a paper," and nothing said as to who gave the invitation.

Since learning what I have of the authorship of the resolution, throwing the address into the middle of our bureau report, and hearing and reading the address itself, and seeing the report of Dr. Wilson in the July *Advance*, accompanied by his March editorial (containing exactly the same sentiment as expressed by Dr. Berridge in relation to Dr. Dunham's "fatal error"), and since I recall the fact that Dr. Lippe had, before that, accused Dr. Dunham of doing great harm by his liberal views, I am forced to the conclusion that *Dr. Berridge was but the imported tool and mouthpiece of others, left sadly in the lurch by them when the time came for administering the prepared dose to the American Institute.*

It is useless, in view of such plain facts, for Dr. Wilson to talk of courtesy violated and freedom of medical opinion trampled under foot, when the American Institute puts its seal of disapprobation upon statements which are devoid of truth in relation to the teachings of Carroll Dunham, and resents the imputation of its special neglect of the primary studies of homœopathy.

It matters not who has conceived the notion and expressed it, that our cause has been injured by the liberal spirit favored by Dunham and generally cherished by our American profession, there is not a particle of foundation for it.

On the other hand, the injury has come more by departures from original homœopathy in the direction of "bottle-washing" and other senseless modes of eliminating drug matter under the pretence of *potentizing medicines.*

But it is not my purpose at this time to pursue the inquiry as to the chief obstacles in the way of the new school.

It is my wish simply to reply to the misstatements and groundless insinuations made by the editor of the *Medical Advance.*

J. P. DAKE.

NASHVILLE, TENN.

THE

HAHNEMANNIAN

MONTHLY.

A HOMŒOPATHIC JOURNAL OF

MEDICINE AND SURGERY.

Editors,

E. A. FARRINGTON, M.D. PEMBERTON DUDLEY, M.D.

Business Manager,

BUSHROD W. JAMES, M.D.

Vol. II. Philadelphia, Pa., August, 1880. No. 8.

Editorial Department.

CONSTANTINE HERING.

SUDDENLY, at half-past ten o'clock, on the evening of July 23d, Dr. Constantine Hering departed this life, in the eighty-first year of his age. During the past decade the doctor has at times suffered quite severely from asthma, though for several years past the attacks have been less severe, so that he has been enabled to attend almost daily upon a large circle of patients. Having spent the early part of the evening of his decease with his family, he retired to his study shortly after eight o'clock, seemingly stronger and more cheery than for some weeks past. Just before ten o'clock he rang for his wife, who, immediately answering, found him suffering from extreme dyspnœa, but perfectly rational. He asked for his old friend and physician, Dr. Charles G. Raue, who was immediately sent for; at the same time Dr. A. W. Koch also, an old and esteemed friend and neighbor, was summoned, but before help could be offered the spirit had departed. Not unexpected nor yet unprepared for, was the call. To one in attendance he remarked: "Now I am dying." Many times during previous illness did his friends despair of his life, but *he* felt his time had not yet come. Now he knew that a change was indeed coming. That undaunted spirit, which for more than fourscore years animated the living clay, was about to leave its abode for realms above. Thus departed one to whom homœopathy in America,—yea, in the whole world,—will ever remain a debtor.

Though called in the ripeness of old age, his death, nevertheless, falls like a heavy pall over the entire profession. We have been called to mourn the departure of others, whose names we must ever revere, but with the death of Hering is broken a connecting link which bound the present to the past, the established, triumphant Homœopathy of our own day to the early struggles and sacrifices of its pioneers.

East, West, North, and South,—Europe and America,—have among their busy practitioners, many who look toward the home of this truly great man as toward the home of a father. Hundreds have shared with him of the wondrous store of knowledge which he possessed. Many came; none were sent empty away. Their capacity to receive, rather than his willingness to give, limited the amount bestowed. Blessings will ever attend his name.

Constantine Hering was born at Oschatz, Saxony, on January 1st, 1800. From earliest childhood he evinced an extreme desire to investigate all things. Apt as a scholar, he soon mastered the preliminary studies, and was prepared at an early age to enter the Classical School at Zittau. Here he continued his studies from 1811 to 1817. Even thus early in life he evinced an aptness for study and an accumulation of knowledge far beyond his years. Besides his familiarity with the classics, his proficiency in mathematics was truly surprising. While thus employed his mind was turned toward medicine, and when opportunity offered, he pursued his studies in that direction, first at the Surgical Academy of Dresden, and later at the University of Leipzig. In the latter institution he was a pupil of the eminent surgeon, Robbi.

About this time his preceptor was requested to write an article against homœopathy,—one which might prove its deathblow. Dr. Robbi declined for want of time, but recommended his young assistant, Hering, who, quite pleased with this mark of confidence, began the work, but meeting much in the writings of Hahnemann which was new to him, and finally reading the expression, "*Machts nach, aber machts recht nach,*" he determined on personal investigation in order that he might the more positively refute the points which Hahnemann had set before the profession.

Calling upon an acquaintance, a druggist of Leipzig, for some Cinchona, he was met by the friendly inquiry: "For what do you want it?" To this he answered, for the purpose of proving it in order the more thoroughly to attack the new folly. To this the druggist replied: "Let it alone, Hering; you are stepping on dangerous ground." Hering's answer was that he feared not the truth. And the result was, the pamphlet was not written, and homœopathy gained an able champion.

Subsequently, while still pursuing his medical studies, Hering received a dissecting-wound, which, under the treatment of his teachers, reached such a degree of severity that amputation of the hand was advised. At the suggestion of a friend who was a student of Hahnemann's, the efficacy of the potentized drug was tried, the result being a complete cure of the wound and a thorough conversion of Hering. So thoroughly was he convinced that the law of cure had indeed been discovered, that he staked thereon even his success at the University. His inaugural thesis, "*De Medicina Futura,*" contained a forcible and unflinching defence of the law of cure. He completed his medical studies and received the degree of Doctor of Medicine from the University of Wurzburg, March 23d, 1826. Soon after his graduation he was appointed by the King of Saxony to accompany the Saxon legation to Dutch Guiana, there to make scientific research and prepare a zoological collection for his government. He continued in this capacity for some years, but his love for the new truth which he had learned impelled him to further study, and finally to the practice of medicine according to Hahnemann's doctrines. Such was his success that he gained great favor with the governor of the province, whose daughter he cured of an affection which the resident physicians had declared incurable.

During his residence at Surinam he was an occasional contributor to the *Homœopathic Archives,* for which journal he had written as early as 1825 while still a student of medicine. The court physician, learning of this, wrought upon the king sufficiently to cause a notice to be sent Hering, directing him to attend to the duties of his appointment, and let medical matters alone.

His independent nature rebelled at such intolerance, and led him promptly to resign his appointment. Dr. George H. Bute, formerly a Moravian missionary at Surinam, and a pupil of Hering, had settled in Philadelphia, and was engaged in the practice of homœopathy. Dr. Hering continued in practice at Paramaribo for a short time after his resignation. Learning, however, from Dr. Bute that Philadelphia offered a good field, Hering left Paramaribo, and landed at Philadelphia January, 1833. Here he remained for a short season, when he was induced by Dr. W. Wesselhœft to assist in the establishment of a homœopathic school at Allentown,—The North American Academy of the Homœopathic Healing Art. He labored in this field until financial embarrassments necessitated the abandonment of the institution.

This led to his return to Philadelphia, where he engaged in practice with Dr. Bute, locating on Vine Street below Fourth. Here he soon acquired a large and lucrative practice. The wide scope of his education naturally offered a ready introduction to scientific and literary circles, while the active interest which he took in our republican form of government led to an acquaintance with many persons of political prominence. Among these may be mentioned Henry Clay, who, as a patient and friend, highly appreciated the services rendered by Dr. Hering, as witness the following extract from a letter, dated December 14th, 1849:

> "Your liberal kindness toward me would not allow you to indulge me in the gratification of testifying my gratitude to you for the successful exercise of your professional skill on me, on two distinct occasions, by the customary compensation; but you cannot prevent the expression of my great obligation to you for the benefit I derived from your obliging prescriptions. I thank you for them most cordially. . . . . With great regard, I am your friend and obedient servant,
>
> "H. CLAY."

Agassiz, Carey, and a host of others, distinguished in politics, art, and science, were among his friends.

Always a student, endowed with indomitable will and untiring industry, he seemed to infuse every one with whom he came in contact with the spirit of work. "Change of occupation is rest," was his oft-repeated expression.

Though conducting a large practice he found time to write much, and to superintend the work of many younger and less experienced. His Saturday-night meetings, held for the instruction of students and young practitioners, were prized as a boon. Here he imparted golden truths reaped from fields of ripe experience, such as but few have enjoyed.

Among the remedies which he proved prior to his departure with the Saxon legation, may be mentioned Mezereum, Sabadilla, Sabina, Colchicum, Plumbum aceticum, Paris quadrifolia, Cantharis, Iodium; also fragmentary provings of Antimonium tartaricum, Argentum metallicum, Aristolochia, Clematis erecta, Belladonna, Caltha palustris, Demantium, Geum rivale, Nostoc, Opium, Ruta, Tanacetum, and Viola tricolor.

During his residence in South America his observations and provings embraced the Lachesis, Theridion, Curassivicum, Askalabotes, Caladium seguinum, Jamboo, Jatropha, Solanum mammosum, Spigelia, Vanilla, Alumina, Phosphoric acid, and Psorinum.

After his arrival at Philadelphia we find him again employed in like work, either proving or superintending the provings of the Mephitis, Ictodes fœtida, Crotalus, Hydrophobinum, Brucea, Calcarea phosph. (both acid and basic), Hippomânes, Castor equorum, Kalmia, Nicandra, Viburnum, Phytolacca, Gelsemium, Gymnocladus, Chlorine, Bromium, Fluoric acid, Ferrum met., Kobalt, Niccolum, Oxalic acid, Oxygen, Ozone, Thallium, Tellurium, Palladium, Platinum, Osmium, Lithium, Glonoine, Apis, Cepa, Aloes, Millefolium, Baryta carb., Nux moschata, and Formica.

Among his other works may be mentioned:

Rise and Progress of Homœopathy; a pamphlet, Philadelphia, 1834, afterwards translated into the Dutch and Swedish languages.

Necessity and Benefits of Homœopathy; a pamphlet, 1835.

Domestic Physician, published in 1835. This work passed through fourteen editions in America, two in England, and thirteen in Germany, and has also been translated into the French, Spanish, Italian, Danish, Hungarian, Russian, and Swedish languages.

The Effects of Snake Poison, 1837.

Homœopathic Hatchels, 1845.

Proposals to Kill Homœopathy; a satire, 1846.

Suggestions for the Provings of Drugs, 1853.

Amerikanische Arzneiprüfungen, 1853–57.

Translation of Gross's *Comparative Materia Medica,* 1866.

Analytical Therapeutics, the first volume only issued, 1875.

Condensed Materia Medica, two editions, 1877–79.

Guiding Symptoms, the third volume of which he completed just prior to his death.*

In addition to these may be mentioned his editorial work connected with the *Homœopathic News,* 1854, and the *American*

---

* The amount of material collected by Dr. Hering, from which his *Analytical Therapeutics* and *Guiding Symptoms* are compiled, is truly marvellous. It is probably the most complete Materia Medica collection extant.

Journal of Homœopathic Materia Medica, 1867–71, besides many miscellaneous writings scattered through the various journals of our school. It may further be added that he assisted in the translation of Jahr's *Manual*, Allentown Edition, 1838.

Dr. Hering was a member of the Academy of Natural Sciences of Philadelphia, to which institution he presented his large zoological collection. He was one of the founders of the American Institute of Homœopathy, and for many years continued in active relationship with it, as well as with the State and county societies. He was one of the originators of the American Provers' Union, instituted August 10th, 1853. He was also one of the founders and a member of the first faculty of the Homœopathic Medical College of Pennsylvania, continuing in this relationship at intervals until 1867, when he assisted in founding the Hahnemann Medical College of Philadelphia, in which he held the Chair of Institutes and Materia Medica, being Emeritus of the same at the time of his death.

It would be difficult to give a proper estimate of Dr. Hering's character, and of his influence upon medical science. His acts are matters of medical history, and the impress of his thought is already made, deep in the medical practice of our age. It is not possible that the memory of his career is one which posterity will willingly let die; for the coming ages, even more than the present, will learn to depend upon LAW as the great governing factor in the production of the facts of natural science, therapeutics included. And so, as homœopathy must become more and more the one only acknowledged therapeutic principle, the brightest names that posterity will cherish, will be those who have done so much to establish it among men, while among the most brilliant of them all, will stand the name of—HERING.

HAHNEMANN CLUB.

ACTION OF THE HOMŒOPATHIC PHYSICIANS OF PHILADELPHIA IN REFERENCE TO THE DECEASE OF DR. HERING.

A MEETING of the homœopathic physicians of Philadelphia was held in the hall of Hahnemann Medical College, on Sunday afternoon, July 25th, at five o'clock. About one hundred and fifty physicians were present.

Dr. John K. Lee presided, and Dr. H. N. Guernsey acted as secretary.

Dr. Adolph Lippe, being called on by the chairman, addressed the meeting as follows:

Mr. President, and fellow-members of the profession: The sad event which has called us together on this occasion, is the unexpected and sudden death of our old and venerable colleague, Constantine Hering. Before I offer for your kind consideration and approval a Preamble and Resolutions drawn up for this occasion, permit me to express my sentiments, and no doubt the sentiments of all those who have known our departed colleague best. Dr. Constantine Hering, deservedly and indisputably, was considered the father of our exclusive school of medicine in the United States. It is now almost half a century since he came here, and, attracted by the institutions of the Republic, he remained here to enjoy for himself, and for the school of medicine he had adopted, the fruits of a republican form of government. Even at that early day the name of Constantine Hering was well known over the world; his contributions towards the homœopathic literature, beginning in the *Archives*, secured him an honored place among the foremost standard bearers of our exclusive law of cure. Fifty years have passed by since this scientist made his first observations on the sick-making properties of the poison of Lachesis trigonocephalus; and these observations, and the deductions drawn from them as to its health-restoring properties,—this alone,—would have made him what he was,—a shining light among medical men. The beginning of a great work was thus made fifty years ago, and we find him giving us the first works on homœopathy in the English language. While engaged in teaching the new healing art at Allentown, in this State, he gave us also, first a translation of our great standard work, *Hahnemann's Organon*, and an abridged *Materia Medica*, with a *Repertory*. Later we find him publishing his *Domestic Physician*, as a textbook for those who could not avail themselves of the assistance of the then few homœopathic practitioners,—a work which was translated into almost all languages.

We find him a large contributor to the homœopathic journals, especially defending the teachings of Hahnemann; protesting against multiplying departures from the methods of the master. We find him among his increasing professional duties continually adding to the homœopathic materia medica; his numerous monograms on old and new remedies he leaves as an heirloom to posterity, to be thereby recollected as the ever faithful worker for the further development of our new resources in the healing art. We find him teaching the principles and practice of the new school in private and in public. The caller on him who earnestly desired to learn found him ever ready to give the wished-for information. We find his enthusiasm not diminished as he became older; his fidelity to our principles was as firm as were the enthusiastic hopes he entertained for the perpetuation of our school of medicine. Always ready to advance the true interests of homœopathy, he took special pleasure in guiding the younger members of the profession, by explaining to them the great results obtainable for the cure of the sick by following strictly, honestly, and persistently the rules and directions to be found in the methods of Hahnemann.

The great joy of his late days was the reading of the address delivered by the President of the American Institute of Homœopathy, in which the methods of Hahnemann, and the immutable principles governing our school, were so earnestly laid before our National Institute, as were also the proceedings of the members of that institute.

As an individual who has known our departed colleague for more than forty years, who profited by his kind instructions and example; who with him, as one of the early pioneers, saw the almost miraculous growth of our school of medicine, I can only faintly express the grief felt, when so noble and so self-sacrificing a member of our school is removed from among us. His works will live after him; coming generations will profit by them, and coming generations, like the present, will honor his memory.

Dr. Lippe then offered the following preamble and resolutions, which were unanimously adopted:

WHEREAS, It has pleased an overruling and allwise Providence to remove from among us our highly-esteemed colleague and co-laborer, Dr. Constantine Hering; and

WHEREAS, We deeply feel the great loss of one who was endeared to us as the father of our school in this country; of one who, for almost half a century, so earnestly, so honestly, so unostentatiously, and so unselfishly devoted himself, aided by an unusually large store of knowledge and by a ripe scholarship, to propagate, advance, and develop the true healing art; of one who added such treasures to our literature; of one so universally known and honored; therefore,

Resolved, By the homœopathic physicians of this city, in which he resided so long, that in the death of Constantine Hering, M.D., we, as well as the whole population throughout the world, have suffered a great loss.

Resolved, That we tender the bereaved family our deep sympathy, and offer them our heartfelt condolence.

Resolved, That the homœopathic physicians of this city will attend his funeral, on the 28th of July, at 11 A.M., from his late residence, in a body.

Resolved, That a copy of this preamble and resolutions be transmitted to the family of our departed friend and colleague.

Dr. O. B. Gause, in seconding the resolutions, said: I had not the pleasure of as intimate acquaintance with Dr. Hering as many who are here. I was associated with him for a number of years while he was actively engaged in the college, and during these years I frequently met him, and in matters educational I found him exceedingly liberal, enthusiastic, energetic, and wise. It was a rare pleasure to hear him discuss the latest developments of science, and their relations to homœopathy. His enthusiasm upon the theme of his life-work never abated. I shall ever cherish the memory of the many interviews with him in connection with the interests of the college. He never advocated any narrow policy. He was in favor of a broad and liberal education in all the sciences and arts, in accordance with the most advanced views of liberal men. I realize as fully as any one that a great and good man has left us, and I rejoice that I can remember him as my friend.

Dr. J. C. Morgan said that during the earlier years of his own studies and practice of homœopathy, he had been prevented from enjoying an intimacy with Dr. Hering by misrepresentations made by those who professed to have a full knowledge of his character. It was said that "Dr. Hering was dogmatic like his master—Hahnemann;—that he was visionary, like his master, Hahnemann; that he was, therefore, unreliable, like his master, Hahnemann." How utterly untrue these statements were, became sufficiently evident to the speaker upon an intimate acquaintance with him. Dr. Hering stood in the front rank of the progressive scientists of our day. He had strong convictions upon subjects related to medicine, because, feeling that he had a mission to fulfil, he bent his best energies to the accomplishment of his work. No one could come in contact with him and remain indifferent to the living questions of the medical science of the day. And men possessed of the progressive spirit of Dr. Hering, cannot be expected to spend precious time in going over the controversies which ignorance may attempt to incite, upon questions which the facts of science have long ago settled to the full satisfaction of intelligent people. Hence the charge of dogmatism, as applied to such men, is what might naturally be expected. Dr. Hering has for many years been an honored teacher among us,—let us revere his teachings; let us emulate his example; let us cherish his memory.

Dr. Aug. Korndœrfer, alluded in feeling terms to his long and intimate relations with Dr. Hering. He felt that words were entirely inadequate to express the depths of our sense at the loss of such a man. He said: "I have been intimately connected with him for more than a decade. From the very first of that connection I knew that he was my friend. He was a man of firm and abiding friendships, and even though it might seem at times as though the warmth of his attachment were withdrawn from one, it was only that he might do him good. Here let me speak more fully of his friendship for the young practitioner. His medical knowledge, his abilities, and his wondrous store of general information, are well known to all of us, and of all these he gave freely to subserve the welfare and progress of the beginner in medicine. His hours were but as minutes,—his labors as pleasures, if he could but render needed assistance to him who sought it.

"I well remember during the early days of my acquaintance with him, how perfectly he abhorred the idea of keeping a secret from the profession; how earnestly he insisted that every new fact which might tend toward the healing of the sick, or render assistance to a sufferer, should be made known—in season and out of season. These phases of his character probably attracted young men to him as strongly as did his ripe and unusual scholarship, or his warm personal interest in their welfare.

"In regard to his work, it has been said by some, as mentioned by Dr. Morgan, that he was unreliable. I can only say, from the deepest and sincerest conviction, that the man who made such a statement did not know Dr. Hering. The truth is, he never put his pen to paper except when he had the fullest conviction of the truthfulness of what he wrote. Every word, every line that he wrote, bears the impress of authority. He accepted the dictum of no man; he received as authoritative no statement, unless it could be verified by subsequent observation. The charge that he made notes and memoranda of the most trivial experiences of physicians, is doubtless true; but all such experiences were thoroughly sifted, and none were accepted finally, unless they were shown to be capable of withstanding the proper test. 'Yes, I do take notes of everything,' said he to me, 'but many of them prove to be fit only for the waste basket.' This exactitude in all his work, and his apparently slow work, was simply the result of a conscientious carefulness, an excessive desire to give all his own observations in their best possible shape to the profession. This I learned from a close and intimate relation with him, continued during a long period of literary labor.

"Dr. Hering lived in faith,—faith in homœopathy, faith in Hahnemann, faith in the divine mission which Hahnemann was called to fill,—faith in the mission to which he himself was called,—the development and promulgation of homœopathy on this continent; and he has passed away from us, feeling that his work was so nearly completed that he could leave it in the hands of others fully competent to carry it on to its perfection and its full fruition. Not long since he expressed himself in that way to me, that there were men in our ranks who were well prepared to go on with the work which he had labored so hard to establish, but which, for want of time, he was compelled to leave unfinished.

"I can only say in conclusion that there is not a brother physician here who will not realize a loss in the departure of our venerated colleague. A good and true, a wise and earnest leader has been taken from our midst."

Dr. W. H. Bigler gave a brief account of the last illness of Dr. Hering and of the observations made at the post-mortem by Dr. A. R. Thomas. These observations, however, included little of interest except an emphysematous condition of the left lung, doubtless connected with the asthmatic attacks, to which the deceased had been subject at times for some years past.

Dr. Pemberton Dudley called the attention of those present to the fact that "Dr. Hering died on the anniversary (the fifty-second) of the day on which the first homœopathic prescription was made in Pennsylvania; also that the day appointed for the interment (July 28th) will be the fifty-second anniversary of the day upon which Dr. Hering secured his first specimen of the Trigonocephalus Lachesis, with which he made those brilliant researches which, even alone, were sufficient to give him a world-wide fame. Speaking of the early champions of Homœopathy, the speaker said that while Hahnemann possessed wondrous capacities for scientific research, Hering superadded to these a remarkable executive and organizing ability, that found its most successful exercise in the permanent establishment of Homœopathy in America. Remembering what Hering was and what he did, it is natural for us to ask, how shall his work be continued and who now shall carry it on? Who shall fill his place? And yet, properly speaking, we do not need a successor to Dr. Hering. Homœopathy will never need to be established in America a second time. That work is done and well done. The rapid development of our materia medica is a fact accomplished. The world does not need another Hering any more than she needs another Newton or another Kepler, another Washington or another Hahnemann. The death of such a man, however, must be felt as a serious loss, unless we, each and all, take up the work where he has laid it down, and endeavor each to perform his own allotted work in the interests of a true medical science. Thus the loss of one like Hering may make us better able and more willing to fulfil the duties and bear the peculiar responsibilities of our position as homœopathists, and our cause may thus make even more rapid advances than ever."

A number of telegrams were read from homœopathic physicians in distant cities, among them being messages of regret and condolence from Drs. A. K. Hills and Samuel Swan, of New York, Dr. J. P. Dake, of Nashville, and Dr. J. H. McClelland, of Pittsburg.

The chairman appointed the following gentlemen to act as pall-bearers: Charles G. Raue, M.D., James Kitchen, M.D., C. Neidhard, M.D., Adolph Lippe, M.D., H. N. Guernsey, M.D., A. W. Koch, M.D., A. R. Thomas, M.D., Philadelphia, Pa.; J. H. Pulte, M.D., Cincinnati, O.; William Wesselhœft, M.D., Boston, Mass.; F. R. McManus, M.D., Baltimore, Md.; Henry Detwiler, M.D., Easton, Pa.; John Romig, M.D., Allentown, Pa.; P. P. Wells, M.D., Brooklyn, N. Y.; Edward Bayard, M.D., John F. Gray, M D., S. Lilienthal, M. D., New York city; J. F. Cooper, M.D., Allegheny City, Pa.

On motion, a resolution was adopted that a memorial meeting be held in honor of the deceased, at which physicians from all parts of the world should be invited to participate either in person or by letter. The following committee was appointed to carry the resolution into effect: Drs. A. Lippe, Edward Bayard, William Wesselhœft, H. N. Guernsey, J. K. Lee.

The meeting then adjourned.

THE OBSEQUIES.

The funeral services took place at the late residence of the deceased, Nos. 112 and 114 North Twelfth Street, at 11 A.M., on Wednesday, July 28th. A large proportion of the homœopathic physicians of Philadelphia were present, besides representatives from New York, Brooklyn, Pittsburg, Allegheny City, Allentown, Easton, West Chester, Wilmington, Camden, and other places. A large concourse of the lay friends and patients of the deceased were also present. The religious services were conducted by Rev. S. S. Seward, of the Swedenborgian Church, of New York city, Dr. Hering being a member of that denomination. Rev. Mr. Seward delivered an address in which he spoke freely of the life, character, and professional labors of the deceased, and of his vast usefulness to the cause of medical science. The interment took place in Laurel Hill Cemetery.

THE LAW OF SIMILARS.—In the *Medical Record* of July 3d, appears an editorial entitled, "The Increased Range of Dosage and the Law of Similars." After illustrating the extension of the therapeutical range of drugs by altering the size of doses, the writer remarks: "Of course, such examples as these are eagerly held up by enthusiasts as proofs of a grand therapeutic law. . . . . We need not look for any great therapeutic triumphs in the *similia similibus* action of the drop posology. There is a physiological law that substances which at first irritate inhibitory centres, when more energetically given, will paralyze them; or what at first constringes a tissue, may, later, relax and destroy it. These new facts in regard to minute dosage, are suggestive, and often useful, but they indicate no mysterious nor universal law."

We are here reminded of a conversation we had with a Dr. ——, at Atlantic City, in reference to the universality of the law upon which homœopathicians base their therapeutics. The doctor admitted a limited application of our "so-called" law, but dubbed us as quacks because we are "so exclusive." We ventured in all humility to inquire if he understood the principles of Hahnemann? He unhesitatingly replied in the affirmative, and began to expound the law of similars in some such words as the following: A drug, which, when taken in large doses, causes certain symptoms (as Ipecac, nausea and vomiting), will, when administered in small quantities for similar symptoms, remove them.

"But," we rejoined, convinced that the doctor, like most critics of his school, had failed to grasp the full meaning of Hahnemann's law, "that is not homœopathy, at least, in its full application. We claim that very minute doses will produce the true therapeutic effects of drugs, which effects these same small doses will remove in the sick.

"Your limitation would confine us to such crude applications of our law as your own textbooks teach. And this would indeed constitute us just such bigots as you denominate us. But the successful practice of our art demands an acquaintance with drug action, compared with which your physiological experiments are coarse and superficial. And this intimate knowledge can never be reached by one who interprets law as you have done. Really, if you will allow me, the narrowness is on the other side."

And, in reply to the *Record*, we may add that no anxiety need be felt lest its interpretation of the subject will lead to any "great therapeutic triumphs in the *similia similibus* action of the drop posology," unless, as happens every year, such experimentation leads students to investigate homœopathy in its entirety, when the delusion of allopathic interpretation of homœopathy will become at once apparent.

THE H. O. AND O. SOCIETY.—Through the kindness of Drs. Beebe and Lewis we are enabled to lay before our readers a report of the fourth annual session of the Homœopathic Ophthalmological and Otological Society, held at Milwaukee in June (see page 508). There is a little matter in the last paragraph of the report to which we invite the notice of physicians not members of the society.

BUSINESS NOTICE.—Will our correspondents do us the favor ALWAYS to send their remittances and other business communications *direct* to the Business Manager, Dr. Bushrod W. James, N. E. corner Eighteenth and Green streets, Philadelphia; the publication office having been removed last January from Messrs. Boericke & Tafel's to the above address.

Book Department.

POST-MORTEM EXAMINATIONS. By Professor Rudolph Virchow, of the Berlin Charité Hospital. Translated from the second German edition by Dr. T. P. Smith. Published by Presley Blakiston, Philadelphia.

The English-reading branch of the medical profession have in the above little work been presented with a really valuable addition to the literature of this department of medicine. Written, as it was, with especial reference to medico-legal practice by one who well knew the needs of the medico-legal witness, it cannot but be received with a hearty welcome. We here find, in a concise form, a systematic method for the conduct of a post-mortem examination; every page giving evidence of its having been written by one who knows whereof he speaks. As an unmethodical examination artificially and prematurely obliterates the existing condition of parts, it becomes of the greatest importance in making an autopsy, either for scientific or medico-legal use, to have a thorough and systematic course to follow; at the same time it is not only desirable but necessary, that the expert be able to give a reason for pursuing a definite order of sequence in every detail of the examination.

Here we have a thoroughly digested order for examination, together with substantial reasons for the order of sequence, step by step.

The closing twenty-six pages are devoted to the REGULATIONS FOR THE GUIDANCE OF MEDICAL JURISTS IN CONDUCTING POST-MORTEM EXAMINATIONS FOR LEGAL PURPOSES. Approved by the Royal Scientific Commission for Medical Affairs.

Typographically the work is good, the paper fair; but for the printing we cannot speak so well, as many pages present a pale appearance most trying to the eyes. Rapidity of presswork is spoiling the good black print so common in old works. Altogether, however, this is a very readable book, and should be in the hands of every one who may be required to act as a medico-legal expert. A. K.

Surgical Therapeutics. By J. C. Gilchrist, M.D. Third edition, rewritten. Published by Duncan Bros., Chicago, 1880.

Comparing this edition with the first, issued in 1873, we find many additions, alterations, and other improvements. Then the book numbered 421 pages, now it has grown to 595 pages. And we feel sure that the additional 174 pages contain valuable matter, which the progressive physician must make his own.

Duncan Bros. have displayed good taste in their part of the work, the type being clear and the printing excellent, with one notable exception. The italics, in which names of remedies and emphatic words are printed, are so irregular in size as to almost make the reader dizzy. Especially is this defect noticeable in the latter half of the book. We hope our energetic Chicago publishers will see to it that their types are better sorted, so that their issues may be typographically above criticism.

Dr. Gilchrist deserves the thanks of the profession for his bold defence of the principles of Hahnemann, especially in their application to a class of diseases too often left to surgical management alone.

So far as time and ability admit we have examined his indications, and find them generally accurate and pointed.

A few inaccuracies have crept in, however, and it will not detract from the value of the work if we mention them. On page 400, symptoms are attributed to Angustura which are now known to belong to Nux vom., such as lips drawn back so as to show the teeth, etc. (see *Guiding Symptoms*, and Allen's *Encyclopædia*, vol. vii.)

Staphysagria, wherever it occurs, should read "Staphisagria." The "y" is a mistake of old authors.

For uniformity Silicea should not be spelled in one place with an "i" in the last syllable and in another with an "e." See pp. 80, 288, etc.

Among omissions we note the following: Graphites should be added to the treatment of ingrowing toe-nails (see Dunham's *Lectures*, vol. i, p. 400). Anthracinum is just as important as the Arsenic in carbuncle. Why omit it? Do not Drosc. and Nat. sulph. deserve a place in the therapeutics of whitlow? But such omissions are the exception.

We cannot close this review without expressing our surprise that Dr. Gilchrist, who is so thorough a student of Hahnemann, can advocate that chancroid is purely local at first, and may be treated with the cautery. True, this is the fashionable doctrine of the day, and is accepted by the great majority; but if the teachings of the *Organon* are correct—and our author will agree with us this far—no disease of contagious origin can remain local. It takes but thirty or forty seconds for a large volume of blood to make the circuit of the body. Consequently infection at any one point must soon affect the whole. Doubtless there is a great difference between chancroid and chancre; but, to say that the former can be cured with the removal of the local sore, is contrary to facts and to reason. We have several times seen cases thus treated in which an antidote to the caustic, such as Hepar, Nat. mer., Sulph., etc., has redeveloped symptoms of the disease.

F.

Gleanings.

A Spurious Tapioca is being manufactured in Germany from potato starch. It may be detected by boiling, for it thus becomes converted into a soft pappy mass.—*Pharm. Journ.*

Sheep Rot is alarmingly present in England. It is, as is known, caused by the Distoma hepaticum and the Distoma lanceolatum. Such sheep, though not fatally poisonous as food, may infect the human system with their entozoa. —See *Journ. of Microscopy*, June, 1880.

Alcohol may aid digestion. For instance, if not more than twenty-five grams of brandy be taken with two hundred of meat, digestion is powerfully assisted. An important requisite, however, is the quality of the spirits. Ethylic or vinous alcohol always yields the best results; and even if taken in excess, injures less than the amylic alcohol, to which latter belong almost all the pernicious symptoms of alcoholism.—See *Boston Journal of Chemistry*, July, 1880.

False Quebracho Bark.—Dr. J. Biel, of St. Petersburg, in the *Pharm. Zeitung*, calls attention to a false white quebracho bark which came to Hamburg. The first lot of white quebracho bark received in Hamburg was a very small quantity, and the second lot consisted of three serons. Dr. Biel, therefore, supposes that what is being used in Germany at present is not the true drug, and therefore sounds this warning note, lest a drug which promises well should be unjustly condemned before it has had a fair trial.

The Cochineal Insects are multiplied by placing the madres in a kind of hothouse, spread out upon shallow wooden boxes. They have neither head nor limbs, but are alive, for they bring forth their young, which look like little white specks. These minute insects, which when closely inspected are seen to have all parts perfect, are transferred to the cactus plants, into which they burrow for a short distance. They at once drop their members and become as inanimate-looking as their parent. Such are the female cochineal insects.—See *New Remedies*, June, 1880.

Arteries are, as is known, generally separated from veins by the interposition of capillaries. Among the exceptions, Hoyer has noted that at the finger tips, matrices of the nails, and tip of the nose, arterioles communicate directly with venules. Other structures are the cornea, the teeth, cartilage, organs of special senses, etc.

This is the "derivative circulation" described in the textbooks. It seems to have been thoroughly studied by Sucquet, who demonstrated its existence in the palmar and plantar surfaces, the knee, elbow, tips of the ears and nose, the forehead, cheeks, lips, etc. These parts, as is well known, are peculiarly liable to congestion under the influence of low temperature and from other causes, and this arrangement of the vascular system therein is held by physiologists to be a provision for preventing undue accumulations of blood.—Eds.

News and Comments.

New Jersey requires her M.D.'s to register their diplomas.

Professor Samuel A. Jones, M.D., has resigned his chair in the Michigan University.

W. T. LAIRD, M.D., has removed from Watertown, N. Y., to become the successor of Dr. James B. Bell at Augusta, Me.

JAMES B. BELL, M.D., has removed to Boston, Mass., and associated with W. P. Wesselhœft, M.D. His address is No. 52 Boylston Street.

S. F. SHANNON, M.D., of Pittsburgh, a student of Dr. J. C. Burgher and a graduate of the Hahnemann College of Philadelphia, has carried off the second prize in Materia Medica, in the London School of Homœopathy.

THE TRANSACTIONS OF THE AMERICAN INSTITUTE OF HOMŒOPATHY for the session of 1880 are in the hands of the printer, and General Secretary Burgher is already "reading proof" of it every day. It bids fair to be in the hands of "paid-up" members within ninety days from date. Dr. Burgher informs us that it will be issued as soon as possible.

A NEW SOCIETY IN CENTRAL OHIO.—All Homœopathic physicians in Central Ohio are requested to meet in Columbus, September 2d, for the purpose of organizing a Central Ohio Homœopathic Medical Society. A large attendance of representive men is already promised. Further particulars will be furnished on request by John C. King, M.D., Circleville, Ohio.

COMMITTEE ON WORLD'S CONVENTION OF 1881.—The American Institute of Homœopathy at its recent session appointed Drs. I. T. Talbot of Boston, E. M. Kellogg of New York, and B. W. James of Philadelphia a committee to devise and carry out measures for promoting the success of the next International Convention of Homœopathic Physicians. This convention is to meet in London in July, 1881. The committee, so we are informed, hope to secure a large attendance of American physicians. The chairman of the committee will doubtless be glad to answer questions on the subject.

THE WORLD'S CONVENTION TRANSACTIONS (2 vols.) and the Transactions of the Institute session of 1879 are in the hands of the former Provisional Secretary, Dr. J. C. Guernsey, and he is hard at work upon them. There is a great deal of labor connected with the World's Convention volumes, on account of the incomplete state of the historical part of the work. But the "missing links" are being supplied, and the unwritten portions will be completed as far as compatible with the limited time that remains. Many other difficulties are being overcome, and the historical volume is being rapidly run through the press.

AMERICAN INSTITUTE OF HOMŒOPATHY—BUREAU OF OBSTETRICS.—The following are the assignments of the Bureau of Obstetrics for the ensuing year:

Puerperal Mortality.

A. MATERNAL. 1. Nervous, Mrs. M. A. Canfield, M.D., Cleveland, O.; 2. Hæmorrhagic, Miss Millie J. Chapman, M.D., Pittsburgh, Pa.; 3. Convulsive, C. Ormes, M.D., Jamestown, N. Y.; 4. Febrile—preventive, C. C. Higbee, M.D., St. Paul, Minn.; 5. Febrile—curative, Mrs. C. T. Canfield, M.D., Titusville, Pa.

B. INFANTILE. 1. Fœtal, J. C. Sanders, M.D., Cleveland, O.; 2. Parturient, O. B. Gause, M.D., Philadelphia, Pa.; 3. Post-partum, L. E. Ober, M.D., Lacrosse, Wis.

The above list will be lengthened and amended as the interests of the theme seem to require. Circulars will soon be issued, which every member of the Institute is desired promptly to answer. The testimony of the humblest practitioner is as important as that of the proudest.

GEO. B. PECK, M.D.,
Chairman.

PROVIDENCE, R. I., July 1st, 1880.

THE SIXTEENTH ANNUAL MEETING OF THE HOMŒOPATHIC MEDICAL SOCIETY OF PENNSYLVANIA will be held at Easton, Pa., September 8th,

1880. The sessions will be held in the parlors of the United States Hotel, the proprietors of which have made arrangements to entertain the members.

We earnestly hope the members will make an effort to be present, as the session bids fair to be an interesting and profitable one. Chairmen of bureaus especially, are requested to make an effort to secure full reports from all the members of their bureaus.

An earnest invitation is extended to homœopathic practitioners in the State, not already members, to unite with the society.

Any information in regard to the meeting will be cheerfully and promptly given by the Corresponding Secretary, Dr. R. E. Caruthers, 107 Arch Street, Allegheny City, Pa.

OUR ADVERTISERS.—We would call attention to the advertisements which appear in our journal from time to time. It will be to the advantage of the journal if our readers will kindly mention the HAHNEMANNIAN MONTHLY when transacting business with any of our advertisers.

Below will be found a list of the advertisements appearing in this number:

Advertising Rates, HAHNEMANN MONTHLY.
Boericke & Tafel, Publications and Homœopathic Pharmacists.
Conover, T. F., M.D., Non-humanized Cow-pox Virus.
Duncan Brothers, Homœopathic Pharmaceutists.
Epps's Cocoa.
Flemming, Otto, Medico-electrical Apparatus.
Gardner, William D., Physicians' Carriages.
Gregg & Bowe, Physicians' Carriages.
Hahnemann Medical College, Philadelphia, Pa.
Homœopathic Hospital College, Cleveland, Ohio.
Hance Brothers & White, Pharmaceutists.
Kern, H. G., Surgical Instruments.
Reeves, Joseph M., Physicians' Obstetrical Register.
Lupus, A., Morocco Medicine Cases.
New York Homœopathic Medical College.
Pettet, J., M.D., Homœopathic Pharmacy.
Pulte Medical College, Cincinnati, Ohio.
Roth, Dr. Theodore, Artificial Eyes.
Snowden, William, Surgical Instruments.
Sherman & Co., Book and Job Printing.
Shoemaker & Co., Johnston's Fluid Beef.
University of Michigan, Ann Arbor, Michigan.
Walker & Everett, Homœopathic Physicians and Surgeons.
Yunck, John A., Homœopathic Vials and Philosophical Glassware.

We have not the slightest hesitation in commending any and all the above advertisers to the confidence of our readers.

ERRATA.—In Dr. A. R. Thomas's paper in the July number on Calcareous Infiltrations, the following corrections should be made:

Page 407, 4th line from top, for "frothy," read *fatty*.
Page 407, 15th line from top, for "pilules," read *plates*.
Page 407, 16th line from top, for "pustules," read *particles*.
Page 408, 6th line from top, for "growth," read *growths*.
Page 409, 3d line from bottom, for "results," read *contents*.

The fault of these mistakes rests with—Well, no matter; our printer is "a biger man than ole Grant."

DECEASED.—DEXTER.—We regret to announce the death of BYRON P. DEXTER, M.D., of Houlton, Me., a graduate of Hahnemann College of Philadelphia, of the class of 1880. The doctor, we learn, contracted diphtheria while attending a case of that disease, and fell a victim after an illness of three days.

THE

HAHNEMANNIAN MONTHLY.

Vol. II., New Series. } Philadelphia, September, 1880. No. 9.

Original Department.

STUDIES IN MATERIA MEDICA.

BY E. A. FARRINGTON, M.D., PHILADELPHIA, PA.

ANIMAL KINGDOM.

(Continued from page 458.)

The SPECIAL SENSES (see August number, p. 450) are usually depressed or perverted by the snake-poisons.

LACHESIS cures the following: Dim vision, worse on awaking; mistiness and flickering.

Blue ring about the light, filled with fiery rays. Flickering, as from sun rays. Zigzag figures.

Pains above the eyes (left), shooting to the temples, top of head, and occiput.

Obstructed feeling in the ears, with roaring, hammering, or chirping; better when inserting finger in external meatus and shaking it.

Tearing from zygoma to ear. Stinging piercing, deep in the left ear, with a disagreeable sensation between ear and throat.

Soreness of the mastoid; swelling between mastoid and ear, with stiffness, pain, and throbbing.

Earwax pale, pap-like; or dryness, want of wax, and hardness of hearing.

Nosebleed, bright red or *dark*, persistent; with the headache before the menses, at climaxis, from blowing the nose; all worse mornings. In diphtheria it is very useful, other symptoms agreeing.

Coryza (see Headache), preceded by obstinate sneezing; becomes dry and suddenly breaks out again; nose sore, remaining so long after discharge ceases; nostrils red; accompanied with stiff neck and sore throat (*q. v.*); worse in weak persons, and especially in the spring.

Ozæna, syphilitic or not, with discharge of blood and pus; and headache.

Redness of the point of the nose.

Of the remaining ophidians, CROTALUS and ELAPS are most similar. The former cures, though less frequently than LACHES., an apoplexy of the retina. Like the last named, it also relieves keratitis, when there are cutting pains around the eye, lids swollen mornings; ciliary neuralgia with these cuttings, worse at menses. Similar, too, is its amblyopia, with colored flames before the vision; the eyes are apt to be yellowish; blood exudes from the eyes.

In the ears CROTALUS causes a stuffed feeling, worse in right ear, with feeling as if hot earwax was trickling out.

ELAPS also causes blue appearances in field of vision; large, red, fiery points, becoming violet, then black, with congestion, as in LACHESIS; blood oozes from eyes.

The ears are subject to catarrh, as in the LACHESIS. In both there are black cerumen, buzzing, etc., in ears, and otorrhœa. In ELAPS the latter is yellow-green, liquid, and bloody. Only LACHESIS seems to have the Eustachian stoppage, better from shaking finger in meatus. ELAPS causes a stuffing of the nostrils, as in babies; must breathe through the mouth; bad smell from the nose; bright blood gushes from the nose and ears.

Related Remedies.—Blue ocular illusions, compare *Bellad.*, Lycop., Stron., Stram., etc.

Misty vision, compare *Caust.*, *Lycop.*, Bell., *Hyosc.*, PHOSPH., etc.

Ciliary pains, compare *Actea rac.*, *Spigelia*, Cedron (over left eye). *Cinnabaris* has pains go round eyeball; hence compare with CROTALUS.

Retinitis apoplectica, compare *Phosph.*, Bellad. (Glon.), Arnica, Hamam.

Blood oozes from eyes, compare Nux vom., Carbo veg., etc.

Yellow color of whites, CROT., *Lachesis*, Con., Iod., Kali bich., Phos. ac., Vipera, Curare, Arsenic, etc.

Mastoid process: NITRIC ACID, AURUM, Hepar, Merc., Capsicum, Silica, etc.

Otorrhœa, compare ELAPS with *Merc.*, Nitric acid, Thuja, Puls., Cinchona (bleeding).

Earwax affected, hard: Puls., Selen., Mur. acid, Elaps, Laches. Pale, pap-like, Laches. Like mouldy paper, Con. In want of wax, compare LACHES. with C. veg., Calc. ostr.

Nosebleed, compare in diphtheria, etc., MERC. CYAN., *Nitric acid*, C. VEG., CINCHONA, ARSENIC. (See Throat, below.) With menses, Puls., Phosph., Hamam., Sec. c., Sep., Bry.

In "snuffles," compare with ELAPS: *Sambuc.*, child arouses smothering; *Sticta*, can't breathe through nose; dry hard cough; NUX VOM.; CHAMOM., nose stuffed and yet water drops; LYCOPOD., AMM. CARB., etc.

In Coryza, compare LACHES. with GELSEM., *Quillaia saponaria*, both of which cause catarrh in spring; MERCUR., which precedes and follows well. It is marked by thick green catarrh, raw, sore throat, worse from exposure to damp evening air, after a warm day; or thin, excoriating coryza, sneezing, bone-pains, and sweat; HEPAR, etc.

In Ozæna, compare AURUM, NITRIC ACID, MERCURIUS, KALI BICH.

For red tip of nose, compare LACHESIS with *Aurum* and PHOSPH., the latter if shining, the nostrils being dry; RHUS TOX., BELLAD., and Hepar, in erysipelas; Nitrum, *Rhus tox.*, and Ruta, in drunkards; NITRIC ACID, HEPAR, *Sulph.*, Carbo anim., all sensitive to touch.

In misty vision, *Causticum* is not unlike LACHES.; the melancholy, weak memory, yellow face, blue lips, paralytic weakness, make it a not improbable choice after the snake-poison in cases of debility.

In dim sight, as an evidence of heart disease and syncope, see above under VERTIGO. LACHESIS leads the list, and may save in apparently hopeless cases. *Laurocer.* or *Hydrocyanic acid* is needed in long-lasting faints; there seems to be no reactive power; face is pale blue, surface cold. If fluids are forced down the throat, they roll audibly into the stomach. If the syncope is attendant upon some poison in the system, as scarlatina, the symptoms are similar, the eruption is livid, and when pressed regains its color very slowly.

DIGITALIS also rivals the ophidians in syncope, with the antecedent dim vision; the pulse is generally very slow, and the patient often complains of nausea and deathly weakness in the epigastrium.

CAMPHOR and VERATRUM ALBUM display coldness, cold sweaty skin; in the latter, the forehead is cold and sweaty. The face may be red while lying, but if raised it turns pale, and the patient faints; pulse thready. CAMPHOR has icy surface, sudden sinking, as in Lauroc., and, although so cold, he throws off clothing so soon as strong enough to move, even though still unconscious.

CARBO VEG. necessarily compares with LACHES. and *Crotalus*, since it suits in cases of torpor, loss of vitality, etc. The charcoal may be aptly termed "a torpid Arsenic," and so stands with the Arsenic as related to snake-poisons. Its points of resemblance are: cold surface, weak pulse, persistent hæmorrhages, as nosebleed for instance, and bleeding from the eyes, gangrenous inflammations, collapse, etc. Both LACHES. and CARBO VEG. have burning of external parts; but the latter, like Arsenic, has it more in inner parts. Mentally they differ widely, the latter not causing marked delirium, excitement, etc. It is, therefore, as observed, in torpidity that they meet, especially in typhoid of drunkards. LACHES. has hot head and cool feet; CARBO VEG. has, very characteristic, feet and legs cold to the knees, oppression of breathing, desires fanning. In severe cases, tongue moist, face hippocratic, breathing rattling, constipation, or, at least, absence of defecation, while in LACHESIS there is usually diarrhœa. In epistaxis, as in diphtheria, metrorrhagia, etc., some of the above will be present as a result of the loss of blood, and then the CARBO is decidedly preferable.

FACE.—As already intimated, the face expresses how seriously the snake-poisons affect the system. Change of complexion shows that the contents of the bloodvessels are altered, while the look of anxiety and the distorted and sunken features complete the picture of suffering and exhaustion.

LACHESIS has: Expression anxious, painful, with the stupor; face disfigured; puffy; looks as after a debauch; hot, red, swollen; sunken features; blue circles around the eyes; earthy gray, with abdominal troubles or ague.

Rush of blood to the face.

Cheeks of a circumscribed yellow-red; also the nose.

Convulsions of the face; lockjaw; distortion. Stretching of the body backwards; screaming; feet cold and itching.

Sudden swelling of the face.

Erysipelas; beating headache on stooping. Face bloated, red, with cerebral symptoms; drowsiness, etc.; or parts bluish-red, gangrenous, pustular. Worse left side. Itches so that it can hardly be endured.

Throbbing in the face, full, slow throbbing of carotids.

Tearing in the zygoma, extending into the ear.

Screwing and digging in the malar bone.

Swelling of the lips; they crack and bleed.

CROTALUS and NAJA claim the same expression and changes in color, as well as the trismic symptoms. CROTALUS causes the same erysipelatous inflammation, and sudden facial puffing.

Elaps develops a similar train of effects, though clinically the CROTALUS and LACHESIS have greatest repute.

Related Remedies.—For swollen face, compare APIS, BELLAD., ARSENIC, *Lycopod.*, Hyosc., RHUS TOX., Pulsat., STRAM., *Kali carb.*, *Phosph.*

For sickly, pale, or earthy complexion: ARSENIC, Bufo, LYCOPOD., Carbo veg., *Rhus tox.*, *Cinchona*, PHOSPH., *Phos. ac.*

Blue about the eyes: ARSENIC, CUPRUM, Phosph., RHUS TOX., *Lycopod.*, *Sec. c.*, *Verat. alb.*

Erysipelatous appearance: *Apis*, BELLAD., Pulsat., *Hepar*, Anac., Euphorb., RHUS TOX., *Ammon. carb.*, Hyosc., Sulph., *Mercur.*, Carbo a.

Debauched look: *Baptisia*, *Hyosc.*, C. VEG., NUX V., *Sulph.* OPIUM, *Nux mosch.*, etc.

Yellow-red cheeks: NUX VOM., Baptisia.

Facial convulsions, etc.: NUX VOM., Hyosc., Bellad., HYDROC. ACID, *Lycopod.*, CICUTA, CAMPH., Phytolacca, *Arsenic.*

Lips crack and bleed: ARSENIC, *Bryon.*, Carbo a.

APIS, ARSENIC, and KALI CARB. agree in puffing of the face, even without any redness. In the first there is also smarting of the eyelids, and a sensation of stiffness. In the second it is noticed about the eyes, glabella, and forehead (also Natrum ars.). KALI has the well-known sacs of upper lids, and also sudden swelling of the cheeks.

The expression, complexion, etc., of ARSENIC are very similar to the snake-poisons. The anxiety and pain are marked by more restlessness and irritability, fear of death, etc., and the sunken face is more completely hippocratic, with pointed features, sunken eyes and cold sweat. When yellow or earthy, it is cachectic.

If trismic symptoms are present the patient will be found lying pale, and as if dead, though yet warm. Suddenly he arouses and goes into severe convulsions, only again to relapse into this sort of cataleptic rigidity. Eyes partly open, with gum on the conjunctiva.

LYCOPODIUM has pale or yellow face, deeply furrowed,

looks elongated. Convulsive movements are unique. All through the provings there is an alternation of contraction and expansion. And in the face we note: tongue pushed out and withdrawn, spasmodic trembling of facial muscles, angles of mouth alternately drawn up and relaxed; alæ nasi alternately expanded and contracted. Eyes may be partly open and covered with mucus,—a bad symptom, generally indicating brain-exhaustion (see Arsenic, above).

PHOSPHORUS has a pale face, but it is distinguished by its ashy, anæmic appearance. This should be remembered, since this remedy, like the class under study, has puffy face, sunken face, blue around eyes, and blue lips.

HYOSCYAMUS is very similar in expression and convulsive phenomena. It has a marked stupid, drunken look; face distorted, blue; face swollen and brown-red; staring; twitchings of single groups of muscles; hunger before attacks.

STRAMONIUM is readily distinguished by its swollen, turgid face, fright on awaking, renewal of spasms from light, and the contracted, gloomy expression, with wrinkling of the forehead.

HYDROCYANIC ACID closely agrees in convulsive symptoms and in color of face. Like the ELAPS, it has fluids roll audibly into the stomach; but the latter has it more as a spasmodic contraction of the sphincters, followed by sudden paretic relaxation. In convulsions the surface in the acid is pale blue and the muscles of the face, jaw, and back are affected. Suddenly a shock is felt, which passes like lightning from head to foot, and then comes the spasm. Here the remedy is more like Cicuta and Helleborus than LACHESIS. But CICUTA has (like snake-poisons) great difficulty in breathing from spasm, and, more than any remedy, it produces staring; the spasm is followed by disproportionately severe weakness.

CAMPHOR is readily distinguished by the coldness, and by the withdrawing of the lip, showing the teeth. (See also Phytolacca, Nux vom.)

In erysipelas BELLADONNA bears no resemblance in its early symptoms. But in the course of the disease, when the inflammation is so intense that the bloated face grows bluish-red, threatening gangrene, or when the brain becomes affected, differentiation may become necessary. Here both have hot head and cold feet, delirium, dry tongue, etc. But, as remarked before, LACHESIS suits when the cerebral symptoms fail to yield to BELLAD.; when the excitement gives way to muttering stupor, the pulse is weak, though rapid, and the cool surface of the limbs is plainly due to fading vitality, rather than to the upward tendency of the blood. CROTALUS holds the same relation to BELLAD.

Metastasis to the brain may also require *Hyosc.* The face will then have assumed a bluish or reddish-brown hue, and the delirium will be of the kind described above under "Mental Symptoms."

APIS develops a pinkish, rosy inflammation; the parts feel bruised, sensitive, or burn and sting. Later the face puffs, becomes œdematous, and the skin may assume a livid or dark-red hue; even sphacelous spots may form. There is, therefore, a similar destructive tendency, and as it is attended with delirium we must separate Apis from the snake-poisons. This is easily effected if we remember that the bee-poison produces a condition of nervous irritation very different from any of its congeners. It is a fidgety, nervous state, a fretted feeling, which deprives the patient of sleep, though he feel sleepy.

RHUS TOX., like the snake-poisons, causes pale swelling of the face, itching, vesication, and even pustulation and gangrene, or, red face. Relatively, the former produces more vesication, and burning-stinging itching; LACHESIS more bluish-red inflammation, with gangrenous tendency. The characteristic color of the RHUS erysipelas is a dark, dingy red; and there is more aching in the limbs and restlessness. If vesicles form in LACHESIS, they quickly fill with pus.

EUPHORBIUM, since it causes dry gangrene with erysipelas, anxiety as from poison, apprehensiveness, dim vision, etc., deserves notice here. The right cheek is of a livid, or dark-red hue; vesicles form as large as peas, and are filled with a yellow liquid. The pains are boring, gnawing, digging from the gum into the ear, with itching and crawling, when pains are relieved.

MOUTH.—The Ophidians affect the mouth and throat, causing stomatitis, copious saliva, loosened or decayed teeth, swollen gums, swelling of the tongue, constriction and burning in the throat. Swollen tongue is very marked under CROTALUS and LACHESIS.

LACHESIS.—Teeth crawling, feel too long, hollow, crumbling, jerking tearing in the roots of lower teeth, through upper jaw to the ear, periodic, always after waking from sleep, soon after eating, also from warm and cold drinks; gum about a hollow tooth swollen, relieved by a discharge of pus.

Gums swollen, spongy, white, bleeding.

Tongue mapped; red, dry, glistening, cracked, especially at

the tip; trembles, catches in the teeth when he tries to put it out; inflamed, swollen, ulcerated; gangrenous; paralyzed.

Talks as one drunk, unintelligibly, after an apoplectic fit.

Aphthous, denuded spots, preceded by burning pain and rawness.

Mouth dry, parched, cracks in various places, which bleed; blisters on the sides of the tongue, burning, with roof sore, mucous membrane feels as if peeling off; offensive odor. Saliva abundant, tenacious; also with the sore throat.

Related Remedies.—In decayed teeth compare: ANT. CRUD., *Staphis.*, Mercur., *Kreos.*, HEPAR, SILICA, Rhodod., *Thuja.*

Ulceration at roots: *Fluor. ac.*, *Petroleum*, Lycopod., Nat. mur., Thuja, MERCUR., HEPAR, SILICA, etc.

Gums spongy: MERCUR., C. VEG., NUX V., *Nat. mur.*, STAPHIS., *Sarsap.*

Tongue red: HYOSC., *Baptis.*, RHUS TOX., Nux v., *Bellad.* Glistening: *Baptis.* (edges), *Kali bichr.* Cracked: Apis, C. veg., ARSENIC, BRYONIA, Stram., *Mur. ac.*, RHUS TOX., *Mercur.*, KALI BICHR., *Phosph.*, *Nitric acid*, *Baptisia*, *Sulph.* Trembling: *Apis*, Gelsem., Bellad., ARSENIC, *Lycopod.*, Secale, *Stram.*, *Hyosc.* Inflamed: APIS, ARSENIC, *Conium*, MERCUR., Bellad. Mapped: ARSENIC, NAT. MUR., Lycopod., *Ran. scel.*, *Tarax.*, *Nitric acid.* Paralyzed: *Baryta c.*, Baptis., Bellad., Dulcam., *Lauroc.*, Hyosc., *Opium*, MUR. AC., Stram., Lycopod. Talks as one drunk: *Baptisia*, Bellad., Stram., Opium, Hyosc., *Rhus tox.*, *Lauroc.*, *Lycop.* Mouth sore: *Apis*, *Arsenic*, *C. veg.*, *Baptisia*, *Con.*, *Kali chlor.*, MERCUR., *Mur. ac.*, NITRIC AC., *Hepar*, *Lycop.*, Nat. mur., *Staphis.*, *Sulph.*, *Sul. ac.*, *Salicylic acid*, *Helleb.*, Phytolacca. Saliva increased or altered: *Arsenic*, *Bellad.*, *C. veg.*, *Lycopod.*, MERCUR., *Rhus.*, STAPHIS., Opium, *Sulph.*, Hepar, *Cinchon.*, Hyosc., Lauroc., *Nitric ac.*, Sul. ac., Stram. Bad smell from mouth: *Arnica*, *Arsenic*, *Baptis.*, *Bellad.*, Carbo a., *Cinchon.*, *Helleb.*, *Hyosc.*, *Kali bich.*, *Lycopod.*, MERCUR., *Nitric acid*, Rhus tox., Sul. ac., Silica, Sulph.

Of the allied remedies in toothache none is so similar as MERCURIUS, which, like LACHES., relieves when the gum is inflamed, tooth decayed, with abscess at the root. It is said to have a direct action on the dentine. The pains are tearing, pulsating, shooting into face and ears. In LACHES. the gum is swollen, and at the same time dark red, livid; or, it is tense, hot, and looks as if it would crack. MERCUR. is markedly worse from warmth of bed. LACHES. often follows the latter, or is needed at once, if the patient has been previously salivated. Only MERCUR. has dirty gums, with white edges.

In sore mouth, aphtha, etc., LACHES. compares with Baptis., Nitric ac., Mur. ac., Arsenic, Apis; while MERCUR. compares more with C. veg., Staphis., Kali chlor., Iod., Sul. ac., Nitric ac.

BAPTISIA has blood oozing from the gums, which looks dark red or purple, salivation, fetor, offensive stools, and thus far is precisely like LACHES. Both, too, are indicated in the stomacace attending the last stages of phthisis. Decide by general differences and also by the tongue, which in the former, is yellow or brown down the centre, with red, shining edges. In the latter it is red, dry, and glistening, especially at the tip, and has its sides and tip covered with blisters.

NITRIC ACID causes an acrid saliva, the pains in the mouth are pricking as from a splinter, aphtha and gums usually whitish, raw places, with shooting pains.

MURIATIC ACID presents deep, bluish ulcers, with dark edges, mucous membrane denuded in places, which latter are dotted with aphtha.

ARSENIC looks very much like LACHES., with livid, bleeding gums, edges of tongue blistered or ulcerated, diarrhœa. The burning is more intense, with restlessness, compelling motion in spite of the weakness. In gangrena oris it causes more acute pain, and heat in the mouth; both have bluish or black sloughing ulcers. ARSENIC has more mental irritability.

APIS has blisters marking the border of the tongue, or in clusters. The mouth is usually rosy red, swollen, and there are marked stinging pains; margin of tongue feels scalded, as does the mouth generally.

Carbo veg., STAPHIS., SUL. AC., agree more with MERCURIUS; the gums are white, spongy, ulcerated, rather than livid. STAPHIS. may cause sores, which look bluish-red or yellow; especially needed after abuse of Mercury or in syphilitic cases, when the general debility is marked with sunken face, blue around eyes, etc. SUL. AC. requires great debility, yellowish-white gums, skin yellow, patient nervous, hasty, constantly complains of trembling, which, however, is not observed by others.

Salicylic acid causes the common canker sores, with burning soreness and fetid breath.

Lycopod. produces these sores near the frænum of the

tongue, LACHESIS at the tip, and *Nitric acid*, Phytolacca, Natrum hypochlor., etc., on inner side of cheeks.

Phytolacca has some symptomatic resemblance to LACHESIS here as well as in the throat (see below). Both cause great weakness, dim vision, sunken face, blue around the eyes, sore mouth, tongue blistered along the edges, tip of tongue red, roof of mouth sore, profuse saliva. The poke-root may be distinguished by the great pain at the root of the tongue when swallowing. These pains are a part of the tired aching and soreness which are general over the body.

Helleborus produces canker in the mouth, but the sores are yellowish, with raised edges.

Returning to the subject of decayed teeth, it may be noted that *Kreosote* cures pains from teeth to left side of face; teeth decay rapidly, gums bleed, the blood being dark; but the accompanying facial pains are burning, and the patient is excitable, nervous, even, as in children, thrown into convulsions.

Thuja causes a decay just at the border of the gums, leaving the crown apparently sound. Gums dark red in streaks. Teeth turn yellow and crumble.

(To be continued.)

FLORIDA AS A HEALTH RESORT FOR CONSUMPTIVES.

BY J. R. TANTUM, M D., WILMINGTON, DEL.

IN the June number of THE HAHNEMANNIAN, I notice an article entitled "*Florida as a Climate Cure*," by A. G. Austin, M.D., of Williamson, N. Y. The writer of that article, from a limited knowledge of the subject, undertakes to condemn the climate of that State as unfitted for persons suffering with exhausting diseases, phthisis included. Actuated solely by a sense of duty to suffering humanity, I feel myself constrained to reply to his article.

It is unnecessary for me to take up in detail each place as he describes it, although I perceive that the rivers and lakes or lagoons were his favorite haunts; he labors hard to make out a case, and almost exhausts the vocabulary of the English language for expletives. He speaks of the inhabitants of these "hell holes" as "pale, lean, hungry individuals, with sunken eyes and hollow cheeks, whose general diet is quinine and bilious pills."

I have spent two winters in the South, visiting most of the places named by Dr. Austin. And to Florida, under the providence of God, I believe I owe my present earthly existence. I left my home in the winter of 1878–79, by the advice of my faithful friend, Dr. Alday, of Philadelphia, who had spent two winters in the South. My left lung was so seriously affected that but few persons expected that I would return alive. Jacksonville was my point of destination. I reached Savannah almost worn out, and halted for a rest. Here I heard stories of Florida similar to those related by Dr. Austin, and had I been as near home as I was to Jacksonville, I would have retraced my steps.

I reached Jacksonville in the morning. As I rode up into the city, the fresh green foliage, the blooming flowers, and the golden orange fruit greeted my vision. The fragrance of the flowers regaled my senses, the plumed songsters of the South warbled their thankful notes to heaven. The surroundings infused new life into my debilitated system. Then I fully realized that I had indeed left the chilling, biting atmosphere of the North, and had entered the "Land of Flowers," the Sunny South. The genial, soothing atmosphere bathed my feverish brow and brought forth the exclamation to my wife, "I will recover here."

The first four weeks spent in Jacksonville added fifteen pounds to my weight. During the winter I visited Palatka, Sanford, and St. Augustine, and other places. In Palatka I met a gentleman from New Jersey, whom I had known for thirty years. Consumption had robbed him of all his family excepting two children. He had been advised by his physician to go to Florida as the only hope of saving his boy. I called at his house and was introduced to his invalid son. The boy looked well and had gained thirty pounds during the first four months of his residence South. The climate of Palatka I found exceedingly pleasant and healthful.

At St. Augustine I called to see a young man, who, far advanced in consumption, had left our city about six years previously. He was in good health, and had taken up the pleasant occupation of undertaker. I also called on a lady whom I had known for many years in the North. She had gone to Florida as a *dernier ressort*, having had several hæmorrhages from the lungs. She, too, I found, enjoying good health. She considered herself cured.

In Jacksonville, where I spent most of my time, I took especial care to note the effect of the climate on consumptives. I studied cases closely, and the improvement in the general health of all those who came under my observation was astonishing. Even those who were sent there by their physicians to die were temporarily improved.

And just here let me say that this custom of sending dying patients from home to Florida, or any other place, is cruel and heartless, and wholly unbecoming the sympathetic and conscientious man and physician. It is absurd to suppose that one's reputation necessarily suffers if a patient dies under treatment. And even if he should lose prestige, what is this to the fate to which he dooms his patients?

It is a sad sight to witness the lonely death of an invalid stranger, far from those who love him most. How his wistful thoughts revert to his distant home, and add to his distress and suffering!

I have made repeated inquiries in Jacksonville, and find that many of the residents were once consumptives, some of them, too, in the advanced stages of the disease, but who now consider themselves fully recovered.

Most of my time I spent on the St. John's River, the piny waters of which are by no means injurious. Still, I would advise those who are seriously affected to go rather inland among the pine groves, the benign influence of which is well known.

My remarks concerning the climatic advantages of Florida refer only to the winter months. Still, though I have but little knowledge of the country during summer, I would not hesitate to recommend St. Augustine or Fort George as suitable localities for consumptives even during hot weather.

Last winter, I should remark, was the most unfavorable season in Florida for thirty years, owing to the unusual mildness of the weather.

A CASE OF RENAL CANCER.

BY W. R. ELDER, M.D., TERRE HAUTE, IND.

(Read at the Fourteenth Annual Session of the Indiana Institute of Homœpathy.)

Some time in March, 1879, my attention was called to a patient who exhibited a tumor in her right side. I examined it and found a hard elongated and movable tumor, just under the floating ribs. When the patient lay upon her back and the tumor was allowed to assume its own position, it presented its long diameter transversely to the abdomen; the anterior end pushing up the abdominal walls so as to make a visible protuberance at a point two inches to the right of and one inch above the navel. By manipulation it could be so crowded down into the right posterior portion of the abdominal cavity as to be scarcely perceptible to the finger.

The patient is a married lady, 27 years of age, and the mother of two children. The youngest was born June 4th, 1878, and about six months later she discovered the existence of the tumor. It was then about the size of a hen's egg. Ten months later, when called to the case, the tumor was about six inches in length, and two to two and a half inches in its short diameter. The only presumable cause which could be assigned was, that previous to the birth of her child she used a patent washing machine, and after each washing suffered from sharp crampy pains in the side.

I made several examinations from time to time, and called in several of my colleagues, all of whom were undecided as to the nature of the disease. Her general health at this time did not seem much impaired, except that pains were sometimes felt in the affected side. Occasionally, too, she had attacks of headache and vomiting. One evening in May, nearly three months after my first knowledge of the tumor, I was summoned to my patient, whom I found flooding. The hæmorrhage was evidently from the urethra, and the attending distress was dysuria, caused by clots in the urethra. I could not tell how much blood had been passed, because it was mixed with a quantity of urine. But I knew it was large, for the bed-vessel was nearly half full of a dirty black mixture of blood and urine. The mystery of the tumor was now solved. It was a movable kidney, increased in size by some neoplastic deposit of a malignant character. Since that time there have been frequent similar attacks, with variable intervals, during which the urine, though seemingly normal, has contained albumen. Latterly the evening passage of urine is normal, while that passed in the morning is bloody.

The tumor has been steadily increasing in size, until at the present time it would apparently measure about eight inches in length by five inches in diameter. It is somewhat pear-shaped, the posterior portion being the largest. She has some aching pain in the right side and frequent pricking, stinging pains in the tumor, especially in the posterior portion. The menses have been entirely suppressed since the first attack of hæmaturia. She has occasional diarrhœa with cramping pains, alternating with constipation. There is also frequent nausea, and sometimes vomiting. The skin has a pale cachectic appearance, and although she suffers to some extent from general weakness, yet she is not confined to her house. In fact she feels best when moving about.

After careful investigation, I have decided the disease to be primary cancer of the kidney, and have been led to this conclusion, mainly, by a careful comparison of the symptoms and conditions, with the etiology and symptoms of that disease, as described in Ziemssen's *Cyclopædia.* Primary cancer of the kidney is there mentioned as a very rare disease, but when it does occur it is almost invariably confined to one kidney, usually the right. The first symptoms are always obscure, owing to their being common to other diseases of the kidneys.

"The most important symptoms to be considered, are, the *renal tumor* and the *hæmaturia.* The latter usually occurs at an early stage of the disease. It is often the very first symptom, and should be regarded with suspicion, although of itself alone, it is no pathognomonic sign of renal cancer, for it is often observed in many diseases of the urinary organs, and especially of the kidneys. But if in connection with hæmaturia, another sign presents itself, viz., a *tumor* of the kidneys, the matter assumes a more definite shape."

Ziemssen further says, "Cancer of the kidneys, like cancer of the liver and testicle, are rich in wide, thin-walled vessels, which often show aneurismal dilatations; consequently extravasations of blood are very likely to take place, as the result of their rupture. It is owing to this pathological condition that the hæmorrhage of renal cancer occurs at irregular intervals, is easily excited by traumatic causes, and is then very profuse. It is never so scanty as to require the microscope for its detection, but the red corpuscles flow intact, and mix intimately with the urine, coloring it from a reddish hue, to a dirty black. There is often considerable pain experienced in voiding this bloody urine, on account of the formation of clots in the urethra, and often in the ureters."

Further, in regard to the tumor, the same author says: "It usually attains considerable size, sometimes excessive. There is on record, one in a child four years old, that weighed between sixteen and seventeen pounds. In the outset the kidney not unfrequently may leave its natural position by reason of its weight, and be felt as a movable tumor beneath the floating ribs, but as it increases in size, it forms adhesions to the neighboring organs, and becomes more or less fixed.

"The amount of urine is almost always normal, and not very much changed in its elements, except that it becomes albuminous."

This synopsis of symptoms corresponds so closely with my

case that I feel assured of the correctness of my diagnosis, in which case it follows as a matter of course, that the prognosis must point to a fatal termination. The recorded history of the duration of this disease, gives it as very variable, the extremes being from five weeks to eighteen years, while the average duration is from one year to two or three years.

Concerning the treatment, the principal thing to be done, is to maintain the strength of the patient as far as possible, by well-selected nutritious food. Medicines are of little avail except to combat dangerous symptoms, such as hæmaturia, vomiting, diarrhœa, etc.

The remaining history of this interesting case, is briefly as follows:

About two weeks after the meeting at Paris, Illinois, for which the first part of this paper was written, my patient was suddenly attacked with what appeared to be a peritoneal inflammation in the right side, and posterior to the tumor. This attack was characterized by high fever, quick wiry pulse, intense pain and soreness in the side, intolerance of the least movement, nausea, vomiting, and hæmaturia. The latter was greatly aggravated by the efforts to vomit. There was also excruciating dysuria, the urine containing many blood-clots mixed with small masses of a grayish-white substance, which I decided to be cancerous matter. Death seemed inevitable, but after five days she recovered rapidly, and was again able to go about the house, though she remained more feeble than before. Subsequently these attacks recurred regularly every four weeks, leading her to surmise that they were connected with the menstrual function. During the intervals, the urine was always more or less bloody, and contained cancerous matter, which was considerably increased in quantity with each succeeding attack. The renal tumor rapidly increased in size, and became more and more firmly attached and immovable. About ten weeks previous to death, œdema of the lower extremities commenced, caused probably by anæmia, and by pressure of the tumor on the inferior vena cava. As the disease advanced, the quantity of fibrinous clots and cancerous matter in the urine increased, and the dysuria was more constant and severe. The latter was relieved by the topical use of warm vinegar. Disturbance of the digestive functions increased, the appetite failed, nausea and vomiting became more frequent, then more frequent attacks of exhausting diarrhœa, the strength rapidly failed, and the patient died from exhaustion on the 12th day of March, 1880, just one year from the time my attention was first called to the tumor.

Dr. Obetz, of Paris, Ills., with Drs. Hyde, Moore, Waters, Wilson, and myself, made a post-mortem examination twelve hours after death. We found considerable effusion into the abdominal cavity, and a large renal tumor in the right side, with a peculiar nodular surface, and weighing four and one-half pounds. The ascending colon was adherent to the whole length of its anterior surface, which, no doubt, protected it from adhesion to the peritoneum in front. At every point of contact with the small intestines and mesentery, there were strong adhesions, and posteriorly, upon and to the right of the spinal column, the adhesions were so firm that it was quite impossible to peel them off, making it necessary to dissect the tumor out with a scalpel. The ureter was greatly enlarged, being a full half inch in diameter. All the other abdominal organs appeared to be normal except the liver, which was thickly studded with secondary cancer nodules. Upon making an incision into the pelvis of the kidney, there flowed out freely a thin, mushy, granular-looking mass of medullary cancerous matter, of a light grayish color and somewhat fetid odor. The cavity of the renal pelvis, and the calyxes, were enormously distended, so that when emptied of their contents, a very material difference was observable in the size of the tumor. I am sorry we did not examine the lungs, for I am quite certain we would have found the secondary cancer nodules there, just as we did in the liver.

I was much gratified with the result of the examination, because it confirmed my previously made diagnosis. These cases are regarded as very difficult of diagnosis, because they are so readily confounded with tumors of neighboring parts.

VERATRUM VIRIDE.

BY W. M'GEORGE, M.D., OF WOODBURY, N. J.

(Read before the New Jersey Homœopathic Medical Society.)

Veratrum viride is called American Hellebore, to distinguish it from *Veratrum album;* the European plant, and yet it is not decided positively that it belongs to the Hellebore family. Gray, in his Manual of Botany, calls *V. viride* the American White Hellebore (*V. album*, being the European White Hellebore), yet he classes the Veratrum family as *False hellebore.* The subject of our paper has many common names. Swamp hellebore, Indian poke, Pokeweed (we must not confound it with Phytolacca decandra, which is also called Pokeroot and Pokeweed), Beanweed, Tickleweed, Itchweed, Devilbit, Wolfbane, etc. Botanically described, it has a "stout stem, very leafy to the top, two to four feet high; leaves broadly oval, pointed, sheath clasping, strongly plaited; panicle pyramidal; the dense spike-like racemes spreading; perianth yellowish-green, moderately spreading; grows in swamps and low grounds; common shrub; flowers in June (too near the V. album of Europe)." Gray, *Manual of Botany*, p. 476.

Although Gray may think that *V. viride* is "too near the *V. album* of Europe," so far as botanical description goes, to distinguish, or separate it from the other, yet we, as physicians, will be able to trace great differences in its pathogenesis, as well as great resemblances.

Both drugs are depressing in their influence on the system, and so are invaluable in weakened and debilitated conditions. Both remedies, if taken in excess, produce emesis and purging; and, consequently, will cure such symptoms when otherwise indicated.

My attention was first strikingly drawn to the Viride, by seeing the effects of it when given as a "sedative" by old-school practitioners. This characteristic is almost wanting in V. album. A few years ago during an epidemic of scarlet fever, in bad cases, when the arterial excitement was intense, and the pulse ran up rapidly, with great congestion of the cerebral vessels, *V. viride* was superior to Aconite or Belladonna. It may be exhibited advantageously as often as every ten minutes. The pulse will soon begin to fall, and when it has been reduced to 100, the time should be lengthened to thirty or sixty minutes; for, if continued too long, it will produce vomiting and great general prostration. *Digitalis,* which also brings down the pulse, does not appear to act for several hours, and then it operates so powerfully and so long, that it is admitted, even by Allopathic practitioners, to be a dangerous agent.

Veratrum viride low, acts promptly; the 500th acts more permanently but less actively than the low. It controls and stops vomiting (other symptoms being similar), more quickly than Bell. or Ipecac, and in many cases of sick headache, with or without vomiting, it has proved curative when Sanguinaria and other remedies have failed. Hence it is also applicable in the emesis of scarlatina.

Another grand sphere of its usefulness is in hæmorrhages from the nose, lungs, bowels or uterus, when the blood is dark red, or when there is any nausea present. Let us not overlook it in these cases, and particularly in metrorrhagia.

THE MILWAUKEE TEST APPLIED IN MILWAUKEE.

BY SAMUEL POTTER, M.D., MILWAUKEE, WIS.

READERS of this journal during the past year will remember me as anything but a believer in the theory of the dynamization of drugs. My position on many subjects in religion, science, morals, etc., has for some years been that of an agnostic, neither believing nor denying, but in all sincerity demanding strict safeguards around all evidence offered in support of all improbable theories. This was the sum of my sinning in my papers on the "Milwaukee Test,"—a measure which has now passed into history.

As a supplement thereto, I desire to make known the result of some experiments in which I have lately borne a part, being an attempt to apply the Milwaukee test to the *low dilutions*, for the purpose of ascertaining whether or not *they* could make their presence manifest under test conditions. The series, of which my work forms a part, was undertaken by Dr. Lewis Sherman, for the Bureau of Materia Medica in the American Institute of Homœopathy. A report has been presented by r. Sherman at the Milwaukee meeting, and will doubtless a ppear in the *Transactions* of that body. In this paper I will only speak of my own share in the experiments, and, under the circumstances, perhaps I may be pardoned if I briefly refer to my qualifications as a witness on such facts as I shall present.

During all the years, from 1862 to 1878, I have been a practitioner of homœopathic medicine more or less. I have devoted more time to the study of drug-action than to any other branch of the science of medicine. Mixing largely with the world, and carrying on the details of the business of extensive engineering works, I am no dreamy theorist, but know something of men and mundane affairs. When, therefore, in the first year of my experience as an actual member of the medical profession, the Milwaukee Test was proposed, I eagerly embraced it as a positive experiment of great value in therapeutical science. One objection, however, made by my friend, Professor Charles Gatchell, impressed me strongly. It was, that we should apply the same test to the 3d as to the 30th, and compare the results, in order to attain to a truly valuable result.

At the request of Dr. Sherman, the Milwaukee Academy of Medicine appointed a committee to place test-conditions around the preparation and dispensing of the agents with which the experiments were to be conducted. This committee, with the other gentlemen mentioned below, had several meetings during the past winter, and did all the work of dilution from the crude substances or the mother tinctures, the *medicating and dispensing* being intrusted wholly to Dr. C. C. Olmsted, formerly of the Cleveland College, for the reason that, although a low potency physician in practice, he unqualifiedly recorded his belief in the efficacy of the 200th Hahnemannian attenuations. Furthermore, being almost a stranger to the experimenters, and a practitioner of many years' standing as a homœopathist, he was, *par excellence*, the most fit gentleman on the committee to do the special work assigned him.

The full committee consisted of the following named persons:

C. C. Olmsted, M.D. (Cleveland Hosp. Coll.), appointed by the chairman of the Bureau of Materia Medica, American Institute of Homœopathy.

Lewis Sherman, A.M. (Union Coll.), M.D. (N. Y. Univ.), representing the aforesaid bureau, of which he is a member.

George W. Peckham, A.M., biologist; teacher of biology, Milwaukee High School.

E. M. Rosenkrans, M.D. (Det. Med. Coll., Hahn. Med. Coll., Chicago).

George C. McDermott, M.D. (Cleveland Hosp. Coll., N. Y. Ophth. Hosp.), now Prof. of Ophth. and Otol., Pulte Med. Coll.

Samuel Potter, M.D. (Hom. Med. Coll., of Mo.).

The last three representing the Milwaukee Academy of Medicine.

Eugene F. Storke, M.D. (Hahn. Med. Coll., Chicago), Secretary of the Wisconsin State Homœopathic Medical Society, and of the Milwaukee Academy of Medicine, was present part of the time.

Professor McDermott would doubtless have proved a valuable experimenter, but for his hurried removal to Cincinnati. He entered upon the test with great enthusiasm, and as he recorded his belief in the efficacy of the very highest potencies of all substances, when prepared in accordance with Hahnemann's directions, his evidence would have been of great value. But higher honors awaited him, and we parted reluctantly.

Each member of the committee stated to the Secretary his position on the potency question. I recorded myself as not believing in the medicinal or pathogenetic efficacy of any drug in any attenuation above the 6th decimal. The utmost care was observed that the safeguards should be entirely scientific in character, as a part of which I was made Secretary, I suppose for the purpose of keeping my myopic eyes off the bottles. The record of which vial in the set of ten was medicated, was made in such a manner, that no one, not even the person who medicated, could possibly know its identity or number, and the record for each set was sealed in a slide box by itself, each member of the committee signing the seals. The experimenters were not allowed to handle these boxes, or the record, until sealed.

To me were handed a set of ten vials for each of the following drugs: Aconite 3^x, Aconite 6^x, Belladonna 3^x, Belladonna 6^x, Arsenicum, 7^x, Phosphorus 5^x, Phosphorus 6_x, Phosphorus 7^x, Phosphorus 8^x, Phosphorus 9^x, Phosphorus 10^x. After several weeks of experimentation, I reported in writing to the committee a number for the medicated vial in each set, with the following result: When the sealed boxes were opened by the committee, *my reports were found to be correct in every instance excepting Phosphorus* 8^x, *and* 10^x. However Dr. Sherman's report on the first of these was correct.

The following is an extract from my journal, written while working with Aconite 6^x:

MILWAUKEE, WISCONSIN, March 17th, 1880.

8 P.M. In my usual health, tired after the day's work but no other condition sensible which I could call abnormal. A young man has just gone whom I have consented to take as a student of medicine. My wife out at a neighbor's. I am writing to-night on the article "Hypochondriasis" for my index, and stop to make this record.

8.35 P.M. Took 3 drops of the fluid in vial No. 1 of the 10 marked Aconite 6^x, given me by the Committee on Tests last night. I was nearly poisoned two years ago by an accidental overdose of this drug taken to produce its physiological effects on the heart. Consequently I feel that I may be somewhat susceptible to the drug.

I cannot find a slip from which I was copying two minutes ago, and feel nervous and put out about it. According to my own views about medicinal action, I ought to get nervous anyway after taking what may be Acon., because I expect it. So I must work and drive this away.

8.48 P.M. Took 3 drops more out of vial No. 1, and will take the same dose every five minutes for the next half hour. No symptoms now except this fidgety, nervous sensation.

9 P.M. Am very nervous, and filled with indefinite apprehensions concerning my wife, who is only two blocks away. Am writing on "Hysteria," and ascribe my sensations to expectancy and the subject of my thoughts. Continue the No. 1 every five minutes.

9.15 P.M. My eyes are getting very sore and tired, my head feels congested, more like Belladonna than Acon. I tried to get up from the desk just now, and was attacked with severe vertigo, so that I had to sit down at once. Some little noises upstairs sound very painful, but then they generally do. The street-car noises sound very loud. My head aches badly.

I smell all the vile scents I can think of, especially that of a dog which has lain in this room, sick for ten days past, a pet of my wife's. Continue the medicine, now only one drop every five minutes.

10 P.M. All of No. 1 gone. I am so nervous that I cannot work. My wife is not yet back, and I have the most intolerable anxiety about her. My head aches fearfully. I put up my books, as I can scarcely see, and go out after her. I have a regular Cactus constricted sensation around my chest. Some one spoke in the alley by my window just now, and I fairly jumped from my seat, but sank back faint with dimness of vision.

11 P.M. Going to bed an hour earlier than usual, reason, I cannot work. All the above symptoms greatly intensified during the last hour.

12. Very restless, cannot go to sleep. Taking a dose of Chloral hydrate.

March 18th, 7 30 P.M. Sit down to work, my wife out again. I will take No. 2 vial to-night of Acon. 6^x in water every five minutes.

11 P.M. Have finished the No. 2. No peculiar symptoms except very heavy eyes.

March 19th, 8 P.M. Began vial No. 3, of Acon 6^x as before.

11.45 P.M. Have taken the medicine steadily all the evening about every five minutes. No unusual symptoms.

March 20th, 12 midnight. I have taken vial No. 4 all evening as before. No unusual symptoms.

March 21st, 2–5 P.M. Have been working and taking No. 5. No unusual symptoms. 8–11 P.M. Working and taking No. 6. No unusual symptoms.

This experiment proves some things and suggests others. It proves that the lower dilutions can vindicate themselves under test conditions. It proves to me that I cannot fix upon the 6^x dilution as the limit of the action of drugs. It forces me to confess that my belief has gone *three degrees higher* during the past winter. It proves that no man is competent to settle the potency question without experiment surrounded by scientific safeguards. Lastly, it suggests that the believers in the 30th were too precipitate in condemning the Milwaukee test, and gently insinuates the hope that they may go and do likewise.

SABADILLA IN MEASLES.

BY EDUARDO FORNIAS, M.D., PHILADELPHIA, PA.

DURING my amateur practice in Cuba I had opportunity to treat several cases of measles, but never found the disease attended with such violent sneezing and pleuritic stitches from the very beginning, as I did during an epidemic which prevailed in the port of Casilda in 1870, and in this city in the early part of the present year. In some of the cases treated in the former place, the stitches disappeared with the rash, undoubtedly under the beneficial influence of our remedies, while in others, they continued later. Diarrhœa, when present, was usually urgent, the stools brown in color, and "fermented," followed by burning, although more frequently, by a severe crawling and itching in the anus, as from ascarides. There was also, frequently, a burning soreness of the abdomen; lassitude, weariness, and inclination to lie down, etc. But the leading characteristics were violent concussive sneezing, often attended with frontal headache, and stitching pains in the chest.

A repetition of these symptoms occurred in three out of the four cases which I treated in this city in February last.

The remedies studied were, Puls., Bryo., Squilla, and Sabad. In almost all cases early in the trouble, Aconite was sufficiently indicated to commence with, but in one single case the moist and hot skin, the sore throat and the character of the sleep called for Bell., which was given with good results. Both Aconite and Bellad. were followed by Sabadilla, which was the similimum in the majority of the cases, and did its work nobly.

As indications for the latter remedy, I found in Calleja's work the following: "Sabadilla is the remedy when, among the catarrhal symptoms, the sneezing is violent and concussive, especially if attended with severe frontal headache, in children nervously ill from worms. When there are stitching pains in the chest, worse when coughing. The cough is dry, short, and spasmodic, with nightly attacks, commencing as soon as the patient lies down. Painful soreness of the abdomen. Repeated epistaxis. Redness of the eyelids and smarting in the eyes, showing the irritated condition of the conjunctiva; eyes suffused and watery, especially when looking to the light, bright objects, sneezing or coughing. The coryza is watery, fluent, with itching of the nose, or alternate obstruction of the right and left nostril. Mouth dry; tongue sore and yellow; throat sore with difficult deglutition and constant sensation of a lump which must be swallowed down. Body hot, and before fever sets in, and sometimes during the whole trouble, there is a marked lassitude and weariness, with inclination to lie down, to yawn and stretch the limbs, which are painful. If diarrhœa is presents the stools are urgent, dark, and fermented, or mixed with blood and mucus; if constipation is present it is with pain in the bowels. In both conditions there are crawling and itching in the anus. The eruption comes out not in patches or groups of concentric form, but in spots and stripes of deep red color."

To these symptoms I would add, that the child may be anxious, restless, starts easily, and feels sick. The periodicity is also well-marked; symptoms returning at precisely the same hour. Fever, with absence of thirst, and alternate coldness of the body, with flushes of heat in the face, etc., is an additional indication for Sabadilla. It must also be borne in mind that Sabadilla antidotes Pulsatilla, and is also suitable to light-haired children of lax fibre.

I do not wish to commend this remedy in measles, guided merely by the pathological name; neither to affirm its absolute efficacy in said affection, as I do not believe in specifics. But I offer it as a neglected remedy, which after a careful study may be made more useful for us. In no other way do I believe that homœopathy can be properly practiced. Next to Sabadilla, the remedy which did me the most good, was Squilla, which differs in having an offensive as well as dark diarrhœa, and in having less marked sneezing and lachrymation. The nasal discharge, although fluent, is corrosive, and the sore throat is less severe than in Sabadilla. The latter has especially absence of thirst; Squilla has absence of sweat, etc. Squilla has the fatigue and general lassitude, with yawning and stretching of the limbs so characteristic of Sabadilla, but without sleepiness. And while speaking of Squilla, I may add, parenthetically, that Squilla is highly recommended by Spanish physicians in pertussis, and I have used it here with success. Its efficacy in diseases of the mucous membranes and their glands is indisputable, and we do wrong to ourselves and our patients if we neglect to verify or confirm it when there are internal cold, together with external heat; or, intense heat, followed by chilliness, so soon as the patient uncovers himself; hardness and tension of the pulse. These febrile symptoms we often observe in advanced catarrhal conditions. It is, besides, well indicated, when the coryza is fluent and corrosive, with constant sneezing, eyes dejected and watery, short cough, dry and violent, or followed by excessive mucous expectoration; the loose morning cough is more fatiguing than the dry evening cough; cough may cause spirting of urine, and is preceded by a sonorous harsh sound; when there is a sensation of painful pressure over the sternum, and painful stitches in different places of the chest, especially in the left side. Finally, Squilla is highly important when the catarrhal stage has great intensity, and the fever so marked as to become synochal. As the majority of these symptoms may be present in measles, this picture will not be out of the way here.

I was greatly pleased to hear Professor Korndörfer, in the February or March meeting of the Homœopathic Medical Society of the County of Philadelphia, speak so favorably of

Squilla in measles, as I had just gone over the symptoms of the drug in this disease.

Bryonia was also sometimes of service, especially for a little girl who had, instead of the sore, moist yellow tongue of Sabad., a dry, white-coated tongue, with a few small blisters on the tip; great thirst for large quantities of cold water; constipation; pains worse from the least motion.

Dr. Valers, of Spain, says, "If we study with care, the effects of measles, localized in the thoracic organs, we will find it characterized by a short dry cough, sometimes spasmodic, and followed by vomiting of drinks; fluent coryza, with nose-bleed; impeded respiration, which is short, anxious, and accompanied by soreness of the chest, caused by the persistency of the cough; rheumatic pains in the limbs; redness and inflammation of the eyelids, with lachrymation; constipation, etc.; for all these symptoms Bryonia[12] is the best indicated agent, quieting them quickly and favoring the development of the exanthema." "This remedy is important in measles for more than one reason, at least I have been able to give it with good results when this trouble has acquired a nervous and typhoid character. It has an efficient action when, by any accidental cause, the rash disappears from the surface of the skin, or when the persistency of thoracic symptoms hinders its development. In both cases we could not find any other agent to take the place of Bryonia."

As Pulsatilla was not used for any of the above cases, I will only say that this drug, especially in my country, is, and has been, the universal panacea of measles; I say panacea, because, unfortunately, it has often been used by our specific seekers indiscriminately. Such practice is unworthy of the school of Hahnemann, and is opposed to the rules laid down by the great masters, but I am inclined to hope, with rational confidence, that these unjustified notions will soon die away, and that such homœopaths, if homœopaths they can be called, will become more careful and industrious. What else could be expected, when we see that even the old school is making such rapid progress in the way of discrimination? We often hear already, allopaths saying, we must treat this case systematically—we must discriminate; even the mental condition of the patient is taken into consideration, and, as Professor Korndörfer says, in his valuable article on Neurasthenia (HAHNEMANNIAN MONTHLY, June, 1880), "The writings of some of the adherents of the old school of medicine, must bring the blush to the cheeks of such of the new faith, who, from lukewarmness, ignorance or fear of ridicule, have buried this one talent, instead of putting it to use."

Of potencies, I have used Sabad.[15] and [16]; Bryonia[6]; Squilla[12], all of Cuban preparation. Of course I don't mean by this to say that higher or lower potencies could not do just as well. In this respect I am very liberal; and if consulted in the matter, I only would say, that just as the best remedy is the indicated one, so I think is the (best) dose, the smallest that can cure.

CARDIAC COMPLICATIONS OF SCARLATINA.

BY W. P. ARMSTRONG, M.D., LAFAYETTE, IND.

AMONG the accompaniments and sequelæ of scarlatina, those which affect the heart are not by any means the least important. With the exception of those speedily or suddenly fatal terminations by heart clot and cardiac paralysis, they are of two kinds,—*inflammatory* and *dropsical.*

Whether the cardiac inflammation is the direct result of the poison of scarlatina, or is merely symptomatic of the rheumatism which so frequently accompanies or follows it, is not known. It is, however, a well-known fact that such inflammation is much more serious than that found in acute rheumatism where there is no scarlatina. It usually first manifests itself during the second week, but may begin earlier or later than this.

Endocarditis, or inflammation of the lining membrane of the heart, attacks by preference the mitral valve and its immediate vicinity, although in rare instances the aortic valve is affected. Pain is not necessarily present, but there is usually faintness, with præcordial anxiety and anxious expression of countenance.

On making a physical examination we find a murmur which is heard loudest at the apex, but somewhat diffused, and which may be *presystolic,* from narrowing of the mitral orifice and consequent obstruction to the blood-stream, but much more frequently is *systolic,* from imperfect closure of the mitral valve and consequent regurgitation. In the latter case, it is heard also to the left for a considerable distance beyond the præcordial limits and often even in the back. It might be confounded with a previously existing mitral, regurgitant murmur, but the latter would be accompanied by more or less enlargement of the left ventricle. A mitral regurgitant murmur might also be produced by inflammation or other cause of extreme debility of that portion of the wall of the left ventricle to which a papillary muscle is attached, *causing the wall to give way at that point and drag the valve down away from the orifice during the systole,* but such instances are rare. Obstruction and regurgitation may both be present at the same time, and here we shall have a double apex murmur, *presystolic* and *systolic.*

Much too often the endocarditis passes entirely unrecognized. Some of the very worst cases of valve diseases originate in scarlatina. According to Hayden such cases rarely survive the period of childhood.

In *pericarditis,* we generally have more or less præcordial pain, which is aggravated by motion and often by taking a deep breath. We also have palpitation, with præcordial anxiety, a sense of constriction about the heart, and commonly a short dry cough. Upon applying the ear or stethoscope to the præcordium, there will be heard at some points a friction-murmur or friction-sound, produced by the rubbing together of the two roughened and sticky pericardial surfaces. This is generally to-and-fro in character, being *systolic* and *post-diastolic,* and, unlike an endocardial murmur, is *not diffused beyond the point of its production.*

When the effusion comes to be predominantly serious, as it often does, and is of considerable quantity, so as not to permit the apex to touch the anterior chest-wall, the friction-sound will be suppressed, and the ventricular impulse can be neither seen nor felt when the patient is lying on the back, for the heart is heavier than the fluid in which it is contained and naturally seeks the lowest point. Turn him on the face, or upon the left side, so as to bring the apex in apposition with the chest-wall again, and the impulse will return, and most likely the murmur also.

A very important physical sign is the dulness on percussion, which is increased in breadth. When the patient is sitting upright, this increased breadth is found especially at the lower part, so that it assumes a *wedge-shape,* with the base downwards.

The effusion of pericarditis of scarlatinal origin is apt to take on a puriform character, in which case the chances of recovery are small.

Extensive inflammation of the heart muscle itself sometimes occurs, and here we have a rapid, feeble, and irregular pulse, with shortness of breath, especially on exertion, anxious expression of countenance, intense præcordial anguish, and fear of impending death. Or we may have two or more of these structures affected at the same time, with a corresponding modification of the symptoms and physical signs.

The *hydropericardium*, met with as a sequelæ of scarlatina, is only a part of the general dropsy which, it is reasonable to suppose, results from the post-scarlatinal nephritis so common in some epidemics. Its physical signs are the same as those of extensive serous effusion in pericarditis, with the exception that there is no friction-sound nor tactile fremitus at any stage, as there is no inflammation and consequently no fibrinous effusion. It usually disappears when the urinary function has been restored.

Time and space forbid more than a few therapeutic hints in an article of this kind. The treatment of these conditions will be found in a more complete form in a forthcoming work.

For *endocarditis*, I would suggest among other remedies, more particularly, Acon., Bry., Naja, and Ars. If these are incapable of entirely removing the inflammation and its consequences, they may at least reduce to the minimum the resulting valvular distortion.

For *pericarditis*, especially Acon., Bry., and Cact., as long as *pain, friction-sound*, and *impulse* are present; that is, as long as the effusion is predominantly fibrinous; but when these cease, and the serum of the effusion comes to predominate, the remedy is more likely to be Apis, Dig., Ars., or Lycopod., according to their respective indications.

Pericardial dropsy will call more especially for such remedies as are capable of acting upon the kidneys, removing the inflammation, and restoring the function of those organs, and here I believe Apis will be found more frequently useful, because more frequently indicated than any other remedy. Many cases will, however, require other medicines, according to the totality of the symptoms of the individual case.

HYOSCYAMUS NIGER.

BY WALLACE M'GEORGE, M.D.

(Read before the West Jersey Homœopathic Medical Society.)

GLANCING over the blackened corks on my medicine bottles, indicating such as are polychrests with me, I notice a well-fingered stopper, showing that it is my trusted preparation of *Hyos. niger*. I ask your attention to the use of this remedy in brain affections, a class of diseases in which, in my opinion, *Hyosc.* is very frequently indicated.

In typhoid and typhus fevers, especially in the form known as typhus centralis, when the brain is active but wandering, when the patient is laboring under hallucinations of various kinds, but all centring in a desire to escape from the room or from those around, *Hyoscyamus* must ever be in our minds. These patients are sometimes able to answer our questions intelligently, and sometimes unable to comprehend our meaning. This remedy is recommended for the versatile as well as the dull and stupid forms, but, in my opinion, it is not very often indicated in the real stupid cases. Nor, indeed, is it the best remedy in the very versatile forms, but rather in the class of cases first described. From the excited condition (not frenzied as in *Belladonna*) we infer that the blood is flowing rapidly to the brain, and that we have patients who require our closest attention. Lilienthal, in his new work on homœopathic therapeutics, recommends it for the first period, or stage of increase, and it is really here that it shows its wonderful power. If well selected and given *alone* it will stop the increase, bring the patient to consciousness, and start him well on the way to recovery. The same writer gives thirty-three good indications under *Hyoscyamus* in typhus and typhoid fevers. But the symptoms that have most impressed themselves on my mind as characteristic of *Hyos.* are: Delirium, with attempt to jump out of bed and run away, sometimes with fear, sometimes without; when spoken to answers correctly in whole or in part, and then is gone again, muttering to himself; loquacity (less marked than under *Lachesis*); talks nonsense continually with his eyes open, but does not pay attention to any one; thinks he is in the wrong place but does not want to go home (like *Bryonia*); picking at the bedclothes and playing with his hands (not grasping for something in the air like *Stramonium*); throws off the bedclothes so as to leave the genitals uncovered; put his hands on the genitals and plays with them. In these cases the patient is entirely unconscious, and it seems that he throws off the clothes to cool the sexual organs, for if the bedclothing is left off a little while he is satisfied. This desire, as well as that of playing with the genitals, shows that the brain is profoundly affected, and that the mental sphere has yielded its supremacy, for the time being, to the animal propensities. And yet in all of these cases I never despair of a cure. I observe under *Hyos.* staring or squinting, either with one or both eyes; involuntary stools in bed and involuntary urination—symptoms that must be soon corrected or the patient will succumb; paralysis of sphincter ani and vesicæ; marked subsultus tendinum. Compare in this last symptom Lycop., Psorin., Rhus tox., Secale, Sulphur, and *Zincum*, but no one has it so violently as Hyoscyamus.

A few brief comparisons may be of interest. Under Hyos. and Apis mellifica we find stupor; but under the latter there are sudden exacerbations and, at times, piercing shrieks, dull, cloudy eyes, with indifference, except during the period of exacerbation. *Arnica* has more stupefaction and terribly offensive breath. *Baptisia* exhibits a besotted look; when questioned the patient presents that uncomfortable symptom just reported by Dr. Bell: "Unable to rest or sleep because she can't get herself together; her head is in one place and her limbs and body in other places; if she could only get together how happy she would be." Under *Gelsemium* we find stupor, but the patient is weaker than under *Hyos.*, as if the vital forces were giving out. Under *Lachesis* we find the stupor and delirium, with an idea that he is dead; great loquacity. We also find, as a grave symptom, dropping of the jaw. This impression that he is dead is of much less serious import than the sensation of being well. Such cases must be closely watched. Lycopodium adds to the stupefaction, delirium, and subsultus tendinum of Hyos. great tympanitis or meteorism and the characteristic fanlike motion of the nostrils. Arnica and Opium have stupor more marked than any others. Opium has also extreme wakefulness, or, as often described, impossibility of going to sleep although very sleepy. Under Stramonium there are stupor and unconsciousness, varying with changeable mood, or violent tossing about, or singing, praying, cursing, or laughing, as the mood takes them. The last symptom is characteristic only of Stramonium. Phosphoric acid, on the other hand, combines great indifference to everything and everybody with the stupefaction.

For the squinting or strabismus so frequently found in brain troubles Belladonna is often given when Hyoscyamus would be more useful and would remove the trouble. In conclusion let me urge a little more attention to this valuable drug in the class of cases alluded to above. And, although I have designated certain well-attested symptoms, do not misunderstand me and neglect other indications, for here, as in all cases, the remedy should cover the totality of the symptoms.

DEMOCRACY IN MEDICINE.

(Read before the Homœopathic Medical Society of Chester, Delaware, and Montgomery Counties.)

BY C. PRESTON, M.D., CHESTER, PA.

By "democracy" we mean simply equality of rights and privileges. "A government of the people, by the people, and for the people," and in the broadest sense of the term. No restrictions should be made by any conditions of caste or circumstances, provided acquirements and merits insure capability for positions assumed. Cultivated intellect, talent and capacity, must, in all free governments, represent the best interests of society, and no one has any right to exert an influence to retard, or in any way hinder the greatest possible development of all the powers of mind which can fully qualify the possessor to meet the responsibilities of his or her calling or profession.

It is not enough that we may arrive at conclusions in regard to the co-education of the sexes, and decide for ourselves which is the better way. Honor to ourselves and justice to all, demand that we should defend the cause of women physicians. Their persistent endeavors to secure the benefits of medical associations have at last been successful, even in the face of strong opposition. And why any member of any medical society at this late day should stand in the way of the free admission of well-qualified women to our medical councils, is a mystery which cannot be understood by the generous, magnanimous, and progressive element of the profession. But if there still remain some amongst us who would close up the avenues of free thought and equal privileges, we should labor earnestly for the removal of this prejudice, knowing that every principle of justice to the opposite sex, and of interest to ourselves, stands boldly out in defence of the cause we espouse.

We can no longer afford to withhold from women the rights which they have so amply qualified themselves to exercise. From the earliest days of homœopathy, women have been among our ablest provers of drugs. Through their zealous and untiring labor in this field, we have acquired our principal knowledge of the abnormal conditions of the female organism and of its treatment. While women are thus needed in perfecting our healing art, any assumption of superiority on the part of the stronger sex must be the result either of ignorance or of prejudice. The shamefulness of an act which appropriates the labor, intelligence and experience of others to enhance our own skill and success, while it throws obstacles in the way of the success of the medium through which this knowledge comes, is too glaring to go unrebuked. Yet our medical colleges and associations have only recently opened their eyes to this fact. Let us hope that acting in full accord with the progressive spirit of our age, this society may not be among the last to open wide its doors to women who may be qualified to assume the responsibilities of medical practice.

AN ATTEMPT TO TRANSPLANT A PIECE OF THE CORNEA OF A DOG TO THE HUMAN EYE.

ENUCLEATION—PATHOLOGICAL CONDITION.

TRANSLATED BY F. PARKE LEWIS, M.D , BUFFALO, N. Y.

On the 24th of March a three-year-old child was brought to our clinic in whose left eye had developed a high degree of staphyloma. The lids could scarcely be closed over the enlarged eyeball, and the parents of the child desired, as they had already been advised from other professional sources, to have the disfiguration relieved by the removal of the globe. In regard to the origin of the trouble, it might be presumed, by putting together the statements of the parents, that in early infancy a conical perforation must have occurred, probably in consequence of blennorrhœa neonatorum. The greater portion of the cornea was occupied by a prominent leucomatous scar, which was sparsely vascularized by single large vessels chiefly running down from above. Above, and toward the temporal side, however, was a small space of stretched and thinned, yet comparatively transparent cornea, under which, and in immediate contact with it, the atrophied iris could be dimly discerned. Enucleation was determined upon. But my assistant, Dr. Angelucci, with Dr. Neelsen, the private instructor, are engaged in experiments in corneal transplantation, and in accordance with their wish, I was quite ready, before removing the eye, to attempt a transplantation. The kerato-plastic results would then be suitable for supplementary histological inquiry. The operation was performed under chloroform narcosis, with a circular trepan, the opening of which had a diameter of 5 mm. The excision was made through the relatively transparent portion of the cornea of which mention has been made. This small operation was performed without difficulty, but in consequence of the loss of a not inconsiderable quantity of vitreous fluid, as was foreseen, a considerable collapse occurred. At the opening thus made, a marked depression took place. Immediately, with the same trepan, a piece of the same size was taken from the cornea of a young dog, and placed in the artificial opening of the staphylomatous eye. The lids were then united with catgut sutures, the arms of the unruly little fellow bound to his side, and an attendant stationed at his bedside to watch him, and, if possible, to control his too violent motions. Concerning the details of the case, little need be said, because the loud crying, and unruly behavior of the strong little patient, on the approach of the physician, rendered a careful examination almost impossible, and in a certain sense, dangerous. It need only be remarked that, after 24 hours the eyeball had again assumed its original form and resistance. The catgut suture had torn its way through before that time, and the place that had been trepanned, without exhibiting any marked appearances of inflammatory reaction, was surrounded by a fine gray band, and it had, moreover, retained a completely transparent appearance. After two or three days this was generally unchanged except that the surrounding gray edge,—which might have been considered a purulent infiltration,—had grown broader and more clearly defined. At the boundaries of the transparent portion, the least diffierence in the evenness of the surface could not be detected. On the fourth day, in order that a complete examination might be made, and in view of a probable enucleation, the boy was put under the influence of chloroform. It could now be seen, that in the surrounding cloudiness, the trepanned place had also become dulled. After an examination the eyeball was enucleated. Although the operation was performed with great care, it unavoidably happened that on cutting the nerve, the scarcely united wound broke open, the vitreous fluid was partially lost, and the globe nearly collapsed. The completion of the operation was thus rendered more difficult if not more important. The histological examination, the results of which increased the value of the work already accomplished, showed the following pathological conditions to have obtained:

"Bulbus filled with blood coagula, in the centre of which was the detached retina. Atrophy of the ciliary body, with enlargement of its vessels. Retina atrophied. In the opening at which the cornea was trepanned, was found the anterior border of the retina, imbedded in a fibrin coagulum, relatively poor in cellular elements and which reached out like a fungoid growth over both edges of the corneal surface. The overhanging edges were thickly infiltrated with round cells. The cut surface of the cornea was covered with new epithelium, which here and there extended a short distance on the coagulum, but at no point reached the centre. In the cornea, surrounding the opening made by the trepan, were small aggregations of round cells."

Although to outward appearances it would seem that union might have occurred, even though it should be followed by some clouding, still there was no trace of the inserted piece to be found in the corneal opening.—(W. Zehnder in the *Klinische Monats blätter für Augenheilkunde.*)

ON THALAMIC EPILEPSY.

Extract from a paper read before the American Neurological Association, and published in the New York *Archives of Medicine.*

BY WILLIAM A. HAMMOND, M.D., SURGEON-GENERAL U. S. ARMY (RETIRED); PROFESSOR OF DISEASES OF THE MIND AND NERVOUS SYSTEM IN THE UNIVERSITY OF NEW YORK, ETC.

WHILST cases of the form of epilepsy I am about to describe have doubtless been not very uncommon, it has happened that they have not hitherto received special attention. Either they have been regarded as something entirely different from epilepsy, or the characteristie phenomena have been overlooked or merged into a general description with little stress being laid upon them. So far as I know, therefore, this is the first attempt to differentiate them and to associate the symptoms by which they are chiefly marked with a definite brain-lesion.

In an interesting paper Dr. Hughlings Jackson specifies the following six varieties of epilepsy, as embracing all known forms of the disease:

1. A sudden and temporary stench in the nose with transient unconsciousness.
2. A sudden and temporary development of blue vision.
3. A spasm of the right side of the face with stoppage of speech.
4. A tingling of the index finger and thumb, followed by spasms of the hand and forearm.
5. A convulsion almost instantly universal, with immediate loss of consciousness.
6. Certain vertiginous attacks.

As is seen, Dr. Jackson does not make loss of consciousness an essential feature of the epileptic paroxysm, and this fact is apparent from his reiterated assertions, not only throughout the paper in question, but in other contributions which he has made to our knowledge of epilepsy. He defines the disease as "an occasional, sudden, and rapid discharge of gray matter of some part of the brain," a bad definition certainly, but I do not quote it now to criticise it further than to call attention to the fact that the element of unconsciousness is not included in its terms.

The more familiar I become with epileptic and epileptiform phenomena, the more convinced I am that there is no true epilepsy without unconsciousness.

Before proceeding, however, to discuss the important questions connected with the physiology and pathology of this form of epilepsy to which I ask attention, it will be well to describe briefly the cases upon which my views are founded.

Case 1.—M. I., a young woman about 22 years of age consulted me July 20th, 1868, to be treated for what her mother informed me were "visions," which she was in the habit of having frequently every day. They occurred to her at the most unexpected times and were of great variety, no two, in fact, ever being exactly alike. While sitting in my waiting-room she had had, as she said, one of these attacks, the principal feature of which was the hallucination of a large crane standing on one leg and attentively looking at her. After a few seconds a period of momentary unconsciousness occurred, on emerging from which there was entire recollections of the hallucination in all its particulars.

Inquiry showed that there were no vertigo or spasms of any kind, nor had there during the whole course of the seizure been any convulsive movements, or, in fact, any essential variation from the peculiar type I have mentioned. As soon as the hallucination appeared, and while still conscious, she conversed about its characteristics and was fully aware of its unreality. Suddenly, a loss of consciousness ensued, but there was no fixing of the eyes, no rigidity. Her head, if she were standing or sitting, fell forward on her chest, her breathing remained normal, there was no acceleration of pulse. In a few seconds she as suddenly raised her head, made a few coherent remarks and was entirely herself.

The next day, July 21st, in company with her mother she came to my residence. A few minutes after entering the consulting-room and while she was conversing in regard to some points in her clinical history, she exclaimed: "It has come, and oh! mother, what do you think it is? A beautiful chair covered with red velvet all spotted with golden stars. It is just such a chair as I suppose is used for a throne. Well, this is the first time I ever had a chair appear to me. I have had rocks and all sorts of animals, but, but, but—" Here her head sank on her breast, her eyes were closed and her respiration became so quiet that it seemed for the moment to be suspended. There was no extraordinary paleness of the countenance and there had not been the slightest convulsive movement. In about three seconds she raised her head, smiled and looked as if nothing of an untoward character had occurred.

I at once formed the opinion that the paroxysm was a fraud, and I was indiscreet enough to say so in very plain terms. I told her that she had attempted to deceive me and I demanded her reasons for so extraordinary a performance. She and her mother both became indignant—justly so, I suppose—and left the house.

I saw nothing more of the case till November 18th, 1878. She then, accompanied as before by her mother, again consulted me. She informed me that the symptoms had continued in an aggravated form; that the "visions" lasted longer; that the period of unconsciousness had been much more severe and prolonged, and that the paroxysms were of more frequent occurrence. Since her last visit to me she had, she said, consulted several practitioners, some of whom thought she was shamming, and others had regarded the attacks as hysterical.

As, during the interval which had elapsed between my interview with her, I had observed a similar case, in regard to which I had formed definite opinions, I determined to study the phenomena with care. I was satisfied, from the case referred to, that my first opinion relative to the present instance was erroneous, and that there was an actual morbid entity with very interesting and characteristic phenomena.

For over a month, therefore, I kept Miss I. under observation, scarcely a day passing that I did not see her. I had the opportunity of witnessing seventeen paroxysms. Sometimes they were preceded by a well-marked aura, and this was always a singular sensation, apparently somewhere within the cranium, but not capable of being exactly localized or described. This was never felt until within the last two years. It lasted only a second or two, and was immediately followed by the "vision."

The first paroxysm of this series which I witnessed was ushered in by the aura. She had hardly time to say, "It's coming," when the hallucination began. She described it as consisting of a large white bear in motion before her on the carpet. It seemed to be walking slowly to and fro, its head bent toward the floor as if scenting something. I closely watched her and could detect no spasm anywhere. She spoke clearly, without hesitation, and with entire distinctness. The pupils were normal.

I had taken out my watch to time the duration of the attack. Thirty-five seconds elapsed, and then her pupils suddenly dilated, her head fell forward, and her left hand, which she was at this instant pointing in the direction of the visional bear, dropped to her side. I pinched the skin of her face, then of each hand, without eliciting any evidence of cutaneous sensibility. I took up a fold of skin on each forearm just above the wrist and stuck a cataract needle which was at hand through it, with a like result. Her pulse—I had not felt it during the existence of the hallucination—was beating at the rate of about sixty per minute, and was full. Her face had not altered in color, nor was there any other change in it except such as was due to relaxation of the muscles—such as is present in sleep. The eyelids were closed, but not spasmodically. She remained in this state exactly twenty-eight seconds, breathing perhaps a little more slowly and deeply than before the accession of the paroxysm. Suddenly she raised her head, looked around inquiringly for a moment, and then, as if becoming aware of a sensation, looked at both her arms where I had pricked them. A drop of blood was oozing from each puncture. She asked what it was, and then, without waiting for an answer, exclaimed, "You have bled me." She was then entirely herself, and talked coherently and without the least excitement about the hallucination.

[The writer here mentions that closing the eyes made no difference in the appearance of the visions. He found that the attacks could be cut short, or at least modified, by inhaling Nitrite of amyl, Ether or Chloroform, by firm pressure upon the jugular veins, or by a band drawn tighly around the head. "A strong volitional effort" also occasionally proved to have an abortive effect on the paroxysm.

Bromide of sodium, 15 grains three times a day, caused the attacks to cease after about a month's treatment. She took the medicine over a year, and then stopped it on account of its effects on the skin.

December 2d, 1879, she was married. December 15th she had a return of the paroxysms in more violent form, with convulsive movements and unconsciousness, and the symptoms were somewhat like those of "epileptic mania and certain forms of what is called morbid impulse." The Bromides of sodium and zinc were resorted to, and under their continuance there has been no recurrence of the attack.]

CASE 2.—Mr. W., a prominent merchant of a neighboring city, consulted me March 1st, 1879, for "nervous attacks," as he called them, with which he had been affected for several months. Upon inquiry I found that these "attacks" consisted of hallucinations of sight, smell, and hearing, accompanied with numbness and tingling on the right side of the body, and followed immediately by periods of unconsciousness. There was no spasm of any kind and the speech was not in the least degree involved. His wife accompanied him and from her I heard many particulars of his clinical history.

Usually, but not always, the sense of hearing was the first to be deranged; at others that of smell took precedence. In whatever way the paroxysms begin, the hallucinations of vision come last.

He was an intelligent man, and I therefore asked him to describe minutely to me all the phenomena of the last seizure. I give his description as nearly as possible in his own words:

"I had risen from bed at about half past seven o'clock, and had just left the bath-tub, when I thought I heard my wife ask me if I had finished my bath; I was at the moment vigorously rubbing myself with a towel, and being in doubt about the exact words, I called out, 'What did you say?' Immediately the words, 'Drown yourself, drown yourself; put your head under the water and hold it there.' I looked out of the bath-room door, but nobody was in the room. The last words, however, convinced me that an attack was coming on, for almost always I am commanded by the voices to inflict some injury on myself which is of a character to be suggested by my occupation at the time. Besides, at this instant I felt a kind of thrill pass through my right side.

"Knowing from experience what was at hand, I lay down on the floor, but not before the smell of fresh blood was perceived. It was a strong, overpowering, sickly smell, being accompanied with a slight sensation of nausea. It only lasted a few seconds, but before it was gone the vision came. I was lying flat on my back, looking up at the ceiling, when suddenly it appeared as though a large basket was descending toward me. It seemed to contain a little old black man, who leaned over the edge and grinned at me. When he got to within a foot of my face the basket began to ascend and another one, similar and with the same sort of old man in it, descended as did the first. It seemed then as though an endless chain were in motion, at regular intervals on which these baskets with little old black men in them, were fixed.

"The movements seemed to continue for an hour or more, and then I lost consciousness. As a matter of fact, the whole seizure, from the beginning to the end, was only about a minute and a half. My wife came in just at the instant I became unconscious, and she is certain this condition did not last over half a minute.

"On regaining my senses I jumped up, took the towel and continued my rubbing as though nothing had happened. I felt as well as I ever had in my life; without, in fact, a single unpleasant feeling in any part of my body."

His wife stated that, hearing him call to her, she came from another room to him, and reached him just as he became unconscious. He lay on the floor perfectly still, without the slightest spasmodic movement anywhere, and when he regained consciousness was perfectly himself, mentally and physically.

I treated this gentleman with the Bromide of sodium in doses of fifteen grains three times a day, with the effect of stopping the seizures on the third day. Since that time till now (June 2d) he has had no paroxysm of any kind. He still continues to take the medicine.

Three other cases, similar in general features, but of which I have no full notes, have come under my observation.

That these are instances of epilepsy will not, I think, be questioned; that they possess peculiar features will be readily admitted. The nearest hitherto described form of epilepsy to this, consists of those paroxysms in which the patient has an hallucination usually of sight and then immediately passes into an ordinary seizure. Many such cases have been reported, and quite a large number have occurred in my experience. I will return to the consideration of these directly.

The main point which it is desired to bring forward in the present communication, relates to the seat of the intracranial disturbance. The title of "Thalamic Epilepsy" which I have given to this paper, sufficiently indicates my view of the matter. My reasons for the opinion held are briefly as follows, and are based as well upon physiology as upon such experiments as disease has made for us:

The relations of the optic thalami to sensibility were first pointed out by Magendie, who ascertained that their irritation in animals produced excessive pain, while the other parts of the brain might be wounded without causing evidences of suffering.

They have also been regarded as specially the centres for vision, as presiding over the movements of the upper extremities, and again, as influencing voluntary movements in both the thoracic and pelvic limbs.

Although Todd, Carpenter, and others have considered the optic thalami as centres for sensorial impression, Luys, more than any other physiologist, has elaborated this idea and has adduced arguments in its support which it is difficult to overlook. His doctrine is that the optic thalami are reservoirs for all sensorial impressions, coming from the periphery of the nervous system, that like other ganglionic masses they elaborate these impressions, and that by means of the fibres of the corona radiata they transmit them to the cortex, to be still further perfectionated by being converted into ideas.

Such being apparently the physiological relations of the optic thalami, we come in the next place to discuss with something more of fulness, the consequences, so far as sensation is concerned, of certain abnormal states of these organs. As I have said, Ritti has collected from various sources, many cases, proving that injury or disease of the optic thalami leads to sensorial derangement, or the entire loss of one or more of the special senses. He has also gathered together from the works of Calmeil, Legardelle, and others, instances tending to establish the fact that hallucinations are the result of disease of one or both optic thalami. Several of the cases were supplied to him by M. Voisin, and had not previously been published. Of these latter I quote the following:

L. A., woman, aged 41, entered the Salpêtrière, January 30th, 1867. Since 1865 she had been subject to hallucinations of sight accompanied at times by some excitement and partial alienation. At her admission, she had hallucinations of sight and hearing, and others connected with the genital organs. There were also delusions of persecution. Latterly the sense of hearing has been impaired. She died April 17th, 1869, of typhoid fever.

Autopsy.—Neither thickening nor adhesions of the membranes; no subarachnoid effusions; cranial nerves normal, with the exception of the eighth pair, which were rotten at the most posterior and internal part of the two lobes of the cerebellum, and in the region nearest to the olivary bodies there were collections of little granulations, such as are seen in the choroid plexus. These were continued as far as the floor of the fourth ventricle, where they covered its cerebellar wall. Nothing was found wrong with the left optic thalamus, but the gray anterior centre of the right thalamus was more than normally vascular, and in the part immediately subjacent to the olfactive centre of gray matter there was a spot, the color of the dregs of wine, due to a globiform extravasation of blood. In the middle region there was a lacuna. Each of these was over a millimeter and a half in diameter.

This case is instructive, not only on account of the situation of the lesion, but for the reason also that there was no other intracranial disease to which the symptoms could have been ascribed.

That the optic thalamus is the centre for perception as the cortex is for intellection is, to say the least, exceedingly probable. Every sense has these two stages in its full action. Something is *perceived*, that is one stage; it is more or less thoroughly *understood*, and that is the other stage.

The intrinsic starting-point of every real sensorial impression is an organ of sense, such as the eye, the ear, or the terminal ramifications of the olfactory nerves. The starting-point of an erroneous or false sensorial impression—illusion or hallucination—may be either the organ of sense concerned therein or the sensory ganglion,—the optic thalamus. The cortex or intellectual centre for any sense cannot form a real or false sensorial impression. It can only elaborate the impressions which reach it from the sensory ganglion, and these are either true or false, real or unreal, according as they come originally from the ganglion, or are transmitted through it, from an organ of sense receiving real impressions from without, and according as the cortex is in a normal or an abnormal condition, will the ideas or beliefs which it forms from these transmitted impressions be normal or abnormal.

In the cases which form the basis of this paper there were hallucinations without intellectual derangement. They differed, therefore, from those cases of epilepsy in which there are hallucinations, and in which these hallucinations are received as realities, and acts, perhaps of violence, committed in logical sequence with the delusions formed. These doubtless have their starting-point in the optic thalamus, as shown by the existence of hallucinations, but the morbid process soon passes to the cortex, and the resultant phenomena are loss of consciousness and intense intellectual and motor disturbance.

I feel warranted, therefore, in concluding that there was in each of my cases no lesion of any of the intellectual sensorial centres situated in the cortex, but that the disease was confined entirely, or nearly so, to the optic thalami. I say nearly so, because the loss of consciousness which ensued showed that there was that necessary cortical disturbance without which there can be, in my opinion, no true epilepsy. Hallucinations without loss of consciousness no more constitute epilepsy than twitching of the hand or a stench in the nostrils, similarly unaccompanied, is epilepsy. Either may become epilepsy by further extension of the morbid intracranial action, but either may exist indefinitely without such extensions occurring.

Dr. Ferrier cites the following case:

The patient, a soldier, was admitted for epileptic insanity. "States that he saw dogs and cats about him; continually trying to tear the bedclothes or to seize hold of his own throat; every five or ten minutes he has epileptiform seizures, during which he grows very violent, requiring restraint.

"Tries to seize the poker or anything else that he may strike those in attendance on him. Endeavored to jump out of the chamber window. He has previously been in the asylum.

"As far as can be ascertained he labors under no delusion, but is decidedly demented. For certain events, such as his former residence here, his memory appears good enough, but for more recent events he possesses not the slightest knowledge.

"But the most peculiar feature in the case is the partial epileptic seizures, which occur every five or ten minutes without any loss of consciousness. The patient is suddenly seized with a convulsion in the left arm, the head is turned to the left as well as the eyes, and occasionally the muscular movements spread to the legs and right arm, but in a very slight degree. Indeed, after each seizure the patient's respiration is heavy, but there is not the least degree of unconsciousness, though he appears inclined to drop off to sleep. The patient is unable to stand, muscular power being entirely lost in left leg and decidedly diminished in left arm."

The patient went on from bad to worse; had long periods of drowsiness and stupor; during one night had ninety fits; spoke of visions of dogs, etc., being in his room all day, and on January 17th, died.

Now, there was a case of epileptiform convulsions attended with paralysis and hallucinations. It was one in which, according to Drs. Jackson's and Ferrier's views, there ought to have been well-defined cortical lesions; it was one in which, according to the views expressed in this paper, there ought to have been lesions of one or both optic thalami. Taking into consideration the facts that the hallucinations in this case were conjoined with left motor spasms and paralysis, I would not have hesitated to diagnosticate the existence of lesion of the right optic thalamus. Now, as a matter of fact, let us see what was revealed by the *post-mortem* examination, which, as Dr. Ferrier tells us, was made with the utmost care and thoroughness.

"*Head.*—The skull is of average thickness and density and is fairly symmetrical. The dura mater is somewhat adherent and the sinuses contain only fluid blood. There is little or no thickening of the arachnoid, but there is a good deal of superficial wasting of the convolutions of the frontal and parietal lobes. The vessels at the base are perfectly normal. There is no visible hyperæmia and pia mater strips with great ease. The gray matter is somewhat pale; it, as well as the white matter is of fair consistence. There is no trace of softening, clot, induration, or other organic change anywhere visible, although the most careful search is made. The ventricles are of average size and contain only a small quantity of fluid. *The optic thalamus on the right side is smaller than its fellow on the left and its posterior end is attenuated.*

"The medullary substance of the brain is perhaps a little firmer than it ought to be. No pathological change can be detected in the cerebellum, pons, or medulla."

Certainly no more striking case in support of the doctrines set forth in this paper could well have been supplied even if it had been made to order.

In conclusion, I think the following deductions may fairly be drawn, at least for the present:

1. That there is a form of epilepsy, the phenomena of which are simply hallucinations and loss of consciousness.
2. That the morbid anatomical basis of this type is seated in the optic thalamus.

PHYSIOLOGICAL EXPERIMENTS WITH THE "POTENTIZED" DRUG.

EXTRACT OF A LETTER FROM W. BOERICKE, M.D.

STUTTGART, August 13th, 1880.

. . . . . I HAD the pleasure of attending the meeting of the Homœopathic Central Verein of Germany. One of the most interesting events of that meeting was the report of Dr. Zöppritz about Professor Jäger's experiments with his "neural apparatus." Though a full account will be published by the Professor himself, I will give you the facts as presented to the society. It seems that Professor Jäger has been experimenting upon the length of time required by the brain to receive impressions; in other words, measuring the interval between irritation of a nerve and conscious perception, and how this interval is affected by inhalation of various odors. The results are interesting and curious, and led Dr. Schlegel, of Stuttgart, to persuade Professor Jäger to try the effect of inhaling homœopathic dilutions, and see whether these small quantities thus taken could affect his "neurometer." Now, Professor Jäger has hitherto been an active opponent of homœopathy; but for the sake of perfecting his experiments in every direction he acquiesced, and selected Aconite 3d, 30th, and 200th.

The normal time required in Professor Jäger's case was 90 to 100 mille seconds. In order to distinguish the action of Aconite from that of the alcohol, the latter was tested alone; but no material change was made in the intervals as recorded by the "neurometer."

When Acon. 3d was inhaled, the rapidity of perception increased, *i. e.*, the interval was shortened. And what is remarkable, it grew in intensity as the higher potencies were inhaled, so that when the 200th was tried Professor Jäger sent for Dr. Schlegel, and acknowledged that he was "dumfounded." He said that he was positive that the result could not possibly be due to any other influence than the Aconite^{200}, as the experiment was conducted with the greatest care, and resulted the same when others tried it. I have seen the diagnostic tracings of the "neurometer," showing the impressions made by the different potencies, and they are certainly very interesting.

The Central Verein is in full sympathy with the experiments, and offers pecuniary support.

W. Boericke, M.D.

EXTRACT OF A LETTER FROM DR. J. E. JAMES.

Luzerne, Switzerland, July 17th, 1880.

Dear Hahnemannian: The compliment tendered me by the Hahnemann Club, upon the eve of my departure from home, is ever fresh in my recollection, and it serves to remind me of the promise I made, to write to you during my absence. First let me say, that my health is very greatly improved; so much so, that I can look forward to the coming winter's work with a feeling of pleasure, and without that sense of weariness that used to come over me at even the thought of work. During my sojourn in England, I looked around me a good deal, and arrived at some conclusions, all of which I trust are fair, even though they may not all be flattering. One of these is that "Listerism," or the use of the antiseptic treatment, as applied to hospital wards, as well as to the patients, is a most fortunate and providential discovery. The long and continuous use of the wards of some of the old hospitals,—wards which are destitute of any efficient system of ventilation,—must naturally be attended with an increased number of cases of septic disease, and an augmented mortality ratio, unlesss some plan can be adopted to overcome the influence of a long-continued use, and the constant presence of a vitiated atmosphere. I have been able to observe instances of this unfavorable tendency in hospitals when the Carbolic spray was not employed. The wave of almost universal opinion in favor of the antiseptic treatment, is beginning, however, to react somewhat; and statistics and the individual experiences of those who are opposed to its universal use are beginning to come to the front. I have little doubt that soon we shall have an array of statistics, and an accumulation of individual observations sufficient to enable us to determine more or less exactly when the "Lister method" is to be regarded as a necessity, and when it may be safely and preferably omitted. But wherever the limit of its usefulness may be found, none the less credit will accrue to its discoverer, especially as he is still pursuing his investigations in the same field; his energies being at this time directed in search of the best possible methods of preparing carbolized gut, that it may not be too rapidly absorbed, nor yet remain sufficiently long to become an irritating foreign substance.

I enjoyed a most pleasant season with many of our brethren of London, and particularly with our old and beloved friend, Dr. A. C. Pope. From our other distinguished friend, Dr. Cooper, the readers of the HAHNEMANNIAN may expect some interesting letters, and some valuable papers bearing upon the treatment of diseases of the ear, and embracing facts and observations gleaned from his own large experience.

I find that the physicians here are looking with great interest upon the rapid growth and progress of homœopathy in America; and while some think we are running to extremes on the subject of symptoms, as against the "physiological action" of drugs, others approve of the methods we have so largely adopted, and all of them are agreed that the steadily increasing advance we are making is cause for universal congratulation.

Many of the homœopathic physicians of England, it seems

to me, are too well content with their present position. Recognizing that they are hemmed in, so to speak, by old customs and landmarks, at least as regards position in society and the chances of public medical preferment, they feel that it is almost useless to make any attempt to secure a change in this respect, at least while so few are coming over to their faith. Hence they go on the even tenor of their way contented; some indeed, even willing to practice in accordance with Hahnemann's law, while unwilling to assume the distinctive title of homœopathists, or in any efficient way to assist in pushing on the cause. There are, however, many faithful and honored men who are ever hard at work, and, as we in America well know, are making their influence favorably felt in the onward march of medical science.

At the annual meeting of the British Homœopathic Society, I had the honor to be present; but the attendance was not large, and the appointed paper failed them, yet a very interesting and profitable discussion took place upon the subject of whooping-cough and its treatment, in which every one present took part, and related personal experiences with the use of various remedies, and the indications for their employment. The address of the retiring President, Dr. Dudgeon, embraced a review of the work of the Society during the past year, with some allusions to the present position and prospects of homœopathy. The address was enjoyed by all present, but as it will doubtless be published, I need not attempt a synopsis of it here.

In Heidelberg I was a little amused to see a sign advertising the proprietor as both an allopathic and homœopathic pharmacist. A brief conversation with him revealed the fact that he was not a very ardent homœopathist, but kept a double shop because of the demand for our medicines. I was glad to find, however, that these latter were kept in a separate room.

There is among homœopathic physicians and pharmacists, but one general opinion regarding their transatlantic brethren. They are all looking to us for the perfecting of our grand system of therapeutics, and the full development and investigation of our medicinal resources, though they themselves are of course doing much to advance this essential work. Though recent "Lecturers" may delight to instruct us how the work is to be done, still all are looking at our own rapid progress under our peculiarly free institutions and forms, for the future of our noble science. The knowledge of this fact, while it adds to our responsibility, should be a stimulus to each of us to do his work well and in full proportion to his abilities and opportunities. No grander achievement could be expected from any one generation, than the purification of our voluminous Materia Medica, sufficiently to render the prescription of every physician a certainty where cure or relief is at all possible.

During my stay in England I observed one fact which impressed me deeply. We have in America our specialists, in every large city, who are the equals, in point of ability and success, of those of the old school. In recognition of this state of things, our governmental and municipal authorities are beginning to concede to us an equal share with them in all public appointments; and any refusal so to do is beginning to be regarded as bigotry of the most offensive kind, which cannot be much longer winked at. It seems to me that if our English brethren, acting in unison, and with a mutual understanding, should assert their claims as the equals or even the superiors of their opponents, not only in general medicine, but also in all the specialties of practice, they might back up their demands for an equal share in public appointments with a force and determination which must eventually insure success.

Another thought which impresses me is, that the homœopathic physicians on opposite sides of the Atlantic see too little of each other. If there could be a free interchange of views and experiences among them, it could hardly fail to exert a wholesome influence upon all. If members of our profession cannot come and go across the Atlantic so frequently as they might wish, there can at least be an increased amount of correspondence, and a wider circulation and interchange of our literature, and especially of our journals, which alone would increase the general stock of knowledge, and strengthen the hands of friendship.

I have for several days enjoyed the companionship of Dr. Pope and family, here, among the beautiful lakes and mighty mountains of Switzerland. Yours truly,

JOHN E. JAMES.

ON VENTILATION.—DEAR HAHNEMANNIAN: The *Medical Tribune*, in its issue of July 15th, referring to my paper on "Ventilation," in the June number of THE HAHNEMANNIAN, calls attention to an article which appeared several years ago in the *American Builder*, in which the same principle is suggested. Since my article was published, I have also learned that the method was patented, some years ago, by a Mr. Durant. So it seems that others, thinking upon the subject of ventilation, have naturally been led to the same conclusions as those urged in my paper. PEMBERTON DUDLEY.

THE

HAHNEMANNIAN MONTHLY.

A HOMŒOPATHIC JOURNAL OF

MEDICINE AND SURGERY.

Editors,

E. A. FARRINGTON, M.D. PEMBERTON DUDLEY, M.D.

Business Manager,

BUSHROD W. JAMES, M.D.

Vol. II. Philadelphia, Pa., September, 1880 No. 9.

☞ The Editors consider themselves responsible for the maintenance of the dignity and courtesy of the journal, but *not* for the opinions expressed by its contributors.

Editorial Department.

"DOES VIVISECTION PAY?"—We commend to our readers an article under the above title in the July number of Scribner's.

The author does not object to the killing of animals for scientific purposes, but protests against the inhuman custom of experimentations without an anæsthetic.

This barbarous method of class demonstration is becoming so prevalent as to demand the intervention of law-makers, as well as the merciful interference of humane societies.

One doctor quoted, coolly and cruelly replies to the question as to whether he had no feeling for his victims: "A man who conducts special research has no time, so to speak, for thinking what the animal will feel or suffer!" Another teaches that "it is not desirable to administer an anæsthetic" in such and such a case, lest it defeat the end in view. And still a third says, "It is much more satisfactory to divide the nerve without etherizing, *as the evidence of pain is an important guide in this delicate operation.*"

A very serious objection to vivisections is the fact that torture-born phenomena, are more often pathological than physiological. The vital domain resists the rude assaults of the experimenter and deceives him with its misinterpreted contortions.

Another still more serious objection, is the degrading influence of the practice. Human sympathy becomes, at first blunted, and then entirely perverted into cruelty. Cruelty, in its turn, whispers direful thoughts into the ambitious ear, suggesting the extension of the practice to *human vivisection.* Nothing but the fear of the law intervenes, and we are not sure but that the fiendish art is already growing under the cover of surgical operations. We do not refer to the legitimate employment of the knife, but to its use in the clandestine study of human physiology. Let the facts, however, be known or not, this is the trend of modern vivisection.

In a letter to the *Medical Record*, August 21st, 1880, Professor Burt G. Wilder suggests the division of vivisection into two classes. The first he would call "callisection;" the second, "sentisection." The former, or *hard*-section, includes all vivisections performed while the animal is under the influence of an anæsthetic; the latter, or *feeling*-section, embraces operations while the unfortunate subject of experimentation is fully conscious.

Whatever may be said of the choice of names for these classes, their division is practical and eminently humanitarian, provided the experimenter is not wanton in his sacrifices.

We cannot, however, subscribe to his concluding words, when he writes: "Sentisection should be the unwelcome prerogative of the very few whose natural and acquired powers of body and mind qualify them above others to determine what experiments should be done, to perform them properly, and to wisely interpret the results. Such men, deserving alike of the highest honor and the deepest pity, should exercise their solemn office not only unrestrained by law, but upheld by the general sentiment of the profession and the public."

Eclecticism.—He is the most popular man of the day, who adopts conservatism in all things, religious, social, and scientific. The man who rigidly adheres to his convictions, is termed radical, and is viewed as the pitiable victim of narrow-mindedness and bigotry. The world has grown to be eclectic, adopting as its plan, the selection of the good from all sources whatsoever. But alas for the sequel! The good is not found, nor can it ever be found, while the seeker deserts law and principle in his foolish search. Religious creeds are crumbling like deserted castles, no longer needed in the warfare of sects. Party lines in science are fading away. And many are gravely considering the union of medical schools upon the broad ground of liberty of thought and action.

But what is this liberty, which is to fraternize all mankind? Is it founded upon sound principles? On the contrary, it discards the narrow path of lawful demands. Laws, as universal as creation itself, are reduced to convenient methods of occasional service. Truths, mistaken for mere opinions, are sacrificed, and what is called liberty, is seen to be but lawlessness.

Eclecticism, in the sense we here employ the term, is no evidence of progress, but rather of decline. Our only safety is in a return to a faithful obedience to laws which have been made known to us. Whatever disputes them, however plausible it may seem, must be false.

Freedom of thought admits of the fullest expression of one's ideas. And though such ideas may be freely discussed, they should never be opposed in the same strenuous manner that violations of law demand.

Hahnemann announced the only known law of cure, but we are not therefore bound to accept also all the theories he propounded. His theory of the itch as a cause of chronic diseases, is insufficient; but the facts which he presents, and the law of consequences from suppression of skin symptoms, are true and ever will be true. Freedom of thought permits A. to differ from B., then, concerning the origin of psoric taint; but it does not extend to either one's denial of Hahnemann's facts, which are based upon the immutable law that disease must be removed from centre to periphery, from more to less vital parts. Calcarea carb. is an antipsoric, not only because it may redevelop and cure itch symptoms, but also because it may act similarly in any suppression of cutaneous disease, other things agreeing. And it possesses this effectiveness, not merely because it reproduces these symptoms, but because it acts surfaceward. Hence Hahnemann's law is indisputable, though his theory is too limited.

So with the grand law of similars; we may differ from its discoverer as to its modus operandi, but to deny it, or limit it in therapeutics, is, in the face of an accumulation of confirmations, inadmissible.

If, then, we would be true physicians, we must be firm advocates of LAW. But this forbids eclecticism. F.

A HINT TO PRECEPTORS AND STUDENTS.—One of the objects which the HAHNEMANNIAN MONTHLY keeps steadily in view, is to discourage the practice sometimes indulged in by homœopathic physicians, of sending their sons and students to allopathic colleges. Whatever may have been expedient ten, twenty, or thirty years ago, there is not *now* the slightest advantage to be gained by such a course, but on the contrary very serious disadvantages do and must result from it. Time was, perhaps, when the facilities for didactic and clinical teaching in allopathic schools were far better than those enjoyed in our own. But to-day it is not so. We now possess opportunities, of whatever kind, equal to theirs. Our clinics are as abundantly supplied, our means for illustrating didactic instruction are as complete, our professors and demonstrators as learned and skilful and experienced as theirs. In addition to all this, our teachers have an incentive to earnest and enthusiastic effort which theirs have not,—the desire and the hope to secure for our system the acknowledgment and support of all intelligent people the world over. This enthusiasm is nowhere more plainly seen and felt than in the lecture-rooms and laboratories of our colleges, and its fruits are apparent in the character, and learning, and skill of the men who are being sent out to carry our standard and promulgate our principles. These young men are going out equipped as the graduates of allopathic schools are not. And these observations apply to all our homœopathic, as set over against all the allopathic colleges.

The term of three years has been designated in the United States as the period necessary for a student to acquire a knowledge of medicine sufficient to enable him to commence medical practice without discredit to himself or his profession, or danger to his patients. When this term was adopted by each of the two schools of medicine, it was not deemed needlessly long for the study of *one* system; but it would have been considered far too short for the acquisition of *two.* It is not possible for any student, however brilliant, to acquire a practical knowledge of both systems in three years; no, nor in four. Whatever, therefore, he learns of one system, must add to his ignorance of the other. Let the homœopathic physician learn all he can of allopathy, of course, but let him not attempt to acquire it during the precious hours of his college career. He can learn all there is of it worth knowing, during the succeeding years, when his practical knowledge of disease and of its treatment shall have taught him how to estimate allopathic principles and methods at their real value, and when the leisure spent in acquiring that knowledge will not be at the cost of more valuable information.

Again, if the son or student of a homœopathist proposes to pursue a complete course and take his degree in an allopathic school, there is now a very serious obstacle in his way. According to the rules of the American Medical College Association, no student is to be allowed to graduate in these colleges unless his preceptor is a "regular (*i. e.*, allopathic) graduate or licentiate," and is also a "regular practitioner." Many a homœopathic student has heretofore avoided this difficulty by taking an allopathic preceptor during his collegiate course. *Now*, however, this plan will not avail him, for the rule requires that the student shall have "studied medicine for at least *three years under a regular practitioner*." (See Articles of Confederation, Section 2, Article III.) Nearly all (over thirty, at least) of the best allopathic schools of the United States have already signed these articles of confederation and *pledged themselves to enforce the above rule.* Homœopathic physicians and students who "lust for the flesh-pots of Egypt" will do well to look carefully into this matter before investing time and money in so doubtful a speculation.

These, then, are the three good reasons why a homœopathic student should not seek his education, in whole or in part, in an allopathic school.

1st. Because he can be as well educated in all the branches, and far better in some, in our homœopathic schools.

2d. Because all that he can learn of allopathy during his student life is so much detracted from his knowledge of homœopathy. He simply swaps off his chances of acquiring valuable knowledge to secure information which will be far less valuable, and with little likelihood of ever regaining what he has lost.

3d. Because at the end of his term of allopathic pupilage he is not hereafter to be allowed to graduate, but will be cheated out of his degree for having studied under a homœopathic preceptor.

"PROFESSIONAL DISHONESTY."—Some three months ago there died in Philadelphia a physician in the very prime of his young manhood, who gave unusual promise of future distinction in his profession. Although the son of a successful homœopathic physician, he studied and graduated in an allopathic institution, and afterwards, notwithstanding the force of parental example and early influence, he announced his adherence to, and accepted honors from, the allopathic school. He came to be regarded by his new-found professional friends as unusually successful in his treatment, and for an allopathist he undoubtedly was; a circumstance by no means astonishing, when the fact is known that a large proportion of his prescriptions bore a very suspicious flavor of homœopathy. Indeed it has been publicly stated in an allopathic journal, that he left some valuable papers upon the use of certain homœopathic remedies.

The editor of the allopathic journal above alluded to, speaks of having known this young physician "ever since he commenced the study of medicine, and watched his triumphant passage through the temptation to professional dishonesty." What the nature of that "temptation" may have been, the editor does not inform us, but from our knowledge of the circumstances we infer it to have been a natural tendency and impulse to *acknowledge* the basis of his homœopathic prescriptions, and the therapeutic law which suggested them. Such a course of conduct *has* been more than once spoken of as "professional dishonesty" by certain allopathic journals whose ideas of professional honesty seem to accord but imperfectly with those held by modern theologians, and by Christian people generally. The abstraction of certain passages, for instance, not to mention whole pages, from homœopathic works, carefully avoiding even the remotest allusion to their origin (see Ringer, Bartholow, Phillips, *et al.*) appears, in allopathic estimation, to be perfectly consonant with the teachings of an exalted morality, if not of a positive religious duty. Other people there are who hold that the eighth commandment protects the property of an opponent as well as that of a friend.

It is quite refreshing, this hot weather, to learn that men who hold such peculiar notions of professional obligations are suddenly beginning to inculcate the principles of professional morals, and to commend their fellows for overcoming the temptation to professional dishonesty. But alas! alas! we learn just a little further on, that this young M.D., whose untimely decease furnishes the occasion for this article, left behind him a series of papers on certain homœopathic remedies, and it is pretty strongly intimated, that if found practicable, these papers will be edited and published for the use and behoof of the allopathic profession. In view of this intimation, all their protestations of professional honesty remind one of Mr. Job Trotter's tears and of Mr. Samuel Weller's remark to that lachrymose gentleman : "Vot an uncommon nice boy you must ha' been to go to school vith."

The decease of the young physician above mentioned is in one respect a sad, sad loss to his allopathic friends. It had been their custom to assert that all homœopathic students educated in allopathic schools came out at the conclusion of their collegiate course with all the homœopathy knocked out of them. When asked to name a few score of such cases they put on their multiplying spectacles and pointed triumphantly at *him*. They seemed to imagine that there were some two or three hundreds of him. And what *will* they do now?

Book Department.

THE SURGERY, SURGICAL PATHOLOGY, AND SURGICAL ANATOMY OF THE FEMALE PELVIC ORGANS. In a series of plates taken from nature, with commentaries, notes, and cases. By Henry Savage, M.D., London, Fellow of the Royal College of Surgeons of England, one of the Consulting Medical Officers of the Samaritan Hospital for Women. Third Edition, revised and greatly extended. 32 plates and 22 wood engravings, with special illustrations of the operations on vesico-vaginal fistula, ovariotomy, and perineal operations. New York. William Wood & Co., 27 Great Jones Street. 1880. 8vo., pp. 129.

This is the sixth number which William Wood & Co. have issued this year in their *Library of Medical Authors;* and although it is not a large volume, yet it is one of the most interesting and valuable works of its kind yet published.

The plates are numerous, well selected, and well executed, and explain quite fully the surgical and general anatomy of the organs and parts that so frequently require surgical procedure at the hands of the gynæcologist.

The relations of all the various structures involved are beautifully brought out, even to the venous plexuses.

The question may be asked, Why be so minute in the anatomical detail of the venous system of this region? My own experience in cases of peritoneal hæmorrhage—which upon several occasions I have observed in post-mortem cases of females that have died suddenly, and where large quantities of coagula and blood have been found in the abdominal cavity—shows that in almost every case it was caused by venous erosion in the process of pathological changes involving the peritoneum in the pelvic region. To my mind there is great importance to be attached to dwelling so carefully upon this portion of his subject, as the author has taken the pains to do.

He reduces the nomenclature of these sanguineous effusions into pelvic-cellular and pelvic-peritoneal sanguineous extravasations; pelvic varices are subperitoneal, necessarily; but sanguineous extravasations frequently take place, and are found in the peritoneal cavity.

He claims that subperitoneal hæmatoma cannot assume a very large size, while a peritoneal hæmatoma may be quite extensive; and he illustrates his position by ten kinds of cases, from practice, as follows:

First. Sudden faintness at a ball; death in half an hour; pelvis full of blood from rupture of subovarian plexus.

Second. Long-standing venous varices in both legs, the right labium, and the vagina of same side; sudden faintness, prostration, pallor; immediate formation of a pelvic hæmatocele, which filled up the left iliac half of the pelvis, and rose to within an inch of the umbilicus; rupture of left subovarian venous plexus.

Third. Sensation of something giving way internally, followed by slowly increasing tumefaction in the lower part of the abdomen, which eventually entirely filled the latter to the navel. Rupture of sanguineous cysts of both ovaries. Some sanguineous effusion beneath the peritoneum.

Fourth. Sudden death at the commencement of a menstrual period, the menstrual fluid not having appeared externally. Intense congestion of genital organs, uterus the size and shape of a large pear. Firm adhesion between right tube and ovary. Rupture of left ovary. Two ounces of blood in the pelvic peritoneum. *The uterine cavity contained a little fluid blood, which when wiped away, may be quickly renewed by slight compression through innumerable vascular orifices.*

Fifth. Sudden cessation of menstruation after the use of the cold bath, followed immediately by the most acute abdominal pains, obstinate constipation, speedy death. Lower part of abdomen filled with blood. The right ovary transformed into a mass resembling a tough coagulum; both Fallopian tubes dilated.

Sixth. Sudden symptoms of peritonitis, with signs of internal hæmorrhage; death in thirty hours. Extensive peritoneal hæmatocele. Rupture of right ovary, enormously increased in size, in structure, and resembling the spleen.

Seventh. Sudden cessation of menstruation after local use of cold water, followed immediately by pain in the left hypogastrium, slowly progressive tumefaction of lower part of abdomen for eight months, then rapid distension of abdomen by ascitic effusion. Ovariotomy. Ovary transformed into a friable mass twice the size of a fœtal head, of a chocolate color, retained by its cortex, much attenuated; two cysts in the interior containing cheesy pus.

Eighth. Signs of peritonitis when in expectation of the menstrual discharge, which did not appear; death in seven days; enormous peritoneal hæmatocele; rupture of left Fallopian tube.

Ninth. Menorrhagia; uterine colic; soon after which, signs of internal hæmorrhage; death in twenty hours. Rupture of Fallopian tube, which was enlarged to the size of the finger.

Tenth. Abortion, with much uterine hæmorrhage; intense pain of abdomen; death in five days. Enormous peritoneal hæmatocele; both Fallopian tubes distended by clots, which projected from their peritoneal terminations.

He then says:

"The above forms of peritoneal hæmatocele are fairly attributed to the uterine system, but instances quite as conspicuous occur which do not admit of such a solution. Blood effusions from any point of the peritoneal surface would gravitate towards the pelvis, forming hæmatomas, presenting physical signs precisely the same as those attending the instances above quoted."

His diagrams show the latest operations for the radical cure of complete prolapsus uteri and lacerated perinæum, and also for vesico-vaginal fistula, and the removal of uterine tumors by gastrotomy. He also represents the various positions of the non-prolapsed uterus, and the relations of the pelvic organs resulting from a uterine prolapsus artificially induced

B. W. J.

MATERIA MEDICA AND THERAPEUTICS ARRANGED UPON A PHYSIOLOGICAL AND PATHOLOGICAL BASIS. By Charles J. Hempel, M.D. Third Edition, revised by the Author, and greatly enlarged by the addition of many new and valuable remedies, personal observations, and numerous clinical contributions from public and private sources, by H. R. Arndt, M.D. Vol. I. 780 pp.

The volume before us is a handsome, well-printed book of about 780 pages. As these excellent qualities at once strike the eye, it is but natural that they should claim recognition here at the start.

In regard to the substance of the work we may remark that it comprises one hundred remedies, alphabetically arranged, embracing the characteristics of each in various pathological conditions. There are numerous quotations from writers of all schools, especially from our own. Whatever may be the preferences of the editors, they have been quite impartial as to the sources whence they have drawn their materials. Clinical cases are given here and there, some of which consist of cures with the high potencies, and some with the low.

It is a question how far it is useful to reduce materia medica to therapeutics. And in reviewing the book before us we would feel like entering an objection to such an arrangement, were it not for a cautionary line in the preface, from the pen, we think, of Dr. Arndt: "To make the best use possible of this edition, it should be read side by side with a reliable work on symptomatology."

With these valuable words before us, then, we may safely advance to the perusal of the several remedies. We shall find each drug introduced with a short account of its history, origin, etc. Then follow its therapeutic applications, with notes and comments, including clinical cases.

Turning to Aconite we find it so fully treated that it occupies eighty-four pages! There are seven hundred and twenty pages of this volume devoted to one hundred drugs, and Aconite is favored with twelve times the average space of a little over seven pages per remedy! Even if we could grant, with Dr. Hempel, that Aconite is the backbone of our materia medica, such partiality is inadmissible in a work like the present. And, besides, it is a pernicious advice which recommends Aconite for so many forms of disease, some of which are entirely foreign to its true range of action, as scrofulous ulcers, adynamic fevers, cholera Asiatica, cancrum oris, stomacace, carbunculous inflammation, tuberculosis, etc. The totality of no one of these maladies compares with that of Aconite, and yet we read in the preface, "As truly as the totality of the symptoms indicates the remedy, so must we carefully study and analyze *all* there is said upon any one remedy." But the two editors may differ here. We hope they do.

Aside from this defect we may recommend the work of Drs. Hempel and Arndt as rich in accumulated facts, containing more than can be found in any other similar work. It is to the whole materia medica what Dr. Hale's books are to the "new remedies."

We should add, too, especially as it is rarely found in first volumes, that there is a copious clinical index. This useful addition renders the work very convenient for reference, and hence eminently practical.

We hope Vol. II will soon be forthcoming. F.

MANAGEMENT OF CHILDREN. By Annie M. Hale, M.D. Published by Presley Blakiston, Philadelphia. 110 pages.

This neat little brochure is written for mothers, but even sage physicians may learn from its practical hints and aphorisms. It comprises thirteen chapters, treating of food, sleep, dress, exercise, air, sunshine, indigestion, croup, etc.; accidents, aphorisms, and several "simple" formulas. The hints concerning dress, food, and exercise are excellent, as are also the remarks on the management of that troublesome accompaniment of babyhood, indigestion. The authoress is an ardent advocate of cleanliness, and insists on the bath. Sound and needful is her advice to give infants water to drink. We have been surprised at the ignorance of mothers in this respect, they thinking that the milk, being fluid, answers as a complete substitute for water. But in summer-time the child may need water, especially if the mother's milk is partially deprived of water by free perspiration.

Many of the trite sayings in the chapter on aphorisms are useful and true. We, however, object to the directions to keep the hair short in both boys and girls until the tenth year (girls).

This section closes with the remark that the common people of Italy are remarkable for beauty of face and symmetry of form. This has been attributed to the pre-natal influence upon the child by the constant presence before mothers, of the pictures of the great masters and the noble structures of antiquity.

We fully believe in the refining and beautifying effects of æsthetics, but we question if the commonalty of Italy possess such taste as the above selection would necessitate.

The chapter on "a few simple formulas" cannot, of course, meet our approbation. For, although the writer discountenances patent and other secret medicines and excessive drugging, nevertheless her recommendations of prescriptions containing Acid. carbolic. (gtt. iv.), Tr. op. camph. (ʒij), Bismuth. subnit. (ʒjss.), Morph. sulph. (gr. j), Quin. sulph. (ʒss.), etc., offends our idea of sanitary safety and legitimate medicine. E. A. F.

CARLSBAD AND ITS NATURAL HEALING AGENTS. By J. Kraus, M.D., with Introductory Notes by Rev. J. T. Walters, A.M. Second edition. London: Turner & Co., Ludgate Hill, 1880.

This neatly printed little book gives full information, topographical, historical, and physiological, concerning the famous springs of Carlsbad.

The analyses of the several springs show that these waters must be possessed of considerable medicinal power.

In view of the importance of the provings, which Dr. Allen has included in his *Encyclopædia*, we advise our readers to procure the Carlsbad salts, which the book under notice advertises. F.

PUBLICATIONS RECEIVED.—Laurie's Homœopathic Domestic Medicine, Twenty-fifth Edition; Laurie's Epitome of Domestic Medicine, Thirtieth Edition; Functional Nervous Diseases; Report of the Board of Health of Philadelphia for 1879; Fox's Illustrations of Skin Diseases; Bulkley's, The Skin in Health and Disease. All these will receive attention in our next issue.

Gleanings.

PODOPHYLLIN, exhibited in repeated small doses, has produced such a condition that the prover could not distinguish one food from another.—*Phila. Med. Times*, July 31st, 1880.

PHLEGMASIA ALBA DOLENS, so long as it remains hard, should never be treated with friction, lest a portion of the thrombus become detached and enter the circulation.—*N. Y. Med. Record*, July 31st, 1880.

SMALL-POX is common in the pigeons and poultry of Europe, and Hindoostan. Out of a dove-cote of 1000, scarcely 100 were unmarked. The poultry-yards of India have been frequently depopulated by it.—*Nat. Health Bulletin*, July 24th, 1880.

POISON FOR RATS AND MICE.—A mixture of one part precipitated barium carbonate, three parts barley flour, and sufficient water to make a mass, is rolled into pills, having the size of beans These are said to be fully as efficacious as Phosphorus pills, and decidedly cheaper.—*Chemist and Druggist*, July 15th, 1880.

TUBERCULOSIS can be transmitted from animal to animal, or from man to animal. Animals' milk sometimes transfers the disease. Cooking is an uncertain security, since flesh is so poor a conductor of heat, and tubercle may be boiled a quarter of an hour without losing its powers of infection. This, however, will admit of some qualifications.—*Nat. Health Bulletin*, July 24th, 1880.

REVOKING DIPLOMAS.—There should exist in every school the right to revoke a diploma, as well as to grant one.—*Homœopathic News*.

Why not authorize our courts of justice to annul a diploma for cause, and upon conviction; especially for gross incompetence, and the perpetration of professional crimes?

Tails in Man was the subject of an interesting study by Virchow and others. Sometimes such an appendage is merely a nævus pilosus. Ornstein, however, reports a case in which there was a genuine elongation from the coccygeal vertebræ. Hair, in considerable quantity, has several times been found upon the sacral region of new-born children, and Michel declares that human embryos always have a distinct tail. Greve, in 1878, reported the case of an infant, whose caudal appendage moved when pricked.—*Phila. Med. Times*, July 31st, 1880.

Vital Statistics of Rhode Island.—In Rhode Island, registration from 1854 to 1878 shows that the proportion of births to American parents is uniformly decreasing, while that from foreign parentage is increasing. Of the whole number of births, only 20 in a hundred were second births of the mother, and only 9 in a hundred were fifth births. There were 7 divorces in every one hundred marriages. Twins occurred once in about ninety-four births, while triplets appeared once in 6871 births.—*National Board of Health Bulletin*, July 3d, 1880.

Ozonwasser.—Ozone water, of English druggists, is the 1 per cent. solution of potassium permanganate.—*Hager.*

Ozonwasser (of Krebs, Kroll & Co., Berlin) contains no trace of ozone, but an extremely small proportion of the oxidation products of hydrogen, nitrogen, and chlorine, which results from the different modes of preparation, and cannot be estimated quantitatively. Hager and Dr. Alb. Kremer found hydroxl, R. Böttger, nitrous acid, Behrens (of Kiel), hypochlorous acid. The latter was probably prepared by treating with sulphuric acid, a potassium permanganate contaminated with perchlorate.—*Chemist and Druggist*, July 15th, 1880.

The Diagnosis of Incipient Phthisis is greatly aided by an examination of the larynx, the mucous membrane covering of which, and also that covering the pharynx, is of an ashy-gray color. The arytenoid cartilages become swollen and pear-shaped. These tumefactions are not œdematous. The loose, submucous tissue is largely infiltrated with a small-celled infiltration, with tendency to the formation of deposits with cheesy centres. Treatment with inhalations, so as to distend the air-cells, and remove the large swollen epithelial cells, which are in various stages of fatty degeneration, promise well. The yellow, viscid sputum soon becomes white and frothy.—Carl Seiler, M.D., in *Philadelphia Med. Times*, July 3d, 1880.

Transverse Depressions on the Nails.—Dr. James Sawyer, in a note to the editor of the *Lancet*, of April 3d, agrees with Dr. Duckworth, that "there is a rather more rapid formation of nail than that of two complete growths in a year." From his own observations, he should say that from three to four months are usually occupied in the passage of a furrow from the lunula to the end of the nail. These grooves are very common. They are sometimes to be seen on all the finger-nails: often they occur only on the thumb-nails. If a person's nails be free from transverse furrows, we may conclude, almost with absolute certainty, that he has not had a serious illness in the last three or four months. He has found three or four of these depressions, equidistant and parallel, on the thumb-nails of women who are the subjects of dysmenorrhœa,—a furrow marking each painful "period."—*Philadelphia Med. Times*, July 3d, 1880.

Hemanthus toxicarius; Order, Amaryllidaceæ, causes in cats drowsiness, weakness, tremors, heightened reflex irritability, impaired sensation, dilated pupils, dim vision, dry mouth, nausea, hurried and shallow breathing, free urination. In frogs the tetanic symptoms are much more marked. Experiments also seem to prove that the poison acts upon the cord.

The Hemanthus paralyzes the vagus and greatly weakens the intercardiac inhibitory apparatus, affecting the heart like Atropia.

In man the drug acts less poisonously, causing general weakness, delirium, dry mouth, increased urine, and, topically applied, dilated pupils.

It antagonizes the action of Muscaria on the heart.

Hemanthus, then, acts similarly to Atropia, Duboisia, Narcissa (from flowering bulk), Hyosc., and Stramon.—Dr. Ringer, *Archiv. of Med.*, June, 1880.

Dr. L. Wolf, of Philadelphia, gives in the *American Journal of Pharmacy*, some fresh hints on the preparation of koumys. Numerous varied experiments, some of them superintended by a Russian who had made koumys in his native country, all failed to produce just the right kind of beverage. Generally the result was sour milk, with a heavy curd, feeble effervescence, and repulsive taste. During a visit to the fermenting-room of a large brewery, the author was struck by the icy coldness of the air, and he was told that if the temperature were allowed to rise the fermentation would prove "wild," that is, acetous. On this hint he acted, with the best results, and the following is the formula he recommends:

Take of grape sugar ½ oz., dissolve in 4 oz. of water; in about 2 oz. of milk dissolve 20 grains of Fleischman's compressed yeast, or else well-washed and pressed-out brewer's yeast. Mix the two in a quart champagne bottle, which is to be filled to within two inches of the top; cork well and secure the cork with strings or a wire, and place in an ice-chest or cellar, at a temperature of 50° F. or less, and agitate three times a day. At the expiration of three or four days the koumys is ready for use, and should not then be kept longer than four or five days. It should be drawn off with a champagne tap.—*Chemist and Druggist*, July 15th, 1880.

The Right of the Insane to Liberty.—Dr. Seguin, the able editor of the *Archives of Medicine*, writing on this subject, quotes the following from Maudsley:

"The true principle to guide our practice should be this, that no one, sane or insane, should ever be entirely deprived of his liberty, unless for his own protection or for the protection of society."

In support of this view, the editor cites illustrative cases of different forms of mental disease, involving no danger either to the life of the patient nor to the lives and property of others. He considers that the holding of such persons under the restraint to which they are usually subjected in our asylums, is "a most singular form of tyranny for any enlightened state to permit to flourish. No matter how scientific or how good a man the superintendent may be, I hold that this degree of authority, of uncontrolled authority over the liberty of citizens ought not to be allowed." Pursuing this subject he expresses his opinions as follows:

"*a.* That a large number of the inmates of asylums could be taken care of with open doors and unbarred windows, and, of course, without restraining apparatus.

"*b.* That many insane now confined in our asylums could be trusted almost implicitly to come and go at will; could be given some nominally remunerative occupation, and above all could be provided with some simple amusement suited to their stations in life.

"*c.* The phases of insanity should be watched more closely with especial reference to early discharge of a patient, to his transfer to another institution, to the amount of liberty allowed him, etc. And I do not think it safe to leave this power wholly in the hands of the superintendent.

"*d.* That the time has come to look around, and attempt in this country, the English and Scotch plan of placing harmless insane persons singly in the families of farmers and of others willing to undertake the task, under frequent and efficient visitation."—*Archives of Medicine.*

News and Comments.

GONE, and almost forgotten,—Tanner.

THOUGH lost to sight, to memory dear,—Professor John Buchanan.

PROFESSOR J. E. JAMES, M.D., has returned from his European tour. His health is fully restored.

PHILADELPHIA contains about two hundred and sixty homœopathic physicians. Twenty years ago she had only about ninety.

REMOVAL.—J. N. Mitchell, M.D., of Philadelphia, has removed from No. 1313 Arch Street, to No. 1733 Chestnut Street.

PROFESSOR R. J. MCCLATCHEY, M.D., has almost entirely recovered from his long and severe illness, and has resumed his professional duties.

SETTLEMENTS—CLASS OF 1880.—L. D. Balliet, M.D., Gloucester City, N. J.; Isaac Crowther, M.D., Upland, Delaware County, Pa.; F. E. Caldwell, M.D., Fort Benton, Montana; Hugh Pitcairn, M.D., Harrisburg, Pa.

DR. J. C. GUERNSEY reports that, up to September 1st, he has printed four hundred pages on the *World's Convention* (1876), and two hundred and fifty pages on the 1879 volume, *Transactions of the American Institute*,—in all six hundred and fifty pages.

MISTAKEN CHARITY.—A physician of Massachusetts, lately deceased, left, it is said, an aggregate of $40,000 of bills receivable outstanding among his patients. He left directions that his poor patients were not to be asked for payment. Such benevolence (?) is not only a fraud upon his professional brethren, but is also a serious injury to public morals.

UNIVERSITY OF MICHIGAN.—Henry C. Allen, M.D., has been elected Professor of Materia Medica and Therapeutics in the above-named institution. Professor Allen was formerly Lecturer on Theory and Practice, and assistant to the chair of Professor Wilson. H. R. Arndt, M.D., editor of the *Medical Counselor*, has been appointed Lecturer on the Therapeutics of Gynæcology and Obstetrics.

PHILADELPHIA DIRECTORY OF HOMŒOPATHIC PHYSICIANS.—Our readers who have received the *Directory of Homœopathic Physicians of Philadelphia*, will confer a favor by immediately forwarding to Charles Mohr, M.D., No. 555 North Sixteenth Street, any additions, erasures, or alterations to be made in the list, as a second edition is about to be issued under the auspices of the Philadelphia County Society.

OMITTED.—The *Homœopathic News* calls attention to the omission, in our report of the sessions of the American Institute, of a paper entitled "The Improvements in the Science and Art of Obstetrics," by G. S. Walker, M.D., of St. Louis. The paper was carefully prepared, and interesting. We hope Dr. Walker will accept our apology for the omission, which was inadvertent, and the *News*, our thanks for directing our notice to it.

INFORMATION WANTED.—A correspondent wishes to know *in which* of "the Eastern States, the legislature and State societies have enacted prohibitory laws, fettering students' desires to go away from home for superior clinical instructions, and imposing a legal fine if they do so," as stated in the announcement of one of our Western colleges. Perhaps some one of our readers can give the desired information.

A Great Water Drinker.—A man named Thomas, who was charged at the Mansion House with being drunk and acting as an unlicensed driver of a hackney carriage, consumed no less than six gallons of water during the twenty-four hours he was in custody. Of this quantity, he drank three and a half gallons—two bucketsful—at the Seething Lane Police Station, and during the four hours he was waiting at the Mansion House, ten quart cans of water were supplied for his consumption.—*Chemist and Druggist*, July 15th, 1880.

"Collary Fantum."—Such is the "cause of death," as given recently in a certificate signed by one of Buchanan's graduates. We once saw a certificate from an equally distinguished source, in which the cause of death was set forth as "tipe-bod fever," and in another, signed by the pre-eminent Buchanan himself, the disease was "necrosis of bone." The dumfounded registrar, on reading it, exclaimed: "If he had only said 'necrosis of *dead* bone,' we should have known what he meant." But Philadelphia still shakes her metaphorical fist at any one who dares deny her claim to be "the centre of medical learning" in America.

Vivisection.—The memorial recently presented to Mr. Gladstone, urging him to do all in his power for the absolute abolition of vivisection, was signed by "one hundred representative men," among them Cardinal Manning, Prince Lucien Bonaparte, Alfred Tennyson, Robert Browning, James Anthony Froude, John Ruskin, the head masters of Rugby, Harrow, and seven other large schools, twenty-one physicians and surgeons, and thirty-seven peers, bishops, and members of Parliament. The memorialists take the ground that vivisection, even with anæsthetics, should by law no longer be allowed, and they quote the opinion of Sir William Fergusson, Sir Charles Bell, and Dr. Syme, that "it has been of no use at all, and has led to error as often as truth." They add that the utility, if proved, would not, in this case, excuse the immorality of the practice.

Women on the Board of Public Charities.—A movement has been begun by a number of distinguished ladies and gentlemen to secure the appointment of one or more women on the Board of Public Charities of Pennsylvania. The duties of the Board are to examine into the condition of charitable, reformatory or correctional institutions within the State, and to have an oversight of their methods of instruction, the government and management of their inmates, the official conduct of their officers, the condition of the buildings and grounds, with all other matters pertaining to their usefulness and good management, etc. In New York and Massachusetts, women have already been placed upon the Boards, and as in Pennsylvania the work of the commission affords so wide a field in which women could be eminently useful, there is little doubt that the movement will be successful.

Locations for Homœopathic Physicians.—Dr. Charles Mohr has received a letter from Dr. F. E. Caldwell, of Fort Benton, Montana, in which the writer says: "Some of our recent graduates may find good openings in Montana. There are a number of towns—small now, but destined to be large ones—in each of which a homœopathic physician could do well. In Helena, Bozeman, Butte, Bannock, Deer Lodge, and Sun River there are old-school physicians who do not amount to much, and only in Helena, one homœopath. These places are filling up very rapidly with a good class of families. Children are plenty, with flattering prospects of more. I will give any information I can to any one desiring it." Dr. B. L. Paine, of Lincoln, Neb., writes: "In Falls City, Nebraska, there is a splendid chance for a homœopath. The place contains 3000 inhabitants, of whom quite a large proportion have homœopathic proclivities. Have you a good man for the place?"

The Homœopathic Medical Society of the State of Pennsylvania will hold its 16th annual session in the parlors of the United States Hotel, Easton, Pa., on Wednesday and Thursday, September 8th and 9th, beginning at 10 o'clock, A.M. The recent meetings of this society have not been so well attended as they should have been, and it is earnestly suggested that we all endeavor to make the coming meeting a grand success in all respects. Philadelphia physicians need be away from home only two days, and we shall not be surprised to see a large delegation from our city.

"The regular summer excursion rates can be secured from all points on the Pennsylvania Central Railroad, buying excursion tickets to Delaware Water-Gap. The rates for the round trip will be: from Philadelphia, $4.40; Lancaster, $7.15; Harrisburg, $8.60; Pittsburg, $18.60. Mr. Hayden, proprietor of the United States Hotel, will entertain physicians, their families, and friends, at $2 per day. A complimentary dinner will be tendered the Society, by our venerable first Vice-President, Dr. Henry Detwiller, on the second day of the meeting."

Vaccination.—The following brief but truthful figures are taken from the report of the Board of Health of Philadelphia for 1872. They embrace the total of cases of variolous disease treated in the Municipal Hospital during the destructive epidemic which raged during the years 1871–1872.

	Admitted.	Died.	Per cent. of deaths.
Vaccinated cases—good cicatrices........	379	40	10.55
Vaccinated cases—fair cicatrices.........	170	21	12.35
Vaccinated cases—poor cicatrices.......	281	87	30.96
Total,................................	830	148	17.83
Unvaccinated cases............................	307	194	63.19

If there is any anti-vaccination fact or argument, that bears a feather's weight in the scale against the above simple statement, we have never yet met with it.

The Bogus Diploma Business.—It is probable that all our readers are already acquainted with the fact that the infamous business of selling medical diplomas to whoever will buy, without any pretence of regard for merit or qualification, has recently been pretty thoroughly broken up, so far as Philadelphia is concerned, at any rate. The notorious "Doctor" John Buchanan, the head and front of the diploma factory, has been driven to flight, or to suicide,—probably the former,—and a list of about nine thousand of his "graduates" has been published by the *Record*—the newspaper through whose exertions the vile traffic has been so effectually suppressed. For some years past, there have been whining inquiries heard in the newspapers, and on the streets, "Why the medical profession did not take steps to prevent the further sale of diplomas," as though this peculiar form of crime was not a proper subject for the constituted legal authorities to deal with. And when our State medical societies, allopathic and homœopathic, did ask for charters of incorporation, and for authority to suppress the practice of unlicensed quackery, our legislators thought proper to deny the request. Indeed the whole history of the bogus diploma business, in its relation to the legal powers of our State, has led to the suspicion that Buchanan or some one of his friends owned somebody high in authority, by that best of titles,—the right of purchase.

The real end, however, has not yet been reached. It remains for the legal authorities everywhere, to ferret out the holders of these bogus diplomas,—who are equally guilty with Buchanan himself,—and compel them to relinquish the practice of the profession they have disgraced. Fortunately, in some of the States this has already been done, and the example thus set will doubtless be speedily followed in other States

THE HOMŒOPATHIC MEDICAL SOCIETY OF THE COUNTY OF PHILADELPHIA.—About a year ago the Philadelphia County Society adopted the "bureau plan" of carrying on its work, and the success of that plan has been most gratifying. Since it went into operation, there have been several papers presented for consideration at each and every meeting. During the months of July and August, no meetings are held, but with the advent of autumn, the regular monthly gatherings of our practicing students of medicine will be resumed. The numerical attendance of physicians has steadily increased until it now reaches nearly or quite half a hundred. We hope to see this number doubled during the coming season. Let it be distinctly understood that physicians *not* on the bureaus, have an equal privilege of presenting papers relating to the various subjects under consideration.

The following is the programme for the coming year, so far as known:

September 2d (*not* 9th), Pædology. B. F. Betts, M.D., chairman.

October 14th, Surgery and Clinical Surgery. W. C. Goodno, M.D., chairman.

November 11th, Ophthalmology, Otology, and Laryngology. C. M. Thomas, M.D., chairman.

December 9th, Zymoses and Dermatology. C. R. Norton, M.D., chairman.

January 13th, Materia Medica, Pharmacy, and Provings. H. N. Martin, M.D., chairman.

February 10th, Clinical Medicine, Diagnosis, and Therapeutics. A. Korndörfer, M.D., chairman.

March 10th, Obstetrics and Gynæcology. J. N. Mitchell, M.D., chairman.

The Secretary is Charles Mohr, M.D., No. 555 North Sixteenth Street.

The meetings are held at the college, Filbert Street above Eleventh, at 8.30 to 10.30 P.M.

DR. TANNER'S FAST, as everybody knows, was persisted in to the close of his "forty days and forty nights," and was terminated by the ingestion of a mixed diet of peaches, melons, apples, wine, beef-steak, and milk, in open violation of all established rules and customs, and with the result of driving his medical advisers—and he had lots of them—to the extreme verge of insanity. Among the other effects may be mentioned the loss of Dr. Tanner's teeth. The experiment has excited a good deal of surprise and some distrust. It has forced physiologists to a modification of some old notions, but it has resulted in little, if any, practical good to mankind. One of the most prominent newspapers of the country, with consummate gravity, expressed the view that the experiment was worthless, because, forsooth, a certain distinguished New York doctor was not in charge of it; and intimated that only by the presence of some *eminent* physician could the doctor's test be guarded against a public suspicion of fraud. That newspaper is old enough to have learned ere this, that there are "eminent physicians" who have acquired their distinction only by a system of judicious lying, and that the testimony of comparatively unknown physicians is as reliable as that of the most distinguished, if not more so. It happens, however, that the men in charge of the experiment are widely known, and their honesty and competency are not questioned by anybody but toadies, ninnies, and rogues.

BUREAU OF GENERAL SANITARY SCIENCE, CLIMATOLOGY, AND HYGIENE.—For the next meeting of the American Institute of Homœopathy, the subject for discussion will be PERSONAL HYGIENE. The papers have been apportioned as follows:

I. Bushrod W. James, M.D., Philadelphia, Pa., Chairman; Progress of Sanitary affairs during the year; Introductory paper on Hygiene and Medication in General.

II. 1. D. H. Beckwith, M.D., Cleveland Ohio; Personal Hygiene as to the Air Breathed.

2. T. S. Verdi, M.D., Washington, D.C.; Personal Hygiene as to Dwellings Occupied.

3. W. H. Holcombe, M.D., New Orleans, Louisiana; Personal Hygiene as to Food Eaten.

4. T. P. Wilson, M.D., Ann Arbor, Michigan; Personal Hygiene as to Habits Formed.

5. E. U. Jones, M.D., Taunton, Massachusetts; Personal Hygiene as to Districts Inhabited.

6. George M. Ockford, M.D., Burlington, Vermont; Personal Hygiene as to Fluids Drank.

7. H. W. Taylor, M.D., Crawfordsville, Indiana; Personal Hygiene as to Business Followed.

8. Lucius D. Morse, M.D., Memphis, Tennessee; Personal Hygiene as to Clothing Worn.

THE HERING MEMORIAL.—PHILADELPHIA, August 14th, 1880: At a meeting of the homœopathic physicians of Philadelphia, held July 25th, 1880, in reference to the decease of Dr. Hering, the following resolution was adopted:

"That a memorial meeting be held in honor of the deceased, at which physicians from all parts of the world should be invited to participate, either in person or by letter."

The following committee was appointed to carry the resolution into effect: Drs. Ad. Lippe, Edward Bayard, William Wesselhœft, H. N. Guernsey, J. K. Lee.

On the 13th of August this committee met at the house of Dr. Ad. Lippe, and the following resolutions were adopted:

To call a memorial meeting of Dr. Hering, to be held in the city of Philadelphia, in the hall of the Hahnemann Medical College, on Sunday, October 10th, 1880, at 8 P.M.

To notify all the homœopathic journals of this memorial meeting, and ask them to so publish it.

To notify the friends of our school and of the deceased in all parts of the world of this proposed memorial meeting, to ask them to hold a memorial meeting on the same day, and forward the report of such meeting to this Committee for incorporation in a memorial volume to be published by the friends of the deceased. By order of the Committee,

AD. LIPPE, Chairman.

THE GUIDING SYMPTOMS.—The executors of the will of the late Constantine Hering, M D., have made arrangements for the publication of *The Guiding Symptoms*. Drs. C. G. Raue, C. B. Knerr, and C. Mohr, who had assisted Dr. Hering in publishing vols. 1 and 2, have been authorized to do the editorial work required on the remaining volumes, and at present are pushing volume 3 through the press as rapidly as is consistent with due care.

MARRIED.—CALDWELL—HORTON.—On Wednesday, August 25th, 1880, Frank E. Caldwell, M.D., of Fort Benton, Montana, to Anna Frances Horton, daughter of Mr. Orlo Horton, of Covert, New York.

THE

HAHNEMANNIAN MONTHLY.

Vol. II., New Series. Philadelphia, October, 1880. No. 10.

Original Department.

STUDIES IN MATERIA MEDICA.

BY E. A. FARRINGTON, M.D., PHILADELPHIA, PA.

ANIMAL KINGDOM.

(Continued from page 522.)

THROAT, LUNGS, HEART.

LACHESIS.—Dryness of the mouth and throat; he awakens choking; can hardly breathe until the dry, shining throat is moistened.

Throat and larynx painful to touch, or when the head is moved.

Pains: Left side of throat to tongue, jaw, ear; rawness and swelling, feels ulcerated, burning; feeling as of a crumb of bread sticking; as from a plug; throat sensitive as if sore from taking cold, with pain in the left side in the evening.

Swallowing: Eating relieves the pain in the throat; liquids cause more difficulty than solids, drinks return through the nose; empty swallowing causes constant pain, food does not. After chewing his food he cannot get it down, because it rests on the back part of the tongue, causing a thrilling there. Deglutition causes a pressure as if a lump was sticking in the throat; causes sharp pain extending into the ear; throat feels ulcerated; throat feels swollen as if two lumps as large as the fist came together; only on empty swallowing.

Sore throat, with deafness; typhoid fever.

Hawking of mucus with rawness, after a nap in the daytime.

Feeling of hollowness as if the pharynx had disappeared.

Throat inflamed, tonsils enlarged; disease travels from left to right. Velum and pharynx inflamed. Mucous membrane looks dark red or purplish, and often has a dull dry appearance. Diphtheritic deposits, spreading from left to right; fetid odor from the mouth. Great debility, especially noticed in cardiac symptoms, such as feeble pulse, cool limbs, fainting; inflammation assumes a malignant type; glands enlarge; cellular tissue of the neck swells and looks blue, with burning; tongue coated thinly white, shading into thick yellow towards the root.

Tonsils enlarged; he hawks up oily whitish lumps.

Ulcers in the throat, extending up into the posterior nares. They often cause a teasing, tickling cough.

Uvula elongated; parts look purplish.

With all the throat and laryngeal symptoms there are intolerance of the least touch or pressure upon the neck; must loosen the clothing; spasmodic contractions, which arouse from sleep or develop as he awakes. Touch provokes them anew. Spasms of the glottis; suddenly something runs from neck to larynx, awakening him and stopping the breathing. Disposition to frequent return of angina of throat.

Feels as if a piece of dry skin was in the pharynx.

Audible beating of the carotids; sometimes they beat slowly.

Larynx: Swollen, sore, raw, scraping; somewhat also when pressing on it; obliged to swallow. Throbbing, narrow sensation, very painful to touch; sensation of a plug, which moves up and down, with short cough; sensation as of something fluttering.

Pain in the pit of the throat, extending to the root of the tongue and into the hyoid and to the left tragus, behind which it shoots out, painful to touch.

Hoarseness, worse evenings; something in the larynx prevents speech, which cannot be hawked up, though mucus is brought up.

Cough: Dry, spasmodic, hacking, tickling. Caused by pressure on the larynx, throwing the head back, eating, drinking, smoke, as from tobacco; ulcers in throat; a tickling in the throat, under sternum or in stomach; heart diseases. Worse after sleep, during sleep without awakening him, from change of temperature, alcoholic drinks, mental emotions, getting wet through, riding in the wind (tickling in left side of larynx caused cough). At every cough, stitch in the hæmorrhoidal tumors.

Expectoration: Mucus and blood as in heart disease, blood

streaked, thick, yellow, as in phthisis pulmonalis; grayish lumps, dislodged with difficulty; a watery, scanty sputum, mixed with mucous lumps; the effort causes vomiting and pain, compelling him to hold the stomach, worse after sleep, after talking.

Breathing: Loud rattling, dyspnœic upon any exertion, in suffocative attacks, arousing from sleep; suffocative feeling during the heat, must loosen clothes about the neck, feels as if they hindered circulation; fits of suffocation, must sit up in bed; constantly obliged to take a deep breath, especially while sitting; shortness of breath, with many affections, difficult and so weak he faints, worse moving around.

Chest so tight evening, after lying down, almost suffocated.

Oppression of the chest, with cold feet; also during sleep. Pressure on the chest as if full of wind; this seems to rise up into the chest; better from eructation.

Constriction of the chest, it feels stuffed.

Stitches in the left chest, with difficult breathing, worse when coughing or on inspiration.

Soreness in the chest and of the sternum.

Burning in the chest at night, with pains in the sternum or deep in the chest.

Hepatization, especially of the left lung; great dyspnœa on waking, heart weak.

Deposition of tubercle after pneumonia, symptoms agreeing.

Purulent dissolution of hepatized lung.

Threatened gangrene of the lungs.

Œdema pulmonum, hydrothorax, etc., when the characteristic respiratory and laryngeal symptoms are present. Better lying on the left side.

Heart: Feels constricted, cramplike pain in the præcordia, causing palpitation, with anxiety.

Feels the beating of the heart, with weakness even to sinking down.

Palpitation: Causing anxiety, fluttering, with weakness to fainting, with nausea and weakness at the stomach, with choking, caused by suppressing old ulcers.

Pressure as if from the stomach or during fever.

Irregular beat of the heart, every intermission accompanied by a strange feeling; sensation as if the circulation were restored by crying a little.

Spasmodic affections of the heart, with a feeling as if the ear-drums would burst.

Cyanosis, with suffocating fits when moving.

Heart feels as if too large; can bear nothing to touch throat or chest; must sit up, slightly bent forwards; aroused suddenly, during acute rheumatism, with smothering and oppression at the heart and palpitation; great anguish; left arm numb; stiff shoulders on taking a deep breath or upon turning to the right side.

Spasmodic pain about the heart.

All the Ophidians affect the throat and cause constriction, dryness, impeded deglutition, hoarseness, sensitive larynx, dyspnœa, cough, blood-spitting; oppression of the chest; palpitation of the heart, with anxiety, etc.

CROTALUS and NAJA, like LACHESIS, have relieved in diphtheria. The former has been selected when the epistaxis is persistent; blood oozes from the mouth, not merely coming from the posterior nares, but escaping from the mucous membrane of the buccal cavity.

NAJA has helped in cases just like LACHESIS, when the larynx is invaded, grasps at the throat, with sensation of choking, fauces dark red, fetid breath, short hoarse cough, with raw feeling in larynx and upper part of trachea.

Vipera torva causes violent chest pains, with chilliness; chest swells, with difficulty of breathing; violent congestion to the chest; he tears his clothes open, with sick sensation in the abdomen; cardiac anguish; upper extremities numb and lame.

In heart affections, LACHESIS suits more accurately the incipiency of rheumatic carditis; NAJA, the after-effects. The last causes a tumultuous fluttering action of the heart; cannot lie on the left side, but great relief lying on right side; nervousness, pain at the heart; sensation as if a hot iron had been run into the chest; temporo-frontal headache, with great depression of spirits. Cardiac cough is prominent in both. NAJA also has palpitation, with crampy pains in the left ovary.

ELAPS causes a constriction of pharynx and œsophagus; liquids are suddenly arrested, and then fall heavily into the stomach, as does also food. It seems as if the spasm suddenly gave way, leaving an opposite, paretic condition. Spasmodic stricture of the œsophagus is found also in LACHESIS and NAJA if not in Crotalus; but if the paretic effect is confirmed, it will help to differentiate; for although not contrary to the genius of the others, it has not yet been recorded for them.

In chest affections, ELAPS is of great service. It, however, affects more the right than the left lung, in which the morning pain is severe enough to prevent the patient's getting up.

Both apices are diseased. There is a feeling of coldness in the chest after drinking. The cough is accompanied with intense pains in the chest, worse in the right apex, as if it were torn out, and the sputum consists of black blood. It also causes a sensation as if the heart was being squeezed. Rush of blood to chest and throat.

Related Remedies.—Mouth and throat dry: Alumina, *Arsenic*,—BELLAD., with moist tongue, or with feeling of a skin on tongue, Bryonia,—Hyosc., burning and dryness of tongue and lips; they look like singed leather—*Cinnabar*, mouth and throat must be moistened every time he awakes; much mucus comes down from the posterior nares; bridge of nose feels as if pressed by a metallic substance. Caustic. Hepar; Kali bich.; Kali carb., evenings without thirst. Lauroc.; *Lycopod.; Mercur.*, palate dry as from heat. *Nux mosch., Natr. mur.; Nux vom.;* Opium, PHOSPH.; Phos. ac.; Plumb.; Rhus tox.; Secale c.; Silica; *Stram.;* Sulph.; Verat. alb., *Wyethia*, etc.

Hoarseness with those who talk much: Lachesis and PHOSPH., Calc. ost., CARB. VEG.

Larynx painful to touch: PHOSPH., *Bellad., Apis, Spongia, Hepar*, Chin. sulph., Bromine, Baryta c. (throat), Bry. (throat), Iod. (pressure on larynx).

Feeling of rawness in throat: Alumina, C. VEG., CAUST., Ignat., *Lyçop.*, MERCUR., *Nitric ac.*, Nux vom., *Phosph.*, etc.

Feeling of a crumb, splinter, etc.: Alumina, Arg. nitric., Canth., HEPAR, Ignat., Kali c., *Merc.*, NIT. AC., Rhus tox.

Feeling of a lump or plug: Alumina, Apis, Arsenic, Baryta c., *Bellad.*, Caust., Carbo v., *Hep.*, Hyosc., *Ignat.*, Kali bich., Kali carb., Kreos., Lycop., Mercur., Nitric ac., *Nux vom.*, Phos. ac., Phytolac., Sepia, Sulph., etc.

Feeling of something rising up like globus hystericus: ASAF., Con., IGNAT., Lycopod., Mercur., *Mosch.*, Nitric ac., Nux mosch., Plumbum, Spig., Sulph., etc.

Worse empty swallowing or swallowing saliva: Baryta c., Bellad., *Bryon., Cocc., Hep.*, Lycop., *Mercur.*, Mercur. corros., *Pulsat., Rhus tox.*

Fluids return through the nose: BELLAD., *Lycopod.*, Aurum, Canth., Cupr., Ignat., Mercur., Phosph., Silica.

Better from swallowing food: Mangan., Ignat.

Pharynx feels hollow: *Phytolac.*, Cinchona.

Ulcers in the throat: Alumina, *Apis, Arg. nit., Arsenic*, Baptis., Carbo v., Hepar, Ignat., Iod., KALI BICH., LYCOP.,

MERCUR., *Merc. corros.*, MERC. CYAN., *Mur. ac.*, NITRIC AC., Phos. ac., Sanguin., etc.

Tonsils suppurate: *Ammon. mur.*, BARYTA C., Bellad., Canth., HEPAR, *Ignat.*, *Lycop.*, MERCUR., *Merc. corros.*, *Phytolac.*, Sabad., SILICA, SULPH.

Hawks up cheesy, oily lumps from follicles in tonsils: Chenop., *Hepar*, *Merc. iod.*

Gangrene of the throat, in addition to LACHESIS: ARSENIC, Bellad., *Silica*, *Conium*, *Kreos.*, *Carbo veg.*, etc. Disposition to frequent return of angina faucium: BARYTA CARB., *Sepia*, *Lycopod.*, SULPH. Uvula elongated: Alum, Alumin., Capsic., Cinchon., HYOSC., Iod., Kali bich., Kali c., Lycopod., Mercur., Phosph., Silica, Sulph.

Diphtheritic deposit: Ailanthus, *Apis*, *Arsenic*, BAPTISIA, Ignat., *Kali bich.*, LYCOPOD., LAC CAN., MERC. CYAN., *Merc. bijod.*, *Merc. proto-jod.*, Mur. ac., *Nitric ac.*, *Phytolac.*, Rhus tox., Sul. ac.

Spasmodic stricture of the œsophagus: Alumin., Arsenic, Arg. nitric., Baptis., BELLAD., Bryon., *Carbo veg.*, Cicuta, Coccul., Hydrophob., Hydroc. ac., Hyosc., Ignat., Kali bich., Kali c., *Naja*, Natr. m., Nit. ac., PHOS., Plumb., Verat. vir.

Throbbing of the carotids: BELLAD., Phosph., etc.

Spasmus glottidis: CHLORINE, *Cupr.*, *Iod.*, Mephitis, *Bromide of camphor*, PLUMB., *Bellad.*, etc.

Dyspnœa on going to sleep or arousing from sleep: *Arsenic*, *Sepia*, *Sulph.*, *Grindelia*, SAMBUC., *C. veg.*; Cough until phlegm is raised, especially *Apis*.

Cardiac cough, especially LAUROC.

Oppression of chest, as if full of wind: C. veg., Cinchon., Lycopod., Sulph., Zinc, etc.

Neglected or badly-treated pneumonia, especially Sulph., LYCOPOD.

Œdema pulmonum; hydrothorax: Ant. tart., Ammon. carb., Apoc. cann., APIS, ARSENIC, Asparagus, C. veg., *Digital.*, *Kali c.*, Kali hyd., Lactüca, LYC., Merc. sul., *Phos.*, Sulph.

Gangrene of lungs: *Arsenic*, *Carbo a.*, *C. veg.* *Cinchon.*, *Kreos.*, Osmium, Secale c.

Heart feels constricted: Arnica, Bufo, Justitia, Kali c., Kali chlor., Lycopus, Cadmium, etc.

Left arm numb, in heart-affections, especially RHUS TOX.

Awakes smothering, with heart-disease, organic or not: ARS., *Digital.*, Grindelia, Kali hyd., Lactuca, Merc. præc. rub.

Cyanosis: Ant. tart. LAUROC., Aconite, *Secale c.*, *Digital.*, *Camph.*, *Op.*, *Cupr.*, Verat. alb.

Heart feels too large, Sulph.
Rheumatism attacks the heart: Apis, ARSENIC, *Bryonia*, *Digital.*, *Kali c.*, Phos., SPIG., Kalmia, Sanguin., Rhus tox.

CARE OF THE MOUTH AND TEETH IN INFANCY AND CHILDHOOD.

BY CHARLES MOHR, M D., PHILADELPHIA, PA.

(Read before the Philadelphia County Homœopathic Medical Society.)

THE subject I here introduce, certainly commands our most serious consideration; not to be given at this hour alone, but during the whole course of our career as physicians. This essay is by no means exhaustive of the subject, but only suggestive, and if it will but open up to us some avenues of thought, which, finally developed, shall be the means of promoting perfect "dentures," we shall be abundantly satisfied.

What is more beautiful and rare than a clean mouth, with thirty-two sound teeth? What is more common than an unclean mouth, with, frequently, no teeth at all? And, for this state of affairs, who is so much to blame as the physician? True, there is a widespread neglect of the mouth and teeth, on the part of parents, but only, I think, because the family doctor does not give timely directions to secure the necessary attention. Later in life the dentist's aid is sought, but all his skill,—and the skill of the American dentist is something of which Americans may well be proud,—is not such as to produce a denture as good as a natural one; his effort to secure comfort, usefulness, and durability (and even the harmony of expression demanded by æsthetics), is in most cases successful, but still, "the best set of artificial teeth that ever was made is so far inferior to an average natural denture, that the two can only be contrasted, not compared."—(J. W. White, D.D.S.)

That the mouth is an expressive and characteristic feature, the teeth maintaining a natural symmetry of the face, you need not be reminded; but, let us for a moment consider what the mouth involves. What portion of the human organism has a more complex structure? Think of its wonderful combination of bones, muscles, arteries, veins, nerves, glands, and membranes. What organ, physiologically, has such diversified functions? Think of gustation, of mastication, of insalivation, and of deglutition! Let us also remember what service the mouth renders in speech and song, and how the teeth, as conservators of the lungs and organs of voice, prevent the breath in speaking or singing from being exhausted too rapidly. Let us bear in mind the direct relation, by continuity of its lining mucous membrane, with the pharynx, œsophagus, stomach, and bowels, as well as with the larynx, trachea, and bronchi; and of its relation by contiguity, as well as by continuity, to the ears, eyes, and nose; and finally, of its relations to all parts of the body, by the nerves.

Physicians know all this, but laymen, as a rule, are ignorant of it. Until teeth decay and ache and are lost, little attention is given by the latter till it is too late to prevent,—the only thing left is to repair, and repair is often a difficult matter. Repair not only requires a careful dentist, but an observing physician. What is to be accomplished? Symmetry of form must be restored; vocalization must be improved; pain must be relieved; dyspepsia and headache, and sometimes protracted derangements of sight and hearing must be cured. The reflex nervous phenomena are legion, and before we pronounce a not well-understood neurological case, "neurasthenia," let the mouth, teeth, and their connections be carefully examined for a possible explanation of symptoms.

Very many of all these troubles may be avoided if the physician will conscientiously do his duty. Remembering that the tooth-pulps are distinguishable in the jaws as early as the seventh week of fetal life; that at the tenth week, the germs of all the temporary teeth are in position; that at the fourth month, the germs of the permanent teeth are already distinguishable; and that, at birth, the jaws contain the deciduous teeth all in a forward state, and the germs of twenty-four of the permanent set in various stages of development, he need not be reminded that much can be done to avoid future mischief, if the child is treated in utero. It is known that medicines given to the pregnant woman will act on the fœtus. If, then, the history of the father or mother, or of former children, shows faulty dentures, the homœopathic medicine, administered to the mother, will correct all abnormalities, and we may have a reasonable hope that, all other things being equal, the child will be born with a fair show for a normal mouth.

I have had some experience in this line, and I speak with certainty. My success has been largely due to the aid furnished by a repertory, published in 1851, by Carl Mohr, of Eisleben, Germany. The title of the book is *Specielles Repertorium der Symptome bei den Zahnkrankheiten, mit Angabe der Homœopatischen Heilmittel*, which I am at present engaged in translating and enlarging, and at no very remote period I hope to be able to place before the English-reading profession a work on the homœopathic treatment of the diseases of the mouth and teeth, that shall assist materially in combating a formidable array of annoying, and ofttimes dangerous affections.

After the birth of the child, the mouth requires careful attention. One of the first things to do is to examine for tongue-tie, cleft palate, or other abnormal development, and to give a few teaspoonsful of cold water, in order to see that the child swallows well, and to begin to teach it to like water as a beverage. If the mouth is kept clean, it will, as a rule, remain healthy, much to the advantage of the teeth to be erupted. The mouth should be washed with cold water several times daily, and each time this is done let the infant swallow a teaspoonful of water; but if, notwithstanding this treatment, sore mouth ensues, besides treating the mother's nipples, if necessary, employ water quite warm for the mouth-wash, or cold water alcoholized. The indicated remedy should be given internally. The usual ones are well known to you, but I desire in this place to call attention to *Kali brom.*, a remedy that is probably as often indicated as the much-abused Borax. In colicky babies, when the intestines under the examining hand seem to roll up into a ball, that can be moved about the abdomen; constipation or diarrhœa, or no special bowel trouble existing; the mouth hot and covered with aphthæ, or thrush, and swallowing liquids causes choking, *Kali brom.* will cure speedily. In cholera infantum with similar symptoms this remedy has proved very efficient. Feeding has very much to do with a healthy mouth. There is such an interdependence between the alimentary canal and the mouth, that if stomach or bowel indigestion results from bad feeding, the mouth is certain to suffer sooner or later. Until after the eruption of the first incisor teeth, the mother's milk is all that is necessary in the way of aliment, excepting cold water, and until the ninth month even, *milk* should be the exclusive diet, except in some special cases.

From the very outset the bad habit of thumb and finger-sucking should be discountenanced. It will certainly result in deformity of the upper jaw.

I need not here give the order of eruption of the teeth. With this every physician is familiar, but he should keep the mother posted, and explain to her, as dentition advances, how the teeth support each other, like the staves of a cask, and how each tooth is met by portions of the surfaces of two teeth. This latter arrangement is a wise provision of nature, so that if a tooth is lost in either jaw, the antagonistic tooth is not rendered useless. And just here it would be well to ask, ought not we, with our God-given intelligence, which enables us to reason, direct, and control, be very zealous in preventing any thwarting of nature's designs? Tooth after tooth is extracted, irrespective of the anatomical arrangement, and in time the grinding surfaces of a whole set is destroyed, much to the detriment of the general health. This is too often the case, and sheer ignorance is the cause. Every deciduous tooth should be retained as long as possible for reasons already intimated, but also because each one exerts some power in the development of the jaw to provide room for the permanent denture. How often does an infringement of this rule occasion the loss of crowded-out permanent teeth, sound in every respect, but destroying the line of the two arches.

While many mothers are careful to keep the mouth of the infant at the breast clean, they think it of no import when the teeth have put in an appearance and the child is weaned. As long as the child is too young to clean its own teeth, it should be done by the mother. A soft linen, wetted and soaped with old Castile soap, must be used every morning, and at evening, before putting the child to bed, the teeth should be carefully cleansed with precipitated chalk, to which a small quantity of the finest sugar of milk has been added, applied with a moistened rag. This will afford so much comfort, that when the child is old enough to cleanse its own mouth, it will never neglect to do so. Then a soft tooth-brush, with long elastic and uneven bristles, may be given it, with directions as to its proper use. From the very beginning prohibit *scrubbing*, so common with adults, who erroneously think the harder the brush, and the more vigorous the application, the better. Teach care, and patience, and gentleness. As dentifrices, old Castile soap for the morning, *Creta præcip. cum sacc. lact.* for the evening, may still be employed. Have the child taught to brush the upper teeth, on both labial and lingual sides downward, and the lower teeth upward, thus preventing the pushing of the gums away from the neck of the teeth. The articulating faces of the teeth must be carefully brushed from side to side, backward and forward, so as to insure a removal of every foreign particle from the depression of the bicuspids; and the same rule will hold good later in life, when the depressions and fissures found in the grinding surfaces of the molars, need the most careful attention to avoid discoloration and decay. A careful rinsing of the mouth after each meal is all that is necessary, if the above rules for the morning and evening cleansing are carried out. This care is not only preventive of caries, but conduces to a healthy condition of the gums and tooth-sockets, by preventing sponginess and recession of the gums, and absorption of the alveolar processes.

About the sixth year, when the first molars are erupted, especial care must be given. Most people suppose them to belong to the milk teeth, and they are generally sacrificed by neglect; being more liable to decay than any of the permanent set, arising from the fact that frequently there is a non-union of the enamel edges, the dentine being thus exposed to the action of acids and decomposing food, these sixth year molars should be examined by a dentist as soon as erupted, and if the dentine is exposed through a fissure, should at once be filled.

It will do no harm to repeat that the deciduous teeth must be retained as long as possible, not only for the part they play in the development of the jaws, but also for the reason that the more healthy they are kept, the more healthy will be the succeeding teeth. Acidity of the mouth must be corrected; if not produced by uncleanness, look to the stomach. Tartar, if it has accumulated and made inroads on the integrity of the structures, must be carefully removed by a dentist, and the cause of its generation be sought, so that the needed remedy can be duly applied. Carious teeth must be carefully cut out and filled. For the deciduous teeth, expensive gold fillings need not be used. The judicious dentist can supply cheaper, but good, fillings.

During the active teething process, careful feeding will be of inestimable benefit. Milk may still be given abundantly; but cracked wheat, oatmeal, and especially lentils, will be needed. These supply the earthy materials of which the teeth are constructed. Of lentils I can speak in the highest terms. Like other leguminosæ, they are difficult of digestion unless properly prepared and cooked. They should be soaked in cold water twelve hours before putting on to boil, and then boiled long enough to become thoroughly softened. Dressed with butter and salt they make a very palatable dish. Lentil flour may be used, made into a soup, when it is a good substitute for beef tea. I have had pregnant women, and women who were nursing infants, fed on lentils, with the effect to produce in the offspring, sound teeth, though all the previous children suffered with carious deciduous and permanent teeth very early in life.

I have said the deciduous teeth must be allowed to remain

in the jaws as long as possible, yet occasionally, extraction of a tooth becomes necessary, and if for any reason a dentist cannot be had to perform the operation, the medical practitioner should know how to do this. The indications for the extraction of temporary teeth are as follows: (1.) When a tooth of replacement is about to emerge from the gums, or has actually made its appearance, either before or behind the corresponding milk teeth. (2.) When the aperture formed by the loss of a temporary tooth is so narrow as to prevent the permanent tooth from acquiring its proper position without the removal of an adjoining temporary tooth. (3.) When dead teeth act as irritants, or have become so loose as to be annoying. (4.) Alveolar abscess, necrosis of the walls of the alveolus, and incurable pain in a temporary tooth.

Two sets of forceps should be among the instruments of the physician: one set (two) adapted for the incisors and cuspids, and one set (two) for the bicuspids and molars. An ordinary, strong, straight forceps may be added, and in most cases these will suffice. I have seen physicians endeavor to remove teeth in children with the ordinary dressing forceps found in surgical pocket cases, much to the annoyance of the child. "What is worth doing at all is worth doing well," and therefore the proper instrument should be employed. The claw of the forceps is usually sharp enough to separate the gum from the neck of the tooth; if not, detach the gum and operate as follows: Grasp the tooth to be extracted firmly at the alveolar edge, but do not compress the handles of the forceps too much, and move the tooth outwards and inwards, in quick succession, until it is loosened, and then draw it from the socket in a line with its normal axis.

Scoring of the gums is, I think, never necessary, but lancing may be. In saying this, I am aware that I may be treading on dangerous ground, but I do not wish to be misunderstood; I do not recommend lancing as a rule. The Hahnemannian has a horror of the knife, and well he may, since homœopathy has replaced the lancet with Aconite. But cases do arise when neither Aconite, nor any other medicine, can do so much good as the knife in the hands of the skilled and intelligent surgeon; and this is sometimes true in cases of faulty dentition. Quite recently I had a case in point. A boy, æt. ten months, was brought to me from out of town. For two months he had been suffering with pain, evidently in the mouth, associated with fever, restlessness, crying or screaming out in sleep, alternate constipation and diarrhœa. His head was abnormally large, and though hydrocephalus had been diagnosed, there was no bulging of the fontanel nor any separation of sutures. The prognosis of the attending physicians was not very encouraging. Latterly he had had treatment from a homœopathist, but notwithstanding, the child grew worse. At the time I saw him the symptoms were not clearly defined for any remedy, in my judgment, though *Belladonna* seemed the nearest similar; but I could not trust it in so grave a case, as it had been prescribed, both low and high, by my predecessor. On examining the mouth I found the upper gums very much tumefied and extremely sensitive. Over the advancing incisor teeth the gums were tense, shining, seeming almost cartilaginous in color and hardness. This condition had been noticed by the mother, and for days the boy was peevish and fretful, requiring to be carried about or rocked constantly, and on two days prior to consulting me he had several convulsions. I might have given *Chamomilla,* or perhaps, *Dolichos,* often useful in these conditions, and I doubted whether the latter had been prescribed, but I dared not depend on it, as the child was to be taken sixty miles away, and could not be seen again for a couple of days. I concluded, therefore, to lance the gums over the incisor teeth, and did so, and before the child left my office he smiled for the first time for weeks, and that night, as I learned afterwards by letter, slept well, and there has been no more trouble up to the present time. The lancet was the remedy for that case. No medicine could have done the work more speedily or more safely. I believe if this boy had received homœopathic treatment during the earliest manifestations of illness the knife would not have been needed.

Allopathic medication has much to answer for in the destruction of teeth, the impairment of the general health, and the inevitable spoiling of cases for successful treatment by the homœopath afterwards. Often symptoms of disease and drug are so intermingled that it is next to impossible, aye, sometimes impossible, to find a remedy to cover the totality, and then it becomes necessary to do the best one can.

I mentioned this case to the late Dr. Hering, who promptly said: "You did right, but never tell it; for if you do, doctors, too lazy to study their cases, will lance gum after gum, simply because a Hahnemannian found it necessary in one case." There may be some truth in this, but my article is not written for the *lazy* doctors, but for those who are honest, who work and can reason, and therefore nothing is hazarded in relating the case. Besides, even the allopaths speak of indiscriminate lancing as barbarous empiricism (West), and state that the circumstances in which the use of the gum-lancet is really indicated are comparatively few. But, admitting, that lancing *sometimes* is a *sine qua non*, how may the operation be performed best? On this subject I know of no teaching better than that given by J. W. White, M.D., D.D.S., editor of the *Dental Cosmos*, in an article on "Pathological Dentition," published April, 1878, in the American Supplement to the *Obstetric Journal of Great Britain and Ireland.* He says: "The operator should be seated directly in front of the assistant, the knees of the two parties corresponding in height. Some direct the child to be held crosswise on the lap of the assistant; others prefer to be behind the head of the child to operate on the left side, and in front to operate on the right side of either jaw; others take the head on their knees when operating on the upper jaw, and placing the head on the knees of the assistant for operations on the lower jaw. In any case, the child should be held with such relation to the window or to the artificial light that the parts to be operated upon may be illuminated to the best advantage. The instrument employed should be a curved double-edged bistoury, so protected by wrapping the blade as to avoid injury to the tongue, lips, or cheek. The left hand of the operator should separate the jaws and protect the tongue and lips of the child in such manner that any unexpected movement may result in injury to his own fingers rather than to the child. In the case of a child disposed to struggle, the insertion of a small cork between the jaws will be of service. This can be held in position by the assistant.

"The manner in which this trifling operation is performed

Fig 1*

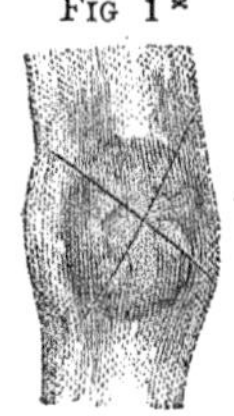

Fig. 2.

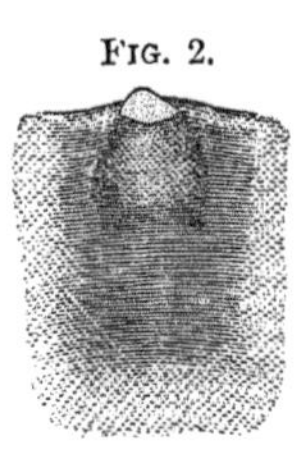

Fig 3.

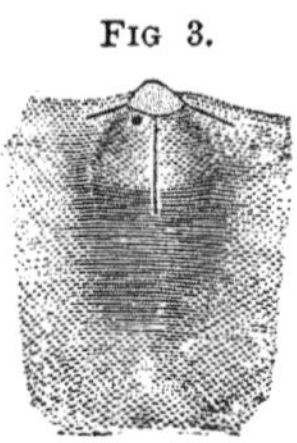

has much to do with its success or failure. . . . . The object is not merely nor chiefly to induce a flow of blood, but to remove tension. The cuts should, therefore, be made with special reference to the form of the presenting tooth. The incisors

---

* The cuts illustrating this paper have been kindly provided by Dr. White.—Mohr.

and cuspids need only a division of the gum in the line of the arch. The molars require a crucial incision, thus ×; — at once easier of performance and more effective than a right-angular division—the centre of the crown, as near as can be determined, indicating the point of decussation. The cuts should, of course, be sufficiently deep to reach the presenting surface, and extend fully up to and a little beyond its boundaries, so as to insure the entire liberation of the tooth. (Fig. 1.) Only an *undue* force will be likely to injure the incompletely solidified enamel of the erupting tooth, or endanger the germs of the developing permanent teeth. It is well always to direct the lance toward the labial instead of the lingual surface of the jaw in lancing over the front teeth, as there is thus less liability to injure the crypts of the permanent teeth, if from any cause the cut should be made deeper than is intended.

"Partial eruption of a tooth is frequently accepted as a solution of the problem—the slightest presentation being considered as definitely deciding against the necessity for lancing. This is generally true in the case of the incisors; far from true of the cuspids and molars. The cone shape of the cuspids insures a persistence of the trouble from pressure of the inclosing ring until fully erupted, as will be seen by reference to Fig. 2. A complete severance of this fibrous ring (on the anterior and posterior as well as lateral surfaces) is indicated, as in Fig. 3, and is even more necessary than before its partial eruption. A cuspid is, indeed, rarely the cause of irritation until after the eruption of its point. All the cusps of a molar may have erupted, and yet strong bands of fibrous integument maintain a resistance as decided as before their appearance, as in Fig. 4. In this case either the boundaries of the tooth should be traced by the lancet, and all such bands surely severed around its outline, or a crucial incision, as in Fig. 5, should be made, so as to insure perfect release from pressure."

FIG. 4.

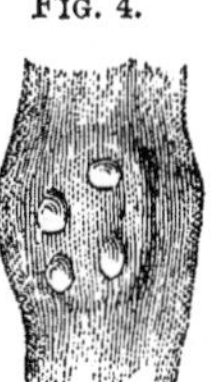

FIG. 5.

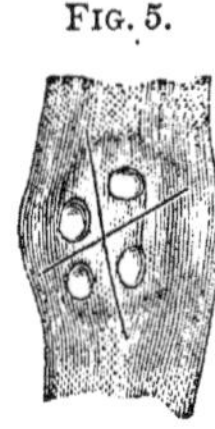

I need hardly say that under no circumstances should the gums be lanced during diphtheritic or erysipelatous inflammations, or when children are subjected to the influences of these poisons.

Finally, let me briefly allude to the necessity of using the utmost care to keep the mouth and teeth clean in children who may be ill with any eruptive fever, notably with measles or scarlatina. Children who contract these diseases, between the fifth and seventh year, unless this precaution is observed, have the permanent teeth, erupted after the illness, disfigured by a furrow across their face. Where the mouth has been properly attended to, however, and homœopathic remedies only administered, I have never found such a sequela.

In closing, let me ask for my paper your earnest consideration. If any of you have been negligent heretofore, let the suggestions herein contained profit you, as well as the little ones placed in your care, and you will lessen suffering and illness, and promote comfort, beauty and health.

EPITHELIOMA OF THE EYELID.

BY W. H. WINSLOW, PH.D., M.D., PITTSBURG, PA.

In October, 1879, W. B. M., a man aged 52 years, was sent to me by Dr. A. P. Bowie, of Uniontown, Pa., for examination of a diseased eyelid.

The gentleman informed me that seven years previous, a suspicious ulceration had appeared upon the right lower eyelid, which an old-school doctor had diagnosed as an epithelioma. The disease extended to the outer canthus, when the eyelid was removed, and a flap brought in from the malar region to close the wound. Recovery followed; the plastic operation was well done, but in healing the new eyelid formed adhesions with the eyeball, and much restricted its motions.

The patient said every time he moved his eyes he experienced a dragging pain in the false symblepharon; the attached eye had failed in vision very rapidly of late, and his sound eye felt weak and watered considerably.

The malignant disease had, however, remained in abeyance until six months before his visit, when he noticed a little crust upon the inner portion of the false eyelid; this had fallen off, a spot of ulceration appeared, and the whole border had become diseased.

I found well-marked epithelioma, extending from the outer canthus along the border of the false lid, around the inner canthus, and one-fourth of an inch along the upper eyelid from within outwards. The palpebral aperture was contracted and small. There was some conjunctivitis, increased lachrymation, and tenderness of the ciliary region. The edges of the ulceration were hard, irregular, and tuberculated; the inner border was firmly attached across the lower third of the cornea, and the subconjunctival and orbital cellular tissue was thickened and infiltrated by inflammatory and cancerous matter. The eyeball had increased tension, was almost immovable, and the cornea showed a haziness at its upper part, which gradually changed to the color of chamois skin below. Vision in this eye was reduced to counting fingers at two feet, and the color of the iris and condition of the deep structures could not be ascertained with certainty. Vision in the left eye was $\frac{20}{30}$ Sn.

The patient was of nervo-bilions temperament, medium size, rather spare build, extremely active, nervous, and irritable. The skin of the face and hands was freckled and blotchy; the general health was excellent, and the man engaged in active business.

In view of the wide extension of the disease, it was decided to abscise the right upper eyelid and the false eyelid below, and to enucleate the globe.

Assisted by Drs. Bowie, Burgher, and Strong, after inducing profound anæsthesia with Ether and Chloroform, I enucleated the eyeball; cleared out the contents of the orbit, except at the apex; removed both eyelids, and the soft tissues upon the side of the nose around the inner canthus; scraped the bone beneath this part, and brushed the wound with pure Carbolic acid. I then dissected up a flap of skin above and below the orbit, trimmed the edges, and brought them together with sutures. So mobile were the parts that I was able to close the whole gaping wound except a round portion at the inner angle not larger than a thumb-nail.

A Carbolic acid and Glycerin dressing was applied, and the patient permitted to return to consciousness. China θ was given for nausea and shock, and the patient made a rapid recovery. The only trouble was to keep his appetite satisfied with the full diet of the hospital.

At the end of five days he insisted upon going home, and I consigned him to the care of Dr. Bowie, with directions to give him *Ars. iod.* 3ˣ continuously for some months. This was faithfully done, and ten months after dismissal the patient came back to show himself. A slight scar and a few hairs of the eyebrow at the outer angle showed the line of union. The skin formed a round depressed pocket in the orbit, about large enough to hold a hickory-nut, and the parts were soft, movable, and healthy. The left eye feels perfectly well; the patient expressed much gratification at being able to see without the dragging pain he had experienced previous to the operation; his health was excellent, and he was hunting up a heavy contract in grain.

ECZEMA CAPITIS.

BY B. FRANK BETTS, M.D., PHILADELPHIA, PA.

(Read before the Philadelphia County Homœopathic Medical Society.)

The appearances presented by this affection are too familiar to require an elaborate description, for we meet the disease quite frequently in practice, either in the acute or chronic form. It has been my experience to be called upon to treat it more frequently in childhood between the second and fourth years than at any other period of life. It generally commences to develop on the vertex first. It may spread to other parts of the scalp afterwards, and extend to the cheeks and face, or be confined to the latter locality exclusively (eczema faciei), but rarely involves the nose and eyelids. When it extends down the neck and back it often manifests itself in a severe form within the axillary folds.

The disease is of constitutional origin; but pediculi may cause an eczema resembling the constitutional variety, or become associated with it. The eczema from pediculi alone, however, is usually confined to the occipital border of the scalp, and associated with such evidences of the presence of the parasites as nits or eggs upon the hair, scratching of apparently healthy portions of the scalp, etc. Syphilitic children have the worst form of eczema. It is attended with greater swelling and induration upon the edges of the eruption, and the scabs are generally darker in color. During the eruption of the teeth, or from any feverish condition of the system, the disease is aggravated.

Vaccination is said to increase the intensity of the chronic form, but not of the acute form. A case, reported in the *Jahrbuch f. Kindheilkunde*, of acute circumscribed eczema on the right cheek and ear, was vaccinated with cow-pox virus, and on the third day afterward the body was covered with a fine papillary eruption, and the eczema seemed worse, but as soon as the vaccine efflorescence appeared, the new eruption and the eczema both subsided. Although other cases of a similar nature have been reported as having been cured in a similar manner, our own predilection has always been in favor of deferring vaccination until all traces of *any* skin disease the child might be affected with, has been cured.

Eczema pustulosum, or impetiginoides, and impetigo capitis, are names applied to eczema in a chronic form, when the vesicles fill with pus. When crusts form, covering the scalp and face like a mask, eczema larvale, impetigo larvalis, and porrigo are names appropriate. As inveterate cases of the disease were formerly believed to be dependent upon some fault in the milk given to the child, the term "milk crust" or "crusta lactea" was much in vogue, and this is the name still used by the laity to designate the affection.

Overfeeding, the habit of feeding the child too frequently, and of allowing children who have passed the milk-diet period to eat frequently of inappropriate food between meals, will prevent the recovery of chronic cases, despite the administration of the well-selected remedy. When the tongue is coated, the breath foul, and the bowels constipated, the diet requires particular attention. Children kept in warm rooms where the air is vitiated, are liable to suffer from this affection, especially if they catch cold easily from the least exposure. Allowing the child to sleep upon a very soft pillow, into which the head becomes buried at night, or feeding "bottle babies" with milk too warm, has seemed to aggravate some cases. Fresh air and sunlight, with attention to hygienic measures, will exert a favorable influence upon this stubborn disease. The use of ointments or medicaments applied externally will prevent the treatment of the case from being conducted homœopathically; therefore, they must be discarded *in toto*.

An eruptive disease manifests itself upon the skin, and we call it a skin disease, but we do not infer that it does not affect other portions of the system as well, or that it is to be treated in a different manner from other diseases, because of its particular location. Eczema capitis has its subjective and objective symptoms, and when we select the remedy according to the indications they give us, we will cure the case homœopathically. If, however, we suppress any of the symptoms by means of external medication, we are adrift, for we have then lost reliable indications for the remedy, and have perhaps developed new symptoms which do not belong to the case proper, and are consequently unreliable guides.

Thick crusts of decomposing material, act as foreign bodies upon the surface, and must be removed just as foreign substances are removed from other sores. This task is quite difficult in some cases, however, and will require persistent effort. When the accumulation has gone on for some time, and the crusts are hard, the hair will have to be cut short and wet cloths or flaxseed-meal poultices inclosed in thin muslin, must be applied at night to soften them.

In such cases an oiled-silk cap should envelop the head, to prevent evaporation as well as to keep the pillows from becoming wet. If the applications become dry and uncomfortable in the night, fresh ones should be substituted. In the morning the part should be washed gently but thoroughly with lukewarm water and white castile soap, or pure German green soap (sapo viridis), made of hempseed oil and potassa. The ordinary green soap made of fats and potassa, with precipitated indigo to give it the color of the sapo viridis, is to be discarded, as well as all scented soaps, medicated soaps, etc.

After the crusts have been removed, the surface needs cleansing only when accumulations commence to re-form into crusts again.

THERAPEUTICS.

Ars. alb.—The eruption upon the scalp or face is dry and scaly. When crusts form they are thick, white, yellow, or made dark-colored from an admixture of blood-cells exuded after scratching. The intense itching is characteristic, and it is not ameliorated by scratching.

When the disease affects the forehead mainly, the scales are thin and dry (branlike), and situated upon an angry excoriated surface, made so by a thin acrid discharge. Little pustules surround the diseased site (Hep., Lach.); these run together, and in this manner the disease spreads. The itching, which is worse at night, is attended with great restlessness and agitation of mind. (Sulph. and Rhus have aggravation of itching at night, with restlessness, but scratching relieves the itching in both remedies, consequently there is less mental anguish; but the itching soon recurs, and thus we have the restlessness developed. Under Sulph. there is often intense pain at the seat of the eruption after scratching, which makes the child cry.)

The discharge from beneath the thick crusts is a thick syrupy fluid. The diseased spots on the scalp are very sensitive to the touch (Hep.) and bleed easily (Sulph.).

The skin, on those parts of the body not affected by the eczema, is often harsh, dry, and parchment-like to the feel. Sulph., which resembles this remedy in so many of its symptoms, has also a harsh, dry, rough, and wrinkled skin, but the mental symptoms may decide between the two, especially when there is a dread of being washed, which is so characteristic of Sulph. Under Hepar it is the dread of being touched that makes them cry from washing. The Arsenic child suffers and becomes emaciated from disturbances in the vegetative sphere. The Sulph. child may have been "runty" from birth.

From the varied nature of the symptoms, it will be seen that Arsenicum is a remedy often called for. It is used extensively by the allopathists, and often with success because of its homœopathicity.

CALC. OS.—Thick, large, yellow scabs form on the occiput first (Calc. phos.), and spread to the face afterwards. The eruption is mostly dry, yet there may be a thick, bland pus beneath the crusts. The itching is not very intense, but after sleep, teething children sometimes scratch their heads impatiently, or pick the scalp and make it bleed. The glands are often swollen. The appetite is mostly very good; urine strong, fetid, and copious (*Cham.*, copious, without smell). Indicated in large, fair, plump children, with open fontanels and large heads, which perspire profusely, especially during sleep. Graph. is similar, but the eruption discharges more, and the discharge is watery and thin but very sticky. Either Calc. os. or Graph. may be indicated for eczema behind the ears.

CICUTA VIROSA.—No itching; exudation dries down to a hard lemon-colored crust. A thick whitish scurf appears on the chin and upper lip, with but slight secretion.

CANTH.—The eruption begins in a small spot, and spreads so as to involve a large surface, with a watery discharge from underneath the scabs. Scales form on the scalp like enormous dandruff. The hair falls out. The child is restless, whining, and complaining; suffers from dysuria.

CAUST.—Eruption on the occipital region (Baryta carb., Calc. phos., Clematis), may extend to the nape of the neck. Itching with burning after scratching (Ars., Sulph., etc.), worse from cold air in evening, and better in warm air or from cold water. Child afraid in the dark; dark-haired children of rigid fibre. Runty children, mentally and physically weak.

CLEMATIS.—The eruption appears on the back part of the head and on the neck. It may extend over the face. It is moist, and discharges an excoriating fluid, which dries into scales. With the itching, there is soreness from the discharge coming in contact with the surrounding surface.

DULCAMARA.—Thick crusts form on the scalp, causing the

hair to fall out. Thick brown or yellowish crusts on the cheeks, forehead, or chin (Lyc.). Oozing of watery fluid from the eruption, with bleeding after scratching. The itching diminishes after the crusts form. The eruption is sensitive to contact.

GRAPHITES.—The eczema affects the folds behind the ears (Calc. os., Hep., Lyc.). It is humid, spreading and scurfy; painful to contact, and may extend to the vertex, and down the sides of the head to the cheeks. After scratching, the watery discharge increases, and the soreness is worse. The discharge may dry up and form thick, white or dirty-looking crusts. At first it is transparent and very sticky, like glue between the finger-tips, and odorless; but may become very offensive afterwards. Blonde children who have a tendency to grow fat, require this remedy most frequently.

HEPAR.—Humid eruption over the whole head; very sensitive and emitting an offensive odor. Intense itching with burning and soreness after scratching. Boils form on the neck and head, very sore to contact. Pustules form around the seat of the disease. The child is chilled from the slightest exposure. Hands and feet are always cold. The remedy is often called for after salves or ointments have been applied.

LAPPA MAJOR.—Moist, badly smelling, grayish-white crusts; most of the hair gone, and the eruption extending to the face. I know of no cures having been effected with the Burdock.

LYCOP.—Moist eczema, with thick, *offensive* discharge. Crusts form, which have deep cracks or clefts running through them. Chronic cases: the occiput, face, neck, and hands are all affected. The eruption bleeds easily. The child is constipated, and has a pale sallow complexion; eyes sunken, with blue rings around them; cervical glands swollen. Brick-dust sediment in the urine; rumbling in the bowels; often indicated after Calc. os.

MERC. VIV.—Humid fetid eruption; thick yellow discharge, or yellow crusts form on the scalp, surrounded by an inflamed border, caused by the excoriating nature of the discharge. Itching worse at night in bed, with pain from scratching, and tendency to bleed (Sulph.). Great tendency to clammy perspiration over the body. The child's thighs feel cold and clammy. It has a green slimy diarrhœa, worse at night, and a dirty yellow or pale clammy skin (Sulph.). Glands are swollen, and there is much salivation.

MEZEREUM.—Head covered with a thick leathery crust,

under which collects pus of an offensive odor. The hairs mat together. The eruption itches, now here, now there, changing place from scratching; it burns after scratching, and the itching increases. Sore boils develop on the head. Scurfy chalk-like scales develop on the scalp with an offensive ichor beneath them.

Nat. mur.—Impetigo on the nape of the neck, or the borders of the hair; the surface is raw, and the discharge corroding. It may develop behind the ears also, and the discharge seem gluey (Graph.), matting the hair, with rawness, soreness, and smarting pain. Herpes about the mouth, the bends of the knees, and folds of the skin generally.

Psorinum.—Dry or humid and fetid eruption. Hair becomes matted (Graph., Lyc., Mezereum, Nat. mur., Sulph.). Itching is worse in bed and from warmth (Merc. viv.). Crusty eruption. When the child is debilitated, with a tendency to profuse perspiration. Diarrhœa watery, dark-colored, and very offensive; worse at night. This remedy should be thought of in cases which do not yield to the well-selected remedy and compared with Sulph.

Rhus tox.—The eruption is generally moist, the surface raw, and the parts swollen. A red, inflamed, swollen rim from subcutaneous infiltration, surrounds every portion of the eruption (Ars., black rim around the eruption). White thick crusts form, which smell offensively, and itch, especially at night. Cheeks and face affected as well as the scalp. The child is restless, wants to be moved continually, especially after midnight, when the itching is intense, but this is relieved for a time by scratching. The cold fresh air is not tolerated on the head; it seems to make the scalp painful; hence the child likes to have its cap on in the open air (compare Sil.).

Sepia.—Itching vesicles or pustules form on the face as well as upon the occiput and vertex. The eruption is dry or soon becomes moist and discharges an offensive pus-like fluid, copiously. This becomes dry, cracks and exfoliates. The eruption terminates abruptly upon the skin. (Rhus tox. has a red rim about the eruption; Hep., Lach., Ars., etc., have little vesicles.) Brown discoloration of the forehead. Face and head itch, and the child jerks its head to and fro, seemingly from the itching. Patient has dark hair, thin delicate skin, and passes putrid urine (compare Calc. os., Benz. ac.).

Silicea.—Eruption on the back part of the head, either moist, or dry and scaly; offensive; scabby; itches; burns; soreness after scratching; pustules form and discharge copiously.

The remedy may be used to limit the suppurative process. Small wounds heal with difficulty (Calc. os., Graph., Hep.). Skin of the child is dry, the face pale and muscles lax. Big-bellied children, with weak ankles; emaciated frame, and irritable tempers, with perspiration about the head towards morning.

This remedy resembles Calc. os. in many respects, but the Silicea child is not fat, although it has a large abdomen. The Calc. os. child is full of mischief. The Silicea child is obstinate, headstrong, and cries when kindly spoken to, and likes to have its cap on and its head wrapped up warmly.

STAPH.—Yellow scabs form on the scalp. The eczema is moist, offensive, and itches violently. A yellow, scaly eruption appears on the cheeks or behind the ears, which discharges from scratching. Face sunken; nose pointed and blue rings encircle the eyes. The child is irritable, and indignantly throws things away from it which were desired but a moment before.

SULPHUR.—Cases of long standing, with much itching, which is worse at night, and attended with pain after scratching. The eczema may extend over the whole body. It is dry or humid, and offensive, discharging thick or thin acrid pus, which forms into yellow crusts and produces itching, followed by pain, bleeding, and a burning sensation. Painful inflamed itching pimples on scalp and forehead. A remedy for colicky babies with dry roughness of the skin of the body, which itches from warmth, and "feels good" from scratching (Silic. feels worse). Lips red, stools excoriating. Soreness between the nates and in the groins (Graph., Lyc., Merc. viv.). The child cannot bear to be washed; is most comfortable when dirty; morning diarrhœa, or bowels moved regularly but always with great pain. (When stools are lumpy and hard, with pain in the rectum, Nitric ac.).

THUYA OCCIDENTALIS.—After vaccination the eczema is worse (Sil.). Aggravation from wet (washing, poulticing, etc.). Eruption is white, scaly, and desquamating. Perspiration on uncovered parts of the body (Sil.). Wants head and face wrapped up warm (Sil.).

VINCA MINOR.—Wintergreen is said to cure a badly smelling eruption on the head, face, and behind the ears. In the provings we find humid eruptions, itching at night, with burning after scratching. Eruptions appearing in spots, moisture oozes therefrom and the hair becomes matted.

VIOLA TRICOLOR.—The eruption burns and itches, especially at night, and discharges tough yellow matter. Thick crusts form.

Dr. W. H. Bigler has used this remedy for the disease in the acute stage, with the eruption confined mainly to the face and having a tendency to rapid pustulation, forming brownish-yellow crusts. Itching temporarily relieved by rubbing. He has found the best results follow the use of an infusion taken three or four times a day.

The late Dr. W. Williamson spoke of its efficacy when involuntary urination was an accompanying symptom.

Compare also the following remedies, viz., Ars. iod., Baryta c., Borax, Bry., Iris, Nitric ac., Oleander, Phytolacca, and Sarsaparilla.

REPERTORY.

Eruption spreading from occiput to face: Calc. os., Clematis, Graph., Lyc., Sep., Sil., Staph., Sulph.

Eruption spreading from occiput down over ears, temples, and cheeks: Psorinum.

Eruption on forehead: Merc. viv., Rhus tox., Sep., Sulph.

Eruption on face: Ars., Baryta c., Calc. os., Cicuta vir., Clematis, Dulc., Fluoric ac., Graph., Hep., Lyc., Merc. viv., Psorinum, Rhus tox., Sep., Staph., Sulph., Vinca minor, Viola tricolor.

Eruption in angles of alæ nasi: Dulc., Millefol., Ledum, Thlaspi.

Eruption in corners of mouth: Arum triph., Graph., Hep., Lyc., Rhus tox., Sil.

Eruption on chin: Borax, Cicuta vir., Graph., Rhus tox., Sep.

Eruption back of auricles: Ars., Calc os., *Graph.*, Hep., Lyc., Nat. mur., Staph.

Eruption on nape of neck and borders of hair: Baryta carb., Clematis, Caust., Hydrastis, Lyc., Nat. mur., Nitric ac., Sulph.

Eruption moist: Calc os., Clematis, Dulc., Graph., Hep., Lyc., Merc. viv., Mezereum, Nat. mur., Phytolacca, Rhus tox., Sep., Sil., Staph., Sulph., Vinca minor.

Eruption dry: Ars., Baryta c., Calc. os., Canth., Fluoric ac., Kali c., Lyc., Sep., Sil., Sulph.

Eruptions raw and angry-looking: Ars., Clematis, Graph., Hep., Merc. viv., Nat. mur., Rhus tox., Sulph.

Discharge corrosive: Ars., Clematis, Graph., Merc. iod., Nat. mur., Sulph.

Hair matted from secretion: Graph., Lyc., Mezer., Nat. mur., Psorinum, Sulph., Vinca minor, Viola tricolor.

White scaly eruption: Ars., Canth., Mezer.

Thick crusts: Ant. crud., Ars., Calc. os., Cicuta, Dulc., Graph., Lyc., Mezer., Rhus tox., Sulph., Viola tricol.

. Branlike scales: Ars., Sulph.

Yellow crusts: Ars., Calc. os., Cicuta vir., Merc. viv., Mezer., Staph., Sulph.

Brownish-yellow crusts: Dulc., Graph., Lyc., Mezer.

Greenish-yellow crusts: Calc. os., Merc. viv., Viola tricol.

Dark-colored eruptions: Ars., Clematis.

Itching eruption: Ars., Calc. os., Caust., Dulc., Hep., Merc. viv., Mezer., Phytolacca, Psorinum, Rhus tox., Sep., Sil., Staph., Sulph., Vinca minor, Viola tricolor.

Bleeding after scratching: Ars., Dulc., Hep., Lyc., Merc. viv., Nitric ac., Sep., Sulph.

Burning after scratching: Ars., Canst., Clematis., Hep., Lyc., Merc. viv., Mezer., Rhus. tox., Sep., Staph., Sulph., Vinca minor., Viola tricol.

Soreness after scratching: Sil., Sulph.

Itching, worse on getting warm in bed: Clematis, Merc. viv., Mezer., Psorinum, Rhus tox., Sulph.

Relief from scratching: Rhus tox., Sulph.

Tingling-itching eruption: Clematis, Mezer., Rhus tox.

Picking the scalp causing it to bleed: Calc. os., Hep.

Sensitiveness of the eruption to touch: Ars., Calc. os., Clematis, Dulc., Graph., Hep., Lyc., Merc. viv., Nitric ac., Sulph.

Sensitiveness of the scalp to open air: Calc. os., Hep., Rhus tox., Sil.

Hair comes out: Ars., Calc. os., Canth., Dulc., Fluor. ac., Graph., Hep., Merc. viv., Rhus tox., Sulph., Vinca minor.

Eruption smells offensive: Ars., Graph., Hep., Lyc., Merc. viv., Mezer., Psorinum, Rhus tox., Sep., Sil., Staph., Sulph., Vinca minor.

Eruption without odor: Clematis, Graph.

Glands swollen: Ars., Baryta carb., Calc. os., Hep, Lyc., Merc. viv., Rhus tox., Staph., Sil., Sulph.

Furuncles on different parts of the body: Hepar, Mezer.

Large head with sweating of same: Calc. os., Calc. phos., Merc. viv., Sil.

Fontanels remain open: Calc. os., Calc. phos., Sil., Sulph.

Face pale, waxen, sallow: Ars. alb., Canst., Sil.

Face pale; hollow eyes, old-looking: Sulph.

Face pale yellowish: Ars., Calc. os., Lyc., Nat. mur.
Face dirty yellow: Merc. viv., Nat. mur., Sil.
Face pale and bloated: Ars., Calc. os., Graph., Lyc.
Face pale and sickly: Ars., Clematis, Nitric ac., Psorinum, Staph.
Face pale; veins show through the skin: Calc. os.
Aggravation from cold: Ars., Calc. os., Canst., Hep., Sil.
Aggravation from cold damp air: Dulc., Mezer., Rhus tox.
Aggravation from going into open air: Ars., Hep., Sarsap.
Aggravation from washing: Calc. os., Clematis, Dulc., Hep., Sep.
Aggravation from hot weather: Lyc., Nat. mur., Sep., Sulph.
Slight injuries suppurate, and abrasions are difficult to heal: Calc. os., Graph., Hep., Sil., Sulph.
Constipation: Ant. crud., Bry., Calc. os., Caust., Graph., Hep., Lyc., Sep., Sil., Sulph.
Stools chalky: Ant. crud., Calc. os.
Stools clay-like, gray, fecal: Calc. os.
Stools hard, causing urging and redness of face: Caust.
Stools hard, difficult: Hep.
Stools difficult; rectum inactive; stools slip back: Sil.
Stools difficult; coated with mucus: Canst., Graph.
Stools scanty with frequent urging: Nux vom.
Diarrhœa: Ars., Calc. os., Canth., Hep., Merc. viv., Mezer., Psorinum, Rhus, Sulph.
Restless at night: Ars., Rhus tox.
Restless day and night: Ars., Caust., Dulc.
Restless anxiety: Ars., Calc. os., Canst.
Irritable temper: Dulc., Canth., Caust.
Fretful and worrisome: Ars., Canth.
Fair plump children: Graph., Hep.
Fair fat children: Calc. os.
Phlegmatic torpid children: Dulc.
Dark-haired children: Caust., Nitric ac., Sep.

IRIS VERSICOLOR.

BY F. F. CASSEDAY, M.D., STEVEN'S POINT, WISCONSIN.

THIS is one of our best proven remedies and a very valuable one. Its range of action includes the gastro-intestinal mucous membrane, and its glandular apparatus and the skin. Its pains are of a sharp cutting character and change often. It is especially useful in gastric or bilious sick-headache, diarrhœa, cholera morbus, cholera infantum, and pustular eruptions. I have found it frequently indicated during the past month, and have used it with uniform success, as the following cases will show.

Case I.—Mrs. H., æt. 60 years. Cholera morbus; complained of severe pain in bowels with much rumbling, constant nausea with vomiting and purging every few moments, limbs and body cold with occasional cramps in the lower extremities. The matter vomited was glairy mucus with some bile at times. The stools were thin and colorless. ℞. Iris 2^x every half hour. It relieved the pain and vomiting instantly and made a complete cure in twenty-four hours.

Case II.—Miss W., æt. 20 years. Cholera morbus. ℞. Iris 2^x every two hours. Cured in twenty-four hours.

Case III.—Baby G., æt. 8 months. Simple diarrhœa of two months' duration. Discharges very green and watery; evacuations, eight to ten in twenty-four hours. ℞. Iris 2^x every three hours. Result, one stool in the next twelve hours, and the patient has been free from diarrhœa ever since.

Case IV.—Baby L., æt. 5 months. Diarrhœa with occasional vomiting, though not amounting to cholera infantum. After trying several remedies with no avail, gave Iris 2^x, which "acted like a charm," and promptly cured the case.

Case V.—Mrs. R. complained of severe headache (frontal), constant nausea, and occasional vomiting. Pain so severe she could not sleep at night. No appetite and great weakness. Iris gave immediate relief.

It is a grand remedy, and has succeeded many times in my hands where carefully chosen remedies, which in my opinion were more clearly indicated, have signally failed. It is certainly a specific in cholera morbus, for I have never seen it fail to relieve a single case, when given on such indications as those above mentioned. Drs. Hale and Kitchen also testify to its efficacy in this distressing complaint. Dr. Hale treated forty-three cases of autumnal diarrhœa and cholera with it, and in no case did it fail to cure, nor was it necessary to continue it longer than twenty-four hours. I commend the drug to every practical physician as deserving of careful study.

A CASE OF PUERPERAL CONVULSIONS.

BY W. M HAINES, M.D , ELLSWORTH, ME.

I WAS called in haste March 21st, 1878, to attend a lady in confinement, living several miles out of town, who, the messenger said, was having "fits." I found her a small, snug-built woman, aged 19, primipara. She was in a dull, listless state, and was only aroused with considerable difficulty sufficiently to answer questions, and soon relapsing into a stupid state again. The attendants stated that she had been expecting to be confined for over a week, and for the last twelve hours seemed to have a fit whenever a pain came on. I administered *Gelsem.* 1^x in water, and waited some time for developments; and finally, as I was on the point of leaving her for a short time, she threw back her head and went into "the most violent convulsion," they said, "that she had had." I was unable to get a towel between her teeth, and she bit her tongue severely, and ground her jaws together so hard that she actually pressed two sound teeth out of the lower jaw, and I removed them from her mouth with my fingers to prevent her swallowing them. During the convulsions, which followed about every twenty minutes, she became black in the face, and rested on her head and heels with every muscle in a condition of extreme rigidity. She passed into a perfectly unconscious state after each paroxysm, the breathing being stertorous in character. I gave her *Gelsem.*, Opium, *Bell.*, and *Stram.*, each during the time occupied by several convulsions, with no perceptible benefit or change. I then determined to deliver with the forceps, and prepared them for use. The os was partially dilated, and the vertex presented. There seemed to be room in the pelvis for the child to pass, but the soft tissues were very tense and unyielding. The membranes were ruptured some time previously. I proceeded to apply the forceps without the administration of *Chloroform*, both on account of the woman being in an unconscious state, and because I have formed the opinion that Chloroform, united with the effects of the shock of delivering by instruments, is often too much for the nervous system to bear, and often the cause of almost immediate death.

I have applied the forceps several times in practice, but never unless absolutely demanded, and have never used any kind of anæsthetic whatever, and have never had any bad results follow such a case, the patients making quick recoveries with proper care and nursing.

In this case it was only with extreme difficulty that I succeeded in applying and locking the long forceps in the superior strait, and during the time of their application she had a severe convulsion, which necessitated a pause in the work. I could not wait for a pain, so with steady and careful traction, following the curve of the pelvis, I gradually drew the child downward. I was obliged to use a great deal of force to complete the delivery; but finally, without the aid of maternal expulsive effort, extracted the child, which, although somewhat asphyxiated, finally came around all right, and the placenta was expelled by a contraction produced by carefully kneading the uterus through the abdominal walls. There was not much hæmorrhage and no convulsions afterwards. The patient seemed to sleep quietly for a couple of hours, and then woke up quite bright and rational, but of course unconscious of what she had passed through. The child was not scarred in the least, and no injuries were received by the mother.

I have since attended the same lady in confinement, when everything came off very nicely, with a short, easy labor. She thought the serious character of her first confinement was caused by her attempting to hide her form by tight lacing, even up to the seventh month, and perhaps she was right.

THE BRITISH HOMŒOPATHIC CONGRESS.

THE annual session of the British Homœopathic Congress was held at the Great Northern Railway Station Hotel, Leeds, on the 9th of September; Dr. Yeldham, of London, presiding:

The President opened the business of the Congress by an address on "The Pursuit of Certainty in Medicine." He remarked that, having accepted the homœopathic system, almost with unquestioning faith in its efficiency for practical purposes, they have expended their surplus energies too exclusively, though perhaps unavoidably, in a kind of life and death struggle in defence of their principles, and to maintain their position as recognized members of the medical body. But they could not always contend. The bitterest foes must sometimes rest upon their arms and take breath. Such an interval of repose, as between themselves and those who professed to differ from them, might, he thought, be said to exist at the present time; and though as opposing parties they had not yet learned to agree, they had, he trusted, learned a calmer and more tolerant spirit than formerly, to bear with, and in some degree to respect, each other. It appeared to him that this lull in the strife offered a fitting opportunity, of which they should avail themselves, to forget for awhile those things which were without, and turn their attention, as statesmen did after fighting for foreign policy, to questions of internal improvement and reform. Excellent as the homœopathic system was as a whole, it was not devoid, in some of its details, of questions of this nature, for much as Hahnemann effected in his own lifetime in giving practical shape to his doctrines, it was inevitable that he should leave so great a work, in many respects, incomplete and imperfect; and whilst they must ever hold in the highest respect, the opinions and teachings of the man who evolved and set in motion a new train of thought and action in medical science, it was also incumbent upon them to realize their own obligations to think, judge, and act for themselves. By comparing the various medical doctrines with homœopathy, he might enforce the fact that the latter, from the admirable simplicity of its principles, partook more largely than any of the older systems of the elements of certainty. Instead of treating the subject of his paper on the ground of practical expediency, he preferred viewing it from the light of a principle—the principle of certainty in medicine. It was needless to state that this principle was an indispensable element in all scientific pursuits, and in none more so than the practice of medicine, since upon the degree of certainty or precision with which they applied their art, the weightiest interests often depended. Whilst it is true that medicine, being a mixed science, could never reach the mathematical exactitude of a pure science, it should be, nevertheless, their constant aim to approximate it, as near as possible, to the highest standard of certainty which any science was capable of. Coming to the consideration of the symptoms recorded in the Materia Medica, and the means by which various defects in it might be rectified, the President said that clearly the task here implied, would involve an amount of labor and responsibility such as no one man, however well qualified for the undertaking, would be justified in assuming. What he would propose was this, that it be undertaken by a committee, to be called "The Materia Medica Committee." This committee should be permanent, being recruited from time to time, as vacancies might occur, and it should be composed of men who, from their practical experience, literary attainments, and widespread acquaintance with homœopathic matters generally, would inspire confidence that whatever they did would be thoroughly well done. Such men were not far to seek. An excellent committee of this kind might be formed from amongst their own body. It might, perhaps, be worth considering whether the co-operation of some of their zealous and accomplished American colleagues might not be enlisted. Should such an idea appear feasible it might be ventilated between the present time and the Congress to be held in London next year, and which, it was to be hoped, would be honored by the presence of many of their transatlantic brethren. The great obstacle to the adoption of this suggestion would be the distance between the two continents, and the consequent difficulty of holding that personal intercourse and interchange of thought which would be almost indispensable to the successful carrying out of such a scheme. But, however, constituted, the labors of such a committee would, he took it, fall almost naturally into three divisions—those of revision, reproving, and rejection. As to the first, he feared such a proposal would fail at the present time on account of its herculean proportions, but such a winnowing should take place as would blow away a cloud of useless symptoms, and would bring out the characteristic features of their remedies in such bold relief that they would be able at once to distinguish them from each other, and judge of their peculiar sphere of curative action; whereas, as they now stood in their books, they looked so much alike, that it was exceedingly difficult to detect their points of difference, and say why any one of them should not equally cure any or all diseases. To the one or the other of the three eliminating processes he had mentioned, every article at the present in their Materia Medica should be rigorously submitted; and as to the future, no medicine should find its way into their Materia Medica that had not undergone such searching and repeated testing as should satisfy the proposed committee, under whose sanction alone it should be recognized as a homœopathic remedy. What was required was a thoroughly good materia medica pura,—pure in the truest sense of the word, setting forth truthfully and honestly those medicines, and those only, that had been proved beyond dispute to be homœopathic, and recording only those symptoms concerning whose genuineness there could be no shadow of doubt. (Applause.)

On the motion of Dr. Pope (London), seconded by Dr. Hughes (Brighton), a vote of thanks was passed to the President for his address.

Dr. Drysdale (Liverpool), moved, "That this meeting of

British homœopathic practitioners has heard with the deepest regret of the recent death of the venerable Constantine Hering, of Philadelphia; that they desire to place upon record the strong sense they entertain of the value of the services that Dr. Hering has rendered to the science of medicine during the whole of his professional career, and of the great zeal and energy he has ever shown in the advance, development, and the propagation of homœopathy; they at the same time desire to express their sympathy with the members of his family, his colleagues in the Hahnemann Medical College, and his professional brethren in Philadelphia at the loss they have sustained by his death, and that the Secretary be instructed to forward a copy of the foregoing resolution to Mrs. Hering, the President of the Homœopathic Medical Society of Pennsylvania, and to the President of the Hahnemann Medical College."

Dr. Dudgeon (London) seconded the motion, which was adopted.

Dr. Burnett (London) read a paper on "The Prevention of Hare-lip, Cleft Palate, and other Congenital Defects, as also of Hereditary Diseases and Constitutional Taints, by the Medicinal and Nutritional Treatment of the Mother during Pregnancy."

A discussion ensued, after which Dr. Gibbs Blake (Birmingham) exhibited some laminated casts of the bronchial tubes from a case of plastic bronchitis.

The Congress then adjourned for luncheon. On resuming, Dr. Drysdale read a paper on "The Need and Requirements of a School of Homœopathy." He stated that there was forced upon them the necessity of founding schools wherein students of medicine might be taught the truth respecting homœopathy before they settled in practice, and were finally, for the most part, withdrawn from all opportunity of learning any new principle of a large and fundamental character. They must remember that although in this country hundreds of qualified medical men were added to the allopathic ranks every year, whilst the homœopathic party could barely claim five or six converts, it must not be supposed that these new practitioners had decided the respective merits of the two methods, and pronounced in favor of the allopath. Nothing of the kind. They had simply believed and adopted what they had been taught, and as they had been taught to use their remedies empirically, whilst the source of them was sedulously concealed from them; and homœopathy, if spoken of at all, was represented in mere caricature; they simply accepted the teaching, and continued through life to assert, and most likely believe, that homœopathy was the absurdity it was stated to be, even when daily using the remedies discovered by means of it. It was obvious that if the teaching of schools were in their hands, the case would be exactly reversed as regarded numbers, although he hoped and trusted they would not exhibit the unfair and persecuting spirit that had been shown to them. Their object being thus to counteract the hindrances which had been put in the way of fair investigation by taking in hand the teaching of young men, let them consider the different ways in which schools for such teaching might be constituted. They might have, first, complete schools or colleges with the title homœopathic, which gave a license to practice; secondly, mixed allopathic and homœopathic schools or colleges, giving a license to practice, in which there were separate lectureships and examinations for the two methods; third, schools or colleges, giving license to practice, in which the professorships were wholly filled by homœopathists, but the name homœopathic was not given to the school, as was expected to be the case when the homœopathic theory was generally received into medicine; fourth, schools with the title homœopathic, in which no general medical education was given, but the distinctive parts of the homœopathic theory and practice were alone taught, and no license to practice was given. The establishment of such schools here and in other European countries would naturally be followed by similar results, and would, of course, be extremely desirable, if practicable, in spite of some defects, even if these could not be obviated. The most important objection to such schools was the difficulty, especially in the early days of homœopathy, of getting the professorships of the neutral branches of medical education filled by competent men. For how could they expect men eminent in chemistry, physics, botany, anatomy, physiology, etc., to accept posts in an apparently sectarian school, whose title was given by a therapeutic doctrine to which they were hostile or indifferent? Homœopathic colleges must, therefore, be restricted in their choice of professors to the comparatively narrow field of homœopathic converts, within which the choice of men eminent in their departments must be limited. The consequence must generally be that these posts would be filled by medical practitioners more or less hastily and imperfectly qualified for the task, and a low standard of general medical education would be the result. In considering the possible plan of improvement which might be suggested by the experience of their American brethren, Dr. Drysdale said there was, first, the establishment of complete homœopathic medical schools giving degrees. A scheme for this purpose was brought forward by Dr. Bayes in the June number of the *Medical Homœopathic Review*, of this year, and he invited the co-operation of medical and lay friends of homœopathy. This was, in the first place, a tacit acknowledgment of failure of the present school, and of the correctness of the arguments for its reform, and implied the destruction of the present school or its amalgamation with some new scheme.

Dr. Bayes read a paper on the same subject, suggesting the possibility of a charter being granted for the establishment of a homœopathic college.

A discussion followed, at the close of which the Congress resolved itself into a committee to transact formal business. Dr. Hamilton (London) was elected President for the ensuing year, and the next meeting of the Congress was fixed to be held in London, in connection with the World's Convention of Homœopaths.

In the evening the members of the Congress dined together at the hotel, the President in the chair. The usual loyal toasts having been proposed,

The President proposed the sentiment of "The Memory of Dr. Hahnemann." He remarked that but for the memory of that great man they would not have been there that evening to celebrate the progress of one of the greatest scientific, and in a certain way social, reforms that were ever proposed to the world. There have been a good many remarks made upon the seemingly slow progress that homœopathy was making in the world. He could not altogether agree with those remarks. It had always appeared to him that reforms were either slow or rapid in their progress, very much in proportion to their magnitude. Small reforms were easily and readily accepted. They interfered but little with men's habits and prejudices; but large reforms such as that which Hahnemann proposed, and which might rather be called a revolution than a reform, was sure to excite an amount of stubborn opposition. It was natural that it should be so. They often found that men could more easily change their habits than they could change their principles or their prejudices; or they might put it in another way, and say their honest convictions. Homœopathy, as they knew, had a great effect upon men's habits. It had influenced in a wonderful degree the practice of the old school. The revolution in that respect had been remarkable. Those who, like himself, had been permitted to grow old enough to have lived through those changes, could appreciate their extent. This was one, and, he thought, the first and the most natural effect of homœopathy upon the medical world, and so surely as day followed night so surely would the destiny of homœopathy be brought about. Men's opinions would change, and homœopathy would be received as one of the great, if not the only leading principle in medicine. (Applause.) Of this he had no doubt. They might wish to see the wheels of progress move more rapidly, but so surely as the oak, though it might live to a thousand years, yielded at length to the blast, it would be brought about. (Applause.) The world knew its great men through their great deeds, and Hahnemann would be known, and was known, by the great work he had done. They would presently bow their heads in reverence and silence to his memory, but before doing so he would refer to two great men who, in their way, were men of considerable mark, and who each did a good work for homœopathy. He alluded in the first instance to Dr. Quin, who was taken from amongst them two years ago, and who, in his peculiar way, did a great work for them. He was a man of high notions of professional honor, of considerable power, of great judgment, and his position in society enabled him to carry homœopathy into a region which it certainly would not have penetrated so thoroughly as it had done but for such a man as he. He kept them together, and in a variety of ways—in the formation of societies and the establishment of an hospital—he did a work which deserved to be held in most respectful memory. (Applause.) The other name he would mention was that of Dr. Constantine Hering. His death had been so recent that they could do no more at present than acknowledge the loss they had sustained with feelings of deep regret. (Applause.)

Dr. Roche proposed "The Homœopathic Hospitals and Dispensaries," coupling with the toast the names of Dr. Dyce Brown and Dr. Bayes.

Dr. Dyce Brown, in reply, said that the hospital in London, with which he had now been connected for some time, was in a very flourishing condition. The management and internal arrangements were very satisfactory, and the institution was a valuable means of teaching the students who went to listen to the lectures. Without it they would not be able to get on half so well as they did, inasmuch as they were able to show the students the practical working-out of what they taught them. (Applause.) The Birmingham Hospital, the Liverpool Dispensaries, and the Bournemouth Convalescent Homes were also in excellent order. (Applause.)

Dr. Bayes also responded. He stated that their first object in the hospital should be to increase their clinical teaching. It was his intention to propose at the next committee meeting that regular clinical instruction should be given once or twice a week. They had abundant means of giving that instruction, and he hoped it would prove an extra object of interest, both as to the hospital and the schools. The two institutions must run together as twin institutions. (Applause.)

Dr. Nankeville (Bournemouth) proposed "The Literature and Societies of Homœopathy," coupling with the toast the name of Dr. Burnett, who responded.

Dr. Pope proposed "The Health of the Readers of the Papers at the Congress."

Dr. Drysdale replied.

Dr. Dudgeon proposed "Success to the International Homœopathic Convention to be held Next Year."

Dr. Hughes responded.

The remaining toasts were "The Visitors," "The Chairman," and "The Secretaries," Dr. Blake and Dr. Ramsbottom.

HOMŒOPATHIC MEDICAL SOCIETY OF PENNSYLVANIA—PROCEEDINGS OF THE SIXTEENTH ANNUAL SESSION.

REPORTED BY PEMBERTON DUDLEY, M.D, PHILADELPHIA.

First Day—Morning Session.—The Sixteenth Annual Session of the Pennsylvania State Society was held in the parlor of the United States Hotel at Easton, September 8th and 9th, 1880. At 10 o'clock the President, Dr. J. K. Lee, of Philadelphia, called the society to order and proceeded to deliver the annual address.

The report of the treasurer, Dr. J. F. Cooper, was received and referred to an auditing committee. Reports were also received from the secretaries and the two committees of publication. These latter show that the *Transactions* of the society have been published, those from 1874 to 1878, inclusive, in a single large volume, and those of 1879 in a small volume, which was issued from the press within six weeks after the session.

The Committee on Legislation reported, recommending that an effort be made to secure an act to define the qualifications for licentiates in medicine, and imposing penalties upon those who practice without being qualified.

The committee also asked the sense of the society as to the expediency of requiring colleges of the Commonwealth to have three courses of lectures previous to graduation.

Dr. A. R. Thomas appreciated the necessity for an extended course in our medical schools. No branch can be sufficiently developed in a course of five months. This term has been in universal use, however, until quite lately. The Hahnemann College of Philadelphia was the first to offer a graded course in this country, and that college expects to make that course obligatory at an early day. He favored the resolution.

Dr. Charles Mohr, delegate from the Philadelphia County Society, stated, on behalf of that body, that it was considered very desirable that some legislation should be secured which might render bogus diplomas nugatory, and protect the public against unqualified practitioners.

Dr. Jones moved that the Legislative Committee be instructed to present resolutions for the adoption of the society expressing its sentiments as to this necessary legislation, which was carried.

On motion, it was resolved to send a message of fraternity to the New York State Society, now in session in Brooklyn.

Dr. J. C. Guernsey, on behalf of the Historical Society, reported the completion of the "History of Homœopathy in Pennsylvania, from July 1828 to 1876," published in the *World's Homœopathic Convention Transactions.* Extra copies have been ordered for members of the society. Dr. Guernsey also read an account of the first homœopathic prescription ever made in Pennsylvania. It was made July 23d, 1828, by Dr. Henry Detwiller, of Easton, the present Vice-President of the society.

Dr. Mohr presented an address from the Board of Managers of the Homœopathic Hospital of Philadelphia, in view of the application to be made for State aid in establishing a large general hospital, and asking the formal indorsement of the society.

Dr. Joseph E. Jones, of West Chester, offered the following:

WHEREAS, This society learns through the report of the Homœopathic Hospital of Philadelphia, just received, that the officers and friends of that institution contemplate a renewal of their application to the legislature for an appropriation for aiding in the erection of a large general hospital in Philadelphia, provided with every modern convenience, and in which patients from every part of the State, and of every color and creed may receive the advantage of homœopathic treatment; therefore,

Resolved, That this society fully appreciates the importance of this enterprise; that it feels the necessity for such an institution in Philadelphia, both for the purpose of maintaining the standard of homœopathy in the State, for the purpose of affording the large and constantly increasing numbers who may desire homœopathic treatment an opportunity for receiving the same, and for the purpose of affording to our medical students opportunities for clinical instruction, as such an institution can only furnish.

Resolved, That the liberal policy which the State has heretofore manifested toward other hospitals of a different practice meets with the approbation of this society, and encourages us to ask with confidence for an extension of the same toward our own institution.

Resolved, That this society urge upon its members, and upon every homœopathic physician of the State the employment of every honorable influence upon the members of the legislature for securing such an appropriation.

Reports were received from the Homœopathic Hospital and Dispensary of Pittsburg, and from the various local societies throughout the State; also from the Missouri Institute of Homœopathy, the New York and Ohio State societies, and various other organizations.

The society, at one o'clock, adjourned until 3 o'clock.

Afternoon Session.—The society re-assembled at 3 P.M.

Dr. A. R. Thomas reported on behalf of the Hahnemann Medical College. There were last year 208 students; graduates, 75. A majority take the graded course. This has not yet been made obligatory, because it would require an increase in the size of our college, and an increased number of rooms. It is hoped that in a little while we shall have a new college building, one in every way adapted to the needs of a large class of students,—all of them taking the graded course. The teaching in the various branches is being made as practical as possible. Anatomy, chemistry, surgery, gynæcology, obstetrics, and microscopy, are all being taught by means of practical exercises, in addition to the didactic lectures. The need of a new college building is fully recognized by the faculty. The chief difficulty in our way as yet is the need of a new hospital for clinical instruction, without which, no course of medical study can at all qualify the student for practice. So soon as the hospital authorities select a site for a large general homœopathic hospital, the college authorities will at once proceed to the securing of ground and the erection of a new college building.

Dr. J. C. Burgher reported on behalf of the Homœopathic Hospital and Dispensary of Pittsburg. The hospital contains forty beds. The report contains a tabulated statement of the cases treated in both departments of the institution.

Dr. W. R. Childs, the necrologist, reported on the death of

Drs. Hahnemann E. Reinhold, of Williamsport, M. Friese, M.D., of Harrisburg, and Constantine Hering, M.D. He recommended that a committee be appointed to prepare a suitable expression of the sense of the society at the death of Dr. Hering. Adopted; and Drs. McClelland, Korndœrfer, and H. Detwiller were appointed the committee.

Dr. Bushrod W. James, Chairman of the Yellow Fever Committee, reported that while the United States had been exempt from the disease during the past summer, the disease had prevailed at Havana all the year round; also, to some extent at some other places, but the ratio of mortality was less than usual, owing doubtless to the improved sanitary precautions exercised.

Reports of bureaus being now in order, Dr. J. J. Detwiller, of Easton, Chairman of the Bureau of Surgery, read a paper on "Recto-vaginal Fistula," by W. D. Hall, M.D., of Altoona.

"Report of Surgical Cases," by W. R. Childs, M.D., of Pittsburg. The paper embraced an account of cases occurring in the Homœopathic Hospital of Pittsburg.

"Lithotrity,"—a case successfully treated, was reported by Dr. J. C. Burgher. It was an oxalate of lime calculus, weighing 310 grains. Bigelow's evacuating apparatus was used as an aid in dislodging the crushed stone.

"On a Modification of the Vance Jacket," by S. C. Scott, M.D., of Pittsburg, giving a description of its construction and its advantages over other forms of spinal supporting apparatus.

"Mammary Sarcoma,"—report of a case treated by H. N. Martin, M.D., and extirpated by Professor J. H. McClelland. The growth weighed five pounds, six ounces. Subsequent to the operation and recovery, Carbolic acid, diluted, had been administered every two hours for the four years that have elapsed since the operation, and there has been no return of the tumor. Dr. J. H. McClelland expressed himself as favorable to the use of Carbolic acid, with the hope of possibly preventing the return of this form of growth,—the spindle-celled sarcoma.

Dr. J. J. Detwiller thought four years not sufficient to test the prophylactic powers of the Carbolic acid.

Dr. McClelland thought the question depended largely upon the stage which the disease had reached at the time of the operation.

Dr. J. J. Detwiller then read a paper on "Senile Gangrene," a report of two cases treated successfully by homœopathic remedies, followed by amputation.

"Extirpation of the Kidney," by J. H. McClelland, M.D., of Pittsburg. Report of a case followed by recovery. But few successful cases are yet on record, and ten years ago the operation was unknown.

Dr. B. W. James mentioned a case of senile gangrene beginning on the tibia and gradually encircling the leg, but not penetrating the deeper tissues. After the integument had sloughed away, skin grafting was successfully tried. An ulcer afterwards formed and continues to exist,—the patient having left the city.

Dr. W. R. Childs alluded to a case of eburnation of the femur, reported at the last meeting.

The Committee on President's Address reported, recommending that the address be published as delivered. Adopted and committee discharged.

The Bureau of Materia Medica and Provings being next in order, Dr. Pemberton Dudley read a paper on "Bryonia and Rhus Tox. in Relation to Motion," by E. A. Farrington, M.D., of Philadelphia. Dr. W. J. Martin, of Pittsburg, presented a paper entitled, "Is there any Rule for Selecting the Potency?"

After discussion the meeting adjourned until 8 o'clock.

Evening Session.—The society re-assembled at 8 o'clock P.M., the President in the chair.

The report of the Bureau of Ophthalmology was presented and embraced the following papers:

"The Ophthalmoscope as an Aid in Diagnosing Special Diseases," by B. W. James, M.D., of Philadelphia.

"Eserine in Glaucoma"—three cases, by C. M. Thomas, M.D., of Philadelphia.

"Arsenicum Iodatum in Scrofulous Ophthalmia," by W. H. Bigler, M.D., of Philadelphia.

"Ophthalmia Neonatorum," by R. E. Caruthers, M.D., of Pittsburg.

Dr. B. W. James objected to keeping a case of infantile ophthalmia in a dark room. They should have some light; and, above all, an abundance of fresh air. If the light is too strong, let the eyes be bandaged. He also objected to the local use of silver nitrate, but would insist on perfect cleanliness.

Dr. J. E. Jones, of West Chester, confirmed the writer of the paper in regard to the internal use of Argentum nitrate,

3d to 12th, with, of course, the proper precautions of cleanliness.

Dr. H. N. Martin spoke of the cases of ophthalmia in a children's home with which he was formerly connected. The cases were cured by cleanliness and the homœopathic remedy, with an abundance of fresh air. One of the best remedies was Asarum, when the patient liked cold air and cold water to the eyes. Dr. Caruthers mentioned a case cured with Argentum nitrate applied locally.

Dr. M. M. Walker had two cases that had come to him from Cape May. He was careful to use water, either cold or warm, according to the child's evident preferences, and gave the indicated remedy.

Dr. Dudley spoke of a contagious ophthalmia in the Northern Home for Friendless Children, in which Dr. James and himself had treated over five hundred cases of the disease without the loss of a single eye. The homœopathic remedies were used in all the cases. The disease, he had been informed, was finally eradicated by the removal of the mattresses of oat-straw and the substitution of some other material.

Dr. Charles Mohr described a case of ophthalmia in which there was evidently a croupous exudation or deposit upon the palpebral conjunctiva, and asked if such deposit should be removed by mechanical means, to which Dr. James answered in the affirmative.

Dr. J. C. Guernsey mentioned Euphrasia, Graphite, and Borax, as frequently indicated remedies.

The Bureau of Gynæcology then reported. Their report included the following papers:

"Pruritus Vulvæ," by F. R. Schmucker, M.D., of Reading.

"Mutilations of the Cervix Uteri," by B. F. Betts, M.D., the paper taking strong grounds against the process as not only needless, but almost always harmful; also suggesting modes of repairing some of the results of these mutilations.

Dr. J. H. McClelland commended the paper of Dr. Betts. Speaking of the incisions of the cervix, he thought the cut should be antero-posterior, as this avoids the eversion which results from the bilateral operation. In some of the operations for uniting lacerations of the cervix he had found it advantageous to unite one side at a time, the contraction of the tissue rendering the remaining portion of the treatment more certain. The doctor said the idea had been suggested to him by Dr. Breyfogle.

Dr. Betts said that much of the difficulty experienced in bringing and retaining the lips in apposition was due to a mass of cicatricial tissue in the angle of the laceration, acting as a wedge to keep the parts asunder. All of this tissue should be cut away.

Dr. C. P. Seip read a paper on "The Treatment of Some Forms of Sterility."

Second Day—Morning Session.—The society re-convened at 10 A.M., President Lee in the chair.

The following additional papers were presented by the Bureau of Gynæcology: "Hot Water Enemata in Congestions and Inflammations of the Pelvic Organs," by H. M. Paine, M.D., of Albany, N. Y.; "Diagnosis of Abdominal Tumors," by J. H. Marsden, M.D., of York Springs, Pa.; "Vaginismus," by H. W. Fulton, M.D., Pittsburg.

The Bureau of Sanitary Science presented its report through Dr. B. W. James. The papers were "Animal Food as a Marketable Product," by W. H. H. Neville, M.D., of Philadelphia; "Transportation and Preparation of Animal Food," by W. F. Edmundson, M.D., of Pittsburg; "Diseased Conditions of Animal Food," by T. M. Strong, M.D., of Pittsburg; "Diseases Resulting from the Use of Animal Food," by J. W. Allen, M.D., of Altoona, Pa.; "Diseases Resulting from the Use of Diseased Animal Food," by B. W. James, M.D., of Philadelphia.

Dr. Betts thought that diseased or tainted meat could not communicate disease to those who eat it, except through some abraded surface. He illustrated his point by the case of a man who, carrying a sheep on his back, was diseased, while those who ate the meat escaped.

Dr. James: It is not true that boiling always destroys the poisonous properties of animal matter, particularly tuberculous meat, which is not always destroyed even by fifteen minutes' boiling.

Dr. J. C. Burgher thought that very little tuberculous meat finds its way to our markets. The careful inspection by experts almost entirely prevents the possibility of meat infected with tubercle ever reaching the consumer.

Dr. A. R. Thomas called attention to the numerous forms of animal and vegetable parasites, and ascribed the safety of the consumer to the solvent and chemical powers of the digestive secretions by which the poisonous properties of these parasites are rendered inert. He considered that all meat-eaters are liable to ingest the larvæ of certain parasites, yet these do not cause disease except in rare instances.

The report of the Bureau of Obstetrics was then presented by its chairman, Dr. R. J. McClatchey. It included the following papers, which were read by title and referred for publication: "Abortion with Retained Placenta," by J. Morgan Maurer, M.D., of Washington, Pa.; "Milk Fever," by Isaac Lefever, of Harrisburg, Pa.; "Neuralgia during Pregnancy," by the same; also, the following, which were read in full by their authors: "Dystocia from Fetal Hydrocephalus," by Mrs. C. T. Canfield, M.D., of Titusville, Pa.; "The Obstetric Forceps," by Pemberton Dudley, M.D., of Philadelphia; "The Vienna Obstetrical School," by M. M. Walker, M.D., of Germantown; "A Case of Placenta Prævia," by C. Vanartsdalen, M.D., of Chelten Hills.

Upon Dr. Canfield's paper a brief discussion was engaged in by Dr. Thomas.

Dr. Dudley's paper was discussed by Dr. Burgher, who thought with the writer that the forceps could be more frequently used with advantage. He now always carries his forceps with him, and did not consider a consultation necessary in ordinary cases. He preferred the instrument recommended by Dr. Dudley.

Dr. Martin was a little conservative in regard to the use of forceps. He thought the labor pain was frequently less than is sometimes imagined. He cited instances in illustration of his point.

Dr. Seip considered the forceps perfectly harmless when properly used, and with the use of an anæsthetic in certain cases, it need not be productive of injury to either mother or child. The talk of "meddlesome midwifery" involved more of poetry than of truth.

Dr. B. W. James did not consider it meddlesome to use the forceps for the alleviation of pain in many cases. It is really a conservative procedure.

Dr. Marsden was of the opinion that the necessity for the use of the forceps is of increasing frequency, though he did not place much value upon the statistics in this line of research. He was sure he had never inflicted any injury on a mother, nor any *serious* injury to a child, by the use of the forceps, yet he was in the habit of using the instrument to alleviate intense pain. The danger from using the forceps depends largely upon the skill of the hand that applies them. Extremely hard pressure upon the handles should be avoided, because such a practice renders the instrument liable to slip, and, moreover, it increases one diameter just in proportion as it diminishes the other. He always carries his forceps with him, and his bottle of chloroform. The use of this agent he has found, thus far, perfectly safe.

Dr. Mohr found truth on both sides of the question under discussion. He alluded to the use of moral influences to aid the woman in bearing her pain, illustrating his point by a ludicrous incident.

Dr. J. C. Guernsey did not know on what ground Dr. Marsden could think that in the future the process will be more frequently needed than in the past.

Dr. Marsden replied that the necessity for an increasing use of the forceps will depend on the increasing weakness—the neurasthenia, if you please, of the human race. If this condition can be better met and prevented by the homœopathic remedy, so much the better, but there are cases to which the use of medicine, homœopathic or allopathic, cannot be applied. The pellet can never take the place of the perforator.

Dr. A. Korndœrfer had always been a friend of the forceps, but objected to any but the most cautious use of chloroform. The carefully selected homœopathic remedy will often prevent the necessity for a resort to either. Cases were cited in illustration.

The committee appointed to prepare a minute in reference to the death of Constantine Hering, M.D., reported as follows, through its chairman, Dr. J. H. McClelland:

The Homœopathic Medical Society of Pennsylvania, in annual session assembled, with unanimous voice adopts the following minute:

The death of Dr. Constantine Hering, of Philadelphia, on the 23d day of July, 1880, is recognized as an event of signal import in the history of medicine. It marks the close of a life remarkable for unflagging and long-sustained industry in the cause of medical science, and in promoting the good of his kind. With full recognition of his prodigious labors in the field of Materia Medica and homœopathic therapeutics, the attainments of Dr. Hering in general science and letters entitle him to a high place among men of learning in this enlightened age.

This society, therefore, records with willing hands, its high appreciation of the distinguished dead, and with sentiments of high regard, offers heartfelt sympathy to the bereaved family.

J. H. McClelland, M.D.,
Aug. Korndœrfer, M.D.,
Henry Detwiller, M D.,
Committee.

The minute was adopted, and a copy was ordered to be

transmitted to the Hering Memorial Meeting, to be held in Philadelphia, October 10th, 1880.

The report and papers of the Bureau of Clinical Medicine were presented by the Chairman, Dr. A. Korndœrfer, as follows: "Purpura Hæmorrhagica," by Henry Detwiller, M.D., of Easton; "Dosage," by J. H. Marsden, M.D., of York Sulphur Springs, Pa.; "Experiences with Scarlatina," by P. S. Duff, M.D., of Great Belt, Pa.; "Cerebro-Spinal Meningitis," by W. D. Hall, M.D., of Altoona, Pa.; "Pancreatic Diseases," by the Philadelphia County Society; "Chorea," by T. C. Williams, M.D., of Philadelphia, Pa.; "Typhoid Fever," by T. C. Williams, M.D., of Philadelphia, Pa.; "A Clinical Case," by T. C. Williams, M.D., of Philadelphia, Pa.; "Ovarian Tumor," by T. C. Williams, M.D., of Philadelphia, Pa.; "Clinical Reflections," by A. Lippe, M.D., of Philadelphia, Pa.; "Solar Neuralgia," by Joseph E. Jones, M.D., of West Chester, Pa.; "Rachitis," by Joseph E. Jones, M.D., of West Chester, Pa.; "Diabetes Mellitus," by John S. Boyd, M.D.; "Chorea," by H. Hoffman. M.D., of Pittsburg, Pa.; "Eczema Pustulosa," by W. J. Guernsey, M.D., of Frankford, Pa. "Clinical Observation," by J. C. Morgan, M.D., of Philadelphia, Pa.; "Pruritus Vulvæ," by E. R. Schmucker, M.D., of Reading, Pa.; "Apis Mel. in Venereal Disease," by J. K. Lee, M.D., of Philadelphia, Pa.; "Typhoid Fever," by Charles Mohr, M.D., of Philadelphia, Pa.; "Eczema," by the Allegheny County Society; "Tuberculosis Mesenterica," by Paz Alvarez, M.D., of Madrid, Spain; "Rheumatic Carditis," by B. W. James, M.D., of Philadelphia, Pa.; "Clinical Notes," by H. Noah Martin, M.D., of Philadelphia, Pa.

After the reading of several of the above papers, the society adjourned at 12.30 for a short recess.

Afternoon Session.—The convention re-assembled at 1.15, President Lee in the chair.

The remaining papers of the report in clinical medicine were presented, and the bureau closed.

The secretaries recommended certain changes in the by-laws of the society, prescribing the duties of those officers. Adopted.

The following was adopted:

Resolved, That the society declares itself unequivocally in favor of a higher medical education, and the protection of the people against incompetent practitioners.

Resolved, Therefore, that the Committee on Legislation be instructed to use all honorable means to secure legislation favorable to that end.

Also the following:

Resolved, That the thanks of this society be tendered to *The Express* and *Free Press*, of Easton, and the *Ledger* and *Press*, of Philadelphia, for publishing the reports of the proceedings of this session.

Ordered that hereafter the sessions be held for three days instead of two, as heretofore; and that the next session be held at West Chester, on the second Tuesday in September, 1881.

The following officers were elected to serve for the ensuing year: President, J. H. McClelland, M.D., of Pittsburg, Pa.; First Vice-President, B. F. Betts, M.D., of Philadelphia, Pa.; Second Vice-President, J. J. Detwiller, M.D., of Easton, Pa.; Recording Secretary, Z. T. Miller, M.D., of Pittsburg, Pa.; Corresponding Secretary, R. E. Caruthers, M.D., Allegheny City, Pa.; Treasurer, J. F. Cooper, M.D., Allegheny City, Pa.; Necrologist, W. R. Childs, M.D., of Pittsburg, Pa.; Censors, Drs. R. J. McClatchey, Joseph E. Jones, and C. T. Canfield.

Committees.—Committee of Arrangements, the Officers of the Society; Committee of Publication, Drs. Z. T. Miller, R. E. Caruthers, T. M. Strong and J. F. Cooper; Committee on Subscription, J. F. Cooper, M.D., Chairman; Committee on Legislation, Drs. J. H. McClelland, J. K. Lee, and H. Pitcairn; Historical Committee, J. C. Guernsey, M.D., Chairman; Delegate to the American Institute of Homœopathy, J. F. Cooper, M.D., Chairman.

Bureaus.—The following is a list of the chairmen of the various bureaus: Bureau of Surgery, C. M. Thomas, M.D., Chairman; Bureau of Materia Medica, C. Mohr, M.D., Chairman; Bureau of Ophthalmology and Otology, W. H. Bigler, M.D., Chairman; Bureau of Gynæcology, J. C. Burgher, M.D., Chairman; Bureau of Obstetrics, C. T. Canfield, M.D., Chairman; Bureau of Clinical Medicine, W. J. Martin, M.D., Chairman; Bureau of General Sanitary Science, Pemberton Dudley, M.D., Chairman.

After the election of officers, general discussion on a variety of subjects was indulged in, in which all pleasantly participated. There was a general feeling of satisfaction at the success of the meeting, which was repeatedly declared to be the most successful that the society had ever held.

The business of the session was over, and at 4 o'clock the society adjourned to the dining-room, to partake of Dr. Detwiller's hospitality.

THE BANQUET.

Dr. Henry Detwiller had invited his relatives and descendants—children and grandchildren—residents in Easton, and vicinity, to meet the doctors at this entertainment. Quite a number of ladies, therefore, lent the grace of their presence to the grand dinner tables. Among those present we noticed, Dr. and Mrs. Detwiller, of Hellertown; Miss Martin, of Allentown; Dr. and Mrs. Porter, of Easton; Dr. and Mrs. Martin, of Philadelphia; Mrs. Charles Hemingway; Dr. and Mrs. W. J. Guernsey; Dr. Henry Detwiller, Jr., and Mrs. Detwiller; Miss Knecht, of Hellertown; Mrs. J. J. Detwiller, of Easton, and others. The Opera House Orchestra provided excellent music during the progress of the dinner. Before taking his seat at the head of the table, Dr. Lee, President, formally, in the name of the State Society, accepted the banquet and, in some well-chosen remarks, alluded to the host's long connection with the science of homœopathy and the pleasure the members of the State Society had experienced in meeting their venerable confrère. Then the attack upon the bill of fare commenced and went on for about an hour, and then the formal toasts were drank.

The first was drank in silence: "To the memory of Samuel Hahnemann and Constantine Hering."

The next was *the* toast of this particular occasion: "Dr. Henry Detwiller, our host and the pioneer of Homœopathy in Pennsylvania." Amid great applause the venerable doctor rose to his feet, and with earnest deliberation and in a clear voice responded as follows:

"*Ladies and Gentlemen, Doctors, Members of the Homœopathic Medical Society of the State of Pennsylvania, Friends, my own Children and Grandchildren*: I embrace this opportunity to give you a short synopsis of my interview with the discoverer of the natural law of cure—*similia similibus curantur*—the illustrious Dr. Samuel Hahnemann, the greatest benefactor of mankind in this nineteenth century. Now past forty-four years, I sailed to Europe and trusted my practice to the care of Dr. H. Wohlfort, a homœopathist, and my family in charge of my brother, then in the village of Hellertown, twelve miles from here. My main object was to interview Dr. Samuel Hahnemann, of Paris, Professor Shoenlein, of Zurich, and Professor Werber, of Freyburg, in the interest of the Allentown Academy of the Homœopathic Healing Art. Dr. Hahnemann and lady received me with marked kindness. He was very much surprised at our enterprise in establishing an institute to teach homœopathy, and more so when I told him that Dr. C. Hering was the pilot of the enterprise. I solicited his advice as to whether it were possible to obtain material aid among our friends in Europe in subscribing stock. To this he answered that he would take the matter into consideration, and he held firmly to the hope of doing something at my next visit. On my next visit in October, 1836, he pleaded his inability to obtain aid or to give any pecuniary aid himself, in subscribing stock, but he would send his life-size marble statue, then in course of sculpture by the famous David, in Paris. He kept his word, but the statue was lost by shipwreck. At my departure he implored God's blessing on our enterprise, and Madame, with a parting kiss, joined in the invocation that the good work begun might prosper and spread, like the Christian religion, all over the world. The result you all know." The doctor sat down amid enthusiastic applause.

The next toast—"Our State Society," was responded to by Dr. Joseph E. Jones, of Westchester; "The Ladies," by Dr. J. H. McClelland, of Pittsburg. "The Press of Easton," by Mr. Emmons, of the Easton *Express*.

A vote of thanks was proposed to Dr. Henry Detwiller, for his complimentary hospitality, and the motion was "carried with a shout," when President Lee addressing the venerable doctor said:

"Dr. Detwiller, I have the pleasure of returning to you the thanks of this society for this entertainment, and of assuring you of its appreciation of the compliment you have paid us in arranging this pleasant social reunion."

The members then separated, with many expressions of pleasure at the unprecedented success of the session, and a hearty hand-shaking with their venerable friend, the pioneer of Homœopathy in Pennsylvania.*

PHILADELPHIA COUNTY HOMŒOPATHIC MEDICAL SOCIETY.

(REPORTED BY CHARLES MOHR, M.D., SECRETARY.)

THE regular monthly meeting of this society was held on Thursday evening, September 2d, in the hall of Hahnemann College. The President, Dr. E. A. Farrington, occupied the chair, and about thirty-five physicians were present. Dr. R. E. Caruthers, Corresponding Secretary of the Pennsylvania State Society, being present, was invited to participate in the discussion.

* I am indebted to Mr. Emmons of the Easton *Express*, for valuable assistance in the preparation of the above report.—P. D.

The president referred to the death of Dr. Constantine Hering, an honorary member of the society, and on motion Drs. J. K. Lee, P. Dudley, and C. R. Norton, were appointed a committee to prepare suitable resolutions and present the same on behalf of the society at the memorial meeting to be held October 10th.

Dr. Charles Mohr was appointed delegate to the Pennsylvania State Society, to convene in annual session at Easton, on September 8th, and was instructed to call the attention of the State Society to the fact that a large number of unqualified persons are practicing medicine throughout the State, many of them in possession of diplomas irregularly obtained, and to urge the necessity of taking such steps as shall eradicate the evil of diploma selling and debar illegal practitioners from carrying on their nefarious calling.

The Bureau of Pædology, through its Chairman, Dr. B. F. Betts, then presented their annual report. It embraced the following papers, which were read by their respective authors, viz.:

a. "Neurasthenia in Childhood," by W. P. Sharkey, M.D.

b. "Care of the Mouth and Teeth in Infancy and Childhood," by C. Mohr, M.D.

c. "Eczema Capitis," by B. Frank Betts, M.D.

The papers were accepted and referred for publication in the HAHNEMANNIAN MONTHLY.

In the discussion which followed, Dr. M. M. Walker thought Dr. Betts placed too low an estimate on Mezereum. He recited three cases cured with that remedy in the 200th potency. Neurasthenia in childhood, he remarked, had its starting-point in defective nutrition, and some cases may be traced to the hobgoblin stories related to children by their nurses. During dentition, children are more liable to these troubles than at other times. As to the care of the teeth, sometimes despite the utmost vigilance the teeth will decay, but probably for the want of the homœopathic remedy.

Dr. W. K. Ingersoll mentioned two cases of eczema capitis cured with Oleander^{200}. The crusts were thick, extending, in one case, over the face, down the chest, and even so low as the hips. Viola tricolor, θ gtt. ij after each meal, cured a case of facial eczema associated with ulcerative keratitis under the care of Dr. W. H. Bigler.

Dr. C. R. Norton also spoke favorably of Mezereum, having cured two cases in which the scalp was covered quite thoroughly, the crusts being thick and cracked, and when raised up, a greenish pus exuded from beneath.

Dr. A. Korndœrfer had used Mezereum[30] for a number of years. He had found it indicated when the scalp was covered with heavy crusts, built up into irregular, brownish, moist-looking scabs, with here and there a portion that assumed a dirty chalklike color, and when the scabs were broken, the exudation was of a thick yellowish or dirty color, approaching a greenish hue, the child's head having quite an unpleasant odor. The child is cross, has more or less itching, scratching being followed by discharge of pus and blood. When the discharge dries it forms more of the black and dirty-looking crusts.

Dr. J. C. Morgan remarked that Oleander was one of the specifics of Teste for eczema capitis. In sore mouth, he had found granulated sugar, moistened to the consistence of an ointment and rubbed on the sores, to be of incalculable value.

Dr. C. Mohr inquired if Dr. Morgan had found the sugar equally valuable in thrush and aphthous sore mouth. To which he replied that the sugar, properly used, *i. e.*, moistened and *rubbed* in, suited both conditions.

Dr. C. Mohr had seen cases of thrush aggravated by the use of sugar, in fact he believed that in thrush, sugar should not be used, on the ground of its tendency to pass into a state of fermentation, thus favoring, rather than preventing, the formation of confervæ.

Dr. Morgan spoke strongly against the indiscriminate use of borax, having seen two cases of aphthous sore mouth prove fatal from its prolonged local use in substance.

Dr. J. C. Morgan was appointed Chairman of the Bureau of Pædology for the ensuing year. The society then adjourned to meet October 14th, when the report of the Bureau of Surgery and Clinical Surgery will be presented and discussed.

THE HOMŒOPATHIC MEDICAL SOCIETY OF CHESTER, DELAWARE AND MONTGOMERY COUNTIES, PENNA.

REPORTED BY L. HOOPES, M.D., SECRETARY.

THIS society held its regular quarterly meeting at the Bingham House, Philadelphia, July 6th, 1880. President, Dr. T. Pratt in the chair. Nineteen members were present.

The committee appointed to prepare a memorial regarding

the relation of women to our colleges, etc., submitted a report,* which after considerable discussion was accepted, and the committee was discharged. Further action on the report was then postponed until the next regular meeting, because of the absence of some of the members who did not know the nature of the memorial and might desire to vote upon it.

Dr. J. B. Wood read a paper entitled, "Is Colocynth a Cure for Diabetes?" in which he described a case of diabetes which recovered while taking Coloc. for colic and diarrhœa.

Dr. C. Preston read a paper entitled, "Democracy in Medicine," relating to the reception of women into our societies and colleges.

Dr. Long read a paper on the treatment and management of the child during and after labor, in which he set forth some ideas differing from those usually taught and practiced.

Dr. Hawley described a case in which the foramen ovale of the heart was evidently not closed, but which was relieved by laying the child on its right side for several days, thus favoring its closure.

Dr. L. Hoopes mentioned two cases in which hæmorrhage from the navel occurred, an hour or two after birth, in consequence of shrinkage of the cord, thereby relaxing the ligature. Dr. Wood also had a child bleed to death from a similar cause. Dr. Williams had a case where hæmorrhage followed ligation of the cord, on the eighth day. Dr. C. Preston held to the view that the cord should not be cut until pulsation had ceased. If this precaution is observed, hæmorrhage will rarely occur, whether the funis is ligated or not. Dr. I. D. Johnson always has the child greased the first day, and wiped off with a woollen cloth, but not washed till the following day.

Dr. Wood moved to appoint Dr. Hawley to prepare a paper for the State society, which was carried.

Dr. Way expressed the hope that at the next meeting the subject of requirements for medical students might be carefully considered.

Dr. C. Preston offered the following resolution:

Resolved, That hereafter the Homœopathic Medical Society of Chester, Delaware, and Montgomery counties will receive female physicians to membership on application, subject to the same qualifications as are required of male members.

---

* A copy of this report is in our hands, but presuming that the society would prefer not to have it published until final action is taken thereon, we withhold it for the present.—Eds.

Some of the members thought the resolution unnecessary, as there was nothing in the Constitution and By-laws prohibiting women from becoming members, and none had ever applied.

On motion of Dr. Way, the subject was laid on the table until next meeting.

Dr. Rossiter presented a patient eighteen years of age, with an affection of the cardiac orifice of the stomach since he was nine years old. Has been treated by a number of old-school doctors with no benefit. He eats until full up to the throat, and then drinks water to force it down, then vomits and eats more. The cardiac orifice is sensitive to the passage of food. Some of the members suggested Nux vom. as a remedy, while others expressed the opinion that Hydrastis was indicated and would prove beneficial.

Drs. Hawley and Wood were appointed delegates to the State society.

Adjourned, to meet at the Bingham House, Philadelphia, on the first Tuesday in October, 1880.

IS COLOCYNTHIS A CURE FOR DIABETES.

BY J. B. WOOD, M D , WEST CHESTER, PA.

(Read before the Homœopathic Medical Society of Chester, Delaware, and Montgomery Counties).

In April, 1878, J. M. F., aged about 40 years, called upon me for relief from severe cutting pain in the region of the umbilicus, and radiating from that point over the entire abdomen. This was also accompanied with diarrhœa with straining at stool.

There was nothing unusual in the appearance of the stool. Nux vom.[2] having failed to relieve him after a fair trial, I substituted Colocynth.[1], which speedily effected a cure.

At the time of my first visit, the patient, who was very much emaciated, though his appetite was good, informed me that he had extreme thirst and drank much, usually taking a pail of water to bed with him, which he drank during the night, and bringing down stairs with him in the morning a vessel of urine, equal to or greater in quantity than the amount of water consumed.

This condition had continued with him for several years, and for which he had applied to several physicians without obtaining any relief, and from which he had been informed that relief could not be obtained.

He is well now, July, 1880, and in the most robust health.

THE

HAHNEMANNIAN

MONTHLY.

A HOMŒOPATHIC JOURNAL OF

MEDICINE AND SURGERY.

Editors,

E. A. Farrington, M.D. Pemberton Dudley, M.D.

Business Manager,

Bushrod W. James, M.D.

Vol. II. Philadelphia, Pa., October, 1880. No. 10.

☞ The Editors consider themselves responsible for the maintenance of the dignity and courtesy of the journal, but *not* for the opinions expressed by its contributors.

Editorial Department.

The Situation in England.—There are few things that would give more sincere gratification to American homœopathists than to see our system of medicine enjoying the same prestige and exerting the same influences in England and on the Continent that it does in this country. We all know, and in some measure appreciate, the nature of the obstacles that lie in the path of medical progress across the Atlantic. The intense conservatism of European thought, and the powerful grip with which the medical authorities hold possession of the universities and clutch the doors of the great hospitals, have thus far been sufficient to prevent effectually any successful invasion of their precincts by the champions of homœopathy. At the same time the legal authorities in Europe, fully as much as in republican America, endeavor to follow the dictates of popular and professional majorities, and fail to appreciate the full force of the doctrine that there are particulars in which the majority has no right to rule, and that men's medical preferences constitute one of them. Springing legitimately from this misconception of men's natural rights, we see an evident indifference to the claims of the homœopathists in England and other countries, simply because they cannot outvote their opponents, who are ever ready in any "lawful" way, to appropriate the belongings of those who disagree with them,—there are so many people in the world, even educated people, who imagine that a legislative enactment can justify even a crime.

There are, it seems to us, two things that our English brethren would do well to force constantly and perseveringly upon the attention of their authorities and people, viz.: First, that *all* the "expert" testimony in reference to homœopathy is in favor of that system. Of all those who, by reason of a thorough knowledge of its principles and practice, and by actual observation of the results of its application in disease, are competent to speak on the subject, not one disputes its claims or doubts its verity. The testimony of its opponents is not expert testimony. Not one of them could pass a graduate's examination in its principles and practice,—not one has a personal knowledge of its effects upon the sick. All the allopathic evidence of any value whatever is favorable to homœopathy, and this evidence consists not in what allopathists may or may not think about it,—that, as we have just said, is of no account either way,—but in the brilliant success which so frequently results even from the bungling use of homœopathic remedies in allopathic hands. ALL THE EVIDENCE, then, *is in favor of homœopathy as one of the settled and established principles of modern medical science,* without a knowledge of which no medical education is complete, and no practitioner qualified for his office.

Secondly, in view of this universal indorsement of homœopathy by those who alone are competent to judge of its merits, the homœopathic taxpayers of England are justified in demanding, with a persistent determination that will accept nothing short of perfect acquiescence, that homœopathy shall, from this time, enjoy in all institutions under the patronage of government equal favors and rights with allopathy. That its practitioners shall have their own colleges, their own hospitals, their own examining and licensing boards, and an equal and due share of governmental preferment.

Of course it must not be expected that such efforts can at once secure a complete or even a partial success. Time, watchfulness, determination, unity, are all-important elements in such an enterprise; but it would be strange, indeed, if the proverbial bull-dog pertinacity of the typical Briton did not eventually triumph over the machinations and the resisting force of the foes of medical progress and the enemies of popular rights. A little banding together of the homœopathic physicians and laymen, for the purpose of defeating candidates for office known to be unfavorable to their claims, would have a wholesome influence upon all officials. It would furnish evidence that these homœopaths did not propose to tolerate any nonsense or any evasion of the question, and would insure to them a more respectful hearing and a speedier acknowledgment of their rights. The mere fact of such an organized opposition to a candidate, even if not a very formidable one, would cause a shaking among the dry bones. Office-seekers know full well that it often takes but a few votes to set aside a majority.

Within quite a recent period an interesting discussion has arisen among the British homœopathists respecting their college and hospital facilities. Apparently some of these men are pretty fully convinced that it is about time for them to have control of the medical education of their own young men, instead of waiting for conversions from the allopathic school, and that the policy of depending for their own leaders upon desertions from the staff of the enemy has prevailed long enough. Some of them are urging the establishment of a completely appointed college and the securing of all needed legal authority to enable them to carry on the work of educating and licensing their own students, thus maintaining an entire independence of the allopathic school. The progress of the movement will be watched with eager interest from this side of the Atlantic, and we suggest that American physicians can give aid and comfort to their English brethren in this movement, by attending in force the World's Homœopathic Convention, to be held next year in London.

Tannerism *v.* Starvation.—A comparison between the condition of a man starving and Dr. Tanner's state, while undergoing a voluntary fast, will show that, in one respect at least, they are widely different. In the first the psychological disturbances operate very deleteriously upon the body. The mind is distressed by the inability to procure nourishment. Suffering, and eventual death, are continually forepictured in the imagination; and, as one by one the mental forebodings are realized, the nerve-force, upon which the integrity of the entire system depends, is greatly impaired, and serious consequences must ensue from this cause. If the faster is compelled to abstain by reason of disease, the mind is necessarily ill at ease. Weakened alike by the malady and by emotional disturbances, we could not expect such a patient to long withstand so exhausting a drain upon his vital powers.

Granting the validity of Dr. Tanner's fast, we must, nevertheless, remember that his mind was in a comparatively calm state. He knew that food was attainable at any time. Though suffering from nervous irritability, dependent upon want of sustenance, he had none of the horrors of starvation looming up before him to urge his nervous irritability forward into actual delirium.

Ambition added its stimulus, and words of encouragement from his physicians spurred on the will to its burdensome work. Further, the body was in a healthy condition, and so better enabled to withstand the drafts made upon it.

In view of these important facts it would be unreasonable to conclude, from his speedy return to a full and varied diet after his long abstinence, that our usual cautionary allowance of food in an ordinary case of partial starvation is necessarily unscientific. The two cases are not parallel, and evidently requires different management.

THE REPORT OF THE BRITISH HOMŒOPATHIC CONGRESS.—Our thanks are due to Dr. Alfred C. Pope, of the *British Monthly Homœopathic Review*, for the above report, which will be found in the present number of this journal.

Book Department.

A PRACTICAL TREATISE ON TUMORS OF THE MAMMARY GLAND. Embracing their histology, pathology, diagnosis, and treatment. By Samuel W. Gross, A.M., M.D., Surgeon to and Lecturer on Clinical Surgery in the Jefferson Medical College Hospital and the Philadelphia Hospital; President of the Pathological Society of Philadelphia; Fellow of and former Mütter Lecturer on Surgical Pathology in the College of Physicians of Philadelphia; Fellow of the Academy of Surgery of Philadelphia, etc. Illustrated by twenty-nine engravings. New York: D. Appleton & Co., 1, 3, and 5 Bond Street. 1880. Octavo, pp. 246.

Surgeons well know what important knowledge has been added to pathology in researches upon morbid growths during the past few years, revolutionizing the histological part of the subject almost as effectually and as thoroughly as the later years of investigation have changed the older ideas in the rapidly expanding field of ophthalmology. The study still goes on, and the microscopic examination of a large number of specimens gives the histologist additional light upon the pathological anatomy of these abnormal structures. The author of this book has penetrated the subject anew, and throwing aside the deductions of older observers, after examining under the microscope many hundreds of specimens has drawn his own conclusions from this personal observation, and by the assistance of well-informed and skilful microscopists.

He believes in the permanent relief of carcinoma by thorough removal in the early stage of its growth, in opposition to the generally accepted ideas upon this point. His diagnoses in the cases on which he bases this belief were confirmed by minute examinations made by expert examiners from the specimens removed. Further, to remove all doubt as to the accuracy of this labor, he has given the distinct features characteristic of these specimens, by drawings made through the aid of the camera, and by photographs of his private and public cases, and introduced them in their proper places through the book. The microscopic showings are thus given in two illustrations of cystic fibromata, the intracanalicular, and one, of a type corresponding to what was formerly known as desmoid or fibroid, taken from a mammary growth of fourteen months, about the size of a walnut. Six plates of sarcoma are shown, giving the small round-celled, lymphoid, small spindle-celled, large spindle-celled, giant-celled, and one unremoved specimen of a myxomatous and telangiectatic, cystic, small spindle-celled sarcoma, one cut of hyaline myxoma, two of cystic adenoma, and thirteen upon carcinoma and scirrhus. To the latter he devotes fifty-eight pages, and with regard to its development he claims that cancer does not appear before puberty, and although Henry records a case, aged twenty-one, he never observed it before the twenty-eighth year. Of 642 cases where the age is given,

18	appeared	between	20 and 30	years of	age.
128	"	"	30 and 40	"	"
245	"	"	40 and 50	"	"
165	"	"	50 and 60	"	"
78	"	"	60 and 70	"	"
8	"	"	70 and 80	"	"

Tumors of the male mammary glands are cut off with about a page and a half, and although very uncommon, still these neoplastic and cystic growths do form in this structure. The average frequency of recurrence in the male is about two, to one hundred in the female mamma.

In reference to treatment he holds out the plan of sponging the exposed surfaces with a strong solution of chloride of zinc, or searing them with the hot iron, and especially if nodules have been removed from the ribs or adjacent muscles the actual cautery should be used. He believes in the use of the knife alone, for that reaches all that caustic applications can. He condemns the practice of medical attendants in waiting, before asking surgical advice, for other manifestations where these growths are once discovered, for patients themselves generally are averse to the knife, and especially so at the period when its best results for success can be had; that is in its incipiency. Physicians should know that the chances of a carcinoma being the result, where a hard mammary tumor comes on after the lady has passed forty years, are as thirteen to one.

The book is a valuable contribution, is well printed and bound, having clear type and paper, and issued in the accustomed good style of the publications of the Appletons. B. W. J.

HEALTH OFFICER'S ANNUAL REPORT OF BIRTHS, MARRIAGES, AND DEATHS, FOR THE CITY OF PHILADELPHIA. 1879. 8vo., pp. 175.

Homœopathic physicians, as a rule, have a higher regard for statistics than do their allopathic brethren, simply because they furnish some pretty solid arguments in favor of Hahnemann's system of therapeutics. The array of figures contained in this volume, however, ought to be of interest to all, particularly because of the lessons they convey to the student of sanitary science. According to these figures, the sum total of deaths in Philadelphia during the year 1879, was 15,473 or one to every 58¼ of the population,—the lowest rate of mortality experienced for at least nineteen years. Of these, 321 were from diphtheria and 336 from scarlet fever. Phthisis claimed 2481 victims; pneumonia, 1003; pleuritis, 19; congestion of the lungs, 178; hæmorrhage from the lungs, 53; hydrothorax (under various names), 27; bronchitis, 297. Total deaths from diseases of the respiratory apparatus, 4058, or over 26 per cent. of the total mortality. Inflammations of the stomach and bowels were fatal in 338 cases; typhoid fever, in 344; dropsy in its various forms, 394. Amongst the infantile population, marasmus swept off 613, and cholera infantum, 804. "Hooping-cough," which, from its evident reference to the cooper's trade, we take to mean *beer drinker's* cough, carried away 103 victims; but we are at a loss to understand why 95 of these deaths should have been infantile cases. "Whooping" cough on the other hand does not appear to have had a single trophy. Croup disposed of 291; craniotomy is responsible for 2; premature birth occasioned 190 deaths, and there were no less than 809 still-births,—a sad, if not a suspicious record. We find that among the total of 362 deaths from cancer, the most frequently involved organs were, the uterus in 82 cases, the stomach in 78, the breasts in 55, the liver in 34, the face in 8, while cases affecting other parts varied in number from 6 to 1. "Debility," that never-failing resource of the inexpert diagnostician, was called upon to explain the "termination" no less than 472 times. (We know a physician who boldly applies to these cases, the more significant title, "Damfino.") Old age closes the record of life's fitful fever with 722 cases, of whom 97 were over 90 years of age, and 15 were over 100. The Registrar, with characteristic generosity, has omitted all mention of deaths occurring from "too much doctor," having probably included them under "debility," though some sarcastic people might consider *that* department too small to hold them.

The total number of births registered for the year was 18,499. The figures vary but little from 1600 per month, except for the months of April, May, and June, when we observe a very marked decrease in the numbers, indicating that conception occurs much less frequently in warm weather than in the colder season. The male births outnumbered the female by nearly 1000.

The volume includes weekly reports of interments and of meteorological states throughout the year, and numerous tables and diagrams of interest to the physician. Our readers can probably obtain copies gratuitously on application at the Health Office. D.

THE HOMŒOPATHIC DOMESTIC MEDICINE. By J. Laurie, M.D. Twenty-fifth edition; edited by R S. Gutteridge, M.D. 1082 pages. Illustrated. 8vo., cloth. Price, 16 shillings.

AN EPITOME OF DOMESTIC MEDICINE. By J. Laurie, M.D. Thirtieth edition, edited by R. S. Gutteridge, M.D. 687 pages. Price, 5 shillings. Both published by Leath & Ross, London.

The fact that Laurie's well-known work has passed through so many editions, is strong evidence of its practical value and widespread reputation.

Dr. Gutteridge, who is the reviser of this twenty-fifth edition, has performed his labor very creditably. It is no easy matter to arrange medicines so as to make them understandable by all classes of the laity. Yet this task the doctor has satisfactorily accomplished.

Among the needed additions to this edition are: "Nursing the Sick," "Change of Air and Scene," "Mineral Baths and Waters," "Ulcer of the Stomach," "Bright's Disease," "Diabetes," "Irritable Bladder," "Gravel," "Calculus," "Stricture," "Hydrocele," "Angina Pectoris," "Diseases of Arteries and Veins," "Pyæmia," "Locomotor Ataxia," "Alcoholism," etc.

The book is full of information, valuable not only to the laity, but also to the professional reader. Indeed, so complete are the various chapters, that we questioned in our mind whether it was not too prolix a work for domestic use. But when we acquainted ourselves with its arrangement, we changed our opinion.

A domestic practice should be full and explicit, especially for travellers and for those who are distantly removed from any physician. And above all, it should give definite directions concerning emergencies. The book under review fulfils all these requirements. For instance, in the chapter on "Domestic Surgery," we find for sprains: Arnica, Calendula, Rhus, Bellis, for external use, and Rhus, Aconite, Sepia, Bryonia, Sulph., Calcarea, Causticum for internal employment. Wounds are carefully described, and the following remedies recommended in their treatment: Hamamelis, Arnica, Calendula, Trillium, Hypericum, Carbolic acid, etc.

Apparent death from drowning is treated of, and the most approved methods of resuscitation are illustrated by woodcuts.

Due attention is also given to the management of fractures, burns, and scalds, and also to the antidoting of poisons.

Part V contains a collection of "The Characteristic Effects of Medicines" mentioned in the book. This is a carefully arranged Materia Medica, covering 170 pages. Then follow a dictionary of medical terms and a copious index.

The epitome is simply an abbreviation of the larger work, and hence is subject to the same criticism. It is recommended by the author for beginners and for those who prefer a small book. F.

A Treatise on Common Forms of Functional Nervous Diseases. By L. Putzel, M.D., Physician to the Clinic for Nervous Diseases, Bellevue Hospital, Outdoor Department; Visiting Physician for Nervous Diseases, Randall's Island Hospital; Pathologist to the Lunatic Asylum, B. I.; Curator to Charity Hospital, etc. New York: William Wood & Co., 27 Great Jones Street. 1880, October. pp. 256.

This volume, just issued by William Wood & Co., in their library of Medical Authors for 1880, is dedicated to Professor E. G. Janeway, M.D., and gives a good insight into the nervous affections, which he terms functional, such as chorea, epilepsy, and neuralgias. The last eighty-six pages are devoted to peripheral paralysis, and a number of cuts are inserted to show the motor points in different portions of the body, and as a guide where to place the anode and cathode in the use of the electric currents.

The important feature of the work is its attention to the diagnostic minutiæ of these diseases, as well as the careful clinical history of the illustrative cases that are so freely thrown in. Differing from him in the use of the medicines to be prescribed in those diseases, we see in the other parts of the subject much that is valuable, and as it brings data up to the present day it is a very useful work to the practitioner. B. W. J.

George P. Rowell & Co.'s American Newspaper Directory, containing accurate lists of all the newspapers and periodicals published in the United States, Territories, and the Dominion of Canada, together with a description of the towns and cities in which they are published. New York. George P. Rowell & Co., publishers. 1880. pp. 1044.

Every journalist knows the importance of saving time in his work. This he does by having his encyclopedias, directories, and other works of reference of the most comprehensive and compact form, and this is just what Rowell's Newspaper Directory accomplishes in its special sphere.

It is, as far as we are able to ascertain, and we have examined the book well, a conscientious and accurate chronicle of the periodicals and newspapers of our country.

An impartial guide in matters where views are so divergent as they are among editors and publishers of newspapers, is no easy task, but we believe this publication has fully accomplished this result, and we take pleasure in commending this toil of years. The fact that this twelfth annual issue comprises 10,250 copies, speaks loudly to its credit. B. W. J.

Photographic Illustrations of Skin Diseases. By George Henry Fox, A.M., M.D., Clinical Professor of Dermatology, Starling Medical College, Columbus, Ohio; Surgeon to the New York Dispensary, Department of Skin and Venereal Diseases; Fellow of the American Academy of Medicine; Member of the New York Dermatological Society, The American Dermatological Association, etc. Forty-eight colored plates taken from Life. New York: E. B. Treat, No. 805 Broadway. Parts 7 to 12, inclusive.

The importance to the physician of a correct appreciation of the diagnostic appearances of the various forms of skin diseases, is sufficiently obvious, and in no other way, perhaps, aside from the actual inspection of cases, can this be obtained so well as by means of colored plates. The object of the author seems to have been well secured in his photographic illustrations, and what is more rare than it should be, the last numbers of the series are, in point of execution, fully up to the promise held out in the initial number. D.

Gleanings.

PHYSIOLOGY OF THE SPHINCTERS.—At a recent meeting of the Société de Biologie (*Le Progrès Méd.*, 1880, p. 472), Dr. Brown-Séquard remarked that Goltz has seen rhythmic movements executed by the anal and vesical sphincters after section of the spinal cord in the dorsal region. Dr. Brown-Séquard has also himself observed exactly similar movements executed by the sphincter vaginæ. He has observed, in addition, that these various rhythmic movements are arrested if one of the great toes is compressed or tickled. This fact agrees with what was long ago demonstrated by Dr. Brown-Séquard, namely, that irritation of the great toe causes the arrest of epileptiform convulsions occurring in certain diseases of the cord.—*Phila. Med. Times.*

INOCULATION.—A correspondent of the *Daily News*, who has been travelling through Persia, gives an interesting account of a curious sort of spider-bug, known scientifically as Arga Persica, and locally as *garrib-gez*, or "bite the stranger." One village is especially infested with this beauty, and the curious fact in reference to it is, that the inhabitants are never stung, or at least if stung are not injured thereby. Experience has shown that when one has been bitten, and has recovered, he is in no further danger. It is a kind of inoculation, and the Persian physicians assert that if the poison be taken into the stomach an equal safety is insured. Consequently, it is usual for strangers going to the particular village referred to, to have some bread with a bug concealed in it, administered to them—decidedly an instance of homœopathic treatment. The bite to strangers is both painful and dangerous.—*The Chemist and Druggist.*

SATURNINE APHASIA.—M. Ernest Gaucher reports to the Société Clinique de Paris the case of a painter, thirty-nine years of age, free from syphilis, alcoholism, and hereditary diathesis, and in good health, who, while working in a white-lead factory, suddenly became unconscious (but without any convulsive symptoms), and continued in this state fifteen minutes. On his removal to the hospital "the only symptom observed besides the blue line on the gums, and the constipation habitual in lead-poisoning, was violent and persistent headache. There was no colic, no vomiting, no nervous symptoms, neither paralysis, anæsthesia, nor trembling. His sight was good; appetite preserved; urine scanty and loaded with salts, but without albumen. Three days later the patient began to suffer with delirium and vertigo, added to the pre-existing cephalalgia. These passed off, however, within twenty-four hours, leaving the headache as bad as ever, but this became slowly better during the succeeding week. Suddenly, however, at the end of that time, the patient was seized with vomiting during the night, and the next morning he was found aphasic.

"The aphasia included also incapacity for writing, and the patient, who instead of '*cette nuit trois heures*,' had written '*ett ar de*,' in a trembling hand, thought he had written correctly. Otherwise his intellectual faculties were preserved. Shortly after the physician's visit the patient fell asleep, and when he awoke in the afternoon the aphasia had disappeared."—*See Phila. Med. Times*, August 28th, 1880); see also *Allen's Encyclopedia*, art. Plumbum, symptoms 163 to 167 inclusive, and 177. EDS. H. M.

Changes in the Seminal Fluid in Connection with Gonorrhœal Epididymitis.—These alterations have already been studied in France, by Gosselin and Godard. Dr. Terrillon has lately given much attention to the subject, and from an analysis of twenty cases, he draws the following conclusions: Epididymitis causes changes in the spermatic fluid, both as regards its color and the nature and interproportion of its anatomical elements. Such alterations vary with the phases of the disease. During the acute stage the semen has a more or less decidedly yellowish-green appearance, resembling pus. This color is due to the presence of a variable quantity of pus-corpuscles. Large granular globules are also found in some number. The spermatozoa may be absent after the first few days, but in some cases they may be found living and well formed in the purulent fluid, but diminished in number. They may continue to be present for a variable period, and may even persist through the course of the disease. The mixture of the pus-corpuscles and granular globules, frequently containing spermatozoa, can only be furnished by the inflamed mucous membrane of the seminal passages, as is shown by its identity with the fluid found in the vas deferens at some autopsies. This fact also shows that a purulent catarrh of the seminal passages takes place in these cases.

After the termination of the acute period of the epididymitis, the same spermatic alterations may still be met with. But the color of the semen is no longer so distinctly purulent, the pus-corpuscles are diminished in number, the spermatozoa are generally absent, and there is a predominance of liquid ingredients. These changes may persist for long periods; sometimes they continue indefinitely long, especially in cases where the spermatozoa fail to reappear. In cases of unilateral epididymitis all these changes are less clearly marked.—*Annales de dermatol. et de syphil.*, July, 1880.

News and Comments.

Professor Charles M. Thomas has removed to No. 1315 Arch Street, Philadelphia, two doors from his former residence.

Chills and fever are prevailing among the people of New England in unaccustomed places.—*Ex.* What nonsense! As if the chills were not already "accustomed" to shake every last inch of a man's body.

Diabolical.—On August 15th and 18th two attempts were made to burn the Massachusetts Homœopathic Hospital. Fortunately, through the exertions of the firemen, the dastardly design was frustrated in both instances.

The Transactions of the Ophthalmological and Otological Society, Vol. III, has been received. Physicians not members of the society, may obtain the three volumes by applying to F. Park Lewis, M.D., Buffalo, N. Y. Price, 1st and 3d vols., fifty cents each; 2d vol., one dollar. Mailed on receipt of price.

The New York Homœopathic Medical College.—Professor J. W. Dowling, who, for the past ten years, has been lecturing on General Practice of Medicine in the New York Homœopathic Medical College has resigned that position, in order to accept the Chair of Physical Diagnosis and Diseases of the Heart and Lungs, recently established in that institution. This is a branch of medicine to which Professor Dowling has long devoted his time, and which will now receive his undivided attention.

Officers of the World's Homœopathic Convention of 1881.—At the recent meeting of the British Homœopathic Congress at Leeds, Eng., the following officers were elected to preside at the Second "World's Homœopathic Convention," which meets next year in London:

President, Dr. Hamilton, of London; Vice-President, Dr. Hughes, of Brighton; Treasurer, Dr. Bayes, of London; General Secretary, Dr. Gibbs Blake, of Birmingham; Local Secretaries, Dr. Burnett, of London, and Dr. Hayward, of Liverpool.

Our State Society.—At the meeting of the Homœopathic Medical Society of Pennsylvania, held September 8th and 9th, 1880, a resolution was adopted to the effect, that hereafter no member, in arrears for dues, shall receive a copy of the *Transactions* until such arrearages are paid.

It is earnestly desired that all members who are indebted to the society will at once settle their accounts with the Treasurer, Dr. J. F. Cooper, of Allegheny City, so that the society may be freed from debt, and the new interest that has been awakened may increase, and the association become, as it should be, a power in the State.

R. E. Caruthers, M.D.,
Secretary.

Hahnemann Medical College of Philadelphia.—The regular session of this college was opened on Monday evening, September 27th, with an introductory address by Professor James. The speaker, in the course of his remarks, drew a comparison between the advantages enjoyed by medical students in the United States and Europe. As a result of his personal observations, he was of opinion that the universities of Europe could claim no preference over our best American colleges, except in the clinical study of the specialties in the large hospitals.

The session of the Philadelphia college opens with every prospect of an excellent class.

Resurrected.—Mr. John Buchanan, late dean, etc., who one night last August, jumped from a ferry-boat into the Delaware River and drowned himself to escape punishment for trafficking in bastard diplomas and begetting illegitimate doctors, was resurrected in September by Gabriel Miller (who thus appears to much better advantage than his predecessor, Joseph), but instead of "going up" in ascension robes, he "went below," which is the Philadelphia lingo for a trip to Moyamensing prison. Notwithstanding the fact that the resurrection was not in all respects a complete success,—the dean having gone down between Pennsylvania and New Jersey, and come up through Michigan,—there are more Millerites in the Quaker City to-day than ever before.

The Claude Bernard Memorial.—The following circular notice was, by inadvertence, omitted from our September issue. We commend the subject to the attention of our readers.

"Having been selected by the Paris Committee (Messrs. Ranvier and Dumontpallier) having charge of the subscription for a monument or memorial to the late Professor Claude Bernard, to represent them in the United States, I beg leave to be allowed to use your columns for the purpose of appealing to the members of the medical profession and all others interested, to subscribe to this worthy object. I need hardly remind your readers of the great debt which every practicing physician owes to the labors of the illustrious physiologist whose memory we are asked to honor in this way. All inquiries and subscriptions in the shape of bank checks or postal money orders should be addressed to me. Trusting that I shall have the advantage of your active personal support in this matter, I remain,

"Yours very respectfully, E. C. Seguin.

"41 West Twentieth Street, New York."

Married.—Egee—Loux.—On the evening of September 15th, 1880, at the residence of the bride's parents, by Rev. John McCron, D.D., J. B. S. Egee, M.D., to Miss Anna M. Loux, both of Philadelphia.

THE

HAHNEMANNIAN MONTHLY.

Vol. II., New Series. } Philadelphia, November, 1880. No. 11.

Original Department.

STUDIES IN MATERIA MEDICA.

BY E. A. FARRINGTON, M.D., PHILADELPHIA, PA.

ANIMAL KINGDOM.

(Continued from page 583.)

THROAT, LUNGS, HEART.

AMONG the **Related Remedies** referred to in our last number, the following are the most important.

Both PHOSPH. and LACHESIS have nervous cough, constriction and sensitiveness of the larynx, hoarseness evenings; cough from tickling in the larynx or trachea. The former has the burning rawness most marked; talking causes severe pain, for the larynx is inflamed, not merely irritated. And, further, the tendency of the inflammation is to extend down the trachea and even to the bronchioles. Tightness across the chest is a prominent symptom and it is accompanied with a sense of weight and oppression, as if the air-vesicles did not fill. Hoarseness is more prominent; but both may meet in membranous croup and require careful discrimination. The hoarseness in LACHESIS is attended by a feeling as if something in the larynx prevented clear speech, it cannot be hawked up. This may be the membrane; or, more likely, a closure of the rima glottidis. It is accompanied with suffocating spells in sleep; the child arouses in agony, as if choking. Now PHOSPH. is needed in croup rather when hoarseness or aphonia remains as a sequel; or, when the nervous system is prostrated and the child lies cold, sweaty, with rattling breathing. It has not the distinctive aggravations after sleep.

Both cause præcordial anxiety; palpitation; feeble pulse; rush of blood to the heart. Only PHOSPH. has the violent beat on the least motion. If it be true that both affect the pneumogastrics, the resulting symptoms are not at all alike. In PHOSPH. there is created a feeling of hunger, demanding food, which relieves; in LACHESIS, the nervous symptoms are choking and constriction of the throat.

The former remedy is not at all comparable with the latter in its many forms of nervous palpitations.

In the after treatment of pneumonia, great care is necessary in the selection of PHOSPH., if there is a deposit of tubercles. LACHESIS, in such an emergency, is often indicated. By thus qualifying the former, it is not intended to teach that this remedy can never be used; but as its imperfect application will result disastrously, we must be sure of its appropriateness before venturing. No one is so skilful in the selection of the similimum that cautionary advice is useless.

PHYTOLACCA depresses the vital powers and causes vomiting and purging. These latter effects are accompanied with coldness and extreme weakness. They are slow in their development, and so resemble the gastro-enteric symptoms attendant on just such blood-poisoning as marks the development of diphtheria. Consequently, we find as characteristic, dizzy and faint when rising in bed, nausea and vomiting. The heart's action is not much weakened at first, though later its beat is feeble. Fatal poisonings do not seem to depend upon paralysis of the heart, but upon that of respiration. Therefore, the cardiac weakness cannot be so important a symptom as it is in LACHESIS. And, further, it is a more acrid drug. The patient complains of chills, followed by fever. The body aches all over as if pounded, with violent pains in forehead, occiput, back, and limbs. LACHESIS has a hard aching all over, necessitating change of position. Both may affect the left side of the throat, with much constriction, swelling, purple color, and with putridity. Only the pokeberry has the feeling as if a hot ball was lodged in the fauces and sensation as after swallowing choke-pears.

In MERCURIUS CYANATUS the corrosive effects of the mercury are manifest in the rapid ulceration of mucous surfaces; while the no less rapidly developed prostration and gangrenous degeneration mark the added effects of the Prussic acid. Other mercurial symptoms are the swollen glands and tenesmus with bloody stools. To the acid are chiefly due the cyanotic face and cold surface, the weakened heart, which post-mortem shows is attended with heart-clot, and the diphtheritic form of inflammation. This remedy holds out some hope when the diphtheritic deposit is also about the anus and in the bowels, with shreddy, bloody, and horribly offensive stools. The systemic poison causes that dangerous symptom, aversion to all food. If the child will not eat and cannot be compelled to, his situation is very critical. In such an emergency the remedy under consideration stands with Mur. ac., Nitric ac., and Liq. calcis chlor. as among the best. The heart is of course weak, so weak that the patient should not be raised to a sitting posture, lest fatal syncope result. Even in the beginning of the disease the fever is adynamic, and the strength sinks before the local deposit in the throat is sufficient to account for the sudden giving way of vital power—a strong indication.

The mouth and fauces are swollen and red, varying from a bright to a dark purple. The deposit is white, opalescent, or grayish; and later, gangrenous and putrid. The tongue has a yellow base; but soon becomes coated with a diphtheritic gray coat, the edges remaining red. As the disease advances, the tongue is dark, probably from changes in its coating. The disease spreads into the posterior and anterior nares and also downwards to the larynx. Profuse epistaxis.

LAC CANINUM has won long-disputed laurels in true diphtheria. It bears many resemblances to LACHESIS, but may be distinguished by the following. The symptoms tend to affect the two sides alternately. Membrane is yellowish-gray or ulcers shine like silver. Mucous membrane red, glistening. Corners of the mouth sore (as in Arum triph.).

Merc. protojod, and *Merc. binjod*, affect characteristically opposite sides of the throat. The former has most effect upon the right and is distinguished by the thick dirty-yellow coating far back on the tongue. In the latter, the patches are numerous on the left tonsil. Both have engorged glands and great prostration. Nosebleed may be a symptom, though it is never so constant as in snake-poisons, rather indicationg congestion than dissolution of the blood.

LYCOPODIUM is an acknowledged complement of LACHESIS. Its symptoms in the sick, move from right to left, or shift about and remain stubbornly fixed in the right side of the throat. Upon swallowing, the throat feels tight; food and drink regurgitate through the nose. Constant inclination to swallow. Fauces deep red, with burning and soreness. Cervical glands swollen and sensitive. The nose is generally involved, with stuffing of the nostrils, compelling the child to breathe with the mouth partly open and tongue protruded. The child has a silly expression, which is a result of this method of getting breath; but also, we believe, dependent upon the relaxed features caused from mental and physical weakness. Early in the case, the child awakens as if frightened; he strikes and kicks any one who attempts to console him. Stupor. If, in addition, the urine, whether passed involuntarily or not, deposits a red, sandy sediment, the choice is certain.

Like Phosph. this remedy may be needed for hoarseness remaining after croup; and like LACHESIS, there may be suffocating spells at night; cough as from tickling in the larynx, constriction of the chest, etc. In the Fern the hoarseness and cough are accompanied with rattling of mucus, worse during sleep, making the breathing difficult and short. The tickling is as if from sulphur fumes.

The chest symptoms are plainly those of catarrh. Râles are heard on both sides, though more on the right. The difficult breathing is in part due to accumulated mucus and is better when the latter is raised. Flatulent distension of the abdomen also contributes to the discomfiture by its upward pressure. But there are two other causes to be observed. One is the already mentioned alternation of contraction and expansion universal in this remedy. The other is the tendency to produce paralytic weakness of organs (see under Mental Symptoms, August issue). The relaxation tends to render the catarrhal and the other chest symptoms persistent, permits the accumulation of mucus and muco-pus and gives rise to the rattling breathing, which is noticed along with the dropped jaw and stupor. Several forms of disease, then, frequently call for the remedy, phthisis pulmonalis, neglected pneumonia, typhoid pneumonia, catarrh of weakly children, etc. And it is in the first three, that the remedy compares with LACHESIS. The latter, however, has alternate chills and flushes, afternoons; spasmodic, gagging cough, compelling patient to sit up and hold his stomach. Finally, he half expectorates and half vomits a purulent, offensive sputum, with some relief. So soon as he sleeps, he sweats, especially about the neck. LYCOPOD. develops a loose, deep cough, as if he were about to expectorate the whole pulmonary parenchyma. Fever worse from 4 to 8 P.M. Sputa are mucous, purulent, lemon-colored, or gray, salt-tasting.

In hydrothorax, the latter is useful when the patient can lie only upon the right side; the former, when only upon the left. Both have accompanying œdema of the limbs. In the Fern the urine deposits a red sediment; in the other the urine is dark, almost black.

Kali bichromicum has choking on lying down, wheezing panting on awaking; dyspnœa in sleep; oppression of the chest, which arouses him suddenly. Oppression at the bifurcation of the trachea into the bronchial tubes. The asthmatic symptoms are worse mornings early and seem to be associated with, if not caused by, a swelling of the bronchial mucous membrane and an accumulation of tough or stringy mucus. The removal of the latter greatly relieves. These sorts of difficult breathing make the bichromate useful as a successor to Lachesis in diphtheria and croup, especially when the disease is spreading downwards. Experience proves that they follow each other well, and profitably.

Baptisia has already been differentiated. All that need be added here is its use in malignant diphtheria. Typhoid symptoms are prominent, and the stupor is decided. The patient can only swallow liquids. Mouth and throat look dark, the membrane is gangrenous, and the breath is horribly putrid. There is great oppression of breathing, which is caused by pulmonary congestion and is relieved when air is freely admitted into the room. Compare *Ailanthus*, which has also drowsiness; livid throat. There is a thin acrid coryza, and the ulcers in the throat discharge an acid fluid. Of the mineral acids, Arsenic, *Mur. ac.*, and *Nitric ac.* present the greatest similarities. The first is distinguished by its general symptoms. The second has developed a gray-white membrane on the fauces, with choking on swallowing; the parts appear dark bluish; rawness and smarting. Dark fetid nasal discharge. Weak, empty feeling at the stomach, with significant loss of appetite; nosebleed; weak, drowsy; pulse weak, intermits every third beat; hoarseness. The third is more acrid than the second; the disease involves the nasal cavities, with excoriation of the lip. This is present in the second also, though less severe. The pulse intermits every fourth beat. Sometimes child complains that a stick or splinter is in his throat.

Nux vomica like Lachesis, has a morning aggravation; but in the former remedy, it is the time of day when many of the Nux symptoms appear; in the latter, it is because of the aggravation from sleep. In the former, sleep helps, unless the patient is suddenly awakened; the throat feels scraped, rough, and though there are fetid ulcers, constriction and sensation of a plug during empty deglutition, yet the throat feels worse during and after solids; while LACHESIS may have relief from solids.

IGNATIA, according to toxic symptoms noticed in India, corresponds very closely to the symptoms of diphtheria. Like LACHESIS, swallowing food relieves; there are ulcers on the tonsils, etc. But in the former the patient has more marked aggravation between the acts of deglutition, and the ulcers are small, flat, and open on the indurated tonsils. The temperament, too, is important; patient is irritable, whining, nervous.

Spasmodic œsophageal stricture often calls for PHOSPH. The cardiac end is especially affected like LACHES., ARG. NITRIC., *Arsenic*. But LACHES. has also spasms of the upper portion, when it more resembles BELLAD., *Hyosc.*, *Stram.*, *Carbo veg.*, Canth., *Alumina*, Ignat., *Lycopod.*, Cicuta, etc. ARSENIC, *Rhus tox.*, and Verat. viride, have the spasm as a symptom of œsophagitis. LACHES., *Ignat.*, *Asaf.*, *Coccul.*, etc., suit in hysterical, nervous patients, when there is also a reverse peristalsis. (See Globus hystericus.)

To distinguish from *Hyosc.*, remember that the latter is worse from cold liquids; solids and warm things give the least trouble; and hiccough is an accompaniment.

Carbo veg. causes a sensation as if the pharynx was contracted or drawn together; food cannot be easily swallowed; throat seems contracted, with spasm, but no pain.

Alumina causes constriction of throat; soreness and constriction. the whole length of the œsophagus, from swallowing a morsel of food; but warm drinks relieve, as does the saliva.

BELLAD. is closely related to LACHESIS, though its faucial and œsophageal spasms are more severe. It causes contraction, frequently recurring, particularly during efforts at swallowing; the whole canal feels narrowed. It may likewise be employed when a large morsel of food or a bone obstructs the œsophagus and incites violent spasmodic contractions. (Compare also Cicuta, Ignat.) LACHESIS has rather a sensation of a crumb or button lodged in the œsophagus; or, the attempt at deglutition produces a gagging and smothering, as if food had gone down "the wrong way."

In sore throat, involving the tonsils, Bellad., Mercur., Hepar, and Laches., form a very interesting group, to which may be added Amygdala persica, Apis, Vespa, Phosph.

BELLAD. has dryness, scraping, burning, stinging; violent and painful constrictions, worse when attempting to swallow fluids. Throat bright red, or when inflammation is intense, deep crimson. Attacks come suddenly and develop rapidly, with throbbing pains, frontal headache, red face. Tonsils rapidly enlarge and threaten to suppurate; cervical glands swollen. Sometimes there is a ropy mucus in the throat. According to the provings, the left side is most affected; clinically, in agreement with the law of direction of symptoms (Hering), they are mostly right-sided.

Even if pus should form, the remedy need not be changed, if the general characteristics of intensity, rapidity, etc., remain. But if, with chills and local throbbing, the faucial color becomes livid, with pains as from splinters sticking, and the external throat is very sensitive, HEPAR is the substitute. Or, again, pus has formed, but will not break forth; much badly-smelling phlegm collects and is hawked out with great pain; throat dark red; sweat aggravates rather than relieves; stitches extend into the ears; drinks regurgitate, then MERCUR. is needed. Now LACHESIS goes farther; the throat is purplish, and the patient very nervous; the least touch is intolerable, more from hyperæsthesia than from inflammatory soreness, as in the others; pus from tonsils is unhealthy, and they tend to degenerate into ulcers. (Compare *Silicia*, *Sulph.*).

AMYGDALA PERSICA causes a dark-red throat and severe pains shooting through the tonsils. The pulse is not as strong as in Bellad. It has been employed when the latter, though seemingly indicated, does not relieve the pains; and also when diphtheritic membrane forms. (Here compare *Merc. iod.* and *biniod.*).

PHOSPHORUS affects tonsils and uvula; the latter is elongated and sometimes œdematous; the pharyngeal wall also looks swollen and glistening; stinging pains, worse in the evening; rawness, worse from talking; hawks mucus, mornings, which has a nasty taste. Worse swallowing fluids, and during and after solids.

APIS MEL. induces a swelling of the mucous lining of the throat, which is rosy, with stinging and a constricted feeling, as if choking; feeling of erosion. The main feature is the tendency of the mucous membrane to puff up or swell, causing the sense of choking and smothering. If ulcers form, they present œdematous borders. VESPA is nearly identical. It may, however, be needed when the symptoms recur periodically.

Among the new aspirants for distinction in throat affections, is *Wyethia helenoides*. As this remedy is said to cause nervousness, apprehensiveness, weakness, slow pulse, pain in left ovary, etc., it may be that its throat symptoms will occasionally need differentiation from LACHESIS. The throat feels dry, with burning; swallows with difficulty; constant desire to swallow, but without relief of the dryness. Hemming to clear the throat, though unsuccessful. Similar dryness, with pricking, in the posterior nares.

Awaking smothering is deservedly considered as an excellent indication for LACHESIS. But in asthma, œdema of lungs, hydrothorax, heart disease, etc., we may be compelled to decide between it and several others.

ARSENIC awakens 12 P.M. or later, with anxiety and smothering; *Kali carb.* and *Kali bich.* towards 3 or 4 A.M.

Lactuca has tightness of lower part of chest; he awakens at night and springs up for breath.

Graphites has a similar symptom, but it is relieved by eating.

SAMBUCUS, starting from sleep with suffocation; head and hands bluish, puffy. So soon as he awakens he begins to sweat, while during sleep he has hot face.

BELLADONNA arouses, choking and frightened; face is red; cries out in sleep.

Sepia and *Sulphur* awake smothering; the latter has marked, sudden jerking of the legs as he drops off to sleep.

PHOSPH. induces suffocation just as the patient drops off to sleep; he is tall, slim, and predisposed to bronchitis. Palpitation and smothering from growing too fast.

Kali hyd., has awakens choking; this indicates it in heart disease, and also in œdema pulmonum; in the latter case, the sputum looks like greenish soap-suds.

Merc. præc. rub., has suffocative fits on the point of falling asleep; he must spring up. It has cured this symptom in cases of simple debility, without organic disease.

Grindelia robusta, oppressed breathing; heart feels too weak to take care of the blood sent to it; on dropping off to sleep, respiration ceases, he awakens smothering.

Baptisia has relieved: awakes with difficult breathing; better when window is opened.

Asparagus should be thought of for dyspnœa of hydrothorax in the aged, with weak heart; pain at the left acromion. Compare *Laches.*, *Apoc. cann.*, DIGITALIS, ARSENIC, *Phosph.*, *Gelsem.* All have weak heart, and the second, like the first, has many symptoms worse on awaking; it also has goneness in the epigastrium, and the heart feels prostrated, flutters now and then, is very feeble, then slow,—all common in hydropericardium. The *Gelsem.* may be distinguished by a feeling as if he must move or his heart will stop.

RHUS. TOX., like LACHESIS, causes numbness of the left arm, and, indeed, more characteristically. If there is any doubt, decide by the restlessness and by the lame and weak feeling about the cardiac walls.

SPIGELIA and LACHESIS have suffocation provoked by moving the arms; and anxiety. But in cardiac rheumatism, the latter is called for when the invasion is announced by a sudden arousing from sleep, with anxiety, oppression, and intolerance of pressure. The former is adapted to undulatory motion of the heart; purring feeling; sharp stitching pains, etc., with anxiety. The intermittent pulse, which both cause, is very characteristic of SPIGELIA. In advanced heart-affection, with dropsy, *Spigelia* has aggravation from sitting bent forwards; LACHESIS, amelioration.

A RARE INSTANCE OF FEMORO-INGUINAL HERNIA, WITH AUTOPSY.

BY JOSEPH V. HOBSON, M.D , RICHMOND, VA.

MISS MAGGIE P., the subject of these notes, was a maiden of 51 years, and member of a family of six persons, three males and three females, all of whom, with one exception, are subjects of hernia. Happening to be visiting a patient in the neighborhood, I was called to see her on the morning of July 3d, ult. I found that she had suffered during the preceding night from what was supposed to be a violent seizure of flatulent colic, a trouble to which she had been subject for more than ten years. She was free of fever and of pain, and was vomiting at intervals of several hours a bitter, yellow fluid. The abdomen was not distended, but felt sore and tender on pressure. Femoral hernia of left side, of the size of a hen's egg, tender, hard, and irreducible. Has had two healthy stools by enemas. Pulse 75. Skin moist and pleasant. Patient tranquil and cheerful. Had been accustomed to wear a truss, but had left it off for a day or two. Prescribed Nux vomica, and did not see her again for four days.

July 7th.—Was sent for to see her again to-day. Found her still vomiting from time to time a bilious fluid with very little retching. No fever, but is quite thirsty, and is eating ice, because water cramps her. Palms of hands rather too warm. The hernia has ceased to be tender, and was reduced by persistent gentle taxis, with an audible gurgle, but leaving behind a slight enlargement, having the feeling of omentum, situated just over the sac, devoid of sensibility, but resists all efforts at reduction. Slight epigastric tenderness. Pulse 75. Patient cheerful, and suffering no pain.

July 8th.—Has not vomited since 3 P.M. yesterday. Is able to take a little iced water, but has taken no food. No stool since 5th inst. Pulse 102. Palms of hands feverish. Feet cool. Temperature of other parts normal. Skin moist.

July 9th.—Condition unchanged. Patient has vomited three or four times. Suffers no pain.

July 10th.—Passed the night right comfortably, and is taking a little milk and beef tea. Had stool by enema yesterday. Audible rumbling in the bowels. No pain. Pulse soft and 104. Has vomited four or five times.

July 11th.—Symptoms generally unchanged. Has just vomited copiously a yellow bilious chymy substance of peculiar odor, faintly suggestive of fæces. Defecating-tube introduced through sigmoid flexure, and bowels feebly distended with warm water, which brought away a small quantity of hardened fæces. No tenderness of hernia, which has returned, and a gurgling sound of passing gas is both felt and heard. Pulse 100. Is cheerful, and takes a little beef tea and some sips of water. Vomits occasionally, without nausea. Is evidently feeling wretchedly, but does not complain. Recognizing now the extreme gravity of the case, I called Dr. Barrett in consultation. We jointly examined the abdomen in the most thorough manner, and reluctantly reached the conclusion that an operation was not advisable.

July 12th.—Stercoraceous vomiting continues. Hernia readily reduced, but the condition of the patient is in the highest degree alarming; indeed she appears to be moribund. Nothing more can be done unless it be by a surgical operation. There is nothing to denote the seat of the obstruction, no tympanitis, no pain, no local tenderness, and nothing to guide us to its seat, unless it be found in the small fleshy mass before spoken of. Perhaps this may be omentum, and the cause of the difficulty. Forced to do something, and with no better indication than this, we proceeded to an immediate operation. Our patient being well chloroformed, the integuments over the visible hernia were divided, exposing the superficial fascia, which was also divided upon the grooved director, bringing into view a small fibrous mass, about an inch in length and three-eighths of an inch thick, which could not be laminated;

but upon passing the finger down to its lower angle, it entered readily into the hernial sac, which was found empty, and of the capacity of about one ounce of water. The little finger passed readily into the crural ring, Gimbernat's ligament being plainly felt on the inner side. An examination of the fibrous mass (which was not divided) demonstrated it to be condensed cellular tissue, produced by the pressure of the truss. With sad hearts we stitched up and closed the wound, feeling that our patient could live but a few hours. But to our great surprise, in about half an hour fecal matter commenced to discharge from the wound, necessitating the removal of the stitches. The vomiting ceased immediately.

July 13th and 14th.—Vomiting has not returned. Fecal matter passes constantly from the wound. No change in symptoms.

July 15th.—No nausea or vomiting. Fecal matter discharging freely as before. Mind clear. No tenderness nor distension of abdomen. Takes a little buttermilk and beef tea. Pulse 102, and feeble. Skin cool and clammy. Temperature of palms of hands 98°. Mind collected. No despondency.

July 16th.—Very feeble during the night, but rallied by use of wine. This morning patient feels more comfortable. Fecal discharge from wound continues, but none from anus. Pulse very feeble. Skin less cold. Feet warm. Occasional slight hiccough. A slight slough discoverable on the fibrous mass within the wound.

July 17th.—Looks to be better. Features more animated. Pulse 100, and very feeble. Skin cool. Feet warm. Slight hiccough occasionally. Urine very scanty. Takes a little food.

July 18th.—Passed a very restless night, and is evidently weaker. During the night and this morning has passed, voluntarily, four liquid stools, fecal in character, and having every appearance of being thorough evacuations. She is very feeble, and life is sustained by wine.

July 19th.—Had no sleep last night, and seems moribund.

July 20th.—Had quiet night, and really seems better. Fecal discharge from wound takes place at intervals of from six to eight hours. There has been no return of the vomiting since the operation.

July 21st.—Patient died this morning at 8 o'clock, nine days after the operation.

Having been informed several days ago that a report was being industriously circulated in the lower part of the city, that our patient had been wounded in the intestines by an unskilful performance of the operation for femoral hernia, Dr. Barrett and I strenuously insisted upon a post-mortem examination of the body, and requested that the family physician (an allopath, living a square off) should be present. The family reluctantly consented, and appointed the next day at 11 o'clock for this purpose, but at the hour indicated the allopath was not at hand. The next day at the same hour was appointed, and on our arrival we were informed that he had flatly refused to be present, and we were invited to proceed with the autopsy in the presence of one of the family.

The body was found in a fair state of preservation, except about the wound, a portion of which had sloughed. Abdomen tympanitic. Rigor mortis incomplete. Countenance placid. Skin and muscular tissues were divided in the usual mode by cross sections, which brought into view the peritoneum, which was found in a healthy condition. This coat being divided, brought into view the cavity of the abdomen, which proved to be free from any extravasation. The large intestine appeared to be in a healthy condition throughout its length. The stomach, duodenum, and jejunum, to its lower extremity, were unchanged, but the ileum, from its jejunal extremity for about two feet was of a dark color, but without adhesions. Crural ring open and in natural condition. On turning back the flap and examining the internal abdominal ring, a very small knuckle of the ileum, near its commencement, was found invaginated, and so closely adherent as not to admit of removal except by dissection. Within the inguinal canal was found the open mouth of the intestine, the discharge from which had found its way through the outer ring and the intervening cellular tissue into the sac of the femoral hernia. Thus it will be seen that the operation prolonged life, and it may safely be assumed that, had the portion of the incarcerated ileum been taken from near the ileo-cœcal valve, life might have been prolonged indefinitely. It appears, too, in every way probable that the strong adhesions to the internal abdominal ring were the result of pressure of the truss on the concealed hernia, and affords a clue to the explanation of the frequent violent attacks of colic to which the deceased was subject.

NEURASTHENIA IN CHILDHOOD.

BY WILLIAM P. SHARKEY, M D., PHILADELPHIA.

(Read before the Philadelphia County Homœopathic Medical Society.)

INTRODUCTORY.—The term *neurasthenia* is etymologically of Greek extraction, and interpreted literally means lack of nerve strength. Although but recently introduced into medical nomenclature, it promises to occupy a conspicuous place in nosology as a suitable title for a family of functional disorders, which have their origin and support in nervous exhaustion.

This disease has been more or less elaborately described by Erb, of Heidelberg, Rosenthal, of Vienna, Grasset, of Paris, Beard, of New York, and other eminent neurologists, but almost without reference to its existence in childhood; neither, so far as I am aware, does the especial mention of neurasthenia occur in any of our standard works on children's diseases. It is nevertheless true that children as well as adults are occasionally real sufferers from nervous debility, and however much the disease may differ in degree or expression comparatively, the essentials are the same, inasmuch as the child is regarded physiologically as the miniature adult in the stage of active development, complete in incompleteness, the nutritive process being assiduously carried on for the double purpose of repair and growth. All the tissues of the delicate and unstable organism are especially noted for refinement, sensibility, and consequent susceptibility to disorder, and this is particularly true of the nervous tissue. From these, as well as other physiological peculiarities of childhood, it is to be inferred that the nervous system of the child is liable to the same pathological conditions and disorders as those which prevail in adult life, some of them possibly even in a more marked degree. Yet owing to the deficiency of cerebral development in infants and children, we would scarcely expect a like quantity or quality of subjective manifestations. Again, the fully developed sexual organs give rise to certain reflex disturbances, from which children are exempt, and thus we find that age, sex, and condition are constant modifiers of disease.

The foregoing observations and conclusions are not entirely at variance with the statements advanced by Beard in his excellent contribution to the literature of neurasthenia, wherein he says: "Infants and children have convulsions, cerebral diseases, spinal complaints, paralysis, chorea, and anæmia, but rarely neurasthenia as he has described." He further remarks:

"Comparatively speaking, neurasthenia is rare and different in its character at the extremes of life."

Etiology.—One of the grand predisposing agencies in the causation of neurasthenia in children is an inherited nervous diathesis; indeed, it is a question whether, to a limited extent, the various neuroses themselves are not transmissible from parent to offspring. Specifically among the exciting causes in infants may be mentioned the irritation of the fifth nerve by the process of dentition, transmitted to an extremely sensitive nerve-centre. Irritation of the stomach and intestinal canal from worms or some indigestible material, may also serve to promote a neurotic condition. So, also, exposure to extremes of temperature, badly ventilated nurseries and school-rooms, improper diet, too much or too little physical or mental exercise, late hours and other indulgences of so-called fashionable life, overstudy as encouraged by the cramming system of education now in vogue, secret vices, certain physical diseases, in short, anything non-hygienic or pathological which is calculated to depreciate nerve-force, must eventually excite and develop nerve-sensitiveness and lead to functional disturbance.

Symptomatology and Diagnosis.—Considering the multitude of neurasthenic symptoms exhibited under so many phases, the limits of this paper will forbid more than a synopsis of them. The following somewhat interesting case of neurasthenia came under my treatment during the autumn of 1879.

Case.—Clara F——, of Plainfield, N. J., aged 3 years, blonde, well nourished, and by a casual observer would have been passed as a healthy child. Both of her parents were of a decidedly nervous temperament and without particular ailments. In company with her mother she came to Philadelphia for the purpose of visiting friends. My attention was first directed to Clara by her peculiar behavior. She had always been esteemed as an amiable, affectionate, obedient, and happy child. Now she was strangely the reverse—irascible, self-willed, morose, easily frightened; commanding, and having others to obey instantly, seemed to her a gratification. The slightest cross or the most trivial circumstance was sufficient to excite one of her characteristic tantrums of screaming and crying, continuing until she tired herself out; and then would follow a whine of an indefinite duration, terminating very often suddenly in a fit of good-humor. Whilst in the act of screaming and crying, however, with manifest tremor, she would jump up and down, dance around on tiptoe, and assume threatening gestures. There was no certainty when or where a paroxysm would take place, or how long it would continue. On one occasion the mother and daughter were preparing to start out to call on a friend; all at once Miss Clara took a stand that her mother should not go, and in her usual tactics carried on for nearly two hours. Indeed, her conduct became so annoying that the mother decided to return home much earlier than was anticipated.

Prior to leaving this city, her parents took me in consultation, and gave the previous history of the case, as follows: The first notice of a change in Clara's nature was observed about three months before. Her behavior then was in a degree similar to what has been described. They consulted a female homœopathic physician, and the medicine then prescribed did her good for a time. A relapse, however, took place, since which time she has been gradually growing worse. To check the paroxysms, all sorts of mild, persuasive means had been resorted to, and whipping and other punishments had been tried without success. Her appetite was sufficient, but her sleep was more or less disturbed by convulsive movements. An examination revealed a slightly irritable heart, but no organic lesion was discoverable.

I gave the parents to understand that the child was not responsible for her strange conduct, as it was, in my belief, the consequence of *nervous exhaustion;* and until the equilibrium of her nervous system could be restored by proper medicine there was little hope of improvement. This opinion was accepted, and arrangements were made to have medicine sent her by mail. The treatment extended over a period of about six weeks, when the child was pronounced by the parents perfectly cured.

A typical case, presenting a rather different array of symptoms, occurred recently in the practice of Professor B. F. Betts, the notes of which, by his kind permission, I have the pleasure of here reporting:

CASE.—Mamie H——, a little girl of three years, was much below the average size of babes at birth, but has grown to be strong and healthy-looking. Her mother and grandmother are both of a nervous temperament.

During a visit to the Academy of Fine Arts with her mother the little girl became very much fatigued. On her way home she suddenly refused to walk, sat down upon the pavement, because very cross and irritable, would not let her mother carry her, and twitched so that the mother feared she would have convulsions. After a time this nervous excitement, which the child had never manifested before, but which was attributed to an outburst of anger, subsided. She was taken home and ate her supper as usual, but passed a very restless night. The next day she appeared languid, timid, and cross; seemed to be afraid of everybody. These symptoms continued for a couple of weeks, when a spasmodic cough supervened, and treatment was solicited. The parents thought she was getting the whooping-cough. She coughed but little at night, but twitched and moaned in her sleep, and was very restless. She had no fever. The cough during the day was harsh, barking, and spasmodic. The lower extremities felt cold. She complained of pain in the limbs and different parts of the body. When walking in the street she would suddenly stop and refuse to go farther, or else sit down upon the pavement and complain of feeling tired, too tired to play. She was accustomed to a drive in the park almost daily before this illness, and seemed to enjoy it; but now she was afraid, and became almost convulsed when riding,—would cry when an attempt was made to put her into the carriage. She refused to go anywhere; was afraid of everything and everybody; complained of being chilly from the slightest exposure.

Bell.^{30} was prescribed without any prompt relief, but in a month the child regained her normal mental and physical condition, without any return of the symptoms. It is worthy of remark in this connection, that the mother of Mamie, at about the same age, was affected in a similar manner.

Children frequently experience abnormal sensations which they are unable to describe in intelligible language. This feature, attributable especially to infancy, becomes a matter of considerable moment, inasmuch as the symptoms of neurasthenia are largely of a subjective character, and the sayings as well as the doings of the patient are invaluable factors in the problem of diagnosis. In many respects, neurasthenic symptoms simulate those of organic or structural diseases of the nervous system. It is, therefore, urged as a preliminary step in making a differential diagnosis, that a critical examination be instituted, particularly of the brain, spinal cord, and peripheral nerves. It may be necessary to carefully distinguish and eliminate certain other allied states, as anæmia, chorea, paralysis, epilepsy, hysteria, etc. For illustration, anæmia is an affection characterized by impoverishment of the blood, from which, also, may arise marked diminution of nerve force. Besides, the origin of anæmia is generally traceable to some malignant or organic disease, and whatever constitutes the cause, if it be removed, the anæmic symptoms usually disappear. Not so, on the other hand, with neurasthenia; it does not depend upon organic disease, or evident change in the constituent elements of the blood. Though the circulation may be disturbed, or the heart be irritable, through the influence of the sympathetic and vasomotor nerves, still there is no positive cardiac murmur or venous hum such as distinguishes anæmia. These are a few of the several distinctive features to be taken into account in establishing a diagnosis.

A glance at hysteria in this relation will suffice. Our ancient medical worthies adopted the word hysteria to designate a certain morbid activity peculiar to the female economy. The very derivation of the word restricts it to the female reproductive organs, which, near and after the time of life known as puberty, evolve a kind of neurosis, having the appearance, though not the identity, of neurasthenia, but from which it may be necessary to differentiate. The hypothesis that man, too, is a victim of hysteria stamps the word as a ludicrous misnomer, and rests upon a very uncertain foundation. And if this hypothesis savors so strongly of the unscientific, how much nearer *reductio ad absurdum* is it to apply the term *hysteria* to young children, whose genital promptings are virtually dormant.

PATHOLOGY.—Aside from the theory, but little can be said concerning the pathology of neurasthenia. Beard views it as an impoverished condition of nerve force, resulting from a bad nutrition of the nerve tissue, on the metamorphosis of which the evolutions of nerve force depends. From this it is reasonably presumed that the nerve force is not only much reduced below the normal, but very inharmoniously distributed. Concerning the pathology, as well as the causation of the disease in question, Hahnemann's theory of *psora* may explain much, and ought under no circumstances to be ignored.

PROGNOSIS.—The prognosis of neurasthenia, as it affects children, can hardly of itself be regarded as unfavorable. Its natural course is progressive, and may be protracted, but when unassociated it can generally be promptly arrested. It should be borne in mind, however, that relapses are not infrequent.

When another disease supervenes, the nervous debility has a tendency to operate seriously towards an aggravation, if not towards a fatal termination. For instance, many of the worst cases of cholera infantum happen upon a neurasthenic basis, just at a period when the child's nervous force has been reduced below par by the extreme summer heat, teething, neglected diarrhœa, or other exciting cause. Here, then, is a dangerous complication, with a correspondingly doubtful prognosis.

TREATMENT.—The treatment of neurasthenia is essentially twofold, hygienic and medicinal. The former includes—first, the entire removal of any and every cause concerned in its initiation and progress; second, the adoption to a proper degree of all means calculated to restore lost energies, particularly rest, exercise, fresh air, sunlight, baths, clothing, nourishing diet, etc.; third, the prohibition of everything over-exciting, stimulating, or in the least degree enervating.

The medical treatment implies the most careful selection and administration of medicines, according to the *magna charta* of homœopathy. Under no other system of therapy are we so well panoplied to battle with this disease. All the symptoms belonging to the disease have a place in our Materia Medica and repertories, to which sources we can resort most confidently in the search for remedies for "neurasthenia in childhood."

ANOTHER WARNING.

BY HENRY C. HOUGHTON, M.D., NEW YORK CITY.

THE profession has so long been accustomed to treat suppurative inflammation of the middle ear as a trivial matter, and some members so continue to resort to questionable expedients in the attempt to remove foreign bodies from the meatus, that it is still well to instance cases in which fatal consequences follow reckless practice.

Under the title, "Contributions to the Pathological Anatomy of the Organ of Hearing," Eugene Frankel, M.D.,* reports five cases which illustrate the relation between otitis media and cerebral diseases. Cases Nos. I and V are specially noteworthy. The first illustrates the consequences of neglect in long-standing disease, and the danger of forcible use of the syringe, the second the danger attending the reckless use of instruments in attempting the removal of a foreign body from the meatus.

The heading of the first case is as follows: "*Otorrhœa of long standing, exacerbation of the inflammation from syringing the ear canal, meningitic symptoms, death in eighteen days.*" A succinct statement of the autopsy follows: "AUTOPSY: *left-*

---

* Archives of Otology, vol. ix, No. 3.

sided purulent otitis media; defect of the membrana tympani; thrombo-phlebitis of the transverse sinus; abscess in subdinal space and in left temporal lobe; purulent lepto-meningitis of the base and the convexity."

The patient, female, aged twenty-three years, had syringed the right ear for years on account of impaired hearing, but two weeks previously she had syringed the left; headache, vertigo, vomiting, and purulent discharge followed. Three days after admission she died.

In commenting on the facts of the autopsy, the writer says: "Among those facts which are deserving of special mention in the discussion of the preceding case, appears to me, in the first place, the *beginning of the exacerbation* of the chronic affection *in connection with a syringing of the ear*. But the possibility of evil consequences of such a nature, in the train of a manipulation which, in medical practice, is mostly left to inferior nurses, imposes the duty upon the physician to bestow sufficient care upon this apparently indifferent assistance.

That there is need for such cautions by those who are in positions to demonstrate the results of such errors, we must admit. It is true that transient vertigo may result from syringing and no evil follow, but my experience is not exceptional in observing cases in which suppurative inflammation has been set up by syringing the ear, the history showing no previous lesion. In chronic suppurative inflammation of the tympanum, with loss of the drumhead, I have seen the most serious cerebral congestion follow forcible syringing, the mastoid cells being first involved. In some cases the history shows an early experience of suppuration, and inspection reveals a cicatrized membrana tympani; in these, the use of the syringe, or even instillation of simple warm water, to relieve an irritation of the canal, has caused a relapse, which proved to be the prelude to serious cerebral congestion.

The heading of case No. V is as follows: "*Pebble in the left external ear canal, attempts at extraction, death from meningitis.*"

"Autopsy: *defect of the membrana tympani; a pebble wedged in the drum-cavity pressing against its labyrinth wall; fissure in the head of the malleus; destruction of the joints between the ossicles; detachment of a piece from the wall of the labyrinth; purulent inflammation of the drum-cavity; purulent convexity; meningitis.*"

The sufferer was a little girl, three years of age, who during play had pushed a pebble into the left ear. A surgeon, and later a physician, had failed to remove the foreign body, the latter placing the patient under chloroform; the following day she was brought to the hospital, attempts at extraction failed, meningitis set in, and on the eighth day she died.

After a minute account of the post-mortem appearances the writer says: "After what has been said it cannot be doubtful that the fatal termination was due to therapeutic attempts at removing the foreign body, whereby the stone was displaced into the drum-cavity through the, at the time, certainly uninjured membrana tympani; and causing, further, an extensive injury to the tympanic mucosa, with consecutive purulent inflammation in the middle ear and adjoining mastoid cells, and a dislocation and partial crushing of the ossicles and the wall of the labyrinth."

Here, then, is another warning, added to those already on record, showing the fatal results likely to follow attempts at extraction of foreign bodies. In a copy of *Pilcher on the Ear*, Philadelphia, 1843, given me by my friend, Henry D. Paine, M.D., I find on page 219 the details of the case quoted by Roosa. A boy, seven years old, put the round head of a nail into the left ear. He was taken to a surgeon, who attempted to remove it, but failed. On Monday, at a public institution, a farther attempt was made with probes, and several pairs of forceps were used; the nail was taken hold of, but not removed; hæmorrhage was so excessive that no more attempts were made, and on the following Thursday the discharge of pus, which succeeded the hæmorrhage, ceased, and pain set in; leeches were applied. On Saturday the severe symptoms had passed, and attempts were renewed. A director was bent, dressing forceps bent; another pair, same result; forceps with hooks bent straight, forceps of various kinds were used. An elevator, and finally a pair of tooth forceps were employed, and three portions of metal, supposed to be parts of the nail, were extracted; the malleus bone followed, then portions of bone, but at last the patient was "nearly exhausted," and operative measures ceased. He had ten drops of Liq. Ant. Tart. every four hours; on Sunday ten grains of Hydrarg. cum creta every eight hours. On Monday he died.

"Post-mortem examination four hours after death. Ear: The temporal bone being removed from the skull, and the soft parts stripped off, the cavity of the tympanum was immediately brought into view, without anything else being done. Not a vestige of the bony portion of the meatus auditorius externus remained, the whole having been removed in the operation, and the floor of the tympanum was also wanting. The remaining portion of the tympanum was covered with pus, which being washed off, the surface of the bone beneath seemed highly inflamed. The nail not being in the tympanum, sections were made through the cochlea, vestibule, semicircular canals, and mastoid cells, but no nail to be found!" Well, may Roosa quote the old saying, "First catch your hare." Be sure you *see* the foreign body before you attempt to remove it.

The experiences of reckless practitioners of forty years ago are commended to the attention of reckless practitioners of to-day.

PSEUDO CONICAL CORNEA.

BY W. H. WINSLOW, PH D, M D., PITTSBURG, PA.

At the recent meeting of our Ophthalmological and Otological Society, I presented a paper upon the above subject, which has just appeared in the *Transactions*. The cases are so rare, remedial measures are generally so useless, the results in this patient are so satisfactory, and the paper as printed contains *such glaring errors*, that I beg leave to present this abstract to those interested in the subject.

Mrs. Blank, aged 35 years, married, had several healthy children; had last confinement in 1876; had fair muscular developments, a stature of 5 feet 4 inches, and weight of 120 pounds.

Her face was clear, bright, and cheerful; her spirits vivacious; she belonged to the upper walks of life, was supplied with moderate luxury, had not suffered from any serious illness, and was a patient of Dr. L. H. Willard. She could not recall any defect of eyesight, or any eye diseases in her brothers or sisters. Two years before applying for treatment, she had passed through a safe and not severe confinement. During convalescence she read too soon and too much, in a dimly-lighted room, and had a little pain in the eyeballs at the time. This pain continued at intervals when she used her eyes, after she was up and about her usual work, so that she was obliged to forbear much reading and sewing.

In a few months the patient noticed that objects at a distance looked a little misty, and when she wished to see any small object close at hand she "squinted" the eyelids together. These symptoms became worse as time passed, till the patient could not recognize people across the street; she became alarmed, and applied to an old-school oculist for treatment. In conjunction with tonic medication, the eyes were kept thoroughly under the influence of Atropia for many months. Attempts were made to correct the refractive anomalies without success; several pairs of glasses were ordered, but they all gave so much discomfort they were abandoned, and an operation by cauterizing the apex of the cornea was hinted at on several occasions.

The treatment relieved the pain, but the discomfort from excess of light entering the eyes, and the non-improvement in vision finally disgusted the patient and she ceased attendance.

During the next few months, use of the eyes brought back the old pain, and the disease continued to advance until January, 1878, when Dr. Willard, of Alleghany City, sent her to me for examination.

The lady was in good general health and spirits, and complained only of defective vision and a tired, aching feeling in the eyes, which became worse after attempting to see small objects.

The eyes appeared normal, except that there was spasmodic action of the orbicularis palpebrarum muscle and continued blinking in attempts to see. There was a slight shrinking from the light, a little frontal headache, and a drawing feeling from the orbits backwards to the base of the brain.

The ophthalmoscope showed healthy tissues as well as I could determine; the plus and minus glasses of the ophthalmoscopic disk brought certain parts of the fundus into view and obscured others, and indicated a great refractive anomaly; but the imperfect images and fitful shadows rendered the examination very unsatisfactory.

Light striking the centre of the cornea was totally reflected like silver, and, using a $+\frac{1}{5}$ spherical lens before my eye, I was able to produce a star of light upon the cornea, surrounded by a red oval band, the transmitted color of the fundus. The profile of the cornea was not altered sufficiently to aid the diagnosis; the test-cards revealed a coarse astigmatism; and I then had recourse to my set of trial-glasses. After much confusion of mind and many contradictory answers on the part of the patient, and much fatigue to myself from an hour's work, I arrived at the following formula:

R. E. $V = \frac{15}{100}$ Sn. With $+\frac{1}{24}$ cy. ax. 180°—$\frac{1}{42}$ cy. ax. 90°, $V = \frac{15}{30}$ Sn., an improvement of about $\frac{1}{3}$.

L. E. $V = \frac{15}{200}$ Sn. With $+\frac{1}{20}$ cy. ax. 180°—$\frac{1}{20}$ cy. ax. 90°, $V = \frac{15}{40}$ Sn., an improvement of $\frac{3}{10}$.

With these glasses combined the patient read No. 2 of Snellen's test-type book at one foot, and had a short range of accommodation within the limit.

The examination was repeated a few days' later under Atropia, with the same results, and spectacles with above glasses ordered to be worn all the time.

On account of the muscular and neurotic symptoms detailed above, the patient was given Physostigma 1^x dilution, on No. 40 pellets, four of these four times a day, and a drop of Eserine solution (1 grain to ℥j of water) was put in the eyes every other day. Relief commenced immediately. In a few days the muscular spasms, blinking, irritation, and pain of the eyes and the frontal headache were much diminished, and the patient went about seeing again. At the end of a fortnight the patient attended a Bazaar of Nations, and spent an entire day looking at the heterogeneous gatherings, and did not feel much discomfort from the imprudence.

The instillation of Eserine was discontinued at the end of a month; the pellets were also stopped, and powders of Silicea 3^x trit., a powder three times daily, were given for two weeks, with an idea of improving the nutrition of the cornea. The Silicea 3^x was used when there were no special symptoms, and the pellets of Physostigma 1^x alone for discomfort and strain of the eyes, and this permissible alternation was continued for six months.

During this period, excessive use of the eyes would awaken an aching, drawing sensation in the eyeballs, but this finally ceased and left the patient free to use vision as much as she pleased, without suffering more than a little discomfort.

For the past year the eyes have been comfortable, and the vision has remained the same as when the glasses were fitted. Mrs. B. keeps a bottle of Physostigma pellets by her, and takes a few when her eyes feel tired.

To all appearances this is a cure, and I claim it as the result of rational therapeutics and the scientific adjustment of spectacles. In looking over some formulæ for glasses for the correction of conical cornea, I was impressed by the fact that the corneas were not conical at all, but that one meridian presented a cylindroid elevation, and the other, at right angles, a cylindroid depression. In nearly all of the cases the plus elevation was in or near the vertical, and the minus depression in or near the horizontal, of course requiring the opposite named glasses for their correction. Now this is exactly the reverse of what we find in congenital astigmatism, and the average normal eye. In these the horizontal meridian has the plus elevation, and the vertical a less degree of plus or a normal curvature.

These peculiar cases must then be regarded as astigmatic, and the history of my case and others, in which the asymmetry came on suddenly from eye strain, would authorize their designation as acquired astigmatism.

In my paper I stated that congenital and hereditary defects may serve to explain conical cornea in youthful persons, but do not suffice for the disease in adults, who, up to middle age, have enjoyed good health and vision. The extra-ocular muscles exercise moderate pressure upon the eyeball; they affect its nutrition and development when they are abnormally shortened, but a wide experience teaches that they do not cause the disease. We are therefore left stranded upon an hypothesis of increased intra-ocular pressure for a cause of idiopathic conical cornea.

The cornea is thinner and less resisting than the sclerotic, and, in case of intra-ocular pressure from disease, it yields, advances forwards, and often ruptures. The contractions of the ciliary muscle for near vision exercise a constricting influence upon the ciliary region like the string of a bag. This diminishes the diameter of the corneo-scleral circle, increases the convexity of the cornea and the antero-posterior pressure, augments the blood in the ciliary vessels, favors serous exudation, makes the lens more convex, and alters the shape of the aqueous and vitreous chambers.

During youth, when the tissues of the eye are soft and yielding, the antero-posterior pressure, resulting from ciliary strain, causes elongated eyeballs, posterior staphylomæ and myopia. In adult life the tissues of the eye are firmer, the cornea is weaker than the sclerotic, and the ciliary muscle more powerful. Efforts of accommodation, then, in impaired health, and without proper illumination, increase the intra-ocular pressure, and this, acting upon the weaker part of the capsule, causes the cornea to bulge forwards.

I would then record my opinion, that acquired astigmatism is a result of abnormal action of the ciliary muscle, and reflection leads me to emphasize the concluding paragraph of my paper. Attempts to see better, call into action the orbicularis palpebrarum and internal recti muscles, these augment the intra-ocular pressure caused by the ciliary muscle, and *influence the direction* the corneal bulge shall take.

In the *Archives of Ophthalmology** for September, 1880, I find this unexpected indorsement of my statements: "Tension of the zonula produces mechanical dilatation of the vessels, as well as irritation of the nerves in the ciliary body, which is followed by increased secretion of blood corpuscles and blood plasma into the vitreous. As long as the capsule of the eye is yielding, no appreciable increase of tension, but dilatation of the eyeball will follow.

"The greater strength of the internal and external recti muscles prevents the globe from expanding as much in the horizontal as in the vertical direction, thus causing astigmatism." The candid reader will conclude that, if I have not made a discovery, I have, at least, brought certain facts to explain acquired astigmatism, falsely called conical cornea, in a manner never before attempted.

NEPHRECTOMY.

BY J. H. M'CLELLAND, M.D , PITTSBURG, PA.

(Read before the Homœopathic Medical Society of Pennsylvania, September, 1880.)

NEPHROTOMY obtained some mention by the older writers, although very few authenticated cases are on record. Troja defines nephrotomy as an operation in which a deep incision is made in the lumbar region, extending into the kidney or renal pelvis in order to remove a calculus situated in these parts. In modern times this operation has been frequently condemned by surgeons, and Malgaigne insisted that it should never be allowed to pass out of the anatomical amphitheatre into surgical practice.

The *extirpation* of the kidney for nephrolithiasis was never seriously thought of before Simon recommended it in 1871. Troja mentioned it as an extraordinary and ridiculous sort of nephrotomy.†

Extirpation of the kidney has received the name of nephrectomy, and, although the operation has been fully described by Simon and others, the standard works on surgery contain little or nothing on the subject.

Marion Sims wrote from Berlin to New York in June,

---

* Archives of Ophthalmology, volume ix, No. 3, page 327, article entitled "On the Common Causes of Glaucoma, Myopia, Astigmatism, and the Majority of Cataracts," by Dr. W. Roeder, Strasburg, Germany; translated by Dr. H. Knapp, New York City.

† Zeimssen's Cyclopædia, vol. xv, p. 739.

1879, as follows: "You remember how we were all electrified, about ten years ago, with the news that the daring, dashing Simon had successfully extirpated the kidney."* Dr. Sims then proceeds to narrate an operation for the removal of a kidney by abdominal section, in which he assisted Dr. Martin, of Berlin. The patient died of peritonitis on the third day. So scarcely more than ten years ago this operation was unknown.

In a historical note by M. Mardual, of Lyons, we find that "since 1869 the operation for extirpation of the kidney has been performed three times in man. The first was performed by Simon, of Heidelberg, on a woman aged 26 years, who had previously undergone ovariotomy, and had consecutive uretero-abdominal fistula, from which the urine from the left kidney escaped. The kidney was extirpated. Six weeks after the operation the patient was able to sit up in bed, and has since done well, making a complete recovery.

"The second was that of a woman 33 years of age, having a displaced, painful kidney, which was extirpated by Dr. Gilmore, of Mobile, Ala.†

"The third case, by Burns, was that of a soldier, wounded by a bullet in the left kidney, which established a reno-lumbar fistula, followed by renal suppuration and purulent infection. As a last hope the kidney was extirpated, but the man died soon after."‡

Professor Czerny, of Heidelberg, reports two cases of extirpation (London *Lancet*, February 21st, 1880). One by abdominal section, which died, and one by lumbar incision, which recovered. He concludes "that both methods of extirpation are justifiable, but that, *cæteris paribus*, the extra-peritoneal operation is the less severe one. It, *i. e.*, lumbar nephrectomy, should be adopted when the organ is not too much enlarged and is fixed. If it be movable, laparotomy may be preferred." In his second case the vertical incision was made along the anterior border of the quadratus lumbo-

---

* New York Medical Record, June 21st, 1879.

† This was a case in which the kidney had been forced up between the muscles of the back (hernia) by the gravid uterus, and was easily reached by an incision down the outer border of the erector spinal muscle. The kidney caught in this position and, constantly compressed by the erector spinal and quadratus muscles, became atrophied, lost its glandular character, and degenerated into a fibrous mass. Only a small vessel fed it, which was ligated after removal. Recovery followed without trouble. (Transactions of the Medical Association of the State of Alabama, 1872.)

‡ Half-Yearly Compendium, January, 1874.

rum, and resection of the rib was had recourse to, in order to enlarge the wound sufficiently to permit the passage of the hand. He points out that all risk from resection is obviated by its being made on the sub-periosteal plan.*

Mr. A. Barker, in a paper read before the Royal Medical and Chirurgical Society (*Lancet*, March 13th, 1880), includes the above mentioned in a list of twenty-eight cases, which he has collected from home and foreign sources. He found that "out of twenty-eight attempted nephrectomies, six were done on a wrong diagnosis, and in two, for neoplasms, the operation was left incompleted, owing to difficulties experienced in the isolation of the organ. Of the remaining twenty undertaken with the distinct object of removing the kidney, and completed, the objects were the following: Two for fistula of the ureter, both successful; two for acute pain in the kidney (cause unknown), one death, one recovery; two for calculus pyelitis, both fatal; three for injury of the organ, two complete recoveries, one fatal; six for acutely painful movable kidney, four complete recoveries, two deaths; four for neoplasms, three recoveries, one death; finally, one for pyonephrosis, perfectly successful. Of the whole twenty-eight there were fourteen deaths and fourteen recoveries, but, excluding the six for wrong diagnosis, there were still thirteen recoveries and nine deaths, two of the latter, however, were desperate and left uncompleted. The causes of death were: peritonitis, four (abdominal section in all); pyæmia, one; in one, cause not given, the patient died sixty-five hours after; in one the cause is stated to have been unexplained by the autopsy, the patient died within a week; two died of shock ten hours after the operation (both desperate cases). Of the thirteen recoveries nine were lumbar sections, four ventral; of the nine fatal cases five were lumbar, four ventral." Mr. Barker concludes: "The lumbar operation appears best suited for the removal of healthy or comparatively healthy kidneys; also when there has been much perinephritic inflammation, old or recent; also for pyo- and hydronephrosis, and perhaps for the smaller new growths of the organ, especially if fixed. The ventral incision appears, on the other hand, best suited for taking away movable kidneys, whether healthy or affected with neoplasms—especially if the latter be large; also for the ordinary cysts of the organ not fixed by inflammation."† Several cases were described at

* The American Journal of Medical Sciences, April, 1880.
† Reported in the Amer. Jour. Med. Sciences, July, 1880.

this meeting by other members, most of which had been included in Mr. Barker's list.

Great stress was laid upon the adoption of the antiseptic method, especially when laparotomy was performed.

An interesting case is reported by Mr. Thomas Savage (*Lancet*, April 17th, 1880), and one by Drs. Day and Thornton (*Lancet*, June 5th, 1880), both by abdominal section and both successful.

The operation of nephrotomy is plainly indicated in nephrolithiasis, and an extremely interesting case of this kind is reported by Professor George A. Hall, of Chicago (*Medical Investigator*, May 15th, 1880); also in some cases of hydronephrosis and pyonephrosis.

Nephrectomy is rapidly coming into favor, although but few cases have as yet been reported in this country. In the early stage of malignant neoplasms, and in non-malignant growths, in hydronephrosis and suppurative pyelitis, in renal and ureteral fistulæ, and in some cases of movable kidney, the extirpation of the organ is a justifiable and even necessary operation. With regard to the merits of the lumbar or abdominal operation, I am unable to speak from my limited experience. The opinions of Simon and Czerny appear in the foregoing. The lumbar operation, where it can be successfully done, I would regard as the less formidable.

With this rather lengthy introduction the following case is appended, that one more may be added to the list of American nephrectomies. The history of this case is obtained from the mother of the patient, and is given somewhat in her own language.

Miss Dora T——, aged 20 years; American; rather short and stout; dark hair and eyes, with light complexion.

She has been ailing ever since she was eight years old. Her attacks would always begin with pain in the bowels and over her left kidney; in one of these "she spit up blood and corruption." She had an unusually severe attack beginning December 29th, 1875, her medical attendant saying it was gallstones. "Her screams were terrifying." This was followed by extreme constipation (probably the effect of opium) and the discharge of "black pieces of flesh" with the urine, so offensive as to be intolerable. The pain and distress continued with greater or less severity, notwithstanding the constant ministrations of physicians, until August, 1876, when an abscess pointed in the back and was opened on the 24th of that month, discharging "matter and water." On October 17th, 1876, "three doctors probed and opened her side to look for rotten bone, but found none;" the bone came away December 13th, 1876; "after this her back gathered and broke in two other places, and matter and water have been running ever since."

Diagnosis.—The above history plainly indicates the following: The case began with nephrolithiasis; the presence of the calculus doubtless produced pyelitis, and this inflammatory action resulted in the pyohydronephrosis, which found relief by the lumbar discharge.

The record says, "the bone came away December 13th, 1876." This bone, so called, is the calculus, which I here show, and which evidently filled the whole pelvis of the kidney. This calculus came away more than three years ago, and since that time pus and urine have been discharged continuously through the lumbar fistula, rendering her condition scarcely tolerable to herself or her friends. The amount flowing from this fistula was at times enormous, keeping her clothes and bedding constantly saturated, the odor arising being almost unbearable.

For two years past she has been in care of Dr. W. J. Martin, who did much to alleviate her suffering and improve her general health. He recommended her admission to the hospital for whatever radical measures might be deemed necessary for her relief. She seemed perfectly willing to submit to an operation, regardless of consequences.

She was admitted to the hospital August 6th, 1880, in very fair condition, except that the pulse was accelerated and temperature a little elevated, owing probably to the presence of another abscess pointing in the left groin, keeping her left leg semiflexed, and she complained of soreness on pressure in the left iliac fossa. This region became gradually more painful until August 12th, when the abscess was opened, discharging about twelve ounces of very offensive pus, *mixed with urine.*

This, then, established another and much more lengthy sinus from the kidney. The discharge of pus gradually decreased during the following week, and the patient's condition improved steadily.

August 19th, 1880, after consultation with the hospital staff, and in the presence of the medical board and others, the operation for extirpation was begun.

The lumbar sinus opened externally just above the crest of the ilium, about five inches from the median line of the vertebral column, penetrating obliquely upward and inward to the kidney, just under the twelfth rib. The track of the sinus was laid open on the director, and then the incision extended from the twelfth rib to the crest of the ilium along the border of the quadratus lumborum. To show the difficulty with which the kidney was reached, I would remark that the lumbar wall at this point was about four inches thick, and the distance between the rib and ilium only about an inch and a half; the patient was "short coupled." The incision, superficially, was about six inches in length. In order to obtain more working space, the deep parts were divided laterally to the extent of an inch.

Passing the finger into the cavity, the kidney was found to be much hollowed out by the long-continued suppuration, and the walls correspondingly thin. The process of enucleation then began, the organ being carefully separated from its bed by the finger. Grasping the mass with a lithotomy forceps, it was drawn through the wound, and with an aneurism-needle a ligature was passed around the pelvis of the organ as close as possible to the exit of the ureter. The vessels were included in this ligature. The removal of the kidney was then completed. Considerable blood was lost by venous oozing, but no large vessels were cut. Hot carbolized water was then thrown into the large cavity remaining, and the wound left gaping, so that complete drainage was secured. The wound was dressed with patent lint soaked in carbolized oil.

After the operation the patient seemed much prostrated; pulse rapid and weak. Toward evening she became restless, having dry mouth, great thirst, and occasional vomiting. ℞. Arsen.[6] every hour.

Second day. Nausea, thirst, and restlessness greatly relieved. Prescription continued.

The weather becoming extremely warm, the utmost care was necessary to prevent septic processes. The flow of serum from the wound was large, wetting the dressings and bedding in the course of a few hours. The wound was thoroughly irrigated with carbolized water twice a day, and all wet clothing and bedding removed and replaced with dry; the bedcovers were also frequently changed. By these unremitting attentions all disagreeable odors were prevented. Arsenicum was continued a number of days, no other remedy being necessary.

The patient's health rapidly improved; nausea, thirst, and restlessness soon subsiding. The urinous odor disappeared from the discharges entirely and at once. Fully double the amount of urine has been voided by the bladder ever since the extirpation. A record of the pulse and temperature is appended, from which it will be seen that the highest temperature was 101$\frac{4}{5}$ degrees. After the first week the temperature scarcely ever rose above 100 degrees. The wound has granulated rapidly, and is now,—twentieth day,—nearly filled up. Patient has gained flesh, and is able to be out of bed.

RECORD OF PULSE AND TEMPERATURE.

DAY.	First.		Second.		Third.		Fourth.		Fifth.	
	A.M.	P.M.	A.M.	P.M.	A.M.	P.M.	A.M.	P.M.	A.M.	
Pulse	140	140	130	110	115	105	105	105	108	
Temp	101	$101\frac{1}{5}$	$101\frac{1}{5}$	$99\frac{1}{2}$	$101\frac{4}{5}$	$99\frac{3}{8}$	$100\frac{1}{5}$	$101\frac{1}{5}$	$100\frac{3}{5}$	

DAY.	Sixth.		Seventh.		Eighth.		Ninth.		Tenth.	
	A.M.	P.M.	A.M.	P.M.	A.M.	P.M.	A.M.	P.M.	A.M.	P.M.
Pulse	115	108	103	100	100	97	96	96	97	96
Temp	$100\frac{4}{5}$	$100\frac{1}{5}$	$100\frac{3}{8}$	$100\frac{1}{5}$	$100\frac{1}{5}$	$99\frac{1}{2}$	$99\frac{2}{5}$	$99\frac{2}{5}$	$99\frac{1}{3}$	$99\frac{4}{5}$

DAY.	Eleventh.		Twelfth.		Thirteenth.		Fourteenth.		Fifteenth.		Sixteenth.	
	A.M.	P.M.	A.M.	P.M.	A.M.	P.M.	A.M.	P.M.	A.M.	P.M.	A.M.	P.M.
Pulse.	97		97	99	96	96	95	97	96	98	99	98
Temp.	$99\frac{4}{5}$		$99\frac{4}{5}$	$99\frac{1}{5}$	$99\frac{1}{5}$	$99\frac{2}{5}$	$99\frac{1}{5}$	99	$99\frac{1}{5}$	$99\frac{1}{5}$	99	99

Up to this time the pulse and temperature have varied but little from the normal.

DRUG ATTENUATION—A REVIEW.

BY H. W. TAYLOR, M.D., CRAWFORDSVILLE, INDIANA.

DRUG ATTENUATION; ITS OBJECTS, MODES, MEANS, AND LIMITS IN HOMŒOPATHIC PHARMACY AND POSOLOGY. BY THE BUREAU OF MATERIA MEDICA, PHARMACY, AND PROVINGS, OF THE AMERICAN INSTITUTE OF HOMŒOPATHY, 1879 AND 1880. J. P. DAKE, A.M., M.D., CHAIRMAN.

THIS report bears evidence of having for its basis an intended "*competitive trial*" of the *low dilutions* and the "*high potencies.*" That this competitive trial has not been so sweeping and comprehensive in its effects as was originally intended and expected, is set forth in the report. The experiments made by the bureau were conducted in a spirit of fairness on the part of the low dilutionists. It was intended to show by a series of fairly conducted trials and tests, which of the two factions in homœopathic posology is most nearly right. And this was done, not to subserve partisan purposes, but in the name and for the sake of *the truth*. It was also contemplated that the enemies of homœopathy might be led to investigate the system through the facts here presented. It was to be shown that there was something in homœopathy for the scientist to take hold of. That the views held by a number of homœopathists regarding drug attenuation are not fairly representative of the belief of the majority of homœopathists, and that the facts and arguments set forth by the bureau in its official capacity are such as may command the respectful attention of educated men of whatever medical belief.

In this view of the aim and scope of the work of the bureau, it is to be regretted that the dynamizationists failed to make their part of the trial as full and complete as it should have been. Why they retired from the contest at the very onset is now a matter for inquiry. Thus far it does not appear that sufficient reasons have been offered to satisfactorily explain and account for this failure. In fact, no reasons, whatever, have been given. Dr. Hawkes's charge, that the test was "not in the hands of representative men," might have been avoided, had Drs. Hawkes and Allen seen fit to carry out in good faith, *their own proposition to test the efficacy of the 30ths*, in a fair and open manner. No low dilutionist will or does say that representative men were not on the bureau. All low dilutionists are satisfied with *their* representation upon the test.

It would appear that the "high potency" challengers to the "Milwaukee test" recanted, and refused to make the test, and afterward used that recantation and refusal as an "argument" against the validity of the test. *In law*, one is not permitted to do an act subversive of the obligations of a contract, and then plead that act in bar of such obligations. The rule of law will hold good in this trial. And thinking men will conclude that henceforth the loud assertions, the invective, and the vituperation of the advocates of "high potencies" are mere fustian. They will no longer regard the cry of "mongrel," "eclectic," and "allopath," when used to designate those who use the low dilutions. These have, in this bureau report, demonstrated their *faith* by their *works*.

The leading papers, by the chairman of the bureau, are models of scholarly writing. It is shown that Hahnemann, through the active part of his life, was a low dilutionist. And further, that at no time was he a dynamizationist, since up to the day of his death he believed that "some of the original drug-matter remained in the highest potency." The question comes up, whether Hahnemann committed himself to the dynamization doctrine in any degree. He was no vacillating time-server. He had strong convictions, and acted upon them. Could such a man have held two views so irreconcilable, so antagonistic? Is it possible that Hahnemann originated the practice (followed by some modern dynamizationists) of making cures with low dilutions, and reporting them as having been achieved with high potencies? Could the man who prescribed the "mother" triturations to his last day, have been a believer in the "minimum dose of the dynamized drug?" His life-work answers these questions with a pronounced negation. It is not difficult to see that Hahnemann's real thoughts and words were misrepresented by that body of his disciples who hoped to duplicate the good fortune of Lutze, and accumulate wealth by adopting his method of "magnetizing" drugs. Thus it is that there runs through the later writings and declarations of Hahnemann a glaring inconsistency,—a blunt contradiction. The "materialistic" and "spiritualistic" explanations of homœopathic pharmacology are as irreconcilable as fire and water. It seems simply impossible that they could have had a common origin in the mind of Hahnemann.

This view is further strengthened in the logical papers of Dr. W. L. Breyfogle. Here it is incontrovertibly proven, that the modern processes of high potency pharmacology were unknown to Hahnemann. How could he have sanctioned that which was not invented until after his death? Would this man, so exact in all his manipulations, have given his sanction to the bottle-washing chimera of Jenichen? Would he, who was a model of neatness in pharmacy, have indorsed the "fluxion potentizer" of Boericke & Tafel, with its dirty Schuylkill water, and its "rubber" channel to the potentizing glass? Would he, who worshipped his new-born science as a god, have submitted to its defilement and profanation by the hydrant water, and single glass tumbler which Fincke borrowed from the Brooklyn bar-room pharmacy? "Cheap and nasty," is the verdict of Dr. Sherman, in which verdict all low-dilution homœopathists will concur.

In every aspect, the tests made by the low dilutionists and chronicled in this "report" are fair, accurate, and scientific. The crucible, the microscope, and the spectroscope, have been interrogated by experts. Their answer is uniformly against the high potencies. The science of mathematics is called upon to disprove the possibility of the presence of drug molecules in the 30th centesimal. And the answer is decisive against the other assumption. In these labors were engaged such well-known men as J. P. Dake, W. L. Breyfogle, C. Wesselhœft, Lewis Sherman, S. A. Jones, and J. Edwards Smith. No bar sinister can be placed against these eminent homœopathists. And the cry of "not representative men" falls upon heedless ears.

But, perhaps, the most signal triumph of the low dilutionists was not in the domain of science—that *terra incognita* of the dynamizationist. Taken all in all, the most telling blow against "high potency" was delivered and received upon its chosen field, the physiological arena. After the bold defiance of the dynamizationists uttered at Lake George, the bureau buckled on its armor in an honest and earnest expectation of the fray. There was no battle—but a slaughter. There was no retreat—but a rout. Words and figures could do no more to overwhelm the dynamizationists.

I may be pardoned for referring to one argument of the defeated party. The experiments of Wurmb and Caspar are again made to do duty as ballast for the high potency craft. These experiments might well have been "freshened" by a repetition under the supervision of Dr. Cowperthwaite. It is, perhaps, sufficient to say, that the average duration of pneumonia under the 30ths, as here reported, would drive any low dilution homœopathist out of practice. Eleven and three-tenths days, may be safely set down as *twice the average duration* of pneumonia in the practice of low dilutionists. Such practice will not begin to compare with "regular" treatment of pneumonia as given by Thomas K. Chambers, in his *Renewal of Life.* It is simply expectancy *v.* the overdosing of allopathy, and is of no significance in a comparison of modern homœopathic methods. Neither is the success of the pioneer homœopathists in America evidence of the efficacy of the 30ths. Their practice was compared solely with the bleeding, blistering, purging practice of the cruder unscientific allopathy of that day. Old Samuel Thomson, with his Lobelia, Capsicum, Bayberry, and steam, achieved "triumphant success" over the barbarous old-school practice of that time. It is fair to assume that no clinical test of the "high potencies" and low dilutions has yet been made, or can be made, except by competitive trial under conditions as just and rigid as those environing the Milwaukee pathogenetic test.

This work of the Bureau of Materia Medica will not prove

a labor in vain. It will demonstrate to reasonable men the fact that the power of the low dilutions is fairly proven, while all tests applied to the 30th have failed to show them possessed of medicinal power; have, in fact, proven them to be without drug-matter, and without drug-power. It only remains to make a competitive trial of the 3d and 30th in a homœopathic hospital, and I earnestly suggest that this be done.

But whether it be done or not, one great good will result to the low dilutionists. They will no longer be under the domination of an oligarchy of self-styled "higher homœopathy." The laugh, as well as the argument, is now all on the side of the low dilutionists. "Cures" with the millionth potency will not obtain that *éclat* that formerly belonged to them. And above all, the man who, out of his experience, dares prescribe Quinine, or Chinoidine, or who in extremity, dares to give a quarter grain dose of Morphia, will henceforth be heard with whatever of respect is due him as a man and a homœopathic physician, instead of the shower of vituperation and abuse which was formerly rained down upon his devoted head. Once more the good old Hahnemannian test of faith will be revived. And belief in the law of similars will again be the sole passport to the cordial recognition and friendly welcome of homœopathic practitioners everywhere.

A DIALOGUE.

Preceptor (who is a Fellow of the Irish College of Surgeons). Well, we've effectually squelched homœopathy and all other forms of quackery, this time.

Student. Ah, indeed! How?

Preceptor. Our learned body met last night and passed a series of resolutions. One need but to read them to be convinced of the wisdom of our proceedings as well as of the flippant nature of modern irregular schools of medicine. Here they are, read them yourself:

"That the ordinance of council of the 22d August, 1861, be and it is hereby rescinded, and instead thereof it be now *resolved*, That it be an ordinance of the council that no Fellow or licentiate of the college shall seek for business through the medium of advertisements or any other disreputable method, or shall consult with, advise, direct, or assist, or have any professional communication with any person who professes to cure disease by the deception called homœopathy, or by the practice called mesmerism, or by any other form of quackery, or who follows any system of practice considered derogatory or dishonorable to physicians and surgeons.

"*And be it furthermore resolved*, That in the opinion of this council it is inconsistent with professional propriety, and derogatory to the reputation, honor, and dignity of the college, to engage in the practice of homœopathy or mesmerism, or any of the forms of quackery as hereinbefore set forth."

Student. These resolutions certainly place your college in positive opposition to all forms of quackery; but may I ask, what do you mean by quackery?

Preceptor. I mean just this. Quackery is derived from the German, quäken; or, as the Dutch have it, kwaaken, and the Danish, qvœkke. It is an onomatopœietic word, whose sound is derived from the well-known noise of the duck; and so becomes a fitting appellation to him who chatters and boasts of his pretended skill, brags loudly of his many cures—in a word a charlatan, a mountebank. You see, the application is patent.

Student (somewhat awed by his preceptor's great learning). Yes, I see, that is, I think I see. But, are these homœopaths such praters? I have a friend, a homœopathic student (preceptor frowns)—an acquaintance, I mean. He boarded at the same house I did, when I was in the States. He was a poor student, who occupied the fourth floor back. I didn't see him very often (frown on preceptor's face fades). He asked me how we in Ireland conducted clinics, and I informed him of your wonderfully successful operations (preceptor's form grows more erect), and how many marvellous cures you report each clinic day. He looked down to the floor for a moment, and then said, mildly, "We don't boast quite so many cures here; but doubtless your professor has a very extensive practice. Come into our clinics some day while you are in Philadelphia. You need have no fear of being hissed or hooted, we don't indulge in that sort of recreation. But it may assist you; for I know no surer way of reaching the truth than to investigate for oneself;" then he bid me "good-morning," and left. Now this doesn't sound like boasting, does it?

Preceptor. He's a ninnyhammer, who is guzzled by the splatterdash of his rascally teachers. Don't have anything to do with him.

Student. No, I will not. Still it's not a little remarkable that his advice is a repetition of your own. When I left you last spring, you advised me to investigate homœopathy for myself, adding that you knew no more certain way of convincing me that the system is fallacious.

Preceptor. Well, are you convinced?

Student (awed). Yes, I'm convinced. But (rallying a little), looking at the matter from a humanitarian point, would you refuse to extend the benefits of your great skill and learning to the patient of a homœopath? I do not now refer to medical advice; for were I a homœopath, if I believed in Hahnemann's law of cure, how could I seek therapeutic assistance from a system which is entirely opposed to that law! I refer to surgical operations for which you are noted; or to the diagnosing of obscure diseases. Could you not lend your aid in such cases, and so extend your usefulness?

Preceptor (emphatically). No, never! These fools who submit to the charlatanry of ignorant impostors don't deserve to get well or to live either. The world would be well rid of them (walks the floor in righteous rage).

Student. But the public are not so fully informed of the deception as you are. I find that the reports of homœopathic hospitals claim a larger percentage of cures than we do. And in Philadelphia, where I was visiting last summer, homœopathic physicians have 200,000 clients. Of course, this is all a part of the deception which the college decries; but are the people to blame? You would require them to dismiss their attendant before you will lend your skill. They respect their physician and fail to see the quackery, which you so sagaciously detect. And so they must die!

Preceptor. And ought to die. Look around you on these four walls, and on the row of book-cases before you. They are all filled with the choicest learning of two thousand years. Think you an obscure Dutchman can subvert all this with a fanciful system, based on a mode of practice known to Hippocrates himself, aye, known to the Chinese for no one knows how long? I tell you, any man who will relinquish all this accumulated lore for the sugar and water of the homœopath, doesn't deserve to be cured. And his infinitesimal portion of brains would never be missed if he should step out. These statistics which you refer to are another proof of the quackery, the empty boasting, to which I alluded a few moments ago.

Student. This is an assertion, but can it be proved?

Preceptor (angrily). Why, you talk like a renegade. Have your investigations tinctured your green pate, too?

Student (with dignity). No, sir; but by every principle of fair play, by the logic you have taught me, by the freedom of thought, which is the prerogative of every man, I claim the right to inquire why this homœopathy is a deception, why you will restrict the benefits of your skill; and, how you and the other members of the Irish College have the boldness to denounce thousands of men as deceivers and quacks—men who are good citizens, upright and moral, and who it would seem would not stoop to anything dishonorable. You call them quacks, but if I can believe the student to whom I referred a few moments ago, many of them are thoroughly educated in every branch of medicine. He showed me the questions which candidates for graduation were required to answer, and I can assure you they were too difficult for me to solve satisfactorily. All this troubles me, and I am determined to investigate for myself. Though confident that the time-honored school of medicine to which you and I belong is the true one, I feel it unbecoming in me to coincide with your college until more acquainted with the facts in the case.

Preceptor. Cease this insolent talk at once, and leave my presence—— But stop. You question my motives in defending science against the invasion of these pretending homœopaths, and you arraign me with "The Royal College of Surgeons of Ireland," as slanderers. Rather than dismiss you uninformed, as you deserve, I will permit you to remain here in my library. I refer you to case N., east wall, in which you will find ample to vindicate my cause and bring the blush of shame to your cheeks. If one day is not sufficient, take a week. The whole library is at your disposal. When your heretical views shall have been dispelled, as they must be if you are the impartial, honest man you pretend, an apology will again ingratiate you into my favor.

Student. Thank you. I will accept your offer. I have been educated after the strictest methods of the regular school. As I said before, I believe its tenets, and have no intention of turning renegade, as you unkindly accuse me. Nevertheless, I await the results of my investigation.

(Two weeks later.) *Preceptor.* Well, sir. What have you to say now in defence of quackery?

Student. Nothing in defence of quackery; but everything in favor of the truth of homœopathy, and of the honor and good repute of its votaries. I followed advice literally, and received my confirmations from your own library.

Preceptor. Impossible, sir, without the grossest perversion. What books do you dare to say confirmed you?

Student. I have the list. I will read it: *Wood's Therapeutics, Materia Medica, and Toxicology; Materia Medica and Therapeutics,* by Phillips; *Handbook of Therapeutics,* by Sidney Ringer; *Graves's Clinical Lectures,* p. 784; *Cyclopædia of Practical Medicine,* vol. i, by Sir John Forbes; *Specific Action of Drugs on the Healthy System, an Index to their Therapeutical Value, as Deduced from Experiments on Men and Animals,* by Alexander G. Burness, M.B.C.M., and T. T. Mavor, M.R.C.V.S.; Trousseau, *Traité de Therapeutique et de Matière*

Médicale, vol. ii, p. 55. Each of these works, sir, openly or inferentially, offers proofs of the genuineness of the system of Hahnemann. On inquiry I find that Professor Wood's work has already converted a dozen or more in America, and I am only happy—

Preceptor. Nonsense; the books you enumerate are, many of them, standard works, true and sound. But I referred you to another case altogether, one containing such exposés of homœopathy as *Palmer's Lectures*, *King's*—

Student. Excuse me; all these I read, but they denounce the homœopathic law of cure, and since the others just mentioned acknowledge that it has a limited application, the absurdity of the former became apparent; therefore—

Preceptor (angrily). 'Tis false. They do not admit—

Student (interrupting). I will read you what Trousseau says. Do not interrupt me, I must be heard. In his *Materia Medica* he writes: "If now Arsenic is employed locally, in very small proportions, it acts homœopathically, that is to say, substitutively."

Preceptor (furious). Leave me forever—do not tarry an instant or you'll tempt me beyond human endurance!

Student (firmly). Stay. I've a word yet to say, and will not be intimidated by threats. You in the "regular school" rush on blindly, changing your prescriptions as do the fashions. You have no law to guide you, but trust to the precarious results of what you term "experience." You do not hesitate to engraft into your therapeutics the choice discoveries of homœopathy, or even to admit the partial application of the law of similars, but it is rarely that you acknowledge the plagiarism. For homœopaths, since they prefer following one of nature's infallible laws, are narrow-minded bigots, whose literary contributions, though adopted by the "regulars," ought not to be acknowledged by so learned a body as "The Royal College of Surgeons of Ireland." These homœopaths are deceivers, disreputable men, and have no rights which you are bound to respect. So filthy are they, that the *Medical Press and Circular* (June 30th, 1880), congratulates you on your determination not to "touch the unclean thing." But—— A shower of epithets, manuscripts, and books, two inkstands, and a bootjack, cut short farther remarks. The wily student successfully dodged the missiles. And the only result was a disordered library, a raging Irish surgeon, and an ugly blot of ink on the last report of "The Royal College of Surgeons of Ireland." TESTIS OCCULATUS.

THE HERING MEMORIAL MEETING.

THE meeting provided for by a resolution adopted by the physicians of Philadelphia, July 25th, was held on Sunday evening, October 10th, in the hall of Hahnemann Medical College. Dr. John K. Lee occupied the chair, and Dr. Henry N. Guernsey acted as secretary.

Dr. J. C. Guernsey read that portion of the minutes of the July meeting, which related to the appointment of a Committee on Memorial Meeting, and Dr. A. Lippe, the chairman of the committee, presented the resolutions under which the meeting was called, and which had been published in the homœopathic journals.

On motion, the report of the Committee on Memorial Meeting was received, and the committee discharged.

Dr. Joseph C. Guernsey then read the "minute" adopted by the Homœopathic Medical Society of Pennsylvania, and resolutions from the Central Society of the State of New York, the College of Physicians and Surgeons of Michigan; also, a paper prepared by Dr. Boyce containing interesting reminiscences of Dr. Hering, and read before the New York State Central Society, a letter from Dr. C. B. Gilbert, of Washington, and a telegram from Dr. W. P. Wesselhœft, of Boston.

Dr. Pemberton Dudley, on behalf of the Philadelphia County Society, read a "minute" from that body, expressive of its sense of the loss sustained in the decease of Dr. Hering.

Dr. Edward Bayard, of New York city, then delivered an eloquent and impressive eulogy on the life, character, and services of the departed, prefacing it with the announcement that he represented his county society as a delegate, and presented on its behalf, an expression of respect for the memory of Dr. Hering, and its sympathy with his family and professional friends.

In the course of his remarks he alluded to Dr. Hering's grand and characteristic reverence for truth. He thought there was some truth everywhere, but complete truth nowhere; that every man holds some truth, and that no man may claim to be the custodian of perfect truth in all things. While expressing his sympathy with the profession in Philadelphia, he yet considered that Hering belonged not to Philadelphia alone, but to the whole world. He cared not for money-getting, but for the interests of humanity and truth; in his labors for these he was indefatigable, and has left behind him as the result of his work, a vast store of materials as a priceless legacy to posterity. He was a true homœopathist. He believed in the law of cure, and he lived up to it. He sought no palliatives, save in homœopathy, and in his closing hours still sought relief only in the principles that he had practiced throughout his long life.

Dr. Clement Pearson, of Washington, D. C., said it was not his fortune to be personally well acquainted with Dr. Hering, yet he felt that he knew him well. He was not surprised that Hering is gone. He had labored earnestly for almost eighty years. Yet he still lives, and a hundred years hence, the child yet to be born will have cause to bless his name for the relief his Lachesis affords.

Fourscore years was a good age to attain, yet far too short to reform a world. And so, the truths promulgated by Hahnemann and Hering should still be jealously guarded by us and the men who shall come after us. It is a pity that knowledge and experience cannot be transmitted to a successor, and that each must dig for himself in the mine of knowledge with few to take him by the hand or wish him God-speed. And it is a sad thing that among all those who strut and fret their brief hour upon the stage, so many of us should be such poor players. The speaker paid a beautiful tribute to the memory of Hering, and closed with the injunction that although a leader had fallen, we who remain must not let the standard be lowered.

Before resuming his seat, Dr. Pearson presented the regrets of Dr. F. R. McManus, of Baltimore, who was unable to be present at the meeting.

Dr. A. Lippe was the next speaker. He said, as mourning children we remember what the departed was to all of us, as an instructor, and as one who added so much to our knowledge of the healing art. Dr. Hering was chosen from among many students at Leipsic, to overthrow, by a pamphlet, the pretensions of the new system. Homœopathy was but slowly gaining ground in those days, and he must have been a fearless man when, in 1824, he avowed himself an advocate of the new art, and was at once made the victim of relentless persecution. Dr. Lippe then alluded briefly to Dr. Hering's experience as a naturalist at Surinam, his dismissal from his post for daring to practice homœopathy, his investigations with Lachesis, his removal to the United States, his connection with the Allentown Academy, his settlement in Philadelphia, and his subsequent labors in organizing and directing the forces of the new system of medicine. He concluded with a sentence from Dr. Hering's last published paper: "If we ever depart from the strict inductive methods of Hahnemann, we are lost."

Dr. H. N. Guernsey gave some interesting reminiscences of his early knowledge of Dr. Hering, of his introduction to him by Housman in the very building in which he was now speaking, and of his continued intimacy and friendship with him from that time till his death. He related an incident of Dr. Hering,—a trip to Frankford to see a case of poisoning by the sting of the bee (*Apis mellifica*), as an evidence of his intense enthusiasm in the study of drug action. As a consultant he was most faithful and earnest, devoting himself with energy to discover the true remedy. He cited numerous instances showing his utmost reliance upon the principle of homœopathy in all cases of disease, from the simplest to the most desperate.

Dr. R. J. McClatchey said he too desired to testify to Dr. Hering's worth as a man, his skill and success as a physician, and to the value of his immense services in the cause of medical science. He considered that one of the most marked characteristics of Dr. Hering was his steadfastness of purpose. He seemed never to lose sight of the one great object of his life. Those of us who knew him well, know what a fascinating conversationalist he was, and how, even the apparently trifling matters of every-day occurrence, were made to contribute to the grand purposes he had in view. Everything that he saw or heard was to him but a part of a completed harmony. His one great thought and theme was to secure the recognition of homœopathy as an established science. He gave full respect to the opinions of others, and hence his own opinions always commanded respect.

Dr. Martin Deschere, of New York, spoke briefly in eulogy of the deceased. He said that we can best honor him by following in the path in which he walked. His mission was to spread the benefits of homœopathy, and though he succeeded in a remarkable degree, yet we must take up the work where he left it and still carry it forward. He alluded to the rapid spread of homœopathy in the United States, and mentioned a letter, lately written by a layman of Germany to Dr. Hering, asking him to prepare a paper on the status of homœopathy in America; one that should encourage the friends of that system in Europe. He appealed to those who should attend the World's Convention in London next year, to exert their utmost influence to advance the cause among our transatlantic brethren.

Dr. John K. Lee felt that any eulogy of Dr. Hering is incomplete which does not include a reflection of his moral nature. And here he needs not the mantle of charity. He related an incident which exhibits Dr. Hering's intense regard for truth. A friend had said to him, "How badly it makes one feel to be convinced of error." The remark made such a profound impression upon Dr. Hering, that, as he afterwards said, he ceased to repose any confidence in him.

Dr. Joseph C. Guernsey spoke of the circumstances of Dr. Hering's graduation in medicine, and his bold avowal of his faith in the system of Hahnemann before the faculty of Wurzburg. He had in his possession a transcript of Dr. Hering's thesis, written fifty-two years ago, on "The Medicine of the Future," of which a translation was being prepared for publication in the Memorial volume.

Dr. Bushrod W. James said: We are not here to erect a monument to the departed; that, his own life has done. His works are known; his virtues need no further inscription. His qualities of heart, his professional skill, his steadfast purpose to benefit mankind are known to all of us.

Every age has its progressive spirits; men who by their labors leave a deep and lasting impress behind them, and truly our departed friend was one of these. Liberal in his methods of homœopathic prescribing, and not bound to excrescent ideas, he read Hahnemann's *Organon* as he read his Bible, testing all therein advanced, and holding firmly to all that proved to be true and valuable.

He was not one to fetter the dose, or to limit its size and repetition. He conceded to all physicians the right of private judgment, while unswervingly exercising his own. Yet while thus liberal, he always adhered strictly to the law of *similars*, and to the selection of the remedy from the totality of the symptoms. The speaker here quoted from Dr. Hering's writings to the effect, that in his view, a thorough and successful practice of homœopathy is not possible without a knowledge of anatomy, physiology, pathology, and chemistry, in addition to a thorough knowledge of the Materia Medica. In reference to his interest in young practitioners and students of homœopathy, the speaker said that no toil was too arduous, no time too precious, no research too burdensome, that might enable him to present to the student clearly, the doctrines of homœopathy. He was earnest in the cause of a higher medical education. He led the followers of Hahnemann to victory, and from his lofty height he saw the promised realization of his hopes,—the world's acknowledgment of the truth of homœopathy, and to-day we place the laurels upon the brow of one of Hahnemann's most trusted and worthy generals.

Dr. Charles Mohr said that from the first time he ever saw Dr. Hering, down to the time of his death, he never once met him without profit to himself and to those within his professional influence. Dr. Hering was earnest in his friendship for the younger members of the profession, and hearty in his efforts for their instruction and advancement. He referred to the *Guiding Symptoms*, as his only adequate monument, and said that upon that monument Dr. Hering had devoted fifty years of labor. It remains for the profession to give completeness to this grand work, and especially so because it is a legacy to the author's family. Dr. Hering, had, on one occasion, said to him: "I shall not be with you until the completion of the *Guiding Symptoms*, but it will be finished by others, and perhaps from my place in heaven I shall be permitted to look down, and to know that the work has been well done."

A committee, consisting of Drs. C. G. Raue, C. B. Knerr, and Charles Mohr, was then appointed to publish the Memorial volume, and it was ordered that all papers received be referred to that committee. Also, that the cost of publishing the volume, and the manner of providing for the same, be referred to the same committee, with power to act.

The meeting then, on motion, adjourned.

THE PHILADELPHIA COUNTY HOMŒOPATHIC MEDICAL SOCIETY.

REPORTED BY CHARLES MOHR, M.D., SECRETARY.

THE regular monthly meeting was held in the hall of the Hahnemann Medical College, on Thursday evening, October 14th, 1880; Dr. W. B. Trites, the Vice-President, in the chair. After reading and approval of the minutes of the September meeting, reports were received from Dr. H. N. Guernsey, delegate "at large," to societies abroad, Dr. B. W. James, delegate to American Institute of Homœopathy, and Dr. C. Mohr, delegate to Pennsylvania State Society.

The committee appointed to prepare a suitable minute on the death of Dr. Constantine Hering made the following report:

Your Committee, appointed to prepare a minute expressive of the sense of this society upon the decease of Dr. Constantine Hering, have prepared the following, which, in accordance with your instructions, was presented to the Memorial Meeting, held October 10th, and will doubtless appear in the Memorial volume:

"The Homœopathic Medical Society of the County of Philadelphia, uniting with the friends of homœopathy and medical progress everywhere in mourning the departure of our late Honorary Member, Constantine Hering, M.D., offers this tribute of respect to his memory.

"We recognize in the decease of Dr. Hering, the loss of one pre-eminently adapted by nature and education to be a leader in the early struggles and sacrifices of a new medical dispensation. Cultured in literature and in general science; learned in all the medical wisdom of the allopathic fathers; careful in the formation of his opinions; zealous for the advancement of his chosen profession, and ambitious to excel in the practice of his art, we yet find him accepting without reserve the overwhelming testimony to the truth of Homœopathy, flinging aside the temptations of professional honor and political preferment; fearlessly asserting his 'liberty of medical opinion and action' in the presence of an arrogant and intolerant profession, and in the face of his king, and deliberately casting his lot with the derided and persecuted pioneers of a new and hated system. Devoting all his talents and energies to the perfection and dissemination of the newly-discovered art of healing; laboring with heart, and hand, and brain for its establishment over a whole continent; unswerving in his adherence to its teachings, unflinching in its defence, and untiring in all labors for its advancement, he seemed ever to realize that he had been raised up for this, his heaven-appointed work. We rejoice that he was permitted to witness the vast results toward which his own vast labors had so largely contributed,—the shaken foundations of the old medical superstructure; the triumphant vindication of the once despised system of Hahnemann; the establishment of its hospitals, its colleges, and its journals; the organization of its societies, and the spread of its beneficent influence by thousands of educated physicians into millions of homes.

"We, his fellow-members of this society, among whom he walked, and taught, and labored for so many years, who enjoyed his intimate personal acquaintance and counsel, are proud to express our appreciation of his personal character, and his abounding services in the cause of progressive medicine,—the cause of suffering humanity. We shall ever hold his name, his work and his worth in warm remembrance, and our posterity will rise up to do him honor."

John K. Lee,
Pemberton Dudley,
Claude R. Norton,
Committee.

Philadelphia, October 10th, 1880.

The Society adopted a resolution of thanks to Messrs. Singerly and Norris of the Philadelphia *Record* for their energy in the suppression of the sale of Bogus Diplomas.

The secretary called attention to the movement on foot in Philadelphia, looking to the formation of a permanent non-sectarian association, for the purpose of securing the observance by each religious body of an Annual Hospital Collection Day, when contributions can be made simultaneously for the benefit of the various hospitals of Philadelphia. A similar plan is in vogue in some of the large European cities, and for several years has been remarkably successful; and in New York city the inaugural step made last year, although only a few churches comparatively had united in the enterprise, resulted in a collection of over $26,000. To secure the immense good such a movement will accomplish in Philadelphia, Dr. Mohr moved that the following be adopted:

"*Resolved*, That the movement on foot in Philadelphia for the establishment of a permanent non-sectarian association, with the object of duly fixing and perpetuating the observance of a yearly Hospital Day, for the purpose of making collections in all the churches and Sunday-schools, and receiving general contributions for the benefit of our hospitals, leaving each church or school and each donor free to indicate the special application of contributions, and providing for a wise distribution of the gifts not designated for any particular hospital, receives the most hearty indorsement of the Homœopathic Medical Society of the County of Philadelphia, and its members agree, individually and collectively, to do all they can to further the object.

"*Resolved*, That the Secretary be instructed to communicate the action of the society to the committee having the matter in charge."

After discussion by Drs. Martin, Johnson, and Mohr, the resolutions were adopted.

The Bureau of Surgery and Clinical Surgery, W. C. Goodno, M.D., *Chairman*, then made its report. The following papers* were presented, read, and referred for publication, viz.:

a. "Rapid Lithotrity," by C. M. Thomas, M.D.

b. "Recent Developments in Surgical Practice," by J. C. Morgan, M.D.

c. "Antiseptic Surgery," by John E. James, M.D.

d. "Colles Fracture," by W. C. Goodno, M.D.

The hour was so late when the reading of the papers was concluded, that no discussion ensued, and on motion the meeting adjourned.

The Bureau of Ophthalmology, Otology, and Laryngology, C. M. Thomas, M.D., *Chairman*, will report November 11th, 1880, when interesting papers will be presented.

A CRITICISM OF THE HERING MEMORIAL MEETING.

MANAYUNK, October 20th, 1880.

EDITORS OF THE HAHNEMANNIAN: I write to express the disappointment I felt when, on Monday morning, the 11th instant, the newspapers announced that the Hering Memorial Meeting had been held the day previous, and that I had been debarred from participating in a meeting held to do honor to one whom I had greatly loved.

But my indignation was aroused when, on inquiry, I learned that no special notice of the meeting had been sent to any of the physicians of Philadelphia and its vicinity, and that the committee had depended solely upon the notice *published nearly*

---

* These papers are deferred on account of the press of matter upon our pages. They will appear in our December number.—EDS.

six weeks previously in the journals. This may have been an oversight; but if so, it was a most unfortunate—I had almost said a criminal one.

Dr. Hering was the leader of no clique, the centre of no ring, and by the liberality of his creed, the honesty of his purpose, and the purity of his life, he had endeared himself to the *whole* profession; and, had proper arrangements been made, two-thirds of the physicians of this city would have assembled to show their respect and veneration for that great man, the leader of homœopathy in America. Instead of this there were, as I am informed, but about twenty Philadelphians in attendance at the meeting. I hope that publicity will be given to the fact, that Dr. Hering's Philadelphia brethren were absent from the meeting, not because of any want of appreciation of his worth, but because their committee failed in one of the duties intrusted to them. Dr. Hering and his fame belonged, in one sense, peculiarly to Philadelphia, and this meeting afforded the only opportunity which most of us could have, to testify our love and esteem and veneration for him. This only opportunity has been allowed to pass unimproved, solely by reason of the committee's neglect to give proper notice; and thus, as I am assured, some most interesting reminiscences of Dr. Hering's life have been lost.

I would like to ask if there was any good excuse for holding the meeting on Sunday,—that one of all the days of the week which should *not* have been selected without some special and incontrovertible reason. In some parts of the world, Sunday might have answered well enough, but in Philadelphia, where the better sort of people do not propose to follow the lead of Berlin and Paris in this respect, the holding of such a meeting on Sunday is both unusual and unpopular.

I write this note, not so much to criticise the committee as to place on record the reasons why the Memorial Meeting was not more largely attended. I know that nothing we may say can add to the fame of Hering; still, his devotion to homœopathy, and the exalted talents he consecrated to her cause, are worthy of some suitable memorial. And since the meeting has proven a failure as a general expression of the sentiments of the profession in Philadelphia, I for one will gladly hail any project that will enduringly testify our admiration and esteem for Dr. Constantine Hering.

Yours fraternally,

W. B. Trites.

PROFESSOR JÆGER'S PHYSIOLOGICAL EXPERIMENTS WITH "POTENTIZED" DRUGS.

It will be remembered that in our September number we called the attention of the profession, through a letter received from Dr. William Boericke, to some experiments made by Professor Jæger, for the purpose of measuring "the length of time required by the brain to receive impressions; in other words, measuring the interval between irritation of a nerve and conscious perception, and how this interval is affected by the inhalation of various odors." Dr. Boericke's letter alluded to some remarkable results obtained by the experimenter with his "neural apparatus" in connection with the use of high attenuations of homœopathic drugs.

We have recently received a copy of a communication published over Professor Jæger's own signature, of which Dr. Korndœrfer has kindly prepared the following translation for the Hahnemannian Monthly. It would be, of course, premature to express an opinion relative to these experiments, but the further publication, promised in the communication of Professor Jæger, will be awaited with intense interest.

Eds. H. M.

Neuralanalysis.

An Introductory Communication by Professor Dr. Gustav Jæger, of Stuttgart.

This chemico-physiological, mathematically exact method of investigation, which was discovered by me, a report of which I presented at the Nat. Phil. Convention held at Baden-Baden last year, has since then received further investigation from me, as well as from my three students, Messrs. Panzer, Schlichter and Göhrum, being followed by the same principal results.

1. The principal conditions, upon which the preliminary physical examination depends, are now known. These are of such character that, with some practice and care, they may easily be complied with. The certainty of neuralanalysis will be still more assured when the new instrument now being constructed is completed.

2. In regard to the penetration power, the following has been established. An alcoholic dilution of Aconit. given by inhalation, in all dilutions up to the 200th dec., may always and with certainty be distinguished from the pure alcohol with

which the dilutions were made. The highest potency gives, in comparison with alcohol, an increase of excitability (according to the individual) of from 18 to 36 per cent. With Thuja^{400} the increase of excitability was still 44 per cent. With Nat. mur.^{100}, 44.6 per cent over against that of pure alcohol.

3. Regarding the power of definition the following was manifest:

(*a.*) The 200th potency of Aconite and the 400th potency of Thuja always give clearly different neuralanalytic curves (osmogram), from which we may infer the possibility of a qualitative analysis of the remaining homœopathic high potencies.

(*b.*) The quality of the osmogram is independent of the quantity of the inhaled fluid, and of the size of the evaporating surface.

(*c.*) The quality and quantity of the osmogram, however, varies with the change of potency, but so gradually that two neighboring potencies cannot with certainty be differentiated. On the other hand widely separated potencies show such clear and constant differences, and nearly related potencies such great similarity, that, in relation to the degree of homœopathic dilution, a quantitative analysis is also possible. With the present remedies, the high, middle, and low potencies are readily distinguished from one another.

(*d.*) Notwithstanding these changes with increasing dilution, the osmogram shows with all potencies of the same substance, some underlying agreement.

4. The differences between the osmograms of different substances and of decidedly different dilutions of the same substance are, when compared with the differences in the osmograms of the same substance, many times greater and more striking than by any of the previous methods of exact investigation.

5. From the physiological standpoint the following results are important:

(*a.*) The physiological action increases with the dilution up to a certain maximum. With Aconite this maximum was found, in three persons, to be undoubtedly between the 12th and 15th potency. With one of these an almost equally high susceptibility was observed in the 30th potency, and with another in the 200th potency.

(*b.*) This maximum may be of a most astonishing height, thus, with one person the sensitiveness to the 15th potency was 39 per cent., and with the 200th potency 36 per cent. To this was added, when the maximum was reached, other physiological indications, such as nosebleed, roaring in the ears, vertigo, headache.

(*c.*) After exceeding the maximum, the physiological action sinks with the increasing dilution, though with all examined individuals it remained as great even in the highest potencies as with the lowest potencies, and especially with the tincture.

(*d.*) The idiosyncratic differences between the four persons, as related to Aconite, are quantitatively small, qualitatively greater. With two persons it was observed that, in consequence of indisposition, a still greater difference in the osmogram was produced, it being a well-known fact that drugs act differently according as the person is well or sick.

From the above it follows: 1. That neuralanalysis reaches far beyond, in analytical power, every other known method of investigation, even spectrum analysis, and with it must begin a new era of exact investigation.

2. Neuralanalysis advances our appreciation of the subdivision of matter even as greatly as the invention of the telescope did our appreciation of the greatness of the starry heavens.

3. The dilution of a soluble material in a liquid vehicle develops, in the first place, a similar change of the molecular motion to that which Crookes has demonstrated in gases which have been extremely rarefied under the air-pump. I look upon this change in the molecular motion as being gained at the cost of actual heat, originating through an elevation of the latent heat, that is to say, a rotation of the molecule around its own axis (in contradistinction from the forward motion of the molecule in space), which rotation I have denominated as the "chemical motion." This it is, which we smell and taste, and which, through neural analysis, is measured.

4. The mathematically constant and mostly readily observed increase of the physiological action of the drug, developed through potentization, raises Homœopathy by one stroke to the rank of an exact physiologically-based method of cure, of equal birthright with Allopathy. The systematic study of Homœopathy, till now impossible even in our high schools, is now, in the light possible through neuralanalysis, placed within the judgment of every man, and by neuralanalysis has been made worthy a position in the universities.

More extended publications with the appropriate tracings and tables will soon be issued. At the same time I would remark that I am prepared to give others practical instruction in the technics of neuralanalysis.

Professor Dr. G. Jæger.

Stuttgart, September 16th, 1880.

THE

HAHNEMANNIAN MONTHLY.

A HOMŒOPATHIC JOURNAL OF

MEDICINE AND SURGERY.

Editors,

E. A. FARRINGTON, M.D. PEMBERTON DUDLEY, M.D.

Business Manager,

BUSHROD W. JAMES, M.D.

Vol. II. Philadelphia, Pa., November, 1880. No. 11.

☞ The Editors consider themselves responsible for the maintenance of the dignity and courtesy of the journal, but *not* for the opinions expressed by its contributors.

Editorial Department.

PROGRESS IN MEDICINE.—The introduction to that valuable book, the *Cypher Repertory*, contains the following significant words: "We have twice the number of weapons to combat with disease that the earlier homœopathic practitioners possessed, and yet with this advantage it is believed by many that our success is inferior to theirs; and it must be admitted that our practical gain has not been equal to the extension of the Materia Medica."

History tells us that all great discoveries and reforms are apt, sooner or later, to become perverted and abused. He to whom the truth comes, preserves his charge with the utmost care, knowing its precious value. For awhile a faithful few cluster around him, eager to learn and to follow. But gradually dissenters arise, and the watchful reformer sees with concern the growth of hurtful factions. Healthful growth is thus seriously impaired, and the new-fledged truth is forced to begin a war of self-defence.

So it has been with homœopathy. For a time Hahnemann's disciples worked arduously and successfully with their teacher. But at length differences arose, and the simple truths of his discovery were assailed on all sides. Fallacies multiplied, and with them a host of supporters. Our literature became such an admixture of truth and falsity, that only the most astute could sift them.

Very early in our history pathology was dragged into service, and misapplied. Physicians tired of the difficult task of fitting remedy to symptoms, and too readily adopted the plan of choosing according to pathology.

So general, nowadays, has become the better plan, that with many the simple tenets of homœopathy are either wholly unknown, or but imperfectly understood. And just here is the sufficient answer to the quotation above. We have wandered far from the principles of true homœopathy, and unless we return, our noble art will be buried in eclecticism.

Happily the number of those who are willing to abide by the plain teachings of the *Organon* is on the increase. And if our practitioners and students will procure such extensive works as the *Cypher Repertory*, and that invaluable addition to our literature, the Index of Allen's *Encyclopedia*,—and both are needed,—we may hope for a speedy return to pure homœopathy. Let every case be studied as an individual. Bring into use all that is true in pathology, physiology, and all other branches of a medical education, and submit the whole to the finding of the indicated remedy, according to the institutes of homœopathy. The excuse can no longer be made that the Materia Medica is too diffuse to be of practical value. Repertories have completely obviated this difficulty. Nothing now stands in the way of success but laziness or incredulity. He who unhappily has both disqualifications should resign. He who possesses the former will be left far behind in the race. He who has not yet outlived the latter belongs without the camp.

Let us learn all we can that is true in Materia Medica; let us work in one common cause, burying all differences, so we agree in how to obtain and use the proper drug. Let us add all the confirmations to the Materia Medica which careful clinical study can afford. But, for integrity's sake, for purity's sake, and for the sake of solid progress, let us admit no new clinical symptoms which are not repeatedly verified and seen to be undoubtedly in accord with the genius of the drug to which they are assigned. The development of provings is a great work, but he who attempts it should publish full particulars of his method. No man's *ipse dixit* is law. Truth is law.

A Tariff on Medical Diplomas.—The State of New York has recently enacted a law (see our news columns) requiring her practitioners of medicine and surgery to be registered by certain officers of the various counties, the registration having the force and effect of a license. The fee for registration, to be paid by the applicant, is twenty-five cents. The law further requires that graduates of colleges outside of the State shall, before commencing practice, submit their diplomas and such other evidences of their medical education as may be required, to the faculty of some one of the New York Medical Colleges, who are authorized to license the applicant to practice, and for said license the applicant is to pay to the dean of said college the sum of twenty dollars.

We are very sure that it is neither necessary nor expedient that the medical colleges of New York should be thus hedged in and "protected" against the competition and rivalry of sister institutions. Equally sure are we that the natural tendency of such a policy of protection will be to keep down their standard of education and graduation. The constant improvement in the character of American medical education is very largely due to the rivalry existing among the colleges, this rivalry having been excited by a desire to meet the plainly expressed demands of the profession for a higher medical education. There may be influences which will prevent this new policy from working actual harm to the colleges, but its natural tendency must and will be precisely as we have stated.

It would be interesting, though not very gratifying, to see what the effect would be, were all the States and Territories to follow the example thus set by New York, adopting at the same time such rules as would make their policy effective. Students would then almost invariably obtain their medical education at home. The great schools of Philadelphia, New York, and other large cities would lose fifty or seventy-five per cent. of their students; some of them would be compelled to close their doors. Our great hospital interests would languish, thorough education in medical and surgical specialties would become next to impossible, and general medical education would rapidly assume a disgracefully low standard. The only way in which American medicine can maintain any sort of respectable comparison with that of Europe is by promoting the prosperity and efficiency of a few large schools, rather than by an indifferent support of the many. The policy of New York can scarcely fail to antagonize the general interests of medical education in America, while towards herself it is simply suicidal.

Even admitting that some sort of protection is advisable and necessary, it seems to us that the fee demanded is exorbitant, while the fact that it is to be paid to the colleges and not to the State treasury will cause it to be regarded as "a tariff for revenue only."

Book Department.

TRANSACTIONS OF THE THIRTY-SECOND SESSION OF THE AMERICAN INSTITUTE OF HOMŒOPATHY, held at Lake George, N. Y., June 24th, 25th, 26th, 27th, 1879. Thirty-sixth Anniversary. Philadelphia: Printed by Sherman & Co., 1880. 8vo., pp. 696.

We have received the advance sheets of the above important work, and by the time this reaches our readers the completed volumes will be ready for distribution to those entitled to receive them. The running of the work through the press has been done as rapidly as was possible in view of the fact that the editor, Dr. Joseph C. Guernsey, has been at the same time pushing rapidly forward the work on the *World's Convention Transactions*, and will soon have one of *these* volumes also ready for distribution.

The work before us is a counterpart of the issues that have preceded it, being arranged and paged in sections like its predecessors. So few of the members of the Institute have any use for this arrangement, and it is withal so inconvenient to those who make but casual reference to these volumes, that we are glad to know that a better plan is to be adopted hereafter. We have not space to enter into an extended review of the volume, but we may be allowed to express our regrets that a work of such vast practical value should be so restricted in its circulation. It will furnish some interesting reading, especially to those members who could not be present at the session at Lake George.

Dr. J. C. Guernsey desires to state, in reference to the above volume, that he was compelled to observe the order of former editions, owing to the fact that the volume had been started in that manner, and nearly 50 pages "set up" before it came to his hands for completion. To have changed its order of arrangement to that of 1880, would have involved the loss of time and money to the Institute, in resetting what had been already put in type. D.

TRANSACTIONS OF THE THIRTY-THIRD SESSION OF THE AMERICAN INSTITUTE OF HOMŒOPATHY, held in Milwaukee, Wisconsin, June 15th, 16th, 17th, 18th, 1880. Thirty-seventh Anniversary. Philadelphia: Printed by Sherman & Co., 1880. 8vo. pp. 738.

This fresh-looking volume comes this year in a neat cloth binding,—a substantial improvement over the Institute's issues of former years. It is paged consecutively throughout, as a well-ordered book should be, and contains a careful "repertorial" index. "The arrangement of the reports and papers of bureaus and committees is similar to that of preceding volumes." The first 140 pages contain a verbatim report of the proceedings of the session, and the reports of various officers and committees. Next comes the report of the Necrologist, in which appears the names of Franklin Bigelow, Abraham C. Burke, Warren Freeman, Michael Friese, William S. Helmuth, Charles J. Hempel, Harrison V. Miller, Erastus A. Munger, Marquis de Nuñez, John A. Ward, W. H. Woodyatt, and others of honored memory. Following this in order, we have the papers presented by the various bureaus, and the discussions thereon, occupying over 500 pages. These papers contain a vast amount of interesting and instructive material, much of which is nowhere else obtainable. The portion of the work which will doubtless excite the greatest degree of professional interest, is the report of the Bureau of Materia Medica, the papers embraced therein being all upon the subject of our homœopathic posology, and both sides of the question at issue being very carefully and clearly presented. All of the other bureau reports, however, include papers of interest and value, some of them involving a large amount of original research.

The volume closes with an account of the origin of the American Institute of Homœopathy, and a list of its officers from its organization until the present time. The list of members contains 835 names. D.

A General Symptom Register of the Homœopathic Materia Medica. By Timothy F. Allen, M.D., being a complete Index to *The Encyclopedia of Pure Materia Medica.* Octavo, 1321 pages. Published by Boericke & Tafel. 1880.

It is with undisguised trepidation that we approach the arduous task of reviewing this stupendous work of Professor Allen. Untiring energy, skill, and, more than all, the almost insuperable difficulties attending the construction of this massive *Encyclopedia*, place it far above ordinary criticism. Petty fault-findings can have no place here. Pedantry fails, however plausibly it may present itself. Only he can fairly criticise who has struggled through the same laborious path that its author has traversed. And even then he must exercise his best judgment, or he will be lost and hopelessly confounded.

Still the would-be purchaser expects some evidence, at least, that his purchase will be useful. And so we must endeavor to gain an insight into its make-up, that we may approximately estimate its value.

Of course it must be understood that the Index does not claim to be a full repertory, embracing all that is known in Materia Medica and Therapeutics. For, as is the *Encyclopedia*, so, of necessity, must be its Index. And as Professor Allen saw fit, whether wisely or not we will discuss presently, to include in the ten volumes only the record of provings, rejecting clinical symptoms, we must expect only the former in the volume under consideration.

As a general symptom register of the *Encyclopedia*, then, the work seems to us well and thoroughly done. We have carefully reviewed many of its pages, comparing them with other standard works, and we feel confident that but few mistakes mar the subject-matter.

Some difficulty is experienced by the compact manner in which the book is necessarily printed; but we find that even a slight familiarity with its plan of construction, aided by a judicious selection of type, materially overcomes this objection.

The reader, accustomed to look for certain leading words, will be annoyed at first on finding that they have in some instances been substituted by others less familiar. But it must be evident that the present undertaking is a departure from all previous methods, and so, if it is to assist in the study of the *Encyclopedia,* its wording must coincide with the provings therein recorded.

No attempt has been made to group symptoms upon any pathological or physiological basis. One of the fairest promises of the INDEX, is that it will compel its readers to discard their favorite routinisms, and submit to the modes of pure homœopathic science. They will find all sorts of drug-effects, subjective and objective; they will find pathological terms here and there, and any number of symptoms detailed under the organs to which they belong. But the names of diseases have only a symptomatic value; they are merely the words used by the prover in explaining the effects of the remedy taken.

A particular feature of the book under notice, one exhibiting the care and precision exercised by its author, is the nicety with which symptoms are separated and arranged. For instance, under "Uterus," the word "weakness" is followed by Abies c.; while Calc. phos. is placed under "Region of uterus," "weakness," because such distinction exists in the text of the proving. Remedies which in some repertories are grouped under one head, as "Obstinacy," are here distributed under two: "Disobedience," and "Obstinacy." Phos. ac. is usually classed, and rightly too, with remedies for "homesickness," but our author arranges it according to its literal rendering: "Lachrymose as in homesickness;" and so inserts it under "Weeping;" sub-heading: "Homesickness, as from." In one repertory Nitric acid is put under "Desire for fish," but in the INDEX it is more correctly recorded as "Desire for herring." In some books Abies c. is included among the drugs causing apathy or indifference but as the symptom reads "quiet, careless, but easily fretted. Irritable," our precise editor quite properly transfers it to "irritability." And so on all through the fourteen hundred pages.

In some instances, however, such an exact method makes it difficult to find what is desired. We think that it would have been better had certain general terms been used, and reference made to the more particular subdivisions. The reader is not always acquainted with the full text; indeed, he very seldom is. And he consults a repertory to learn which remedies may be studied for an especial symptom. If, now, he can find a general heading he will thus be enabled to complete his search; but if he is obliged to hunt through a dozen pages he will soon become annoyed, and perhaps abandon the search, and eventually the book itself. For instance, if we are seeking to find remedies for a case of erysipelas, and turn to that word in the INDEX, page 372, we will find mentioned thirteen drugs—by no means a complete list. Now if we examine pages 426, 403, 832, 715, etc., we shall become acquainted with eight not included in page 372. Why, then, were all not comprised under one general head, as well as scattered under "Face," "Eyelids," "Nose," and "Limbs?" Again, music aggravates, and we turn to that word in the INDEX, page 796. Two remedies are mentioned, neither of which, however, has aggravation therefrom.' Unless our patient can particularize just what is made worse from music, the book fails to aid us. Under "Aversion," page 132, we note six remedies arranged under "Music," but they are not distinguished.

The INDEX, so far as we have been able to determine, and we have studied it closely for hours, is singularly free from typographical errors. And considering the slight differences between the abbreviations of some medicines and the great variety of type employed, this is a fact which throws credit upon him or them who undertook the tedious task of proof-reading. Two or three mistakes we observed, which we record as exceptional. On page 305, line 11 from foot, "*Arg. m.*" should be "*Arg. n.*," and on page 96, line 25 from top, Colc. c. should be Calc. c.

Of omissions we have found but few. We record them here in compliance with Professor Allen's request to inform him of errors, and not in any spirit of fault-finding. Cina is omitted under "Indifference," page 659. Aloes belongs under "Speech," page 996, and under "Mischievousness," page 784. Natr. nitricum is to be added to remedies, having aversion to coffee. Also add to "Desire for cheese," Arg. nitric. We cannot find the symptom of Lactuca v.: "Appetite for bread and meat fails." Medusa seems to be omitted under "Milk," as is also Secale c. On page 771, line 22 from the foot, $>$ should be $<$. To "Easy conception," page 265, should not Mercurius sol. be added? And, too, Canthar. is said to have favored conception in a woman who had not been pregnant for fourteen years. See *Encyclopedia*, volume ii, page 527. Morphinum should at least be mentioned under sterility; for this symptom is recorded in volume vi. of the *Encyclopedia:* "Conception has never been noticed in amenorrhœic women," etc. On page 778 of the INDEX, Morphinum is mentioned under suppressed menses, but no reference is made to sterility that we have found. Calc. carb. caused profuse menses and the bringing away of a small fœtus. Why omit it from among remedies for abortion? Under "Tonsils" Belladonna is included in the list of remedies causing suppuration and swelling (see page 1214), but is forgotten under inflammation. The provings, however, read: "*Tonsils inflamed.*" See *Encyclopedia*, volume ii, page 95. The well-known symptom of Hepar: "Sticking in the throat, as from a splinter on swallowing," etc., we cannot find either under "throat" or "swallowing." The nearest approach to it is under "stitches," page 1171.

It is probable that this insertion of Hepar under "stitches" was intended to include "splinter" and "sticking;" for it is stated in the introduction, that "what may seem to one only a *sharp pain*, may by another be distinguished as a *cutting* or *sticking*," etc.

Still it is not in keeping with the usual precision of our author to fail to separate such different sensations as "stitches" and "sticking as from a splinter." And especially, we think, is this applicable, since on page 1170, he has already designated Acon., Iod., Sang., and Alum., under the heading, "Sharp, sticking in, sensation of something."

The sign $>$ before Zinc., page 568, line 30, should be $<$. Eup. per., pp. 170, 171, under "Fulness," "Pressure," "Smarting," "Tension," should be, Eup. pur. Kali iod. ought to be included under diminished milk, page 784. The first part of the symptom, emaciated mammæ, occurs on page 770; but the second part deserves recording too. The "excessive coryza" of Merc. c. has been forgotten. Mucus in the nares, Merc. c., line 11, page 797, is not in the provings—at least not under the symptoms of the nose in *Encyclopedia*, Volume VI.

Other similar mistakes no doubt exist; for in such a work they could not be prevented. It should be the pleasant duty of each physician to acquaint the editor with such errors as he may encounter, that another edition—and may it soon be needed—may correct them.

No physician attempting to practice homœopathy should be without the INDEX. And this advice holds good, even if he do not possess the other ten volumes; for it is so rich in suggestions, that he may use it with smaller works on Materia Medica. Every graduate from the respective colleges should see to it, that he carries home with him not only his diploma, but also Allen's INDEX. So much for this great work, which will, we predict, go far towards re-establishing the purity of homœopathic practice.

But we would be unjust to the founder of homœopathy, to his contemporaries, and to our science itself, if we neglected to mention what to us seems a serious error. We refer to the following lines, contained in the introduction to the INDEX: "As long as our knowledge of the action of drugs upon the healthy is imperfect, so long we are obliged at times (*though rarely*) to rely upon clinical indications, and to this end we recommend the use of *repertories* which contain such indications."

We fully agree with Professor Allen that clinical indications should never be used to the disparaging of pathogenetic indications. We, too, look with anxiety upon the rapid increase of cured symptoms, which writers too readily incorporate into textbooks. And above all, do we, with Professor Allen, lament the introduction of isopathic symptoms, which never have, and never can be, produced on the healthy. If this is all our author means by his remarks, we take no issue with him. But there is another interpretation to his words. The weak side of the *Encyclopedia* is a result of the exclusion of all symptoms not strictly in the words of the original provings. Thus is wiped out unceremoniously all the experience of homœopathic physicians, except that which is expressed in the dictum of the original provings themselves. This is, in our estimation, a serious mistake. Provings, the best of them, contain many imperfectly developed symptoms, which clinical experience often elaborates. And so far from such indications being "rarely" of use, they form a large and indispensable portion of every-day practice. Let the reader consult the INDEX, turning to "Erysipelas of the face," page 416. Belladonna is not mentioned, because, forsooth, it is a clinical symptom. And yet neither Professor Allen, nor any other homœopathician, will deny its use in such a case. Now, it may be retorted that the characteristic facial symptoms, by means of which Bellad. should be selected, are given, and that these are sufficient. *All* such characteristics are not given, however, and even if they were, such a piece of clinical development as this use of Bellad. deserves a prominent place in any pure Materia Medica; deserves it, because it is an evidence of the growth and expansion of the drug beyond its mere literal rendering. Hepar has long been employed in suppurations, with certain well-defined conditions. And yet, since it is not so described in the provings, this invaluable fact is set aside as "rarely" needed.

Hahnemann himself, could he speak, would cry out against the slight offered to his contributions from clinical sources.

So far from "rarely" needing these clinical symptoms, we require them so often, that they form at least thirty per cent. of *Positive Materia Medica.* Let the reader but compare his textbooks with the original provings as rendered in the *Encyclopedia*, and he will be assured of the truth of the proportion named.

We reiterate the statement, then, that we regard with no little concern, the indiscriminate or careless introduction of clinical or cured symptoms, *unless they have been confirmed over and over again.* But if confirmed, they frequently become more important than the original symptom, which they more or less resemble.

Every symptom, which disappears or lessens after the taking of a drug, does not therefore become an effect of this drug. The main symptoms removed, others follow also. But when a prominent symptom, over and over again disappears after the administration of a certain drug, with the genius of which the symptom agrees, we unhesitatingly consider it as pathogenetic of the drug, and as often of great value.

We are sorry, then, that Professor Allen changed his mind after publishing Volume I; for in that issue he promised to incorporate well-verified clinical symptoms.

We would be negligent of duty did we forget, in closing this review, to congratulate the publishers as well as the editor. Boericke & Tafel deserve the unqualified encomiums of every member of the profession, for their enterprise in consummating the grandest literary attempt ever made in the history of homœopathy. And this great enterprise was successfully conducted through the most trying period of our country's financial difficulties, and despite many other serious obstacles.

To Professor Allen we extend our warmest congratulations. We know something of the time and energy and expense to which his work has subjected him. We know how patiently he has toiled over tables stacked with confusing symptom-slips, and this at an hour when most of us prefer to sleep. We know, too, how conscientiously he has striven to free his books from errors, and to give to his colleagues a faithful record of the provings of drugs.

F.

OTHER PUBLICATIONS RECEIVED.—Lincoln's School and Industrial Hygiene; Hoyne's Clinical Therapeutics; Bastian's The Brain as an Organ of Mind; American Institute's Report on Homœopathy in Pennsylvania, advance sheets; American Institute's Report of the Bureau of General Sanitary Science, etc.; Leggs, On the Bile, Jaundice, and Liver Diseases; Transactions of the American Homœopathic Ophthalmological and Otological Society, Fourth Annual Meeting; American Institute's Report of the Bureau of Organization, Registration and Statistics; Eaton's Medical and Surgical Diseases of Women; Annals of the British Homœopathic Society and London Homœopathic Hospitals, No. LI; Lincoln's Treatise on Therapeutics; Nichols's Homemade Treatment; Mackenzie's Diseases of the Pharynx, Larynx and Trachea.

Gleanings.

GLYCERIN IN ACIDITY OF THE STOMACH.—A drachm or two of glycerin in water, coffee, tea, or lemonade, taken before a meal, prevents acidity and the formation of wind. It probably acts by checking fermentation. It in no way hinders digestion, and so becomes a valuable palliative in dyspepsia. —Drs. Ringer and Murrill, *Lancet.*

EXTIRPATION OF THE KIDNEY.—The patient recently subjected to this operation by Dr. J. H. McClelland, of Pittsburg, and reported by him at the last meeting of the State Medical Society, is making a rapid and complete recovery. The remaining kidney is "working on double time," and may be expected to undergo some degree of hypertrophy.

AFFECTIONS OF THE MIDDLE EAR may occur early in syphilis, or in connection with mucous patches of the pharynx. The symptoms are pain of a dull character, with occasional sharp twinges and marked periodicity. Sometimes the otitis media does not appear until the eruptions on the skin and mucous membranes have passed off.—*N. Y. Med. Journ.*, October, 1880.

THE CHORDA TYMPANI NERVE is now found to be distinct from the facial. It is derived from the nerve of Wrisberg. If the latter is cut in the aqueduct behind the ganglion, the sense of taste will be entirely destroyed; but if the facial is severed behind the origin of the chorda tympani, the sense of taste will be lost only after a lapse of time.—*N. Y. Med. Journ.*, October, 1880.

MÉNIÈRE'S DISEASE includes every case of vertigo caused by abnormal irritation of the nervous apparatus of the semicircular canals. In a more restricted sense it is an inflammatory state either of these canals or of the middle ear. The vertigo is accompanied or preceded by a sense of rotation. This begins by a sense of rotation around a vertical axis, always in the sense of the diseased organ; next follows a sense of rotation around a frontal axis, forward and backward; then the vertigo becomes general and the patient falls.—*N. Y. Med. Journ.*, October, 1880.

ECZEMA CAPITIS.—Dr. H. Taylor, of Boston, writes us: "I have treated with unfailing success the above disorder by the administration of Petroleum[3] internally, and the simple application externally of Myro-petroleum soap, dissolved in hot water, washing the head frequently with it. This destroys the disagreeable odor, and soon the crust ceases to form. I never remove the crusts, as recommended by Dr. B. F. Betts in his paper published in your October issue.

"I wish also to add my testimony to the great value of Iris versicolor in cholera infantum. It has not failed me in any instance of these derangements of the bowels, where its employment seemed indicated."

REMEDIES FOR SPERMATORRHŒA.—Joseph W. Kerr, M.D., in the *N. Y. Med. and Surg. Journal*, mentions the following among other medicaments:

Tinct. Gelsemium, 30 drops, three times a day, has an excellent effect in checking nocturnal lopes.

Helonias dioica, Senecio gracilis, Cannabis ind., Ergot, Digitalis, Lactucarium, Collinsonia, etc.

He recommends the following preventive measures: 1. Avoid all sources of sexual excitement. 2. Bathe the parts with cold water, ten minutes night and morning. 3. Evacuate the urine before going to bed. 4. Sleep on a hard bed with light covering, lying on the right side. 5. Arise at the first awakening in the morning. 6. Avoid the use of stimulants, tea, coffee, tobacco, and medicines or drinks of a diuretic nature.

News and Comments.

PROFESSOR HENRY C. HOUGHTON, M.D., the well-known aurist of New York city, has changed his residence to No. 44 West Thirty-fourth Street.

CHR. SANDERS, M.D., of the Class "80," has located in New Orleans, La., where, as we learn through Messrs. Boericke & Tafel, he is already doing well.

HERBERT C. CLAPP, M.D., of Boston, has just finished a new book entitled "*Is Consumption Contagious, and can it be Transmitted by Means of Food?*" Otis Clapp & Son will publish it in November.

LOCATION FOR A HOMŒOPATHIC PHYSICIAN.—Fredericksburg, Va. No homœopathist there. Population in 1870 about 5000. Write for particulars to Dr. C. S. Middleton, 646 North Tenth Street, Philadelphia.

COLLEGE CHARTERS ANNULLED.—The courts have annulled the charters of the two colleges of which John Buchanan was the head and front, that individual having confessed judgment and thus saved the county some trouble and expense.

DR. W. H. WINSLOW, our editorial predecessor, has recently had a severe attack of hay asthma. He celebrates his recovery by sending us a most valuable paper on "Pseudo Conical Cornea," which our readers will find in the present number.

ANOTHER BOGUS DIPLOMA SHOP has been discovered, this time in New England. Our readers need have no fear of any disgrace to the homœopathic cause from such agencies. The business seems to be getting entirely too "regular" for that.

THE ANATOMICAL SOCIETY of Pittsburg, Pa., at a recent meeting elected the following officers for the ensuing year: President, Dr. W. H. Winslow; Demonstrator, Dr. John B. McClelland; Secretary and Treasurer, Dr. W. J. Martin; Executive Committee, Drs. W. R. Childs and J. F. Cooper.

The organization is in a flourishing condition, and the next course of lectures will include the following subjects: Histology and physiology of bone, cartilage, fibrous tissue, voluntary and involuntary muscles, nerves and ganglia of the cerebro-spinal system, nerves and ganglia of the sympathetic system, heart and bloodvessels, lymphatic system, lungs, liver, spleen, and kidneys. The lectures are distributed among the members, are carefully prepared, and handsomely illustrated by charts, drawings, and microscopic slides of rare beauty.

THE LONDON HOMŒOPATHIC HOSPITAL.—At this institution there were treated during the year 1879, 494 in-patients and 6903 out-patients, making a total of 7397 patients.

Miss J. Durning Smith has expressed her desire, through Dr. D. Dyce Brown, to maintain six beds at her sole cost for accommodating cases which, according to the rules of the hospital, would be refused as in-patients on account of the nature of the illness requiring treatment for a longer period than two months. She has further intimated that, on being satisfied that the experiment proves satisfactory, it is her intention to permanently endow six beds.

AMERICAN INSTITUTE OF HOMŒOPATHY—BUREAU OF MATERIA MEDICA, PHARMACY, AND PROVINGS.

DEAR DOCTOR: Your attention is hereby directed to the plan adopted for the work of this bureau, the present year, to be reported upon at the session of the Institute, in June, 1881.

The bureau will pursue a systematic study of the following named drugs: Caladium seguinum, Papaya vulgaris, and Viburnum opulus.

These drugs will be studied with special relation to their (1) *History*, (2) *Pharmacology*, (3) *Toxicology*, (4) *Provings*, (5) *Mode of Action*, (6) *Clinical Application.*

To facilitate the work of provings, each drug will be placed in the hands of a sub-committee, under whose direction the provings of that drug will be conducted. These sub-committees are constituted as follows:

Caladium seguinum.—E. A. Farrington, M.D., T. F. Allen, M.D., A. C. Cowperthwaite, M.D.

Papaya vulgaris.—E. M. Hale, M.D., W. H. Leonard, M.D., J. Heber Smith, M.D., L. D. Morse, M.D.

Viburnum opulus.—W. J. Hawkes, M.D., O. S. Wood, M.D., with the invited co-operation of Professor H. C. Allen, M.D., of Michigan University.

In addition to these committees, Miss Kate Parsons, M.D., has been selected to obtain provings of each of the above-named drugs upon women.

The profession at large are cordially invited to participate in the important work of proving these remedies. Those willing to do so, and those who may be in possession of any items of information concerning the history, pathogenesis, or therapeusis of either of these drugs, are requested to communicate at once with the chairman of the bureau. Reliable preparations of both Caladium and Papaya will be obtained by the chairman direct from the Island of Jamaica, and furnished to those who signify their willingness to assist in the provings. Reliable preparations of Viburnum may be obtained at any homœopathic pharmacy. No standard of quantity or potency has been adopted, the preparations used being left entirely to the individual preference of the prover.

Your attention is especially directed to the fact that the final reports of all provings must be in the hands of the chairman prior to the 1st day of March, 1881, and *no attention will be paid to any reports arriving after that date.* This becomes necessary from the fact, that such reports must be printed and in the hands of each member of the bureau before the 15th of March, in order that they may be able to prepare from these reports their special papers as hereinafter designated.

The reports of provings in full will not be read before the Institute, but will be printed and distributed to members, and will appear in the printed *Transactions.*

Special papers relating to the drugs proven will be presented for discussion, as follows:

History and Pharmacology, E. M. Hale, M.D., and J. Heber Smith, M.D.

Toxicology, L. D. Morse, M.D., and O. S. Wood, M.D.

Critical Examination of Provings, T. F. Allen, M.D.

Differential Diagnosis, E. A. Farrington, M.D.

Arrangements of Schema, A. C. Cowperthwaite, M.D.

Mode of Action, Pathogenetic and Therapeutic, William Owens, M.D., and W. J. Hawkes, M.D.

Primary and Secondary Action, and Action on Genito-Urinary System, W. H. Leonard, M.D., and E. M. Hale, M.D.

Action on Female Generative System, Kate Parsons, M.D.

It is needless for me to urge upon the profession, and especially upon the members of the bureau, the great importance of the work here undertaken, and I confidently rely upon the cordial co-operation and active assistance of every lover of a complete and pure Materia Medica.

Fraternally yours,

A. C. COWPERTHWAITE,
Chairman.

IOWA CITY, IA., September, 1880.

MARRIED.—BUCHMAN—LEARY.—October 5th, 1880, at the Church of the Immaculate Conception, by Rev. M. A. Filan, Dr. F. Buchman and Miss Ella M. Leary, both of Philadelphia.

LEFFERTS—FENTON.—At the residence of the bride's parents, Churchville, Bucks County, Pa., October 7th, 1880, by Rev. B. C. Lippincott, Dr. Frank P. Lefferts, of Belvidere, N. J., and Miss Anna Fenton, daughter of John Fenton, Esq.

DIED.—SORG—September 15th, 1880, at his residence, Harrisburg, Pa., John F. Sorg., M.D., in the sixty-fifth year of his age. His death was the result of cystitis superinduced by a calculus, and the fever and prostration following an operation for its removal.

OBITUARY.

W. J. SIMON, M.D.

DR. W. JACKSON SIMON, of Philadelphia, departed this life, after an illness of five days, on the morning of October 7th, 1880, in the sixty-seventh year of his age. He was born in Baltimore, Maryland, on the 22d of August, 1814. His father, David Simon, was at that time superintendent and professor of a large classical academy in that city, which he himself had founded. He removed to Harrisburg, Pa., in 1820. He received an English education at that place in his father's academy. W. Jackson Simon removed to Philadelphia in the year 1842, and commenced the study of medicine at the Pennsylvania Medical College (allopathic), from which he graduated in 1845. He entered upon the practice of medicine on the allopathic system in the State of New Jersey, but becoming convinced by experience of the merits and the great superiority of the homœopathic system, he was led to adopt it; and accordingly, in the year 1851, he matriculated at the Homœopathic Medical College of Pennsylvania, and graduated in the class of 1853. In the same year he removed his residence to Philadelphia, where he has since been engaged in active practice up to the time of his death, beloved and respected by those who knew him. He was very active and skilful in his profession, and labored faithfully in response to the demands of a large practice. S. H. S.

A. O. H. HARDENSTEIN, M.D.

WE are pained to chronicle the death of Dr. A. O. H. Hardenstein, which occurred at his residence, Vicksburg, Mississippi, at 4.05 o'clock, on Friday evening, October 15th, after an illness of several weeks, his disease being gastro-enteritis. He died in the seventy-fourth year of his age, leaving behind the memory of a life filled with deeds of benevolence, charity, and worth. From Cleave's *Biographical Cyclopedia of Homœopathic Physicians and Surgeons* we clip the following regarding the deceased:

"Dr. A. O. H. Hardenstein was born in Greece, January 12th, 1807. His father was by birth a German, and a man of large and varied culture; his mother a Grecian lady of proud and ancient lineage. At an early age he was placed at the best schools, successively at Berlin, Bonn, and Marsburg, where he received a classical education. In the Medical Department of the University of Berlin he became a graduate of the allopathic system of practice.

"In 1828, his first duties led him to Russia, to study the treatment of cholera, and a full investigation of the system of allopathy applied to the disease proved that more than seventy-five per cent. of the cases were fatal. While in Russia he was first led to investigate the theories of homœopathy by close observation of cures wrought by the skill of a lady, the wife of a missionary and a pupil of Hahnemann. Astonished at her wonderful success in the treatment of cholera, he, on his return to Prussia, became a student of Hahnemann, and thoroughly impressed with faith in the new school, surrendered his allopathic theories of practice, and with all zeal adopted the Hahnemann system.

"In 1830, desiring to see the world, he for five years extended his travels over Egypt, Asia Minor, Persia, Afghanistan; also in South America and Mexico. In 1836 he settled in New Orleans. In 1840, through the persuasion of friends, he removed to Kentucky, and there, in 1843, distinguished himself by his treatment of typhoid pneumonia, then an epidemic. The same year he married Miss H. E. Haven, of Cincinnati.

"In 1849, concluding to visit California, he started West over the plains. He was detained in his journey at St. Joseph, where, with infinite success, he administered to the many attacked by the cholera epidemic then raging. In California he displayed skill in combating the same disease.

"Having returned East, he, in 1854, located at Cincinnati, where he remained until, in 1858, induced by the Hon. William L. Sharkey, he removed to Jackson, Mississippi, and there became the pioneer of homœopathy. He thence removed to Vicksburg, where he established a large practice."

His refinement and amiability have won for him the esteem and affection of his patients, as well as of a large circle of friends. He was one of the very few remaining pupils of Hahnemann. His remarkable success in the treatment of yellow fever, during the great epidemic of 1878, is doubtless known to all our readers.

And so, another of our venerable standard-bearers has fallen; and this time it leaves a vacancy at a point where the highest order of talent and skill and the most untiring energy are imperatively needed. His place will be hard to fill.

OFFICE OF THE HAHNEMANNIAN MONTHLY, *N. E. corner Eighteenth and Green streets,* Philadelphia.

Send all business communications direct to our office.

THE

HAHNEMANNIAN MONTHLY.

Vol. II., New Series. Philadelphia, December, 1880. No. 12.

Original Department.

STUDIES IN MATERIA MEDICA.

BY E. A. FARRINGTON, M.D., PHILADELPHIA, PA.

ANIMAL KINGDOM.

(Continued from page 649.)

DIGESTIVE ORGANS, ETC.

THE Ophidians weaken digestion, cause bitter or sour taste; sour or acrid eructations, bilious or bloody vomit; colic, flatulency; swollen abdomen; diarrhœa, bilious, slimy, bloody.

LACHESIS.—Taste: salt; sourish and saltish taste of mucus and saliva; bitter, also early in the morning and at night; food tastes bitter; metallic, with dry mouth.

Thirst.

Appetite: lost in many complaints. At one time good, at another, absent. Hunger, cannot wait for food; face pale, he feels faint. Aversion to food; to warm things. Craves oysters, which agree; wine, but it disagrees; coffee, which agrees; milk, but it causes nausea.

Worse from: brandy; fruits; tobacco. Acids cause diarrhœa, feverishness, or retard the case.

Before eating: languid, can scarely move, drowsy.

After eating: drowsy, with repletion; indolence, desires to lie down; heaviness after every copious meal; nausea and vomiting, pressure in the stomach, with weak feeling in the knees; raises a sour water; regurgitation of ingesta. Eating relieves gnawing in stomach for awhile.

Eructations: sour; feels very ill until he eructates, then is better.

Nausea with faintness, must loosen the clothing.

Nausea and paroxysm. Nausea after drinking.

Inclination to vomit, with sensation of illness rousing him from a sound sleep—also in the morning in bed, as with drunkards or during pregnancy.

Vomits ingesta, bile, especially mornings, with mucus.

Spasmodic vomiting, with diarrhœa.

Vomits mucus with relief; worse mornings, as in drunkards.

Vomits blood.

Vomiting renewed by the slightest motion; nausea, with great flow of saliva.

Stomach.—Pressure as from a load after eating, feels relieved by eructations of wind; worse after siesta.

Feeling as if something was gnawing, though without pain; then same in both sides and across ribs, deep in abdomen.

Pit of stomach very painful to touch.

Great discomfort from having the clothes tight around the waist.

Stitching extending from stomach to chest.

Great weakness of digestion; with many eructations; scarcely any sort of food agrees. Accompanying symptoms are pale, sunken face, vertigo. Causes are abuse of cinchona, mercury, alcohol, etc. Feels badly immediately after eating. Very costive.

Digestive derangements, with hypochondriasis; thinks he is an object of dislike, suspicion, or hatred to his friends.

Liver.—Violent pains in the hepatic region; clothing annoys.

Pain as if something had lodged in the right side, with stinging, and a sensation as if forming into a lump moving towards the stomach.

Ulcerative pain in the liver, especially when coughing.

Suppuration of the liver. Burning pains.

Abdomen, Rectum, Stools.—Pain across the abdomen, after walking.

Sensation of a ball rolling in the abdomen.

Tearing in the abdomen. Cutting, lacerating, and burning pains.

Enteritis, peritonitis, when general symptoms agree; especially during suppuration.

Burning in the abdomen, mounting towards the chest and descending to the thighs. Burning and sensitiveness. Burning with pressure extending to throat, with scanty menses. Burning about the navel.

Cramplike pain in the abdomen; which is hot and very sensitive.

Incarcerated flatus. Eructations relieve; pit of stomach painful to touch.

Abdomen distended and hard. Distended, must loosen clothing and remove all pressure, however slight.

Cutting pain in right side of abdomen, throwing her into fainting attacks.

Hernia, with strangulation; skin mottled, bluish.

Griping pains, left to right; feels as if diarrhœa would set in.

Painful stiffness from the loins down the thighs.

Drawing from the anus to the navel.

Typhlitis, must lie on the back with knees drawn up.

Burning in the anus during and after stool.

Prolapsus ani followed by painful constriction of anus.

Spasmodic pains in the anus, internally, shortly before and after stool.

Beating in the anus as from little hammers, as in piles, and also after the evening diarrhœa.

Piles protruding and strangulated; every cough or sneeze causes stitches; worse in drunkards; at climaxis; with scanty menses, etc.

Tormenting, constant urging in the rectum, but it increases the pain so he must desist without a stool.

Stools hard, like sheep's dung. Unsuccessful urging, the anus feels closed.

Constipation of years' standing, with hard, distended abdomen.

The stool lies in the rectum, down to the anus, without any urging.

After great straining, discharges offensive, croupous masses.

Soft, bright-yellow stools.

The desire continues after the evacuation of a paplike, offensive stool.

Sudden diarrhœa, with great urging about 12 P.M.; movements excessively offensive.

Even formed stools are horribly offensive.

Watery stools, with burning in the anus, in the evening.

Bloody, purulent discharges. Dark, chocolate-colored or looking like charred straw and very offensive.

Diarrhœa in the spring; from acids; of drunkards; at the climaxis; evening or night; during typhoid; after sleep.

Alternate diarrhœa and constipation.

Hæmorrhage from the bowels; blood decomposed.

Of the remaining Ophidians, ELAPS is the best confirmed here. It may be distinguished by the fact that cold drinks feel like ice in the stomach. There are also a sinking feeling at the pit of the stomach, relieved by lying on the abdomen; burning in the stomach; desire for sweetened buttermilk. The stools resemble the others, but it is particularly called for when the diarrhœa consists of black frothy blood, with twisting in the bowels. Useful for consumptives.

CROTALUS has burning thirst; violent, greenish or bloody vomit; black vomit. Stomach so irritable it can retain nothing but brandy or gelatin. Cannot bear the clothing to touch the epigastrium. Irregular stools with pimples on the face, headache and nausea, worse in spring weather. Colic after dinner and early in the morning. Hæmorrhages from the anus, as from every other orifice. Fetid diarrhœa. Sore pain from pit of stomach to hepatic region, with qualmishness, nausea, and greenish vomit. Mouldy smell from the mouth.

Naja has similar symptoms, but as yet they are not confirmed.

Related Remedies.—Craves oysters: Lycopod., Brom., Rhus tox.

Longs for wine or brandy: STAPHIS., *Sulph.*, *Selen.*, *Hepar*, SUL. AC., etc.

Coffee agrees: Angustura, Arsenic.

Complaints of drunkards: ARSENIC, Actea rac. (see Mind), *C. veg.*, *Nux mosch.*, *Cinchon.*, *Hyosc.*, *Opium*, *Stram.*, *Cannab. indica.*

Must loosen clothing: *Nux v.*, LYCOP., *C. veg.*, Kreos., Sulph., Amm. c., *Graphites*, Kali bich., Phos. ac., Stram., Aurum, *Cinchon.*, Bovista.

Vomiting bile, black vomit: ARSENIC, Curare, CADMIUM, *Phosph.*, *Plumb.*, Opium, *Verat. alb.*, etc.

Eating relieves stomach: *Petrol.*, *Chelid.*, ANAC. (while eating), Mezer., *Graph.*, etc.

Acids cause diarrhœa: *Ant. crud.*, *Arsenic.*, Phos. ac., Apis.

Digestion weak: HEPAR, CINCHON., LYCOPOD., Arg. nitric., *Mercur.*, SUL. AC., PULSAT., KREOS., NUX VOM., *Digital.*, CARBO. VEG., *Arnica*, *Nat. mur.*, *Nat. carb.*, Graph.

Before eating face pale, lassitude, see Kali carb. Zinc has weakness, trembling, legs weak. SULPH., Phosph., Natr.

carb., have gone, hungry feeling, 10 to 11 A.M. Pale, sunken countenance: ARSENIC, VERAT. ALB., *Nux vom.*

Nausea with faintness: Alumin., ARSENIC, Cinchon., *Hepar, Phosph., Tabac., Verat. alb.*, Kali carb., Kali bich.

Pressure as from a load, after eating: NUX VOM., *Abies nigra, Lobelia* (like a plug), BRYON., ARSENIC, *Calc ostr., Kali carb.*, LYCOP., *Mercur.*, Pulsat., Plumb., *Phosph.* (cardia), Sepia (before and after), Opium (as from too hard food).

Cold sensation in the stomach: Lachesis less than ELAPS. Compare: *Arsenic*, Camph., Cinchon., *Colchic.*, Kali bich., Nat. mur., Phos. ac., Sabad., Sulph., Sul. ac., Verat. alb.

Stomach worse on awaking: *Arg. nitric*, Kali bich., Kali carb., *Lycopod.*, Natr. mur., Pulsat., Oxalic acid, *Staphis., Sulph., Nux vom.*

Hypochondriasis: NUX VOM., *Cinchon., Sepia, Aurum*, SULPH., *Silica, Nat. carb., Nitric acid*, etc.

Pit of stomach sensitive, with weak digestion: *Arnica, Nux vom.*, CALC. OSTR., *Pulsat., Cinchon., Arsenic, Sulph., Phosph.*, Secale c., *Mercur., Bryon., Carbo veg.*, Graph., *Sepia.*

Liver sensitive: *Phosph.*, Sulph., MERCUR., *Bellad.*, Lycopod., *Arsenic, Rhus tox., Carbo veg.*

Burning pains in liver: *Mercur.*, ARSENIC, Bryonia, Anac., Kali carb., Phos. ac., Sulph., Phosph., etc.

Abdomen sensitive to touch: APIS, NITRIC AC., *Phosph.*, Phos. ac.

Pains across upper abdomen chiefly: LYCOPOD., IPECAC., Carbo veg., Sepia, Stannum, Arnica.

Inflammatory conditions, especially with exudation, suppuration, or with typhoid symptoms: MERCUR., *Bryon.*, RHUS TOX., *Merc. corros., Lycopod.*, Plumb., ARSENIC, BAPTIS., *Apis, Hyosc., Canthar., Oxalic ac.*

Typhlitis: BELLAD., MERCUR., Ginseng, Opium, Plumb., *Rhus tox.*, etc.

Burning in the abdomen: Apis, ARSENIC, Bellad., CARBO VEG., *Colchic., Kali bich.*, MERCUR., PHOSPH., Arnica, Phos. ac., Secale c., Silica.

Incarcerated flatus: *Arnica*, CARBO VEG., COCCUL., GRAPH., LYCOPOD., PLUMB., STAPHIS., Anilin sulph., SULPH., Phosph.

Faint, with pains in abdomen: Alumin., Ammon. carb., Calc. ostr., *Cinchon.*, Sepia, Sul. ac.

Strangulated hernia and gangrene: ARSENIC, *Carbo veg.*, Plumb.

Prolapsus ani, with painful constriction: *Mezer.*, *Nitric acid*, Sepia.

Spasmodic pains in the anus: Lauroc.

Beating at the anus: Berberis, Caustic., Apis, Alumin., *Nat. mur.*, etc.

Constriction of the anus: BELLAD., Alumin., CAUST., *Colchic.*, *Kali bich.*, *Lycopod.*, NATR. MUR., *Nitric ac.*, NUX VOM., PLUMB, Sepia, Silica, IGNAT., Staphis., Coccul., *Mezer.*, Sarsap., Secale c.

Constriction after stool: IGNAT., Sepia, Sulph., Kali bich., *Nitric ac.*, *Colchic.*

Constipation, abdomen distended: Bellad., *Graph.*, Hyosc., *Sulph.*, Phosph., *Lycopod.*

Costive, urine retained: Laches., Hyosc., Lauroc., OPIUM, Morphia acet.

Stool lies in rectum, no urging: OPIUM, ALUMIN., *Lycopod.*, Hyosc., Carbo veg., Sepia, Kali carb., Nux mosch., SILICA, VERAT. ALB., *Cinchona*, *Graph.*

Piles, with stitches at every cough: *Ignat.*

Piles protrude and become strangulated: Silica, Nux vom., Ignat.

Varices hinder stool: Laches., Caustic., Sul. ac.

Hæmorrhages from the bowels, blood dark: *Alumen*, ALUMIN., HAMAM., MERCUR., Ant. crud., *Pulsat.*, SECALE C., Mur. ac., *Carbo veg.*, NITRIC ACID (black, offensive, or bright), Terebinth.

Diarrhœa sudden: Apis, Kali bich., CROTON TIG., PODOPH., etc.

Stool involuntary: Opium, *Mur. ac.*, RHUS TOX., Colchic., *Hyosc.*, Baptis., Carbo veg., *Arnica*, Phos. ac., *Apis*, etc.

Offensive: BAPTIS., CINCHON., ARSENIC, GRAPH., *Colchic.*, Lycopod., Kreos., Nitric acid, *Opium*, PODOPH., RHUS TOX., SECALE C., *Arg. nitric*, CARBO VEG., *Stram.*, SILICA, *Sulph.*, Arnica.

Bright yellow, papescent: CHELIDON., Apis (orange), *Podoph.*, *Gelsem.*, Nuphar, Yucca, GAMBOGE, *Hepar*, Rhus tox., *Natr. sulph.*, *Aloes*, *Sul. ac.*, *Colchic.*

Watery: APIS, Apoc. cann., ARSENIC, *Arnica*, CINCHON., CROTON TIG., *Colchic.*, *Chelidon.*, *Elaterium*, *Gamboge*, *Hyosc.*, *Kali bich.*, *Magn. carb.*, Mur. ac., PODOPH., PHOSPH., PHOS. AC., *Secale c.*, SULPH. AC., VERAT. ALB., *Rhus tox.*

Purulent: *Arnica*, ARSENIC, Bellad., Apis, Calc. ost., *Carbo veg.*, *Calc. phos.*, CANTH., Cinchon., Kali carb., *Lycopod.*, MERCUR., *Pulsat.*, SULPH., SILICA.

Croupous: MERC. CYAN., *Arg. nitric.*

Of the drugs enumerated above, only a very few bear more than a partial similarity to the especial remedies under study. A succinct account of the action of LACHESIS here shows that it relieves when digestion is weakened from want of vitality. And with this, there are always hypersensitiveness to touch, aggravation after sleep, and either obstinate constipation or offensive stools. Contractions and constrictions are here, as everywhere, predominant. So can we explain the difficult stool and colic. The sphincter ani tends to this constriction; and, in the one case, holds back the fæces, despite the urging; in the other, threatens the protruding piles with strangulation. Inflammations in the abdomen or in its parietes partake of the low grade so characteristic of snake-poison.

Examining, now, analogous remedies, in the light of these essentials, we find the following of especial interest: LYCOPOD., NUX VOM., HEPAR, CINCHON., MERCUR., SUL. AC., ARSENIC, CARBO VEG., *Baptisia, Opium, Hyosc., Rhus tox., Natr. mur., Nitric ac.*, Kali bich., Phosph., Alumin., Silica. We shall consider these in detail, with an occasional reference to others.

LYCOPOD. requires that food have its natural flavor. There may, however, be sour taste, and, in the morning, bitter taste. Eructations relieve the sense of repletion, but not the feeling of illness. The smallest quantity of food fills to bursting, and then the clothing must be loosened. There are waterbrash, oppression of the chest, heat in the abdomen, and cold face, oppressed breathing from flatulency, not from constriction of the throat. Distended abdomen, with rumbling, worse in region of splenic flexure, and pains in consequence. Constipation predominates; urging is frequent enough, but the anus constricts and thus retards defecation; but the rectal urging is less painful.

In hepatic abscess the one often follows the other. LACHESIS has a contractive feeling; LYCOPOD., a feeling as of a cord constricting the hypochondria. In the former the urine is black, frothy, or rarely turbid, with red sediment; in the latter it deposits a red sand. Though both have gastralgia, it is far more marked in LYCOPOD., and only the snake-poison has temporary relief from eating.

NUX VOM. materially alters the taste; it is, particularly in the morning, sour, or putrid, or bitter after raising mucus from the throat. Hunger is usually wanting, except sometimes as a precursor of gastric disorder. Worse generally after meals, especially after dinner. Very marked is an aggravation, one to two hours after eating (duodenal digestion). Nausea is attended with a faintness and illness, as in LACHESIS, and the pressure of the clothing is annoying. When these symptoms result from abuse of alcohol, the choice from merely local symptoms is difficult. Usually NUX suits when there are mental and bodily over-impressibility; LACHESIS, when the sufferer is greatly weakened by repeated debauchery. If constipation obtains, the urging in the former is spasmodic, fitful, and ineffectual; in the latter, painful and fruitless from constriction of the anus; and this, with large purplish piles, increases with the amount of alcoholic abuse.

The abdomen is distended by the action of NUX, but the principal sensation, as we understand it, is a tense feeling out of proportion to the objective swelling; and the characteristic irritability of the remedy is displayed in the griping colic, feeling of a load in the abdomen, sensitiveness to touch, and, withal, irregular urgings to stool. Constipation prevails; but diarrhœa may be present, when it is usually scanty, with straining; bloody, slimy, with tenesmus.

HEPAR resembles LACHESIS in weak digestion; the plainest food disagrees. The cravings are unique. As if knowing instinctively what will "tone up" the stomach, the patient longs for condiments or wine. Eating relieves the relaxed feeling, but food annoys so soon as the digestive process begins its slow and imperfect work. The bowels move very sluggishly, even when the stools are soft.

CINCHONA, too, enfeebles digestion, and induces great weakness and languor after meals. It also has a craving for coffee beans. Fruits induce diarrhœa with abdominal fermentation. Both cause fulness after eating; but only CINCHONA has sense of fulness to hurting, with little or no relief from belching. Bitter eructations, bitter taste, belong to each; the latter has the altered taste after swallowing, food retaining its normal taste while being masticated.

The discharges from the bowels are offensive, as is the flatus; yellow, watery stools, undigested. But the marked aggravation at night, after a meal, and the resulting prostration, are not at all like LACHESIS. In dysentery, etc., when putrid or gangrenous changes occur, the choice is more difficult. Both have cadaverous-smelling discharges of a chocolate color, with coldness and great debility. And although the CINCHONA is far preferable if the disease is of malarial origin, such a complication does not contraindicate the snake-poison. The apparently close similarity is also enhanced by the nervous excitability in both. Light touch is distressing, the epigastrium is sensitive, and clothing annoys in each remedy. But this in CINCHONA is an increased general sensibility, while in LACHESIS there is general torpor, with hyperæsthesia of the cutaneous nerves. The former is suitable when the offensive discharges follow a severe, rapidly exhausting inflammation; or, when the frequency and quantity of the evacuations have greatly reduced the vitality, thus favoring retrogressive changes. If symptoms of hectic are present, the choice is rendered more certain. In addition we may also refer to the well-known anæmic symptoms of CINCHONA, paleness, ringing in the ears, easy fainting, etc., which show at once how it affects the blood.

In hypochondriasis the patient is peevish, unhappy, and tormented with anxious dreams.

MERCURIUS presents many points of similarity with LACHESIS. The latter frequently follows the former, and also antidotes its abuse. There are loss of appetite, coated tongue, nausea, with oppression, and epigastric tenderness. Pressure in the pit of the stomach produces a deadly faintness. The stomach hangs heavily, even after a light meal of food of ordinary digestibility. The sensitiveness of the stomach to the clothing is a part of a symptom which is completed by a similar tenderness over both hypochondria, with fulness and upward pressure from the abdomen. Patient cannot lie on the right side.

If hypochondriacal he is suspicious, anxious, and restless at night, with vascular erethism and sweat. In fact this erethism is directly contrary to the torpid LACHESIS.

In abdominal inflammations with suppuration, as in typhlitis, both remedies are useful and follow each other well. MERCURIUS has its ever-present perspiration without relief; stools slimy, or much straining, with or without stool. LACHESIS follows when the symptoms threaten a typhoid condition. Can lie only on the back with the knees drawn up; if he turns on to the left side, a ball seems to roll over in the abdomen.

In rectum and anus MERCURIUS has more persistent tenesmus; protrusion of the rectum, which looks inflamed and blackish; LACHESIS, more spasmodic tenesmus, with constriction of the anus, which tightly constricts the prolapsed rectum. Both have chronic constipation. The former induces much straining, with tenacious or crumbling stools; chilliness during defecation.

ARSENICUM intensifies the gastric and systemic weakness, to which we referred in the remedies just considered. While it is true that the patient does not fully realize his want of strength, and hence does not so much care to lie quietly, yet, nevertheless, his actual amount of vitality is seriously reduced. In a word, he is excessively weak, without *feeling* so fatigued. Any exertion induces fainting. Taste is lost, or is bitter, sour, putrid. Stomach feels swollen as if full of water. Craving for acids and for coffee; the latter, as in LACHESIS, agrees with the patient. There are burning feelings, red, rough tongue, and anxiety and distress after eating, as in subacute gastritis, which no remedy better pictures. Nausea is frequent, often periodical (12 P.M.), and is accompanied with great prostration. Vomiting is of many kinds, but is distinguished from the bilious, slimy, or bloody emesis of LACHESIS by its irregular convulsive character, indicative of gastric irritability. LACHESIS is adapted to the nervous weakness and trembling of drunkards; spasms of the stomach, spasmodic constrictions, relieved temporarily by eating; vomiting of bile or mucus; ARSENIC, to burning periodical pains, with acrid, sour vomit, violent thirst, but vomits the water; *Cadmium sulph.* to nausea, yellowish or black vomit, saltish, rancid belching, cold sweat of the face, burning cutting in the stomach; gripings in the lower bowels; cramps after beer. Both induce marked sensitiveness to touch upon stomach or abdomen, spots of burning soreness here and there over the swollen abdomen (peritonitis); offensive, bloody, chocolate-colored discharges, as in dysentery, with constriction in the bowels, cutting pains in bowels. But in ARSENIC there is more lamenting with agonized expression; restless moving despite the pains. The constriction of the intestines is torturing, the patient declares he cannot stand it, and rolls about in agony, despairing of his life. The extreme tenderness of the pit of the stomach denotes a more positive state of acute inflammation than LACHESIS causes.

In the vomiting of yellow fever, LACHESIS has, in addition, brown coating on the teeth, abdominal tenderness.

ARSENIC has also spasmodic protrusion of the rectum, very painful; tenesmus, with burning. Hæmorrhoids, especially in drunkards; they protrude at stool, with burning. Alvine discharges are offensive, dark, sometimes involuntary, with great weakness and coldness. But LACHESIS has less tenesmus recti, the distress there being attributable to a constriction of the anus not found in the other drug. ARSENIC, moreover, causes more acridity of the stools, with rawness and excoriation of the anus.

All that is here stated might be tersely described as a difference between two drugs, of which one causes intense irritability and acute inflammation of tissue, mental anguish and extreme prostration; the other, torpidity, with the loss of vitality, but associated with nervous excitability, constrictions, and cutaneous hyperæsthesia. Still, some minds require more attention to detail; and every one retains general mental impressions more accurately, if they are formed with due attention to particulars.

When there is ulceration of the bowels, tendency to sloughing, with offensive, purulent, or bloody discharges, the two remedies are very nearly allied. Vitality is at a very low ebb, blood oozes from the cracked lips and tongue, and the extremities are cold. But even here, the best distinctions are the mental irritability of ARSENIC, and the intolerance of pressure of LACHESIS.

CARBO VEGETABILIS resembles LACHESIS in weak digestion, complaints of drunkards, flatulent asthma, constriction of the œsophagus, annoyance from clothing about the waist, offensive, bloody, decomposed, purulent stools, collapse, etc.

There is craving for coffee, but it does not relieve. Milk disagrees in both remedies; but only the snake-poison has craving for it. The CARBO has aggravation from fats, tainted meats, or fish, oysters, foods causing flatulency, ices, vinegar, and sour cabbage—the latter principally on account of the flatulency it causes. Eructations are sour, rancid. Both drugs have relief from flatulent dissention from belching, but LACHESIS has an ill feeling in addition, which is relieved. Both drugs experience freer breathing after belching. In CARBO VEG. this is expressed as the lessening of a tension and upward drawing which marks the costal attachments of the diaphragm; in LACHESIS, there is a relief after eructations, which seem to suffocate him. They come rapidly, and induce the ever-present Lachesis constriction of the throat. The latter remedy also has empty eructations, which intensify the pains.

CARBO VEG. has heaviness, fulness, sleepiness, after eating, with fulness of the abdomen almost to bursting. Burning in the stomach is also increased. This heaviness is very characteristic and is noted likewise in the abdomen, which seems to hang heavily; also in the head, which feels as heavy as lead. The burning is attended with a creeping feeling up to the throat. In LACHESIS the fulness and pressure is as from a load, and the sense of repletion induces lowness of spirits. There is, too, a feeling as if a lump was accumulating in the stomach and also in the bowels; burning, with hard abdominal distension, and a feeling as if a stone was descending, he must stand still or step cautiously. This lumping is presumably a part of the Lachesis constriction, which we have so often designated as highly characteristic. In CARBO VEG., the flatus is more rancid, putrid, or when passed per anum, burning, moist, offensive. Its incarceration with burning is a cause of many of the symptoms, and is more in quantity than in the snake-poison. It also causes a bearing down upon bladder and sacral region. LACHESIS relieves a gnawing gastralgia, when eating, lessens the pain; CARBO cures when there are burning, with a contractive cramp bending him double; the pains are paroxysmal and take his breath. The burning spreads up to the chest and down into the abdomen, seemingly following the sympathetic.

Tenesmus recti is most prominent in the CARBO, anal constriction in the LACHESIS. It is this latter symptom which explains, as we have before observed, the ineffectual urging to stool; while in CARBO the urging is fruitless on account of the pressure of flatus. Both have bluish, protruding piles, as after debauchery. This constriction distinguishes them, as do also the headache and diarrhœa. In each there is throbbing headache; but CARBO has more of the heaviness, and the diarrhœa is thin.

In typhoid forms, whether the specific fever, or as a sequel to peritonitis, dysentery, etc., the CARBO causes the more perfect picture of collapse, while in LACHESIS the cardiac debility, drowsiness, cool extremities, etc., indicate failing vitality, but not so near death as the following belonging to the former: tympany; legs cold, especially to the knees; pulse filiform; breath cool; absence of discharges from the bowels; or, involuntary, putrid, bloody, purulent diarrhœa.

In hernia CARBO VEG. has anxiety, as in Arsenic, but with uneasiness rather than restless change of place; and it resembles LACHESIS in the annoyance of the clothing, foulness of parts if strangulated, etc. There is, however, more meteorism and fetid flatus.

GRAPHITES has anxiety, melancholy; tip of tongue blistered; feeling of a lump in the left side of the throat, over which the food seems to pass with difficulty; on empty deglutition a constrictive retching from œsophagus up to larynx. Must loosen the clothing after eating. Gastralgia, relieved by eating. Chronic gastritis, especially after abuse of alcoholic drinks. Sensation of a lump in the stomach. Flatulent distension of the abdomen, with congestion to the head. Fetid flatus. Suffocative spells arousing from sleep, must jump out of bed; compelled to eat something. Offensive stools.

But this remedy causes more flatulency than LACHESIS. The gastralgic pains are burning and griping; and the feeling of a lump in the stomach is accompanied with a constant beating; the heartburn is rancid. The suffocative spells are usually worse after 12 P.M.; instead of during or after a sleep at any time. And the constriction noticed on falling asleep is of the chest instead of the larynx. The offensive movements from the bowels are half digested, dark and pappy, indicating the imperfect digestion which is so characteristic of this remedy.

There is some resemblance in the constitutional symptoms of GRAPH. and LACHESIS, since both are needed at times in the phlegmatic. But the former has as a distinguishing group: fat, cold, and costive; skin herpetic, rough, and disposed to crack and ooze a glutinous fluid.

Aside, then, from a few resemblances to the snake-poison, GRAPHITES belongs more with Arsenic, Nux vom., and Lycopodium. The first two it resembles in gastritis and gastralgia; the latter, in flatulency.

SULPHURIC ACID somewhat resembles the snake-poisons, especially in the ailments of drunkards. Its corrosive effects, however, are distinctively prominent, as shown in the violent inflammation of the alimentary canal. But the nervous system is so involved that several symptoms look like those of LACHESIS; as, epigastrium sensitive, constrictive feeling in the bowels, griping, cutting, twisting, with faintlike nausea; trembling, pale face, apprehensiveness; fluttering pulse; cramps in the pharynx; he cannot swallow; œsophageal stricture; great weakness, etc. Both likewise crave brandy.

The ACID acts well when the patient is weak, emaciated, complains of trembling, but it is more subjective than objective. He is anxious and restless, must do everything hurriedly. The face is pale, and sometimes presents dry, shrivelled spots, especially when the hæmorrhoids are worse. Eructations are sour. The stomach feels relaxed and cold. Wine may palliate and spirituous liquors aggravate as in LACHESIS. But the peculiarity of the ACID is, that the stomach rejects cold water, unless it is mixed with brandy. The abdominal muscles are spasmodically retracted. Stools are yellow, like LACHESIS, but present a chopped appearance, and are stringy. The watery diarrhœa is very offensive. Piles are moist, burn, and may prevent defecation.

As the ACID causes croupous formations, it should be remembered with LACHESIS when the stools indicate such a condition in the intestine.

The ACID also resembles ELAPS: drinks chill the stomach. But only the former has the relief from the admixture of spirit.

COLCHICUM deserves mention here, especially since, like LACHESIS, it causes coldness or cold feeling in the stomach (ELAPS), intolerance of pressure of clothing (in provings, but not confirmed), burning in stomach, vomiting and purging, *spasms of sphincter ani,* urging to stool, offensive flatus, offensive diarrhœa, sensitiveness to least touch, very much exhausted, slow breathing, feeble pulse. But there is generally present nausea, worse from the smell of food; if the patient sits or lies very quietly, the vomiting is suppressed (like Veratrum). Senses too acute; a bright light, touch, or *strong odors* irritate him (like Nux vom.). Vomiting and purging as in cholera morbus; the sphincter ani contracts after each stool, with fruitless urging. The similarity, then, exists chiefly in the sensitiveness to touch and constrictions of sphincters with weakness, other symptoms being so different as to render a choice easy. (See also below.)

In cholera, LACHESIS has been employed when the vomiting was renewed by the least motion, and the nausea was attended with a great flow of saliva. As COLCHIC. has precisely the same symptoms, other indications must decide.

In reflex irritation, as convulsions, with variegated, slimy stools in teething children, and rolling of the head, COLCHIC. resembles PODOPHYL.

Belladon., Lachesis, Rhus tox., and Baptisia, constitute a group serviceable in peritonitis, enteritis, etc.

BELLADON. differs from all in the character of the inflammation. It is only when the affection becomes asthenic that the others are needed. LACHESIS follows BELLADON. when, especially in children with inflammatory diarrhœa, constipation suddenly sets in with abdominal swelling and tenderness, particularly at one spot. Or, if suppuration ensues and Mercurius fails. Or, again, if gangrene threatens.

RHUS TOX. requires drowsiness, the fever remaining high or increasing; restlessness; tongue dry, parched, brown, with red triangular tips; diarrhœa slimy, watery or putrid, yellowish-brown and bloody, involuntary during sleep; generally it is accompanied with tearing down the thighs, while LACHESIS has painful stiffness from loins into thighs. In typhlitis, in which affection either may follow BELLAD., RHUS TOX. has relief from pressing the swelling gently from below upwards; LACHESIS, intolerance of touch.

In periproctitis, RHUS TOX. may be needed if the inflammation was of traumatic origin; LACHESIS, if an abscess forms and fails to point, the surrounding tissues presenting a purplish hue.

In typhoid conditions, when the abdominal symptoms are severe, with involuntary stools, sopor, dropping of the jaw, compare LACHESIS with OPIUM when the stertor is marked; with HYOSCY. if the apathy is complete, with mucous râles in the chest, stools watery, sphincters paralyzed (compare August No., p. 454); with *Apis*, when the watery, yellow, diarrhœa escapes from the open anus at every movement of the body; and with MURIATIC ACID, when the patient slides down in bed and the involuntary diarrhœa is fetid and often accompanied with profuse hæmorrhages.

COLCHICUM compares with LACHESIS when the prostration is extreme, with coma, hot abdomen and cold extremities; thready pulse; if raised, the head falls back and the jaw drops; the face is hippocratic, the tongue is protruded with difficulty, and the bowels move involuntarily. But the tympany is more marked in the former; and the stools contain white flakes or shreds; the tongue is either thickly coated brown, or it is bright red, except at the root, where it is coated. According to provings and cases of poisoning, Colchicum does not cause sensitive abdomen below the epigastrium.

Arnica develops a profound stupor, with blowing respiration, dry tongue, brown down the middle, distended abdomen, and involuntary fæces and urine. It may be distinguished by the ecchymoses, and the bruised aching, inducing restlessness, which latter is relieved if the patient's clothing is smoothed down and his position changed.

Among the remedies causing constriction of the anus, the following are worthy of notice: Bellad., Caustic., Nitric ac., Nat. mur., Ignat., Kali bich., Opium, Plumbum, Mezereum, Coccul.

The first has: pressing and urging toward anus and genitals, alternating with contractions of the anus; spasmodic constriction of anus as in dysentery.

The second, CAUSTICUM, causes fruitless urging to stool, with anxiety and red face.

Nitric acid causes sticking in the rectum as from a splinter; the constriction occurs during stool and lasts for hours afterwards, the rectum feels as if torn.

NATRUM MUR. has sensation of contraction in the rectum during stool, the fæces tear the anus; frequent ineffectual urging; spasmodic constriction of the anus.

Ignatia induces a proctalgia; contraction, with cutting, shooting pains; contraction of anus worse after stool. Symptoms are inconsistent, irregular, fitful as in hysteria.

Kali bich., has sensation of a plug, similar to LACHESIS; diarrhœa of a brown, frothy water, spirting out in the early morning and followed by tenesmus ani.

Opium, anus is spasmodically closed during the colic, with obstinate constipation. *Plumbum* is very similar.

But all these are readily distinguished from the characteristic symptoms of LACHESIS: tormenting urging in the rectum, but on account of constriction of the anus it becomes so painful he must desist. Protruded piles, with constricted anus.

Much nearer, and indeed almost identical here, is MEZEREUM; after the stool, the anus is constricted around the protruded rectum. In other respects, however, the two remedies are widely different.

KALI BICHROMICUM must also be remembered as a relative of LACHESIS in dysentery. Both have red, cracked, smooth tongue; blackish stools; hence in severe or typhoid cases; and, further, they follow each other well. The offensive odor of the discharges distinguishes the latter; the jellylike mucus, sometimes stringy, the former.

A peculiar feature of *Cocculus* is tenesmus recti after stool, with faintness and yet peristalsis is lessened. (Compare Ignatia.)

GETTYSBURG SALT IN RACHITIS.*

BY C. F. NICHOLS, M.D., BOSTON, MASS.

I. 1878, October 3d. Willie V., aged 7 years; old-faced, yellow; since infancy sickly and deformed. Probably the place of curvature was determined by a blow on the nape. The fifth and sixth cervical vertebræ project, and are most sensitive, while the bodies of all above are thickened sufficiently to force the head forwards. His shoulderblades push upwards. He usually forces his head up and looks forwards; is energetic; seems "*better after he gets started*" *in the morning.* Is

---

* Prepared and proved by Dr. M. McFarlan. See also Allen's Encyclopedia. "Pott's disease. Little children with curvature. *Abscesses each side of curvature.* Soreness of joints. Brown or muddy urine. Changes of weather much felt."—M. F.

emaciated; legs and neck especially weak and thin. Falls often, striking the head.

Has sudden attacks of nervous trembling. *Starts and screams in sleep.* Is always peevish and restless.

Constant thirst, with hectic heat, in A.M.

The *abdomen tense, tympanitic,* and sensitive to touch for weeks at a time; it then softens, with *painless,* watery, blood-streaked, yellow, offensive stools, accompanied by complete jaundice. Wind breaks with stool. Is *awakened* by pain in *left* hypochondrium. Eats only meat and bread. Sweets cause diarrhœa. Urine slimy (no albumen).

Wears a brace, which, frequently adapted, seems to give much relief. Palpitation and dyspnœa when the brace is not worn.

Usually cries *when touched anywhere,* particularly upper back. *Suffers if jarred,* and has been severely jarred. Is better in open air. Axillary and parotid glands swell.

October 3d. *Phosphorus*^{dm}, dry.

October 15th. Grows very weak, with ascites persisting. (Eighth week.) *Sulphur*^{dm}, dry.

October 20th and 23d. Abdomen drumlike. Three doses of Chamomilla^{cm}, in water, were given at each of the above dates.

October 26th. The condition was not ameliorated. *Silicea*^{dm}, dry. Shortly after *exostosis appeared* on metacarpals and finger-ends. He *drooled much* in sleep. *Plugs* aud constant nasal catarrh occurred (never before). The abdomen remained soft, with occasional diarrhœa. Still very feeble, sensitive, emaciated, with hectic flushes.

December 13th. Fell violently, striking head. *Arnica*^{dm}, dry, and two days later, *Bryonia*^{cm}, dry.

1879, January 5th. *Gettysburg salt*^{cm}, four doses, in water, was given under circumstances of doubtful improvement. Also *Gettysburg salt*^{mm}, dry, February 11th.

Thereafter the gain was gradual, but constant. Unfortunately, it seemed necessary occasionally throughout the following summer to atone for imprudences in diet, causing diarrhœa, and during the winter season, for severe colds. *Aconite, Calcarea, Pulsatilla,* and *Spigelia* were given. *Gettysburg salt* was, however, twice repeated (after *Calcarea* and *Spigelia*).

1880, June 10th. The curvature decreases, and the attitude is more nearly erect, with an apparent gain of four inches in height since October, 1878. But little sensitiveness to touch is discovered. Nervousness, emaciation, bloated abdomen, etc., no longer present their first distressing picture. The brace is worn, lightly applied.

II.—1877, January 3d. A mulatto boy, two years old, has a curvature which *has worked upwards* from lower lumbar vertebræ to last dorsal; also laterally towards right. He is pigeon-breasted, asthmatic (mother has phthisis). The child has a loose cough, painless diarrhœa; abdomen bloats; emaciated. Right leg seems numb and powerless. Two doses of *Gettysburg salt*^{cm}, dry, were given, four weeks apart, with gradual improvement.

1880, February 20th. The child appears well, and no curvature is discoverable. No brace has been worn.

III.—1879, May 24th. M. W., a boy of fourteen years, has taken homœopathic remedies and vegetine during two years past for scrofulous enlargements of bones.

Previously "pneumonia, erysipelas, abscesses," and an eruption, suppressed, on the scalp. Relatives have died with spinal disease. Both tibiæ (especially the right) are bent outward and the shafts enlarged trebly. All night sharp pains are intensified and keep him awake, darting upward and downward from the exostoses. Flushes through the legs before the pains. Cold sweat on the legs day and night. Motion or rubbing usually relieves. Sometimes the swollen parts are sensitive to touch, when throbbing is experienced. The elbow, knee and ankle-joints are loose; the ankle-joints lame. He is emaciated, thirsty, without appetite. Despondent and peevish. His pains and other symptoms have become much worse within two months, so that he is seldom quiet, day or night. Given *Gettysburg salt*^{cm}, three doses in water, May 24th.

August 6th. Legs are increasingly sensitive, but the swelling grows softer. The hectic symptoms have disappeared and he seems strong and happy.

1880, January 17th. The remedy was repeated in the ^{mm} potency, pains having returned in the right leg.

June 11th. The enlargement of the bones is much diminished, while general improvement continues.

IV.—In addition to the above pronounced cases of rachitis, the following may be of interest:

A married woman, æt. twenty-eight, had been well until her back was injured, in 1870, by a fall which produced a miscarriage. She forthwith suffered from symptoms of cerebro-spinal irritation. The body was bent backward with clonic contractions of the limbs.

When examined, October, 1878, the last three dorsal and two upper lumbar vertebræ were prominent; their spinous processes could be detected by motion, and *could be pushed two inches laterally or horizontally.* Great pain ensued, its intensity relieved by pushing the fragments back into place. She had the distressing sensation "as if maggots were crawling along the spine." Was *relieved by hard pressure,* lying on her back across a chair, or over the end of a lounge. *Objects appeared double.* There were other less persistent exhibitions of spinal irritation, appearing from time to time. Her sufferings had been increased of late by using a crutch for a sprain. Wore a tight waist for relief. *Worse from all jarring.* The position of the womb was normal. There was copious purulent expectoration, with loose cough; dulness through the left chest, with râles, sibilant and mucous.

1878, October 12th. *Belladonna*^{cmm}, dry.

October 17th. *Coffea*^{cm}, four doses, in water.

October 27th. *Phosphorus*^{dm}, dry.

November 30th. *Chamomilla*^{cm}, six doses, in water.

December 5th. *Lachesis*^{cm}, twice, in water.

December 12th. *Rhus tox.*^{cm}, twice, in water.

1879, January 9th. *Bryonia*^{cm}, twice, dry.

January 17th. *Calc. phos.*^{cm}. six doses, in water.

February 4th. *Rhus*^{dm}, dry.

February 21st. *Theridion*^{dm}, dry.

March 22d. *Nat. mur.*^{dm}, dry.

April 12th. *Sulphur*^{dm}, dry.

July 14th. *Arnica*^{dm}, dry.

She had seemed better after *Calc. phos.*, and after *Theridion*, yet the cough was persistent. Examination of chest discovered little improvement, and the spinal symptoms often recurred.

July 21st. *Gettysburg salt*^{cm}, dry, was followed by diminished pain.

October 9th. Another dose, ^{cm}, dry, was given.

1880, October 10th. The sufferings in the back have much decreased during the past year, and she seems better, subjectively and objectively.

FRACTURES OF THE LOWER END OF THE RADIUS, OR COLLES'S FRACTURE.

BY W. C. GOODNO, M D, PHILADELPHIA, PA.

(Read before the Philadelphia County Homœopathic Medical Society.)

SIXTY-SIX years ago the eminent Irish surgeon whose name this fracture bears, wrote the first clear account of its nature.

Although his observations were ignored and passed over in silence for a time, they at last received the attention they merited, and to-day constitute the essence of our knowledge concerning this subject. A notable exception existed in Dr. R. W. Smith, of Dublin, who wrote a treatise on *Fractures in the Neighborhood of Joints*, and who did Colles full justice. Even the late Sir William Fergusson passes the matter over with a bare mention. As compared with other fractures of similar importance, its literature is insignificant. Aside from the short descriptions given in the standard textbooks, the best of which is by Hamilton in his book on fractures, there are only a few productions in English and American literature possessing merit. Sir Astley Cooper, who wrote extensively upon fractures, does not mention Colles's name, although he describes the fracture in question. Dr. E. M. Moore, of Rochester, N. Y., wrote an interesting article, which was published in the *Transactions of the New York State Medical Society* for 1870. In the same *Transactions* for 1874 was a prize essay by Dr. Thomas K. Cruse, of New York. In the *Transactions of the King's County Medical Society* is an article by Dr. Pilcher, of Brooklyn. In the *American Journal of the Medical Sciences* for January, 1879, is an article by Dr. Packard, of Philadelphia. The first American contribution was by the celebrated Philadelphia surgeon, Dr. John Rhea Barton, who attempted to establish a variety of this fracture called by his name, but which has not been sustained.

Upon the pathology of Colles's fracture I have nothing to offer. I have never made nor witnessed a post-mortem examination, opportunities for which are exceedingly rare. In the absence of sufficient opportunities, experimentation upon the cadaver has been extensively conducted, especially by Sir A. Cooper, Gordon of Belfast, Cruse of New York, Pilcher of Brooklyn, and Packard of Philadelphia, as well as by many others. The results of these experiments are fully set forth in the papers referred to, but are too lengthy for consideration upon this occasion, and in a limited paper, particularly as there is such a diversity of opinion among the writers, viz., Dr. Packard in his paper says: "Concerning impaction we find very opposite views expressed." Gordon says that in Colles's fracture it is impossible. Callender says that thirty-six specimens in the various museums in London show deformity, in all clearly due to "the impaction of the proximal into the distal end of the bone." Voillemier thought the impaction so marked a feature of the injury, that he would rank it among what he called "fractures by penetration." R. W. Smith argues that the appearances which led Voillemier to this opinion were due to deposits of new bone. The diagnosis is usually sufficiently easy; the deformity is characteristic, but especial care is to be exercised at times to obviate mistaking this fracture for a sprain, which has frequently occurred. The difficulties, however, are at times considerable, particularly to one of little surgical experience. The proximity of the fracture to the joint, which is surrounded by a large number of tendons and firm dense fascia and ligaments, bridging over and obscuring inequalities, and assisting by their firm contraction in preserving deformity; also dislocation of the ulna and certain tendons, the rapid swelling and pain, all assist in obscuring the diagnosis.

In the treatment of Colles's fracture I do not think that we need depart from the great surgical axioms which have been handed down for our guidance in the treatment of all fractures in the neighborhood of joints, and which have grown out of the combined experience of surgeons of all ages. These are substantially as follows: 1st. Replacement of the fragments as nearly as possible in their normal position. 2d. Retentive means to preserve this relation. 3d. Complete quiet of the fractured joint, as well as the nearest proximal and distal joint, except at such times as passive motion of these joints becomes necessary. If these principles are complied with we shall preserve coaptation, prevent spasm and inflammation, and usually get a good result. In the treatment of any fracture presenting unusual difficulty, we should scan our list of principles with great care, and ascertain whether we have complied thoroughly with all their requirements; unless we have, it is unnecessary to jump to new conclusions and procedures.

Reduction.—The difficulties attending reduction of this fracture are attributed by various authorities to various causes, each considering the cause given by himself as the principal one. Colles taught that by extension, a reduction could be secured, the deformity recurring upon its removal.

Mr. Callender, *in St. George's Hospital Reports*, states the difficulty to be impaction, it being impossible in many instances to separate the fragments, the upper one usually being driven into the terminal one.

Pilcher lays stress upon the fact that in many cases the periosteum upon the dorsal surface remains intact, and that extension will not bring down the lower fragment unless it be strong enough to lacerate this periosteal band; that the hand must be carried into extreme extension and the fragment pressed forward with the fingers.

Dr. E. M. Moore, of Rochester, N. Y., in the very interesting article in the *Transactions of the New York State Medical Society* for 1870, already referred to, states his opinion that luxation of the ulna is the usual impediment to reduction. This opinion is founded upon two post-mortem examinations, and Dr. Moore concludes that "all difficulty in treatment disappears when the luxation is restored." These varying opinions teach us, says Dr. Packard, that "cases differ," which it seems to me is a fact of great importance to remember when commencing the treatment of a case of Colles's fracture. The mechanical treatment is evidently not easy. There is no *splint* which is a royal highway to a cure. It has been well said "that the multiplicity of methods recommended for the cure of any given diseased condition indicates the poverty of our reliable resources for such treatment," and such I suspect must be our opinion in reference to the subject under consideration. So many methods have been lauded, to be in a little time discarded, that we are forced to the conclusion that there must be some radical defect existing in our past methods. Too much confidence, I fear, is reposed in apparatus in the treatment of Colles's as well as many other fractures. Mechanical contrivances are expected to do that which nothing but the skill of a good surgeon can accomplish; rather a good surgeon with poor apparatus than a poor surgeon with the most perfected dressings. In no fracture are good results more dependent upon assiduous attention to the details of treatment. I am satisfied from my own experience and my observation of the practice of others, that the fear of displacement prevents the frequent examinations necessary during the first week. It is safer to remove the bandage every day and carefully inspect the parts, and in most cases all the dressings, to make passive motion of the wrist-joint, and gently shampoo the surface with soap lather or vasoline in cases where much swelling or inflammation exists. This plan of procedure causes a good deal of trouble for the surgeon, but it has repaid me well in the cases in which I have tried it. I will not spend time discussing the great variety of splints that have been used in the treatment of this fracture. The use of two straight splints, the pistol splint of Nélaton, Bond's, Gordon's, Carr's, and lastly the zinc splint of Dr. Levis, of this city, have all enjoyed considerable popularity. Undoubtedly good cures have been made by all these splints, in the hands of careful surgeons. I have used the two straight splints and Bond's with a good deal of satisfaction. Nélaton's pistol splint is an abomination. Gordon's, Carr's, and Levis's splints are constructed with more reference to the anatomical characteristics of the region. I have heard Professor Pancoast say, in reference to the surgical or dissecting forceps that they consisted of the "bite," that is, the terminal serrations of the instrument, and that all the rest was handle, even if it were a mile long. I think we may say of a splint for this fracture, that the splint proper is that portion in immediate relation with the lower end of the radius and all the rest is handle. This handle is serviceable for quieting muscular action, and keeping the hand at rest; but the proper relation of the fragments is preserved by that portion of the splint in contact with the immediate vicinity of the fracture. Any one who will carefully examine the subject will find that the ingenuity of surgeons has been spent in perfecting the handle, not the splint.

I believe the plastic splints to be superior to all others in the treatment of fractures of the lower extremity of the radius. For over three years I have used them in most of the cases that have come under my care, as have also several friends to whom I have recommended them. I am not cognizant of the fact that they have been used by others. My success has been very much more satisfactory since their adoption, although it may be somewhat due to increased interest in the subject. My first trials were with plaster of Paris. A plaster roller of suitable width having been damped, six to eight folds are rapidly laid upon each other upon the table at the patient's side, the table being upon the side of the patient corresponding to the injured limb; the folds should be long enough to extend from the middle of the first row of phalangeal bones to just below the elbow. The surface of the skin should be protected from the bandage by a single layer of cotton; beneath the lower extremity of the bandage should be now placed a ball of yarn, or some similar substance. By the aid of an assistant give an anæsthetic, if necessary, and prepare the limb for the dressing. When proper coaptation of fragments has been attained the arm is placed upon the splint, the patient instructed to grasp the terminal extremity of the dressing (if an anæsthetic is not used), and with it the ball; in the meantime the surgeon can with the fingers mould the splint to the concave surface of the radius. A very good method of moulding to the inequalities of the forearm is also by placing in proper position cotton or some similar substance, which will adapt itself to these inequalities. When the plaster has acquired some stiffness the arm may be lifted from the table, for the better completion of the moulding. When the splint has become rather firm we may adopt one of several plans: *a*, apply immediately a roller with a quantity of oakum, cotton, tow, or other similar substance, to keep the splint well up into the inequalities of the region, leaving the ball in position for a day or two, or until the plaster will preserve the form given to it; or, *b*, apply the same dressing with a compress over the back of the lower fragment, if the tendency to displacement is considerable; or, what is better, a strip of firm adhesive plaster, which takes the place of a posterior splint. Gutta-percha I now give the preference; it is cleaner, pleasanter to apply, and its moulding qualities are greater, but it is more expensive; it comes in sheets of varying thickness, which can be cut with a sharp, strong knife into any desired shape and size; when cut, it is to be surrounded by a piece of stout muslin and placed in hot water, for the purpose of softening it. When sufficiently pliable it is removed from the water and moulded to the limb. The proper softening of the gutta-percha requires care.

RAPID LITHOTRITY.

WITH A REPORT OF TWO CASES.

BY CHARLES M. THOMAS, M.D.

(Read before the Philadelphia County Homœopathic Medical Society.)

It is now about two years since Professor Bigelow, of Boston, first gave to the profession, in an article published in the *American Journal of Medical Sciences*, an account of a modified method of lithotrity, to which he has applied the term *Litholapaxy*, meaning the crushing of a vesical stone with an immediate evacuation of the fragments.

The removal of a calculus by crushing is, comparatively speaking, a modern operation. It was first performed by Civiale, in France, in the year 1824, and, although carried out by means of very crude instruments, it was considered, and properly so, a great triumph in operative surgery. Since that time, this method of dealing with stone has been variously modified and improved, both by the originator and others, Civiale having had the pleasure of watching and participating in the progress of this most valuable operation for a period of more than forty years.

The most important changes during that time were in the

construction of the crushing instruments, there having been no effort made until recent years toward a mechanical assistance in relieving the bladder of the fragments produced. The aim in each modification was therefore to so construct the lithotrite as to enable the operator to shorten the duration of the sitting and diminish the risk of injury to the bladder and related organs.

Sir Henry Thompson, in his delightful treatise on the diseases of the urinary organs, says: "What is the problem to be solved by lithotrity? It is the removal of a stone without injury to the urinary passages; and injury can occur by two means only: either in the employment of the instruments, or by the action of the calculus fragments which are produced."

So great was the intolerance of the bladder to contact with instruments supposed to be, that even at the hands of the most skilful operators it was not considered safe for an instrument to remain in the organ during the act of crushing for a longer average time than two minutes.

In this way the complete breaking up of a stone of any size, necessitated the subjection of the patient to from three, to a dozen or more sittings, and required for its entire removal, in many cases, a period of several weeks.

Since the introduction of general anæsthetics, however, there has been a gradual leaning, even among the strong advocates of the "cautious" or many-sitting style of operating, to prolong the time and so increase the amount of work done by the lithotrite at each sitting.

Since the early days of lithotrity, the danger of inflammation of the bladder and other urinary organs from the irritation produced by sharp fragments of crushed stone has been fully realized, but, singularly enough, little has been done to overcome this, except by careful attention to the parts while the fragments are lying within the organ, awaiting their expulsion with the urine. There has been at all times a marked difference in opinion as to the manner in which the fragments should be dealt with, in order to insure the least possible irritation, the great majority of surgeons agreeing with Sir Henry Thompson, who, as late as 1863, laid down the rule that on no account should the fragments after the first crushing be disturbed, but be left for spontaneous expulsion by the bladder, his object being to avoid the necessarily additional use of instruments for that purpose. Of late years, however, there has been a tendency among some operators to remove more and more of the débris at the time of crushing, in spite of the supposed additional risk run from instrumentation, and a Mr. Clover, of England, invented an apparatus for this purpose, consisting of a rubber exhausting-bottle attached to a large-sized catheter. Hence it will be seen that injury to the bladder through manipulation with instruments was more dreaded than the irritation produced by the rough particles of stone left by the crushing.

Although the later history of lithotrity shows an increasing tendency towards prolonging the sittings, and by doing more work, thus lessening their number, still the early teachings of Civiale and his followers as to the excessive sensitiveness of the bladder and urethra to prolonged manipulation held full sway up to the very time in which Professor Bigelow brought forward his radical change in the operation.

This method is founded upon an entirely different understanding of the endurance of the bladder and urethra under instrumentation, and involves principles in the performance of the operation entirely at variance with the older method. In his brochure on the subject, published in 1878; he says: "That the average bladder and urethra have *no* extreme susceptibility, is attested by the general favorable results of lithotrity, and even of catheterism, which are practiced with varying skill everywhere; also by the singularly innocuous results of laceration of the contracted urethra, by an instrument like that of Voillemier, for example; so, too, by the recovery of these organs from the considerable injury inflicted during the extraction of a large and rough stone in lithotomy. The bladder is often also, to an extraordinary degree, tolerant of the presence even of a mulberry calculus. If we remember that, in this case, it clasps the stone at every micturition, often with a persistent gripe, the comparative immunity of its tender mucous membrane is quite remarkable. But when, after an operation, sharp fragments are thus embraced, presenting acute angles, which do not soon become blunted, and to which the bladder is unaccustomed, it is still more remarkable that serious consequences are the exception and not the rule in lithotrity. Polished metal surfaces, carefully manipulated, can hardly do such damage as the other agencies here mentioned."

Hence the object of Professor Bigelow is to rapidly relieve the bladder, if possible, at one sitting, of all sharp pieces of stone, even under what would formerly have been considered an extremely dangerous prolongation of instrumental manipulation. Thus, in one of the cases reported by him, he occupied 3¾ hours in crushing and removing 706 grains. Under the common mode of operating, stones were never attacked which measured over two inches in diameter, but were relegated to the more dangerous operation of lithotomy. In Bigelow's operation the size of the stone is only limited by the grasping capacity of the lithotrite.

Professor Bigelow employs a scoop lithotrite, considerably heavier than those in ordinary use, with a modification in the catch, so that the sliding of the blades is turned into a screw motion by a movement of the wrist, instead of by a push of the thumb, as in that of the Thompson pattern. The male blade is also so modified as to better cast out the fragments as they are formed, and thereby, as it is claimed, avoid the clogging or impaction of the blades.

His apparatus for evacuating the bladder I show you here in its latest modification. It consists of a rubber bulb, holding from eight to ten ounces, at the lower end of which is attached, by a bayonet joint, a glass chamber. From the other end runs a large rubber tube about a foot long, which is in connection with the evacuating catheters or tubes. These latter should be of as large a size as the urethra will accommodate, *i. e.*, from No. 28 to 31 F., as recommended by Bigelow, and preferably straight in shape, although curved ones may be employed. The eyélet is not placed upon the side, as in ordinary catheters, but in front and at the end, and is very much larger, being nearly, if not quite, the size of the calibre of the tube.

The calculus having been crushed, or as much of it as may be deemed prudent, the bulb and tubes are filled with warm water, the catheter is introduced and attached to the rubber-pipe. The bulb being now compressed, it drives the water into and distends the bladder, and, upon the relaxation of the pressure, it expands and sucks the water back again, bringing with it more or less of the débris, which immediately falls into the glass chamber below.

The shower of fragments into the trap having ceased, the bulb is detached, the catheter withdrawn, and any remaining larger fragments, broken by the lithotrite; after which the evacuation is repeated, and in this way the operation goes on to completion. When, during the working of the evacuator, the sound or clicking of fragments upon the end of the catheter entirely stops, it is fair to suppose, unless there be an encysted stone present, that the bladder is empty. Indeed, the absence of this sound is probably now the best test we have of the completion of the operation.

CASE 1.—*Removal of eleven hundred and sixty grains of*

Vesical Calculi by Bigelow's Method.—M. S., æt. 65 years, consulted me at the suggestion of Dr. Wareheim, of Glenrock, Pennsylvania, in September, 1879. He had always been in good health up to about 1875, when he began to be troubled with frequent and painful urination. These urinary symptoms increased rapidly, so that within a year he suffered almost constant pain both at the neck of the bladder and end of penis, made very much worse in walking or riding over a rough road and immediately after urinating. The pain and urging to urinate were so constant as to entirely deprive him of sleep for nights in succession. Had occasionally passed some small particles of sand-like substance. Had lately had frequent incontinence of urine. His father and a brother had suffered for years with the gravel.

Examination at my office showed a capacious but irritable urethra; hypertrophied prostate; moderate-sized, extremely sensitive bladder, holding at least two good-sized stones. Kidneys and heart apparently normal. During the first week in October I crushed and removed in two sittings of about a half hour each 510 grains of mainly uric acid fragments.

This being my first case of lithotrity after Bigelow's method I had much hesitation in prolonging the operation to even a half hour, never having before allowed my lithotrite to remain in the bladder in any case longer then five minutes. After neither of these sittings was there more than a degree's elevation in temperature, and no suffering or uncomfortable sensation whatever.

The vesical sphincter became quite competent immediately after the first operation, and the intervals between urinations increased from a few minutes to three hours. Indeed the patient felt so well two days after the second sitting that he insisted upon going home, although I felt sure that his stone was not completely removed.

Early in January, 1880, I was therefore not surprised on again finding him in my office, presenting his old symptom in a milder form. He had experienced complete relief for only about a fortnight after the operation. On January 13th, 1880, I crushed and removed two hundred grains, leaving apparently nothing in the bladder. At this sitting I made a trial of Bigelow's lithotrite, but finding that it clogged with débris equally as much as my Thompson instrument, and was to me clumsier to handle, I was not encouraged to continue its use.

On the first of last month I received a third visit from my patient, who stated that for many weeks following the operation in January last, he had entire relief from his old symptoms, but that ever since, he had experienced a gradually increasing, heavy, dull aching in the perinæum or about the neck of the bladder, and a sharp pain at the same place during the end of urinating, always of the same character, and in the same situation, with more frequent calls to urination, which he accomplished with much difficulty. He felt sure there must be "a stone sticking fast in his pipe." My exploring sound, as it entered the bladder, seemed to strike with its under surface a rather broad calculus, lying apparently back of and to the left of the prostate, and as it was not changed from this position either by injections into the bladder or in any position of the patient, I was led to suspect a partially encysted stone. On September 9th I introduced a lithotrite with the patient under Ether, and by turning the blades well to the left grasped a stone about an inch and a quarter in diameter, but could not rotate it from its position; nor could I satisfy myself that a fold of mucous membrane was not included with the stone within the jaws of the lithotrite.

I therefore refrained from any attempt at crushing, and fully distended the bladder with warm water in order to displace what mucous folds might overlap the surface of the calculus. Then grasping it again, I succeeded after a time in rotating the instrument with the stone in its jaws. After this there was little further difficulty, but as in the first washings some blood and threads, apparently of mucous membrane, appeared in the trap, I did not push the operation to complete removal of the stone, not knowing how much damage I might have already done the bladder in the dislodgment of the stone. After drying, the débris from this sitting weighed 200 grains.

No troublesome symptoms following, I again etherized him on the 14th, six days later, and crushed without difficulty; but as the working of the evacuator became defective through a leak, by which air was admitted to the bladder, I again was obliged to stop the operation before completion, after washing out 200 grains more. On the 20th, no sign of irritation having shown itself from the operation, 50 grains were removed in a few minutes by crushing and washing, and without giving rise to the least inflammatory disturbance either locally or generally. At the end of the last sitting, as no sign of stone could be made out, either with the sound or by free circulation of water through the bladder and evacuating apparatus, he was dismissed as cured, and feeling, as he said, just as well as ever in his life. Two days later he left for his home, and has within a week notified me of his perfect health.

CASE 2.—*One hundred and sixty grains of Uric Acid Calculus removed at One Sitting.*—J. G., æt. 52 years, a patient of Dr. Korndœrfer, presented himself at my office in June last, complaining of the usual symptoms attending stone in the bladder. Examination showed the presence of two calculi, one of which was about a half inch in diameter. He desired an early operation. From June 26th to 29th he was kept quietly in bed on a light diet, and directed to drink freely of Vichy water, in order, by dilution, to render his urine as unirritating as possible. Arnica 30^x was administered twice daily.

Before operation his heart and kidneys were examined and found normal.

At 11 o'clock A.M., on the 29th of June, litholapaxy was performed, and 160 grains of calcular fragments removed. The whole procedure lasted 45 minutes. Immediately after, the patient was placed in a warm bed and hot fomentations applied to perinæum and over bladder. At 5 P.M. temperature 101.3°; Arnica and light diet continued. At 7.30 P.M. temperature 100.4°. As there was no sign of vomiting, a liberal supply of Vichy water and flaxseed tea was ordered.

June 30th (2d day), 8 A.M., temperature 99° scant, pulse 84. Had slept during night, and had no pain; slight stain of blood in urine; passages much less frequent than before operation. Poultices removed; diet to be mainly broths of beef or mutton and plenty of raw milk.

2 P.M., urine clear, passed with little pain; temperature 99.7° full; slightly flushed; stopped Arn. and gave Acon. 3^x. 7.45 P.M., temperature 98.4°; stopped Acon.

From this time on he made an almost uninterruptedly good recovery. Three days after the operation felt well in every way, could retain urine two to three hours, and pass it without pain.

On July 7th (nine days after operation) I directed him to take a ride in a street-car over a rough road, which he did without experiencing the slightest annoyance. July 8th examined the bladder very carefully with sound, and failed to find a trace of stone, nor has he since, to my knowledge, shown any evidence of the disease.

Although the total number of cases in which this method of lithotrity has been employed is still too small to enable us to judge fairly as to its ultimate position in surgical procedures, yet from the universally favorable reception it has received, both in this country and in Europe, it evidently bids fair to take a higher rank than would ever have been attained by lithotrity as performed according to the older method.

OBSERVATIONS UPON FIFTY ANALYSES OF URINE.

BY CLIFFORD MITCHELL, M.D., PROFESSOR OF CHEMISTRY, CHICAGO HOMŒOPATHIC COLLEGE.

TWENTY-SEVEN specimens out of the fifty showed a specific gravity of 1030, or upwards; ten of these twenty-seven contained sugar and two albumen, the latter, however, being due to the presence of blood.

The highest specific gravity *without* sugar was 1037; the highest *with* sugar, 1044.

Seventeen specimens were between 1015 and 1030 in specific gravity, only one of these containing any abnormal constituent.

The remaining six cases were below 1015, the lowest being 1007, and in all of them albumen was found.

Thirty-four per cent. of the specimens, then, were of a high specific gravity *without* sugar; this should warn the hasty generalizer not to conclude that his patient has *diabetes mellitus* from the fact that the specific gravity of his urine is above 1030. Of the seventeen cases of high specific gravity *without* sugar ten were given me to test for sugar, the foregone conclusion having been that, because the specific gravity was above 1030, sugar must *necessarily* be present, although there were no other indications of the presence of saccharine matter. Very many excellent textbooks have been written upon the urine, such as Neubauer and Vogel, Hofman and Ultzman, Beale, Hurley, Thudichum, Flint, Roberts, etc., and every work on diagnosis contains a chapter on this subject, yet in spite of the presence of such works, or some one of them, in the library of the average practitioner, the unread physician finds the specific gravity of a sample of urine to be 1035, and says, with equally great "specific gravity," "Sugar."

Increase in specific gravity simply means increase of solids. Now there are something like *sixty* solids, normal and abnormal, to be found in the urine besides sugar. Hence it is not to be supposed that sugar is the only substance which can, by its presence, raise the specific gravity.

In most febrile conditions, the normal constituents of urine—urea, phosphates, sulphates, and urates—are increased in amount, such increase being necessarily accompanied by increased specific gravity. A knowledge of this fact is important, for I have seen patients unnecessarily terrified by a diagnosis of diabetes mellitus made from a urinometer test alone. In one of the specimens analyzed by myself, the specific gravity was 1037 without sugar being present; the urine was loaded with earthy phosphates, which had been mistaken for sugar by a painstaking practitioner, who took the trouble to test the specimen with Trommer's test,—caustic potash, and sulphate of copper. This suggests another point of great importance: when urine contains an increased amount of earthy phosphates, the addition of an alkali like caustic potash causes them to be precipitated in abundance, and the inexperienced in applying Trommer's test, and perceiving this flocculent mass of dirty-white phosphates, are apt to deem it the rich red of the sugar test, although why dirty white should be mistaken for red is a question for the oculist. The words of Carl Neubauer are: "If a solution of sugar is treated with a little caustic potash and a few drops of a solution of sulphate of copper, either no precipitate occurs, or that which takes place dissolves again to a beautiful blue fluid. If this mixture be heated the fluid is first colored orange-yellow, soon becomes cloudy, and finally a beautiful red precipitate of cuprous oxide separates." This, then, is what happens when sugar is actually present; when sugar is *absent*, the addition of caustic potash solution causes, perhaps, a cloudiness to appear; then, when the sulphate of copper is added, the beautiful blue color may or may not be present according to the quantity of copper sulphate added, but when *heat* is applied, there results either (1) a liquid, generally of a color slightly darker than normal urine, containing dirty-white flocks of phosphates, or else (2) a bluish liquid containing these same flocks of phosphates; when there appears *no "orange-yellow, which soon becomes cloudy, ending in a beautiful red precipitate," there is no sugar present.*

In case of any doubt in regard to colors, the practitioner should take a fresh sample of the urine and add to it caustic potash (solution), heat, and then add nitric acid. Neubauer says: "If a solution of grape-sugar be warmed with potassic hydrate (caustic potash) it becomes a beautiful brown-red color; if nitric acid is then added, a piercing sweetish odor is evolved, which reminds one of caramel or of formic acid."

In the case of urine containing sugar then, caustic potash solution added, heat applied, and further nitric acid added, converts the liquid into a substance strongly resembling molasses. I have known patients to diagnose their own cases upon being shown test-tubes containing their urine which had been subjected to the treatment above mentioned,—the universal verdict was "molasses!"

Lastly, the filtration of urine containing sugar, through animal charcoal four or five times, will cause the liquid to become colorless, and the application of Trommer's test will then leave no room for doubt, as no color can result which even the inexperienced would mistake for "orange-yellow turning to beautiful red."

When the specific gravity is 1040, or upwards, we are very sure of finding sugar without much trouble.

Ninety-four per cent of the above-mentioned cases, where the specific gravity ranged from 1015 to 1030, contained neither albumen nor sugar, and in general we do not expect to find either of these ingredients in urines having this range of specific gravity. Nevertheless we may find blood or pus in urine when the specific gravity is within the normal limits, 1015 to 1025, and if such urine be tested for albumen, the latter will be found, and the diagnosis "Bright's disease" may be given by the incautious physician, to the consternation of the patient, who was only aware of a bad case of gonorrhœa! The moral is, examine albuminous urine for tube-casts also, in order to distinguish true kidney albumen from simple blood or pus albumen.

One hundred per cent. of the specimens whose specific gravity was below 1015 were found to contain albumen, and in all these cases tube-casts were also discovered.

If, then, the urine contains neither blood nor pus, yet responds to the test for albumen, we diagnose *true albuminuria*, and disease of the kidney itself is indicated. If, together with the albumen (when pus and blood are not responsible for the same), we find a lowered specific gravity, we have to distinguish between (i) desquamative nephritis, (ii) chronic parenchymatous nephritis and secondary atrophy, (iii) interstitial nephritis, and (iv) amyloid kidney. The differential diagnosis of these four conditions may be made with the microscope.

In case the albumen present is not due to blood or pus, and we find the specific gravity to be *higher* than normal, we may infer either (i) renal stasis or (ii) acute parenchymatous nephritis, and the microscope will differentiate here, renal stasis not having cellular forms nor granular casts in its sediments.

In general, then, when we find the specific gravity persistently below 1015 we are warranted in looking for albumen.

One of these last cases referred to was of especial interest. The urine was colorless, of a specific gravity of 1007, contained albumen, and was remarkable for the almost entire absence of the normal sulphates and earthy phosphates.

The attending physician had diagnosed the disease to be chronic morbus Brightii, and the patient died not long after I first made my analysis of the urine.

The importance of the case is evident. Heller has claimed that in chronic renal diseases, as well as in some others, the sulphates are diminished. Lehmann and Gruner doubt it, and Vogel is non-committal.

Inasmuch as in several different analyses I was only able to detect traces of the sulphates in considerable amounts of urine, the views of Heller would seem to be confirmed so far as this one case is concerned, and the obscure subject of the sulphates in urine of renal diseases cleared up in one small particular, inasmuch as we may now say without hesitation, "In some cases of chronic renal disease the amount of sulphates in the urine is diminished." I may add that care was taken to give me the urine of twenty-four hours.*

There were but slight amounts of earthy phosphates found, confirming the views of Brattler on the urine in renal diseases. The chlorides were tolerably abundant.

Twenty specimens of the fifty contained heavy deposits. Of these, eight were of urates, seven of phosphates, and five chiefly of free uric acid with urates.

Nothing seems to alarm the laity more than "blood-red" urine, which on standing deposits large amounts of "brick-dust." A distinction must be made between occasional and persistent deposits of urates. In my pamphlet on the *Clinical Significance of Urine*, pp. 20 and 21, I have given the causes of sediments of urates as follows:

"An *occasional* sediment of urates may be due to:

"(i) Over-eating or over-drinking.

"(ii) Great exertion, revelry, or excitement.

"(iii) Hard study.

"(iv) Fright.

"(v) Change in manner of living."

Again, on pp. 22 and 24:

"The *persistent* presence of uric acid and of urates in the urine in the form of deposits is one of the most constant signs of functional derangements of the liver.—*W. H. Draper*."

---

* This case would at least show that if Sulphuric acid were present at all it was in such a form as not to be detected by Barium chloride.

In this Western country, nothing is more common than persistent urate deposits due to hepatic disorders. Heavy phosphatic deposits may be due to nervous disorders. Especially is the Ammonic magnesium deposit due to diseases of the spinal cord *if present in freshly passed urine of an alkaline reaction and putrid odor.* The distinction between *fresh* and *stale* urine is of importance here, since the earthy phosphates are precipitated in perfectly normal urine as soon as it is old enough to become alkaline in reaction.

Drinks containing lime or magnesia will increase the earthy phosphates, and we must not be surprised to see occasional phosphatic deposits in districts where lime-water is used.

HOMATROPIN.

BY WILLIAM H. BIGLER, M.D., AND CLARENCE BARTLETT, M D.

(Read before the Philadelphia County Homœopathic Medical Society, Philadelphia, November 11th, 1880.)

THE use of mydriatics being acknowledged by oculists to be a necessity in various conditions and diseases of the eye, for the purpose either of diagnosis, prognosis, or treatment, it becomes a matter of importance to discover one whose use shall be attended with the greatest advantages and the fewest inconveniences and dangers.

A good mydriatic should possess the following characteristics:

1. Its mydriatic effects should be promptly produced. 2. These effects should not be too persistent, since it is easier to repeat the application than to limit its action. 3. When continued use becomes necessary, it should exert no irritating action on the tissues with which it comes in immediate contact. 4. Its effect on the tension of the eyeball should be a minimum. 5. Its use should produce no constitutional disturbances.

In some one or more of these requirements, each of the substances hitherto found capable of producing mydriasis has been found wanting; thus, in most of them, the local and constitutional effects were so closely connected as to render their use unadvisable if not positively dangerous. Until quite recently the Sulphate of atropia has been almost exclusively employed. Although in the majority of cases perfectly satisfactory, yet there were certain disadvantages connected with its use that rendered some other mydriatic desirable. In the case of some, who possess an idiosyncrasy of constitution fortunately rare, the general symptoms of even a weak solution, used locally, are so distressing as to contraindicate its application. When used for the purpose of paralyzing the ciliary muscle in order to test the refraction, its effects are so persistent as to be a source of great inconvenience. Its alleged increase in tension posteriorly forbids its employment in glaucoma, and where its constant and long-continued use is indicated for therapeutic purposes, an irritation and almost granular condition of the tarsal conjunctiva are very frequently produced.

No wonder then that the announcement of the discovery of a new mydriatic, the Sulphate of Duboisia, possessing all of the advantages and none of the disadvantages of Atropia, was received with enthusiasm by oculists everywhere. But here, too, not all the expectations raised were realized. Although its mydriatic effects are prompt and not quite so persistent as those of Atropia, yet in its action on the ciliary muscle we have not found it reliable when used in the strength that we consider safe, viz., two grains to the ounce of distilled water. Intense vertigo and delirium, lasting for twenty-four hours, have been known to follow the instillation of a solution of four grains to the ounce.

Again, its therapeutic application is neither so extended nor so reliable as that of Atropia, and in some cases where a mydriatic was demanded, this latter has had to be used after the complete failure of Duboisia to act.

Another claimant for favor has but lately made its appearance, and it is the purpose of the present paper to prepare the way for a proper estimation of its properties as a mydriatic.

Oxytoluyl-tropein or Homatropin was discovered by Ladenberg, of Kiel. The fact that Atropia could be split into Tropia and Tropic acid had been found out some years ago; but Ladenberg further discovered that by organic acids and Hydrochloric acid a number of new bases, to which he gave the generic name Tropeins, could be obtained. Of these, Oxytoluyl-tropein or Homatropin (called so from its similarity to Atropia) is one, and is prepared from Tropin by Amygdalic and dilute Hydrochloric acids. It forms regular, colorless, transparent crystals, hygroscopic but not readily soluble in water. The mydriatic we employ is the Hydrobromate of homatropin, and is readily soluble in ten parts of water. It is manufactured by Merck, of Darmstadt, and was imported for us by Wyeth & Brother of this city. The literature on the subject of its mydriatic properties is as yet but scant. In the *Centralblatt für pracktische augenheilkunde*, iv, 182–184, there is an article, "Homatropinum Hydrobromatum," by E. Fuchs. In the

London *Lancet* for August of this year, Tweedie and Ringer have a contribution on the mydriatic properties of Homatropin or Oxytoluyl-tropein, with an account of its general physiological action, and Drs. Schell and Keyser of this city give short notices of it, with illustrative cases, in the October number of the Philadelphia *Medical Times*.

As to its general physiological action, Ringer gives the following as one of the results of his experiments: "Homatropin appears to possess many of the properties of Atropia, but in a weaker degree. On the heart, however, their effect is very different, for Atropia accelerates and strengthens the heart's contractions in man, whereas Homatropin slows the beats and renders them irregular in force and rhythm."

During the past two months we have been making use of the Hydrobromate of homatropin, and have applied it in sixty-five cases, among which were not only cases of the various anomalies of refraction, but also of a number of diseases of the eye, including among others the following: conjunctivitis; traumatic, scrofulous, and phlyctenular keratitis; iritis, choroiditis, retinitis, neuro-retinitis, chronic glaucoma, and atrophy of the optic nerve. Our experiments seem to favor the following conclusions:

1. As a mydriatic, we have found Homatropin to be prompt in its action. Under its influence the pupil begins to dilate in the course of fifteen minutes, and attains its maximum size in from forty minutes to one hour in the case of the stronger solutions (grs. viij and xvj–℥j), a much longer time being required where the weaker solutions have been employed. Thus, while in the case of the one and two grain solutions, the pupil commences to dilate in a quarter of an hour, the maximum degree of dilatation is not reached until nearly three hours after the instillation of the drops. Occasionally we meet with a patient more susceptible than others to the action of the drug, and in whose case dilatation of the pupil commences as early as five minutes after the application of a solution no stronger than four grains to the ounce of distilled water. The weakest solution which we employed, was one of an eighth of a grain to the ounce. This we found to produce a very slight dilatation of the pupil and an equally slight effect on the ciliary muscle. These effects passed away so soon that we failed to note their duration. The effect of the weaker solutions on the accommodation was found to vary with the patient's peculiarities. Thus, where the ciliary muscle had been weakened from long-continued strain, a nearly complete paralysis of the ac-

commodation ensued after the instillation of three drops of a four-grain solution. But where the ciliary muscle was in a vigorous condition this quantity of a four-grain solution would not be so effectual. By repeatedly instilling the four-grain solution until from ten to sixteen drops had been used the accommodation was completely paralyzed in the course of an hour or an hour and a quarter. A much better effect from the drug may be obtained by using more concentrated solutions, such as eight or sixteen grains to the ounce. From three to six drops of the latter were found to paralyze the accommodation completely in from forty minutes to an hour.

2. The principal advantage attending the use of Homatropin as a mydriatic, lies in the fact that its effects are evanescent. Thus the effects from the one and two grain solutions were found to pass away in the course of twelve or twenty-four hours, and those of a four-grain solution in from eighteen to thirty-six hours. A longer time, however, was required for the entire disappearance of the mydriasis and paralysis of the accommodation produced by a sixteen-grain solution. The patient was always able to read his newspaper the next day, but it was not until twenty-four or thirty hours later that the accommodation had regained its wonted vigor.

3. We have found Homatropin to produce but slight irritation of the tissues with which it comes in contact, excepting in occasional instances, in which it might readily be ascribed to the idiosyncrasies of the patient. In all the sixty-five cases to which we applied Homatropin, there were but half a dozen in which any but the most transient irritation was produced; this, too, notwithstanding the fact that we instilled the mydriatic in eyes suffering from violent acute and chronic inflammations of the more important tunics. The cases in which a marked irritation was observed, were two in number, and were both cases of hypermetropia. A four-grain solution was employed in both instances. In one, eight drops were used, and in the other, fourteen. In the latter, the injection of the eye was not only conjunctival, but subconjunctival also. The ophthalmoscope too, revealed only an occasional case in which any hyperæmia was produced. In both of the abovementioned cases the irritation was of short duration, lasting but a quarter of an hour in either case. It is barely possible that the instillation of an equally large number of drops of distilled water might have produced nearly the same effect. Where a smaller number of drops and a stronger solution were employed, none but a barely perceptible irritation was produced,

and that in but a single case, where six drops of a sixteen-grain solution were used.

4. We found that in several of our patients the intraocular tension had been increased after the instillation of Homatropin. Other instances were reported to us in which the patient, after leaving for his home, was troubled with a bursting sensation in the eye. This warns us to use every precautionary measure before using Homatropin in patients in whom a glaucomatous tendency is suspected. Our patient with chronic glaucoma, however, observed no inconvenience from its use. He was a German, cabinetmaker by trade, and was fifty-six years of age. About two and a half years ago the vision of his right eye began to gradually disappear, and in nine months had progressed to blindness to everything but perception of light. The aqueous humor was somewhat cloudy, as it occasionally is in that disease; the pupil was of normal size, but reacted very sluggishly to light, T + 2. At no time did he suffer from any severe pain, but he was frequently annoyed by a squeezing, pressing sensation in the glaucomatous eye. Homatropin was used in his case to facilitate an examination of the fundus, when a marked glaucomatous excavation of the disk, together with violent pulsation of the retinal arteries, was observed. The solution employed was one of four grains to the ounce. This, however, is but one case.

5. In none of our experiments have we observed a single case in which any constitutional symptoms whatever were produced. Even an infant, two and a half years of age, only obtained from it its mydriatic effects (and that, too, without any local irritation), although we instilled in his eye six drops of a four-grain solution.

In comparing the action of Homatropin with solutions of Duboisia and Atropia of equal strength, we found Homatropin to be the weakest drug of the three. As compared with Atropia its strength was as one to two; with Duboisia, as one to four. When, however, we used a very strong solution of Homatropin (gr. xvj–℥j), we were enabled to get a much more complete and more rapid effect than was obtainable from the solutions of Duboisia and Atropia ammon., employed particularly in paralyzing the accommodation. The greatest difference between it and the other mydriatics was observed in the evanescent nature of its action.

While, after the instillation of Atropia, the patient was unable to read for ten days, and after Duboisia for three to four days, he was able to read on the following day after the instillation of Homatropin, although accommodation was not restored to its normal condition until a day later. Although we found a few cases in which irritation of the eye was produced by Homatropin, it was no more, but much less, than we had observed after the instillation of Atropia. We have not observed any case in which irritation of the eye ensued from Duboisia, but Dr. T. D. Risley, of this city,* reports a case in which both Atropia and Duboisia excited a smart conjunctivitis. In producing an apparent increase of the intraocular tension, Homatropin does not stand alone among the mydriatics. The same effect has frequently been observed to follow the use of Atropia by some authorities, although this has been denied by others. Increased tension, we believe, has not been known as yet to follow the use of Duboisia. Both Atropia and Duboisia, particularly the latter, have produced constitutional disturbances when applied to the eye. Dr. Little, in a recent number of the *Medical Times*, reports two instances in which a two-grain solution of Duboisia applied to the eye produced incontinence of urine.

Intense headaches, delirium, etc., have also been observed to follow the use of Duboisia. Similar symptoms, but of a less violent nature, have frequently followed the instillation into the eye of a few drops of Atropia. None of these symptoms have, as yet, been produced by the local use of Homatropin.

Our experiments have led us to the following conclusions respecting the use of Homatropin:

1. As a therapeutic agent to be used for mechanical purposes in effecting a forcible dilatation of the pupil, it will be of but slight utility, not so much because of the irritation it might produce as on account of the ephemeral nature of its action.

2. It will be a very valuable agent for producing a temporary mydriasis when necessary to a thorough examination of the fundus. Here the weaker solutions will be the most useful.

3. The stronger solutions (gr. viij and xvj–℥j) furnish us with the most prompt means for producing paralysis of the accommodation when testing the refraction of the eye.

4. The apparently increased intraocular tension would admonish us to use the drug with discretion in the case of patients in whom a glaucomatous tendency was known to exist.

---

* American Journal of Medical Sciences, January, 1880.

CASES FROM PRACTICE.

BY L. HOOPES, M.D., DOWNINGTOWN, PA.

(Read before the Homœopathic Medical Society of Chester, Delaware, and Montgomery Counties.)

CASE I.—Mrs. N., aged forty-eight years; short and heavy; dark complexion; at the climacteric period; suffers a great deal from mental depression, almost amounting to melancholy; great disposition to weep; thinks everything is working against her; her mind constantly dwells on suicide, and it requires a great effort of the will to refrain from throwing herself out of the window; is in constant fear of doing it in some unguarded moment; constant inclination to talk of her troubles to others. Leucorrhœa; the menses reappeared after being absent nine months. One prescription of Aur. met.^{30}, repeated three times daily for one week, removed all the mental symptoms, but as the patient removed to the West, I am unable to say whether the other symptoms were removed or not.

CASE II.—Sarah D., aged about sixty years; leucophlegmatic temperament; eyelid swollen and red, with profuse acrid lachrymation; itching very much evening and night; most soreness in the canthi; worse from heat of the fire; headache in the evening. Puls.^{30}, five powders, taken one each day; cured.

CASE III.—Was called, July 30th, 1880, to attend Mrs. P. in her third confinement. I found a breech presentation, and labor was tedious. The child was finally delivered with the blunt hook, and delivery was immediately followed by a very profuse and exhausting hæmorrhage. The blood pouring away as from a hydrant, so that in a few minutes the patient was pulseless and almost breathless; the slightest motion, even breathing, as it came in irregular gasps, seemed to aggravate the flow of bright-red blood, and I thought my patient about to expire. Erigeron^{3} in water, a few doses repeated at intervals of from three to five minutes, completely checked the hæmorrhage and there was nothing more than the normal lochia thereafter. The patient made a good recovery.

AMERICAN HOMŒOPATHIC PUBLISHING SOCIETY.

REPORTED BY CHARLES MOHR, M.D., SECRETARY.

THE third annual meeting of the stockholders was held on Monday, November 8th, 1880, at the residence of A. R. Thomas, M.D., Philadelphia.

Dr. Thomas was called on to preside, and Isaac G. Smedley, M.D., acted as Secretary.

The secretary of the retiring Board of Directors submitted the following annual report:

"Since the report submitted one year ago, the society has issued Volume II of Hering's *Guiding Symptoms,* which was more favorably received even than Volume I, and soon after its appearance many new subscribers were secured for the whole work, some of them (35) becoming stockholders in the Publishing Society.

"The death of the venerable author necessarily delayed for a time the labor required to put Volume III on the market. The literary executors,* however, are now busily engaged on this volume, and it will be placed in the hands of the subscribers at no distant day. Our agents, Messrs. J. M. Stoddart & Co., who have a large experience in the sale of subscription books, assure us that it only requires that one or two more volumes shall be issued to insure a very large addition to the list of subscribers. This consummation will be much more speedily reached if more of the profession can be induced to purchase stock and Volumes I and II *at once.* This will encourage the editors, who, it must be understood, are laboring without any remuneration, and are willing to do all they can to publish the whole work, *if the profession wants it.* Dr. Hering labored incessantly on the *Guiding Symptoms* for fifty years, sacrificing ease and money, hoping some day to give to the world the best and most complete Materia Medica ever published. His hope may be realized if the homœopathic profession wills it so. The MSS. are in such shape as will enable the editors to do their appointed work. It should, therefore, be the endeavor and pleasure of every homœopath, who feels any gratitude for what Hering was to Homœopathy, to become a holder of at least one share of stock, costing $10, and a purchaser of the volumes as they appear. This work is Dr. Hering's self-erected monument, one that does him more honor than any that may be reared of stone, and more enduring and endearing, and, being a legacy to his family, can only be made a source of revenue by its publication and *sale.* Our recommendation, therefore, is that each stockholder will further interest himself to the extent of inducing other members of the profession to become subscribers.

"During the year no work has been offered for publication. This is to be deprecated. The publication of some small books that would meet with a ready sale would be the means

* Drs. Charles G. Raue, C. B. Knerr, and C. Mohr.

of rapidly increasing the interest of the profession in the Society and its objects.

"The Treasurer's report, hereunto annexed, shows in detail the receipts ($1357.33) and expenditures ($1310.10.)"

This report was accepted and ordered to be printed.

The annual election for a Board of Directors was then held, and resulted in the choice of the following: A. R. Thomas, M.D., President; W. C. Goodno, M.D , Treasurer; C. Mohr, M.D., Secretary; B. F. Betts, M.D., M. M. Walker, M.D., C. B. Knerr, M.D., C. R. Norton, M.D.

After some discussion, during which the stockholders expressed a desire that the newly elected Board of Directors should do everything possible to secure the early completion of the *Guiding Symptoms*, the Society adjourned.

HOMŒOPATHIC MEDICAL SOCIETY OF THE COUNTY OF PHILADELPHIA.

REPORTED BY CHARLES MOHR, M D., SECRETARY.

THE regular meeting was held in the hall of the Hahnemann Medical College on Thursday evening, November 11th, 1880, Dr. E. A. Farrington presiding. Nearly fifty physicians were present.

Dr. Horace J. Shinkle was elected to membership, and the applications of Drs. J. P. Birch, R. Straube and F. D. Mount were received and referred to the censors, under the rule.

The President appointed Dr. W. B. Trites chairman of the Bureau of Surgery and Clinical Surgery for the ensuing year, to report in October, 1881.

In order to make the fees of newly elected members more equitable, the following amendment to the by-laws was submitted, action to be taken at the December meeting:

"SEC. I. The initiation fee shall be one dollar, payable within one month after election. Besides the initiation fee, the newly elected members shall pay dues at the rate of one dollar per annum, proportioned according to the unexpired time of the fiscal year.

"SEC. II. Each member shall pay annually the sum of one dollar at the meeting in April."

Dr. Charles M. Thomas, chairman of the Bureau of Ophthalmology, Otology and Laryngology, then submitted a report embracing the following papers, which were read, accepted, and referred for publication in the HAHNEMANNIAN MONTHLY, viz.:

a. Anisometropia, by Bushrod W. James, M.D.

b. Mydriatics: Their Action and Uses, by C. M. Thomas, M.D.

c. Homatropin, by W. H. Bigler, M.D., and C. Bartlett, M.D.

A discussion then ensued, in which Dr. J. C. Morgan said, on the question of mydriatics interfering with the action of potentized medicines, he had not quite made up his mind, but he had settled to his own satisfaction that carbolic acid used locally in surgical diseases as an antiseptic did not mar the action of the indicated homœopathic remedy. It interferes no more than does coffee, tea, or salt. So, too, after the use of anæsthetics, potentized drugs act. He believed the potentized remedy more often antidoted the crude drug and prevented its proper action. He called attention to the fact that formerly it was taught that presbyopia and farsight were one and the same thing; but now it is taught that in presbyopia there is loss of flexibility of the lens, and therefore loss of the power of accommodation, whether the patient is nearsighted or farsighted. He mentioned a case of anisometropia in a lady who had such severe headaches that she had to cover the windows with shawls, bury her face in her hands, and lie perfectly quiet. Glasses $+ \frac{1}{42}$ gave partial relief. The *Lac defloratum* 1^{m} removed the headaches until the following spring, when she was fitted for glasses again. For anisometropia, $China^{200}$ (when there is hypermetropia), *Magnesia phos.* (in the myopic), and *Pulsatilla* (when mental symptoms correspond) had been found useful. Von Graefe had observed that Atropia diminished the intraocular tension, others that it increased it; but old-school physicians seem capable of observing but one effect. From an old-school standpoint, mydriatics are necessary in iritis to prevent posterior synechia. He (Dr. Morgan) had treated rheumatic iritis without Atropia. One patient was put into a darkened room and on Ferrum phos., and was cured; still he would not say that mydriatics must never be used in iritis. In prolapse of the iris Atropia may be used. Physostigma, according to the late Dr. Woodyatt, has been found useful in progressive myopia. The irritation produced by Atropia is frequently the result of a badly prepared or a spoiled solution. He had cured a case of glaucoma, so diagnosed by himself and Dr. C. M. Thomas, with $Pulsatilla^{200}$, there being now no impairment of the visual field.

Dr. J. K. Lee thought Dr. Morgan's position, that crude drugs did not interfere with potentized medicine, untenable, and desired to enter a protest to any such teaching. He believed that the proper sphere for mydriatics was for the dilatation of the pupil for mechanical purposes.

Dr. A. Korndœrfer's experience led him to disagree with Dr. Morgan, and related a sad experience he had twelve years ago with Carbolic acid, used as a disinfectant in scarlatina. He had three cases of this disease in one family; two were doing very well, but the third child had some dangerous symptoms. Dr. Lippe was called in consultation, and in a couple of days the children were all in a fair way to recovery, when a new nurse was employed, who sprinkled the room of the two lighter cases with Carbolic acid, and the next morning both children were dead. Dr. Hering had told him that Carbolic acid so used was devilish stuff, and worthy only of condemnation. He related a case of neuralgia treated by *Spigelia*, well indicated, but an instillation of Atropia sulph. interfered with its curative powers.

Dr. W. H. Bigler said he had often antidoted the bad effects of instillations of Atropia in the eye, with Atropia $\frac{1}{1000}$ gr. given internally.

Dr. Harriet J. Sartain confirmed the views set forth that the potentized drug was more likely to antidote the crude drug, than the crude drug, the potentized. *Hyoscyamus* had frequently acted antidotally to Sulphate of atropia in her practice.

Dr. B. W. James was in the habit of using Eserine locally where Atropia was acting too powerfully. He questioned the cure of Dr. Morgan's case of glaucoma. Time would decide however.

Discussion closed, and Dr. W. H. Bigler was appointed chairman for the ensuing year.

The Bureau of Zymoses and Dermatology will report December 9th, 1880.

THE HOMŒOPATHIC MEDICAL SOCIETY OF CHESTER, DELAWARE AND MONTGOMERY COUNTIES.

REPORTED BY L. HOOPES, M.D., SECRETARY.

This society, at its regular quarterly session, at the Bingham House, Philadelphia, elected the following officers to serve for the ensuing year: President, Dr. J. B. Wood; Vice-President, Dr. J. H. Way; Secretary, Dr. L. Hoopes, of Downingtown; Corresponding Secretary, Dr. R. P. Mercer, of Chester; Treasurer, Dr. C. Preston.

A memorial to the trustees and faculty of Hahnemann Medical College of Philadelphia, urging the admission of women, was adopted by a vote of six yeas to four nays, and Drs. I. D. Johnson, J. B. Wood, C. Preston, and L. B. Hawley were appointed a committee to present it.

On motion, it was agreed that the society admit women to membership on the same conditions as men.

Dr. J. B. Wood read a paper on the "Medical Education of Women." Dr. L. Hoopes reported some interesting "Cases from Practice."

The next meeting of the society will be held at the same place on the first Tuesday in January, 1881.

REVIEW OF A REVIEW.

DEAR EDITORS: Dr. Taylor, in his "Review," in your issue of November, page 671, is so much in the "facetious vein," that one cannot but wonder how the author, who dealt telling facetiæ upon the Milwaukee's devoted head, has come to grief; but evidently he has met Lewis Sherman, and "he is his."

To prove this, one need only read "Spirit of Fairness on the part of Low Dilutionists." "'Cheap and nasty,' is the verdict of Dr. Sherman, in which verdict all low dilution homœopathists will concur;" "no battle, but a slaughter; no retreat, but a rout;" "all tests applied to the 30ths have . . . . proved them to be without drug matter, and without drug power;" "the laugh, as well as the argument, is now all on the side of the low dilutionists," etc. Shade of Carroll Dunham! thou of the *suaviter in modo, fortiter in re,* is this the salute which thy lovers fire over thy grave, in honor of thy brave and true championship of "freedom of medical opinion and action?" Wast thou but a blockhead after all? Thy editorship, thy professorship, thy experience, thy testimony,—were all these a grand self-deception at best, or, worse, an ignoble fraud? Who are these that defend thy good name, who build and adorn thy sepulchre?

Well, Messrs. Editors, such lapses carry within themselves the assurance of vital reaction, just as do all other pathogeneses. Moderate men will revolt, and weak men, if men at all, will become strong, in resentment of these tirades, as well as of certain papers entertained by the American Institute, and which Dr. T. praises.

Just here let me assure Dr. Taylor, and your readers, that not all the "eminent homœopathists" are content, as he very improperly implies, to be "counted in" with the opponents of the 30ths. I speak by the card when I repudiate such use of the name of my friend, Professor J. Edwards Smith, M.D., of Cleveland, a microscopist, too, of the very first rank, as admitted by both schools of medicine, and of whom our own is justly proud. Publicly and privately Professor Smith loses no opportunity to insist that it is not in the mathematics of the microscope, as *now* conditioned, to settle the potency question, nor to decide anything in regard to "the ultimate divisibility of matter." Both his papers on Gold triturations expressly so declare. Even Professor C. Wesselhoeft, with his present light, may be reasonably expected to admit the same. I leave other gentlemen to speak for themselves, but you will permit me to add that the cheeks of the scholarly chairman of the bureau must burn with shame as he reads the lucubrations of certain of his associates and admirers, now gone abroad as samples of American homœopathic erudition! J. C. M.

"DRUG ATTENUATION."

LETTER FROM MESSRS. BOERICKE & TAFEL.

PHILADELPHIA, November 15th, 1880.

EDITORS OF THE HAHNEMANNIAN MONTHLY.

GENTLEMEN: Our attention has been called to an article in your last number, which contains a misstatement which needs prompt correction.

The writer of the article "Drug Attenuation" makes the following remark:

> "Would he (Hahnemann), who was a model of neatness in pharmacy, have indorsed the 'fluxion potentizer' of Boericke & Tafel, with its dirty Schuylkill water and its rubber channel, to the potentizing glass?"

As this remark stands and reads, it is decidedly misleading to your readers, and it seems that the writer did not take proper care about informing himself.

The facts about a fluxion potentizer (to start with, *not* Boericke & Tafel's, *but* Boericke's) are the following, and we are sure that yourselves can readily recall the facts, as you at the time saw the working of it.

About seven years ago when the subject of high potencies by the fluxion process was much talked of in Philadelphia, our Dr. Boericke made some experiments with five remedies, and at last constructed a little machine which both measured and potentized (*i. e.*, shook) the liquid. This we made known through our *Bulletin*, but we were careful enough to state that certain (five mentioned) remedies were potentized to the millionth, and "*these remedies we regard as an* EXPERIMENT *toward* TRYING *to* DEFINE THE LIMITS *of* POTENTATION, *and to that effect, these potencies are offered gratis to such as choose to try their efficacy.*" . . . .

These potencies were never advertised for sale; no further remedies were ever made by it; in fact, the matter was not mentioned again, and dropped of itself out of existence. To refer to it now in the manner the writer has done, we regard as a gross misstatement, and is simply doing us injustice.

As an experiment, however, "*to try to define the limits of potentation,*" we regard it as a perfectly legitimate one, as legitimate as any other test; nor can we see that any one, not even Hahnemann himself, could object to experimentation, if all the facts about it are given.

We remain, very truly yours,
BOERICKE & TAFEL.

TRACHEOTOMY SUPERSEDED.

IN the *British Medical Journal*, July 24th–31st, Dr. McEwen, of the Glasgow Royal Infirmary, advocates the use of tracheal tubes by the mouth instead of tracheotomy. He gives three cases in which he had recourse to the tubes, and their use was attended with very good results. Two were for the relief of œdema glottidis, and one to occlude hæmorrhage from the larynx during an operation. The practical conclusions which he draws from these cases are as follows: 1. Tubes may be passed through the mouth into the trachea, not only in chronic but also in acute affections, such as œdema glottidis. 2. They can be introduced without placing the patient under an anæsthetic. 3. The respirations can be perfectly carried on through them. 4. The expectoration can be expelled through them. 5. Deglutition can be carried on during the time the tube is in the trachea. 6. Though the patient at first suffers from a painful sensation, yet this passes off, and the parts soon become tolerant of the presence of the tube. 7. The patient can sleep with the tube *in situ*. 8. The tubes, in these cases at least, were harmless. 9. The ultimate results were rapid, complete, and satisfactory. 10. Such tubes may be introduced in operations on the face and mouth in order to keep blood from gaining access to the trachea, and for the purpose of administering the anæsthetic, and they answer this purpose admirably.—*Independent Practitioner*.

THE

HAHNEMANNIAN MONTHLY.

A HOMŒOPATHIC JOURNAL OF

MEDICINE AND SURGERY.

Editors,

E. A. Farrington, M.D. Pemberton Dudley, M.D.

Business Manager,

Bushrod W. James, M.D.

Vol. II. Philadelphia, Pa., December, 1880. No. 12.

☞ The Editors consider themselves responsible for the maintenance of the dignity and courtesy of the journal, but *not* for the opinions expressed by its contributors.

Editorial Department.

Our Threescore and Ten Contributors.—As the fifteenth volume of the journal is about closing, the publishers desire to express their obligations to those who, with no interest in its success above that of any other homœopathic periodical, have yet done so much to make it acceptable and profitable to its readers. From the numerous kindly and encouraging expressions received from our readers, and from our rapidly increasing subscription list, we are convinced that the year's issue is regarded as a success, and for this we have to thank our contributors.

The first few numbers of the volume were furnished almost entirely by Philadelphia contributors. Undesirable as this was, it seemed to be unavoidable. Now, however, we are in receipt of first-class articles from eminent writers of our school in all parts of the country, and have the promise of papers for next year from some whose names do not appear in the list of contributors to this volume. And we hope to retain every one of those who have favored us in the past.

The Magnet in Therapeutics.—The November issue of the *New York Medical Journal* contains an interesting article by Dr. W. A. Hammond, entitled "The Therapeutical Use of the Magnet."

While the doctor gives due credit to the experiments of Reichenbach, Vansant, Charcot and Volpicelli, he fails to even mention the extensive studies of Hahnemann, which antedate the oldest observations quoted. In these days, when it is fashionable to adorn literary contributions with numerous references to writers on the subject treated, and even to subjoin more or less lengthy bibliographical tables, such an omission as that referred to above is highly significant of the bias of Dr. Hammond.

Hahnemann and his followers are so generally ostracized by the old school of physicians that their contributions to medical literature are either wholly disregarded or are clandestinely appropriated without any acknowledgment of their source. As an illustration of the first we have Dr. Hammond's neglect of Hahnemann's experiments with the magnet. Illustrations of the second are very numerous. We will merely refer to one or two of its more recent plagiarisms. Copper is now recommended as a prophylactic against cholera. Homœopathic literature is replete with such recommendations from the time of Hahnemann to the present day. Quite recently Nitroglycerin is advertised as a specific for congestive headaches! Homœopaths also employ this drug for similar conditions. This would be a remarkable coincidence were it not for the fact that the new school has used the remedy ever since 1848! Prejudice and bigotry are selfish masters, and so can have no part with honesty. How is it that we are never shown the steps by which allopaths are led to these "discoveries?"

The Cloven Foot.—The *Homœopathic World* for November 1st, 1880, contains an article by Dr. E. W. Berridge entitled "Reminiscences of the late Constantine Hering, M.D.," which would be highly amusing if it were not intensely disgusting. It seems that the writer of that article made a series of visits to Dr. Hering just previous and subsequent to the meeting of the American Institute in Milwaukee, and from a careful reading of his paper, the object of those interviews appears to have been to secure the sanction and influence of Dr. Hering to a dastardly scheme for dividing the homœopathic profession into two distinct and opposing factions. The writer, who evidently has not learned as much as he might from the lesson he received at Milwaukee, has so far mistaken the temper of honest homœopathists as to assert boldly that he has for years been laboring for the destruction of homœopathic influence and prestige. Of course the profession cares nothing for what Dr. Berridge's opinion may or may not be, but all true homœopathists will be glad to know, even from his lips, that Dr. Hering was unalterably opposed to the villainous project. "There is nothing more horrible than a split," wrote the stanch old hero. "When I asked him," says Berridge, "to join our new Hahnemannian Association, he said, 'I will do it if a clause is inserted to the effect that *your sole object is to help those who stand half way.*'" Whether this assurance was given we do not know, but Hering's name was not secured. At any rate Dr. Berridge now hopes that this Hahnemannian Association "will prove the thin edge of the wedge" for effecting "a clean separation" from those who will not allow ignorant pretenders to be the sole interpreters of the principles and facts of medical science, nor tolerate their impudent interference in the conscientious exercise of professional prerogatives. We shall be greatly surprised if the Hahnemannian Association as a body does not at the very first opportunity place the seal of its condemnation upon Dr. Berridge's little game, and very plainly inform him that here in America, at least, the notoriety he craves cannot be purchased at so low a price.

Even the civilization of this nineteenth century has not proved sufficient to prevent the growth of the usual crop of mountebanks. Every age has produced its quacks in religion, in morals and in science,—men who, with unblushing impudence, have claimed not only the ability but the right to fix the creeds of other men, to determine a world's belief, and decide its practice. The world to-day is administering to these impostors some pretty sharp lessons, but every little while it becomes necessary to place an iron heel upon their necks and crush them into a little "decent respect for the opinions of mankind."

So far from being apprehensive of any serious inroads upon the integrity and solidity of the homœopathic profession by the machinations of its enemies, we believe that this last and most impotent assault will only make its members draw closer together,—like sheep, when wolves are prowling around. The few men bad enough to engage in such a nefarious undertaking are, fortunately, not possessed of sufficient ability and influence to make it successful.

"THE LEGION OF HONOR."—The energetic editors of *The Organon* have secured a list of names, comprising such homœopathic physicians as are willing to subscribe to a specified creed, which has been derived from the principles of medicine as expounded by Hahnemann. This list is denominated "The Legion of Honor." As a firm believer in Hahnemann's method of treating the sick, we added our name to the list when solicited. But in so doing, we claimed the right to use any external application which was employed in accordance with the law of similars; and, further, we protested against some of the company we were called upon to keep. We recognized the names of quite a number in the Legion who we know are not practicing as they claim to. One name in the list before us is singularly out of place, since we know that its possessor has treated his patients with extravagant doses of crude drugs, and has used pounds of purgative medicine, and this, too, since signing the roll.

If, then, *The Organon* wishes to publish a list of such practitioners as desire to openly express their allegiance to Hahnemannianism let there be a conscientious revision of the list as published. This can be done, because one of the editors has already been informed of several on the roll who are violating their contract. Either this, or drop the title of "Legion of *Honor*."

PETTY JEALOUSY.—In the New York *Medical Record*, October 30th, 1880, are the following words: "Dr. Austin Flint, Jr., has declined an invitation to accept the chair of Physiology in the Jefferson Medical College of Philadelphia. The Bellevue Hospital Medical College is to be congratulated on this decision. But we wonder what Philadelphia had to offer which New York has not—outside of Dr. Buchanan?"

Aside from the egotism evinced, the *Record*, since it knows full well the unsullied reputation of all Philadelphia colleges, —the diploma-shops being now defunct,—displays a spirit of petty jealousy and even malignancy. In politics such littleness is so common as to be expected, but when professional men stoop so low, one cannot but express his mortification and chagrin.

A doctor's calling should make him cosmopolitan. He should know no limit to his possible usefulness; and, if he really loves his office, that of healing the sick, he should extend a helping hand or cheering word whenever and wherever he can. If his colleague's reputation is at stake, he should assist in its preservation rather than add his personal influence to aid in the accomplishment of an evil purpose.

If our New York contemporary should but remember that many of Dr. Buchanan's co-conspirators came from the State of New York, perhaps it might make that journal a little more just towards the reputable colleges of Philadelphia; and then again, perhaps it mightn't.

THE NEW VOLUME.—The HAHNEMANNIAN MONTHLY will enter upon the sixteenth year of its existence with brighter prospects than would have been deemed possible one year ago. During the past year it has been fortunate enough to gain a large number of friends, and to lose very few. Its list of subscribers grows steadily and rapidly, and its contributors are of a class of which any journal might well be proud. With such opportunities as are opening before us, a failure to make a good journal would evince only the grossest incompetence or the most culpable indifference on the part of its managers.

The opening number of the new volume will furnish, we think, a most acceptable treat to our readers. It will contain articles by James B. Bell, M.D., John C. Morgan, M.D., John E. James, M.D., Morris Weinor, M.D., E. A. Farrington, M.D., George B. Peck, M.D., Charles M. Thomas, M.D., Bushrod W. James, M.D., Henry C. Houghton, M.D., F. F. Casseday, M.D., the late A. O. H. Hardenstein, M.D., and perhaps others, besides the usual array of book reviews, gleanings, news, personal items, etc. These papers, one and all, are of a purely practical character, designed to help us in our daily practice, and we are very sure that our readers will enjoy their perusal and derive profit from them.

NOT A SPLIT BUT A SPLINTER.—It takes a true aim, a steady nerve and a strong muscle to split a giant of the forest. If these be lacking, the axe glances and strikes the shins of the too conceited young woodman. So will it be with any attempt to rive asunder the members of our noble profession. It will only take off a shaving from the outside—where the excrescences grow, and the parasites crawl, and the dirt collects,—and it will leave the trunk smoother and whiter, and cleaner and healthier than ever. A little, just a little, of the good wood may be splintered off, but the heart of oak will not be disturbed. Spirit of Hering, rest in peace!

MISPRINT.—In our last number, page 692, line 11, "better" should be *latter*. The error makes the writer say just the opposite of what he intended.

Book Department.

A MANUAL OF PHARMACODYNAMICS. Fourth edition, revised and augmented; being the course of Materia Medica and Therapeutics delivered at the London School of Homœopathy, 1877 to 1880. By Richard Hughes, L.R.C.P., Ed. Published at London by Leath & Ross. Octavo, 945 pages.

The volume before us is, as the author himself states, a revised and augmented issue of the third edition. The framework on which the former edition was constructed is substantially unaltered; "but it has been filled in with a liberal hand, so as to make the volume more than one-fourth larger than its predecessor."

The first seven lectures, embracing 106 pages, are devoted to introductory remarks and various interesting matters connected with the principles of homœopathy, its posology, etc. The remaining lectures, exclusive of an appendix and two indexes, one to the medicines and the other clinical, are devoted to the description, etc., of drugs.

If we counted correctly, the book treats more or less fully of 281 remedies.

Of the general qualifications of the work we can speak in the highest terms. Clothed in excellent English, and composed in an easy style, it becomes a pleasure to peruse its pages, rather than a mental strain needed to grasp the full meaning of the text.

The book is to be commended, too, for the immense amount of labor it represents. Our author has read very extensively, as his abundant quotations show, and his research into the source of homœopathic drugs is in itself worth the price of the book. There is no one volume in our literature which contains so much general information concerning homœopathic materia medica as the one under review.

In treating of the general principles of drug action, Dr. Hughes introduces a theory which we most emphatically object to. "All on one side of our organism," he says, "is life; on the other it is non-life. Now this white corpuscle, which I have taken as the type of living matter, is a structureless, transparent, colorless, semifluid substance, ... and in continued spontaneous movement. Such is living matter everywhere. . . . . The cell-wall may be taken as a type of this other substance. In it there is the beginning of structure, of rigidity. . . . It is 'formed material,' and so far has passed from life to death, and has become the subject of chemical and mechanical laws, of which, in its living state, it was independent."

The protoplasmic theory of life is absurd; at least so it seems to us. But when the human organism is described as alive and dead, as life dying into nerve, muscle, bone, etc., as a *living corpse*, reason and common-sense are outraged. Why protoplasm itself is dead. It is only a convenient resting-place whereon the very scientist, groping in the darkness of materialism, rests in his insane search. Our author would have us believe that whatever modifications may be required in the protoplasmic theory, "in the time to come as to details, there can be no doubt as to its substantial truth." Life is the Lord's, and he distributes its bounty to all created forms, human, merely animal, vegetable, and mineral. It is manifested in one way in rational man, in another in the brute, in another in the vegetable, and in still another in the mineral world. Life does not cease, even if, for the sake of argument, we grant protoplasm to be its synonym, when we descend into the chemical and mechanical laws of matter. The observer of nature sees life in the wonderful movings of the planetary systems, in the formation and dissolution of the clouds, in the course of the winds, and, no less, in the miracles of the chemical laboratory. In the human organism the soul lives, not protoplasm. And every bodily function, be it ideation, respiration, digestion, or locomotion, is a manifestation of the soul in a material body, which is constructed for its habitation, and by and in which, it is present in this nether world. Therefore there must be mediate forms far more subtle than protoplasm. Nature is not plain and structureless in her microscopic work; and in her hypermicroscopic productions, as she rises and deepens towards her origin, her wonders multiply instead of growing more simple.

In regard to the vexed subject of dosage Dr. Hughes places himself on record as favorable to low attenuations, though he by no means denies the efficacy of the 30th or 200th potency. In fact his language is emphatic when he states that "the testimony in favor of the high is overwhelming." His own experience with the 6th, 12th, and 30th is such as to make him "join with unquestioning acclamation in their praise." But how inconsistent do these words seem when we read them in connection with the following, taken from the same page: "Much as I regret the necessity of employing the higher infinitesimals, I cannot but acknowledge it." These are an echo of Watzke's strange remarks: "I am, alas! (I say, alas! for I would much rather have upheld the larger doses which accord with current views) I am compelled to declare myself for the higher dilutions." Why should the seeker after truth regret the necessity of abandoning his mistaken opinions? Should he not rather rejoice?

But such an admission as this of the efficacy of the 30th and 200th potencies, is a terrible blow against so crude a life-substance as protoplasm. Protoplasm is comparatively tangible. It may be seen and described; but the 200th! who may measure it? Who see it? The 200th tells of a more subtle subdivision of matter than the molecule or the spherical particles of protoplasm.

We notice that Dr. Hughes, though admitting the superiority of, as he chooses to term it, the homœopathic *rule* of practice, claims the right to employ antipathic palliatives. Hence he speaks of Amyl nitrosum in angina pectoris, epilepsy, etc.; Iron in anæmia, and so on. This is perfectly consistent with his teachings concerning homœopathy, and is broad enough to invite many followers. But, believing that homœopathy is a law, rather than a rule, the subject of palliation assumes with us a different aspect. All adjuvant treatment not in accord with the law of similars is so much evidence of our ignorance of the science we profess. Such ignorance may arise from imperfect study, or it may depend upon the present state of homœopathic development. We could not say conscientiously with Dr. Hughes: "We are as free as others to use antipathic palliatives."

In reference to Iron as a food we are not prepared to deny the statement; but to regard it as the one great remedy for anæmia is too bold and general an assertion, and is altogether foreign to the genius of true medicine. Unquestionably ferruginous preparations deepen the color of the blood and increase the number of corpuscles, red and white. But the causes of anæmia are numerous, and can be reached permanently only when sought for in the legitimate method. To use a drug merely because it is a hæmatic stimulus, is no more scientific treatment than to treat other affections with specifics.

On page 808, we read: "It does not appear what led Hahnemann to introduce the juice of the cuttle-fish into medicine." We learned from the lamented Dr. Hering, that Hahnemann first obtained its symptoms from an artist who, while using Sepia, frequently moistened his brush with his lips, and so became slowly poisoned. Failing to cure his patient of symptoms, the source of which Hahnemann was then ignorant of, he persuaded the artist to desist from wetting his brush with his saliva, when, lo! he began at once to improve. His symptoms were carefully collated, and subsequent provings confirmed them as belonging to Sepia.

There are some omissions of symptoms in the book before us which we would have been better pleased to see inserted. These exclusions, we think, are of a kind to set forth the profounder operations of the soul in its body. They tell of the emotions and their material effects. They describe disturbances in the most hidden and refined particles of the body, and tend to lift the thought above the crudities of modern physiology and pathology, and suggest the construction of a new science. They are not at enmity with their coarser allies. They do not refute pathology and kindred sciences; nor do they forbid a settling down into physiological and pathological terms, as Dr. Hughes has done. But they wonderfully expand the view, and show how much too small are our terms to fully hold them. And, above all, they assert their essentialness in the just and effective application of Hahnemann's rules concerning mental symptoms, direction of symptoms, etc. They are the inevitables of an untrammelled homœopathy.

Still, as we stated before, the work as a whole is well worthy a place in every physician's library. It contains a vast store of facts, so entertainingly told, that we would we could have been present when they were delivered. But the next best thing is to read them. F.

Index Catalogue of the Library of the Surgeon-General's Office, United States Army. Authors and Subjects. Vol. I, A to Berlinski. With a list of Abbreviations of Titles of Periodicals indexed. Washington: Government Printing Office, 1880. Royal Octavo, pp. 888.

To essay a review of this magnificent work, would be somewhat like attempting the same impossible task upon a Webster's Unabridged. The book is just what it professes to be,—not only a *catalogue of the books* but an *index of the subjects* treated of in the books, yes, and in the periodicals and pamphlets contained in that vast storehouse,—the library of the surgeon-general's office. As a sample of what the book is, or rather of what the library contains, the article "Aneurisms" includes no less than one hundred and thirty-two closely printed columns of references, yet Dr. Billings, in his preface to the work, is careful to call attention to the fact that "this is not a complete medical bibliography, and that any one who relies upon it as such, will commit a serious error."

The general arrangement of the work is the one preferred by the large majority of physicians to whom a "specimen fasciculus" was sent in 1876. The present volume includes 9090 authorities, representing 8031 volumes, and 6398 pamphlets. It also includes 9000 subject-titles of separate books and pamphlets, and 34,604 titles of articles in periodicals. The volume (I) embraces A to Berlinski, so that a dozen similar issues will probably be required to complete this vast work. D.

The Skin in Health and Disease. By L. Duncan Bulkley, M.D., Attending Physician for Skin and Venereal Diseases at the New York Hospital, Out-Patient Department; late Physician to the Skin Department, Demilt Dispensary, New York, etc. Philadelphia: Presley Blakiston, 1012 Walnut Street. 1880. 16mo., pp. 148. Price, 50 cents.

This is another of the Health Primer Series issued by the above house under the editorial direction of Dr. W. W. Keen. It includes chapters on the "Anatomy and Physiology of the Skin," "The Care of the Skin in Health," "Diseases of the Skin," "Diet and Hygiene in Diseases of the Skin," and a very complete "Index." It is also well illustrated. The work ought to interest the profession, as well as the laity, for whom it is specially intended. D.

Treatise on Therapeutics. Translated by D. F. Lincoln, M.D., from the French of A. Trousseau, Professor of Therapeutics in the Faculty of Medicine of Paris, Physician to the Hôtel Dieu, Member of the Academy of Medicine, Commander of the Legion of Honor, Ex-representative of the people in the Constituent Assembly, etc., and H. Pidoux, Member of the Academy of Medicine, Honorary Physician to the Hospitals, Inspector of Eaux Bonnes, Honorary Member of the Royal Belgian Academy of Medicine, Honorary President of the Société de Thérapeutique, etc. Ninth edition, revised and enlarged, with the assistance of Constantine Paul, Professeur Agrigé in the Faculty of Medicine of Paris, Physician to the Hospital Saint-Antoine, Sécrétaire General of the Société de Thérapeutique. Volume II. New York: William Wood & Company, 27 Great Jones Street, 1880. Pp. 299.

This is the second volume of the work we noted in the July number of our journal, and contains four chapters, as follows: 5, Antiphlogistic treatment; 6, Evacuants; 7, Musculo-motor excitants, or excito-motors; 8, Narcotics. Under the latter, in speaking of Aconite, he says of it in regard to erysipelas and neuralgia:

"Aconite has been recommended in erysipelas, whether spontaneous or traumatic. The English surgeon, Liston, seems to be the first, according to M. Imbert-Gourbeyre, who used this remedy in this disease. According to his observations the use of the extract of Aconite in erysipelas and other inflammatory affections, is often followed by a notable diminution of vascular excitement, which makes bloodletting needless. Fleming quotes several cases of erysipelas of internal origin, located in the limbs, and accompanied by very acute inflammation, which yielded very quickly to a few doses of Aconite. But M. Teissier, of Lyons, first insisted very strongly on the value of this remedy in the treatment of traumatic erysipelas. 'I have repeatedly seen,' says this distinguished observer, 'erysipelas appear in the neighborhood of wounds or ulcers, and accompanied by general symptoms, as burning fever, chills, desire to vomit, delirium, fugax, etc., which improved with remarkable promptitude under the administration of ten or twenty drops of tincture of Aconite per diem. I particularly remember,' he adds, 'two patients who had extremely painful traumatic erysipelas, with febrile symptoms so marked as to make me anxious, but who were relieved in a truly astonishing way in the space of twenty-four hours.'"

We will add that Aconite, the value of which in certain neuralgias, especially those of the face, cannot be questioned, is one of the best remedies (according to Addington Symonds) for nervous cephalalgia. It would seem most useful in cases where cephalalgia affects a chronic form, in which there is a continual malaise or a constant disposition to headache. Three drops of the tincture are given three times a day, alone or in combination with some tonic.

Hahnemann, long before Trousseau issued his notable work, was using Aconite, not only in erysipelatous and neuralgic diseases, but made it a hinge upon which turned the door against the antiphlogistic treatment so much in vogue at that time.

Hahnemann, in his *Materia Medica Pura*, under Aconite, says: "It is precisely in the cases in which the partisans of allopathy pride themselves most on their method; it is in the violent acute inflammatory fevers where they expect to save their patients alone by excessive and frequent bloodlettings, and hereby exceed so far the powers of homœopathy that they most grossly deceive themselves. Here, more than ever, in fact, homœopathy exhibits her universal superiority, for she has no necessity for shedding a drop of that precious fluid, of which allopathy is so dangerously profuse, in order to triumph over those fatal fevers, and restore health sometimes in as few hours as the ordinary practice requires months, completely to re-establish those whom their violent remedies have not, it is true, conducted to the tomb, but have left a prey to those chronic sufferings which are their natural consequences." B. W. J.

HOMEMADE TREATMENT, copyrighted by C. F. Nichols, 1879,

Is a unique little brochure, without any title-page—only a P with an M in it, standing forth in the middle of an otherwise blank page. *Homemade Treatment* is printed in gilded letters diagonally across the pasteboard cover; so possibly *this* is meant for the title-page.

Turning to the substance-matter of the book we find forty pages just as oddly arranged as is the title. While the entire page is perhaps forty square inches, the printed matter covers an area of only eight or ten square inches.

But when we proceed to read this book we are pleased with its contents. It is like a fruit with a thick rind, the centre of which, though small, is rich in flavor and wholesome. In a commonplace style the author has given plain directions for the use of nineteen of our oft-indicated remedies.

In the quaintest way possible he tells the reader how to apply the principles of homœopathy and avoid mere names of diseases. Some M.D.s might learn a lesson here, and prune themselves of a useless and pedantic display of weighty words—so weighty that they crush out all the meaning and sense of pure homœopathy. Truth, like beauty, needs but little adornment.

Part second of the work is not introduced with the usual heading, but with an epitaph, inclosed between two diagonal heavy black lines. It consists of a pithy extract from *Pilgrim's Progress*, and is really a paraphrase on the failing power of the old giant, allopathy, instead of an epitaph. It serves, however, to preface a series of extracts, the purport of which is to show the efficacy of homœopathy and the ineffective assaults of its adversaries. This is excellent, and we advise physicians to procure several copies of the queer little book and distribute them among the laity, after they have first enjoyed it themselves. F.

PROCEEDINGS OF THE HOMŒOPATHIC MEDICAL SOCIETY OF OHIO. Sixth Annual Session: Cincinnati, May 18th and 19th, 1880.

This is a neatly printed pamphlet of 100 pages, containing, in addition to the usual minutes, list of members, etc., several interesting reports from the various bureaus appointed by the society.

After a brief and well-rounded welcoming address by Dr. J. D. Buck, of Cincinnati, the President, Dr. E. B. Gaylord, of Toledo, delivered his official address. His remarks were pointed and instructive, embracing an interesting account of the gigantic strides which have been made in one year in the scientific world.

Dr. Eaton, who has lately so ably edited a work on gynæcology, contributes an article on Dysmenorrhœa. The Bureau of Surgery is favored with a lecture on Catheterism, by Dr. D. W. Hartshorn.

Dr. J. A. Gann writes concerning The Relation of Food to Physiology and Pathology.

The pathology of convulsions is described, with numerous references to standard authors, by Dr. M. H. Parmalee.

Sanitary science claims the attention of Dr. Eggleston, who furnishes two papers, the latter of which examines into the now fashionable germ theory.

Clinical medicine comprises three papers. The first, on Diphtheria, by Dr. R. B. Johnson, discusses the nature of the disease and details the treatment. The second, on Clinical Thermometry, by Dr. H. E. Beebe, concludes with a list of remedies, during the action of which, their respective temperatures have been noted. Dr. Gillard is the author of the third paper, which is very brief, and contains his belief that the typhoid poison is essentially miasmatic.

Dr. R. B. Rush enters a plea for an institution in which the insane may have the advantage of homœopathic treatment, and Dr. E. C. Beckwith seconds the plea with a similar article.

In the obstetrical department, Dr. J. C. Sanders comes to the conclusion that it is our bounden duly to tie the cord of the neonatus.

The concluding article of the report is one on Strabismus, by Dr. F. H. Schell.

The next meeting of the society will be held at Toledo, on the second Thursday of May, 1881. F.

TRANSACTIONS OF THE ELEVENTH ANNUAL SESSION OF THE HOMŒOPATHIC MEDICAL SOCIETY OF THE STATE OF MICHIGAN; Vol. I, No. 2.

The *Transactions* is a creditable record of a very active society. In addition to business reports, constitution, list of members, etc., we notice several interesting and instructive papers.

Among these are: "The Ophthalmoscope in General Medicine," by Dr. McGuire; "Corneal Ulcers," by Dr. Brown; "Diagnosis and Semeiology of Urethral Strictures," by Dr. Gilchrist; "Spasmodic Stricture," by Dr. Whitworth; "Urethrotomy," by Dr. Franklin; "Treatment of Stricture by Electrolysis," by Dr. Nelson; "Comparative Study of Belladonna and Atropia," by Dr. Arndt; "Advantages of the Single Remedy," by Dr. Grant; "Catarrh," by Dr. Brigham; "Colchicum in Malignant Dysentery," by Dr. Jones; "Masturbation of Women," by Dr. Arndt, a paper which we fear is but too true; "Provings of Viburnum Opulus," by Dr H. C Allen, etc.

Were it for nothing else than these Viburnum provings, the *Transactions* would be a valuable addition to the library; and we advise our readers to procure it at once. The secretary is R. B. House, M.D., of Tecumseh, who would no doubt be glad to supply copies at a reasonable figure. F.

DISEASES OF THE PHARYNX, LARYNX, AND TRACHEA. By Morell Mackenzie, M.D., London, Senior Physician to the Hospital for Diseases of the Throat and Chest, Lecturer on Diseases of the Throat at the London Medical College, and Corresponding Member of the Imperial Royal Society of Physicians of Vienna. New York, William Wood & Co., 27 Great Jones Street. 1880. pp. 440.

Another welcome volume of Wood's Medical Library presents itself in its promised time. Dr. Mackenzie has selected a theme that deeply interests the profession of the temperate zone, where the most obstinate and inveterate cases of catarrhal and other inflammations of these passages occur. His strongest and best points are found in the department of laryngoscopy, laryngeal diseases, and their medical and surgical treatment; he gives numerous wood-cut illustrations, to show the best instruments in present use, as well as the more approved methods of operating. B. W. J.

Gleanings.

Hereditary Syphilis is said to depend upon maternal and not paternal inheritance (?).—*Philadelphia Medical Times*, October 23d, 1880.

The Cost of Homatropin.—At present this valuable medicine is retailed to physicians at the rate of one dollar per grain. According to *New Remedies* for November, 1880, a cheaper method of manufacturing Amygdalic acid must be discovered before it can be sold at much lower prices.

Ergot is considered a dangerous drug in obstetrical practice. Chloroform increases the danger of post-partum hæmorrhage, and should not be used during the employment of forceps. In placenta prævia, divide the placenta with the fingers, rupture the membranes, and allow the head to descend. Experience in 800 obstetrical cases.—Dr. W. J. Kelly, *Medical Record,* October 23d, 1880.

A new acarus has been found on barley, which is of an oblong-oval shape, yellowish-white in color, with a round head and four pairs of feet. It causes, when handled, burning, itching urticaria; delicate skins are raised into papules, vesicles, and finally pustules; frequently, too, loss of appetite, sleeplessness, and febrile symptoms run over four or six days.—*Philadelphia Medical Times*, October 23d, 1880.

Paræsthesia of the Hands, consisting of an annoying, and sometimes painful numbness, was observed in 31 patients. These were not cases of organic nervous disease, at least so far as could be determined. The numbness was worse in the winter, and recurred periodically, at night or early in the morning. Sometimes the fingers were stiff, and the skin either pale or red.—James J. Putnam, *Archives of Medicine*, October, 1880.

Chian Turpentine, if genuine, has a fragrant odor, not at all like turpentine oil, little or no taste, and is very fragile, though it may be rolled into pills without adhering to the fingers. It will not dissolve in alcohol, but will leave a glutinous residue. Placed between two warm pieces of clean glass, if it contain Venice turpentine, it will look like water; if Canada balsam, a gentle heat will cause the latter to seek the circumference, for it melts more quickly than the Chian turpentine.—Professor Clay, *London Lancet;* see *Philadelphia Medical Times*, October 23d, 1880.

The Fate of Midwifery.—Professor Barker says: "When the chemist shall succeed in producing a mass constitutionally identical with protoplasmic albumen, there is every reason to expect that it will exhibit all the phenomena which characterize its life."—*Popular Science Monthly*, October, 1880.

Then the savans will begin to construct plants and animals, put vivacity into statuary, and finally fashion man himself. Obstetrics will then be a horror of the past, and Helmholtz and others who disparage the perfection of several of the organs of the body can construct them on the strictest principles of human art.—Eds.

Alcohol, in small doses, causes increased pulse-rate and cardiac force; but, if oft repeated, the pulse becomes rapid, feeble, and irregular, with diminished arterial pressure, and finally the heart is arrested in diastole. Large doses cause an immediate fall of the pulse-rate with irregular pulsations; the rate then returns to or goes above normal, but the blood-pressure diminishes. If while this increase exists another dose is given, the rate may be still further increased, but the arterial pressure is diminished, or it may immediately sink, the heart being arrested in diastole. After experimenting on animals, in which the vagi and cervical spinal cord were cut, it was found that the heart was still affected by the alcohol. Hence, alcohol must act on the heart itself.—J. D. Castillo, M.D., *Philadelphia Medical Times*, October 23d, 1880.

CHRONIC RHEUMATISM is frequently complicated with neuritis, caused by an extension of the inflammation to the nerve sheaths. Especially is this observed in rheumatism of the shoulder-joint and deltoid. The pains are usually worse at night and from motion. Pressure with the finger along the course of the brachial plexus reveals tenderness. Adhesive inflammation in the joint occurs, producing false anchylosis. In the treatment of such cases, as well as similar anchylosis elsewhere, and also stiff, deformed, joints in rheumatoid arthritis, massage and persistent movement of the joints are employed, no matter how painful such manipulation may be. By a systematic moving of the stiffened joint, mobility may be generally restored. In enlarged joints from synovial effusion, however, rest is essential, as manipulation would aggravate. And since anchylosis does not occur while the effusion lasts, such a procedure is superfluous.—W. Pepper, M.D., *Archives of Medicine*, October, 1880.

DIPHTHERITIC MEMBRANE was inoculated into thirty-two animals, with the result of causing six deaths. In no case was anything like diphtheria caused. These experiments dispute those of Oertel, who stated that such inoculated animals were infested with micrococci. The post-mortem revealed, in every case, tubercular disease. This state, at least in the rabbit, may be produced by simple local inflammation. And in the cases referred to, the inoculation was followed by local inflammation with the formation of large cheesy lumps, so the tubercles were secondary.

In the lower animals, as well as in man, chemical irritants will produce pseudo-membranous trachitis. There seems to be no anatomical difference between the lesions of true croup and of diphtheritic angina.

It is believed that the contagious material of diphtheria is really of the nature of a septic poison, which, when brought in contact with the mucous membrane, produces intense inflammation by a local action. Or, it may be absorbed, and then act locally by transmission through the blood to the membranes. Hence the writers believe the disease may be local.—*Philadelphia Medical Times*, October 23d, 1880.

Strictly speaking, this is an impossibility. No poison can attack merely a circumscribed part of so harmonious and sympathetic a mechanism as the human body.—EDS.

News and Comments.

DR. S. F. SHANNON has returned from Europe, and taken an office with his old preceptor, Dr. J. C. Burgher, 332 Penn Avenue, Pittsburg, Pa.

SETTLEMENTS—CLASS OF 1880.—Albert Rice, M.D., Columbus, Ind.; T. L Adams, M.D., Berwyn, Chester County, Pa.; W. H. Baker, M.D., Fernwood, Delaware County, Pa.

REMOVALS.—Dr. S. H. Quint, to 43 North Third Street, Camden, N. J.; Dr. Joseph M. Reeves, to 1619 Mt. Vernon Street, Philadelphia.

J. H. ENLOE, M.D., has removed from McLemoresville, Tenn., to Rome, Ga.

GREAT EXPECTATIONS.—"After many days" we are now almost able to promise our readers a paper from our friend, Dr. J. Edwards Smith, of Cleveland. It will come when the professor has time to prepare a good one, and not before.

PROFESSOR H. C. HOUGHTON has sent us an excellent paper on his specialty for our January number. By the way, we made a mistake last month in announcing his change of residence. It should be No. 44 *West Thirty-fifth Street*, New York—*not Thirty-fourth Street*, as we stated.

PETTET'S COW-POX VIRUS is reputed to be the best out, and the Philadelphia agent, Dr. T. H. Conover, 1721 Jefferson Street, receives fresh supplies almost daily. It sells at 10 points for $1, or extra heavily charged points, 5 for $1, and warranted. (See advertisement.)

THE TRANSACTIONS OF THE HOMŒOPATHIC MEDICAL SOCIETY OF PENNSYLVANIA FOR 1880,—a handsome cloth-bound volume of about 400 pages, is just issued. Members who have not received them will write at once to the Treasurer, Dr. J. F. Cooper, Allegheny, Pa. The book contains about fifty-five papers on various medical topics.

MINERAL WATERS OF CALIFORNIA.—Dr. W. Jefferson Guernsey, of Frankford, Pa, calls attention to a property of certain mineral waters of California, of "inducing blennorrhœal symptoms" (see Dunglison's *Medical Dictionary*), and asks if any provings have ever been made of these waters. Will some of our California physicians interest themselves in this important matter?

THE INTERNATIONAL HOMŒOPATHIC CONVENTION IN 1881 will assemble in London on July 11th, and a cordial invitation has been extended to American physicians to attend. The undersigned were appointed by the American Institute of Homœopathy a committee, with full powers to make arrangements. In order to do this in the most satisfactory manner, it is important to know the approximate number of those who will attend. By communicating at once to one of this committee the names of such physicians as now intend to go, and the number to accompany them, the work will be facilitated.

I. T. TALBOT, 66 Marlborough Street, Boston,
WILLIAM TOD HELMUTH, 299 Madison Avenue, New York,
BUSHROD W. JAMES, 18th and Green streets, Philadelphia,
Committee.

TRANSACTIONS OF THE WORLD'S HOMŒOPATHIC CONVENTION, 1876.—Dr. J. C. Guernsey writes us that he is hard at work upon the above volumes, and that one of them, the Historic, is all in type excepting only the chapter on "Literature."

He fully expected this volume would be issued by December 1st, but it has taken a much longer time to procure and complete the many missing links in this important work than he anticipated. Meanwhile he has had 705 pages of proof struck from the stereotyped plates of the remaining volume.

The profession will thus see that the work is well forwarded, and that the volumes will in due time be ready for distribution to all those who are square in their accounts with the Treasurer of the American Institute of Homœopathy.

ANSWER TO A CORRESPONDENT.—In our September issue a correspondent asks, "In which of the Eastern States, the legislature and State societies have enacted prohibitory laws, fettering students' desires to go away from home for (medical) instruction, and imposing a legal fine if they do so?" The answer to the question will probably be found in "An Act to Regulate the Licensing of Physicians and Surgeons," passed by the legislature of the State of New York, May 29th, 1880.

The following extracts will convey an idea of its general scope and purpose:

"§ 2. Every person now lawfully engaged in the practice of physic and surgery within the State shall, on or before the first day of October, eighteen hundred and eighty, and every person hereafter duly authorized to practice physic and surgery shall, before commencing to practice, register in the clerk's office of the county where he is practicing, or intends to commence the practice of physic and surgery, in a book to be kept by said clerk, his name, residence, and place of birth, together with his authority for so practicing physic and surgery as prescribed in this act. The person so registering shall subscribe and verify by oath or affirmation, before a person duly qualified to administer oaths under the laws of the State, an affidavit containing such facts, and whether such authority is by diploma or license, and the date of the same and by whom granted, which, if wilfully false, shall subject the affiant to conviction and punishment for perjury. *The county clerk to receive a fee of twenty-five cents for such registration*, to be paid by the person so registering.

* * * *

"§ 4. A person coming to the State from without the State may be licensed to practice physic and surgery, or either, within the State, in the following manner: If he has a diploma conferring upon him the degree of doctor of medicine, issued by an incorporated university, medical college, or medical school without the State, he shall exhibit the same to the faculty of some incorporated medical college or medical school of this State, with satisfactory evidence of his good moral character, and such other evidence, if any, of his qualifications as a physician or surgeon, as said faculty may require. If his diploma and qualifications are approved by them, then they shall indorse said diploma, which shall make it for the purpose of his license to practice medicine and surgery within this State the same as if issued by them. *The applicant shall pay to the dean of said faculty the sum of twenty dollars for such examination and indorsement.* This indorsed diploma shall authorize him to practice physic and surgery within the State upon his complying with the provisions of section two of this act.

"§ 5. The degree of doctor of medicine lawfully conferred by any incorporated medical college or university in this State shall be a license to practice physic and surgery within the State after the person to whom it is granted shall have complied with section two of this act."

MARRIED.—HARRIS—CRAWFORD —On Tuesday, November 16th, 1880, David R. Harris, M.D , to Mrs. Mary Crawford, both of New Castle, Pa.

QUINT—PIERSON.—On Wednesday evening, November 3d, 1880, by Rev. William J. Purington, of Hopewell, N. J., S. H. Quint, M D., and Miss Katie M. Pierson, both of Camden, N. J.

REEVES—LEWRY.—On Thursday, November 4th, 1880, at St. Mark's Lutheran Church, by Rev. S. Laird, Joseph M. Reeves, M.D., and Josephine Lewry, both of Philadelphia.

DECEASED.—Francis Sims, M.D., the first Professor of Surgery in the old Homœopathic Medical College of Pennsylvania, died November 29th, 1880. A more extended notice of the deceased will appear in our next issue.

OFFICE OF THE HAHNEMANNIAN MONTHLY, *N. E. corner Eighteenth and Green streets*, Philadelphia.

Send all business communications direct to our office.

Lightning Source UK Ltd.
Milton Keynes UK
UKHW012001110219
337098UK00012B/547/P